Current Topics in Microbiology and Immunology

Volume 386

More information about this series at http://www.springer.com/series/82

Michael B. A. Oldstone · Richard W. Compans
Editors

Influenza Pathogenesis and Control - Volume II

Responsible Series Editors: Michael B. A. Oldstone and Richard W. Compans

Springer

Editors
Michael B. A. Oldstone
Department of Immunology
and Microbial Science
The Scripps Research Institute
La Jolla, CA
USA

Richard W. Compans
Department of Microbiology
and Immunology
Emory University
Atlanta, GA
USA

ISSN 0070-217X
ISSN 2196-9965 (electronic)
ISBN 978-3-319-11157-5
ISBN 978-3-319-11158-2 (eBook)
DOI 10.1007/978-3-319-11158-2

Library of Congress Control Number: 2014951138

Springer Cham Heidelberg New York Dordrecht London

Printed on acid-free paper

Springer is part of Springer Science+Business Media (www.springer.com)

Preface

Perhaps first described in the Bible in Numbers 11:31–34 and later by the poet W.H. Auden:

Little birds with scarlet legs,
Sitting on their speckled eggs,
Eye each flu-infected city

Influenza has over the course of human experience been defined by the suffering, illness, and death rates it caused and causes of epidemics and pandemics worldwide.

Influenza virus belongs to the orthomyxovirus family and comes in three flavors, types A, B, and C, with type A and B viruses being important causes of disease in humans, with the majority of cases due to type A. These viruses have a negative strand sense, segmented RNA genome with eight genes that can code for up to 11 proteins. Because of the segmented genome and permissive infection of several animal species (primarily humans, birds, and pigs) influenza virus can easily reassort differing RNA segments between human and animal viruses. Such an event leads to antigenic shift, and possible new pandemic strains. Further, as with other RNA viruses, influenza's RNA-dependent RNA polymerase is error-prone such that mutations occur frequently, and in the absence of a proofreading frame that eliminates and thus fails to control fit mutated viruses from evolving. The fitness of such mutated virus is suggested by their fidelity during replication. They undergo further selection because of antibody responses and immune escape, termed antigenic drift.

This work consisting of two volumes explores influenza pathogenesis and control from basic structure, binding, entry, replication, and release of influenza virus to its spread, the results of its interaction with animal models, the innate and adaptive immune systems, and current epidemiologic efforts at rapid recognition and antiviral, anti-host cytokine storm therapies as well as vaccine strategies to control and prevent influenza virus infections.

Volume I provides overviews of current information on molecular determinants of viral pathogenicity, virus entry and cell tropism, pandemic risk assessment, transmission and pathogenesis in animal species, viral evolution, ecology, and antigenic variation. Leading investigators who provide current information on these topics include Hans-Dieter Klenk and colleagues on the influenza hemagglutinin, Guelsah Gabriel and Ervin Fodor on the polymerase complex, David Steinhauer and John McCauley on receptor binding, and Charles Russell on membrane fusion activity of the hemagglutinin protein. Nancy Cox and colleagues describe the influenza risk assessment tool (IRAT) to evaluate pandemic potential of novel influenza viruses. Yoshi Kawaoka, Ron Fouchier, Anice Lowen, John Steel, Hualan Chen, Juergen Richt, and their colleagues provide overviews of studies on viral transmission in animal hosts. Monique Franca, Jacqueline Katz, Ian York, Terrence Tumpey, Amy Vincent, and colleagues review studies on pathogenesis in avian and mammalian hosts. Amber Smith and Jon McCullers describe the significance of secondary bacterial infection in viral pathogenesis. Viral ecology, evolution, and antigenic variation are discussed in chapters by Sun-Woo Yoon, Robert Webster, Richard Webby, Anice Lowen, John Steel, and Ruben Donis.

The second volume in this series, Volume II is concerned with innate immunity and adaptive immunity, vaccines, and antivirals. Experts in these various areas including John Teijaro, Adolfo Garcia-Sastre, Bali Pulendran, Stacey Shultz-Cherry, Paul Thomas, and colleagues have contributed chapters on specific aspects of innate immunity, while Tom Braciale, Rafi Ahmed, Donna Farber, and colleagues describe B and T cell adaptive immunity. Chapters on vaccines and vaccination include those contributed by Rino Rappuoli, Ian Wilson, Peter Palese, John Steel, Kanta Subbarao, Daniel Perez, Philip Dormitzer, Hongquan Wan, Maryna Eichelberger, Hiroshi Kida, Hideki Hasegawa, Richard Compans, Ioanna Skountzou, and their colleagues. Lastly, Ralph Tripp and S. Mark Tompkins discuss new antiviral discoveries, while John Teijaro writes about the use of sphingosine-1-phosphate receptor 1 agonist to control the resultant cytokine storm caused by influenza virus infection.

La Jolla, USA — Michael B. A. Oldstone
Atlanta, USA — Richard W. Compans

Contents

Part I
Innate Immunity

The Role of Cytokine Responses During Influenza Virus Pathogenesis and Potential Therapeutic Options

John R. Teijaro

Abstract Aberrant pulmonary immune responses are linked to the pathogenesis of multiple human respiratory viral infections. Elevated cytokine and chemokine production "cytokine storm" has been continuously associated with poor clinical outcome and pathogenesis during influenza virus infection in humans and animal models. Initial trials using global immune suppression with corticosteroids or targeted neutralization of single inflammatory mediators proved ineffective to ameliorate pathology during pathogenic influenza virus infection. Thus, it was believed that cytokine storm was either chemically intractable or not causal in the pathology observed. During this review, we will discuss the history of research assessing the roles various cytokines, chemokines, and innate immune cells play in promoting pathology or protection during influenza virus infection. Several promising new strategies modulating lipid signaling have been recently uncovered for global blunting, but not ablation, of innate immune responses following influenza virus infection. Importantly, modulating lipid signaling through various means has proven effective at curbing morbidity and mortality in animal models and may be useful for curbing influenza virus induced pathology in humans. Finally, we highlight future research directions for mechanistically dissecting how modulation of lipid signaling pathways results in favorable outcomes following influenza virus infection.

J.R. Teijaro (✉)
Department of Immunology and Microbial Science, The Scripps Research Institute, La Jolla, San Diego, CA 92037, USA
e-mail: teijaro@scripps.edu

J.R. Teijaro
Department of Chemical Physiology, The Scripps Research Institute, La Jolla, San Diego, CA 92037, USA

Current Topics in Microbiology and Immunology (2015) 386: 3–22
DOI: 10.1007/82_2014_411

Published Online: 30 September 2014

Contents

1 Introduction

The morbidity and mortality of severe influenza infections reflects properties intrinsic to the virus strain, including the ability to enter, replicate, and lyse respiratory epithelial cells (Garcia-Sastre 2010; Tscherne and Garcia-Sastre 2011). Host-intrinsic properties reflect both susceptibilities to infection as well as the double-edged sword of host immune responses that may ameliorate or exacerbate both infection and clinical outcome. The correlation of an aggressive immune response and severe disease following influenza virus infection in humans and animal models has been discussed previously (La Gruta et al. 2007). An aggressive innate response, with elevated recruitment of inflammatory leukocytes to lung, likely contributed to the morbidity of the 1918 influenza infection (Ahmed et al. 2007; Kobasa et al. 2007). In fact, lung injury during infection of macaques with the 1918 H1N1 influenza virus strain directly correlated with early dysregulated inflammatory gene expression (Cilloniz et al. 2009; Kobasa et al. 2007). More recently, clinical studies on avian H5N1 infected humans documented a significant association between excessive early cytokine responses and immune cell recruitment as predictive of poor outcome (de Jong et al. 2006). Moreover, an aberrant cytokine/chemokine response was observed in patients with severe disease during the most recent H1N1 pandemic in 2009 (Arankalle et al. 2010).

Thus far, public health approaches to influenza pandemics have relied primarily on preventative vaccine strategies and supportive measures including extensive use of various antiviral therapies. Nevertheless, the speed at which the 2009 H1N1 influenza virus pandemic spread coupled with increased morbidity associated with infection made evident the need to identify additional therapeutic strategies for the amelioration of influenza virus associated pathologies (Openshaw and Dunning

2010). While antiviral drugs that inhibit virus replication run the risk of mutational escape rendering the therapy ineffective, modulating the host immune response is less susceptible to selective pressure and drug resistance. Moreover, the current vaccine platforms require bi- or triennial modification to anticipate newly-emerging viral strains. Thus, uncovering novel therapies that can blunt the pathogenic immune response without compromising viral clearance could save countless lives and economic losses when the next lethal influenza virus pandemic emerges. Because of the strong connection between pathogenic influenza virus infection and excessive cytokine/chemokine production, this review will focus exclusively on the role various cytokines, chemokines, and innate immune cells play in promoting influenza virus protection versus pathogenesis. While it is recognized that some animal models have reported enhanced cytokine responses, control of influenza virus replication and reduced morbidity during influenza virus infection (Maelfait et al. 2012; Strutt et al. 2010), the majority of clinical and animal model studies overwhelmingly support that aberrant immune responses play a commanding role during influenza virus pathogenesis (La Gruta et al. 2007; Salomon and Webster 2009; Tisoncik et al. 2012).

For this reason, the focus of this chapter will be to evaluate the role innate immune cytokines, chemokines, and leukocytes play in protection and pathology during influenza virus infection.

2 Role of Cytokines and Chemokines in Immunopathology Versus Protection

2.1 Interferon

Type I interferon signaling is well-known to inhibit influenza virus replication and spread (Garcia-Sastre and Biron 2006). In fact, a major function of the viral NS1 protein, one of 11 viral proteins, is to inhibit type 1 interferon production and signaling (Hale et al. 2008). Deletion or mutation of the NS1 gene results in significant increases in the levels of type 1 interferon in infected cells and significantly lower virus titers both in vitro and in vivo (Garcia-Sastre et al. 1998; Jiao et al. 2008; Kochs et al. 2007). Despite strong evidence demonstrating extensive antiviral properties of type 1 interferon, several studies also suggest pathogenic roles for IFN-α during influenza virus infection. The production of several pro-inflammatory cytokines and chemokines are known to be amplified by type I interferon receptor signaling. Moreover, symptom onset correlates directly with the local appearance of IFN-α in respiratory lavage fluid in humans (Hayden et al. 1998; Van Reeth 2000). Thus, type I interferon signaling has dual roles in virus control and pathogenesis. Infection of IFNAR1$^{-/-}$ mice with the PR8 strain of influenza virus resulted in altered recruitment of Ly6C^{hi} versus Ly6C^{int} monocytes in the lung, translating into increased production of the neutrophil chemoattractant,

KC (CXCL8), elevated numbers of neutrophils in the lung and increased morbidity and mortality (Seo et al. 2011). Therefore, modulation of type 1 interferon signaling and production needs to be balanced to have enough to control virus infection but not promote excessive inflammation.

Type II interferon, made up of IFN-γ, is produced throughout influenza virus infection. Early levels of IFN-γ (within the first 3 days of infection) are made by macrophages and natural killer (NK) cells. While later on during infection (days 5–10 postinfection) IFN-γ is produced primarily by antiviral CD4 and CD8 T cells in the lung and secondary lymphoid tissues. Administration of IFN-γ early following influenza virus infection has been demonstrated to exert antiviral properties and is protective (Weiss et al. 2010). The protective role of IFN-γ is supported by the use of proteinase-activated receptor 2 (PAR2) agonist in vivo, which increased IFN-γ production, reduced influenza virus titers, and improved survival (Khoufache et al. 2009). However, a subsequent study demonstrated that following high-dose influenza virus infection, the absence of PAR2 resulted in improved survival (Nhu et al. 2010). Enhanced survival was also observed following lethal influenza virus infection in protease-activated receptor-1 (PAR1)-deficient mice or wild-type mice treated with PAR1 antagonist peptide, which correlated with a decrease in early influenza virus titers though the levels of IFN-γ were not assessed in this study (Khoufache et al. 2013). Protective memory CD4 T cell responses are correlated with the elevated numbers of lung CD4 T cells producing IFN-γ (McKinstry et al. 2012; Teijaro et al. 2010, 2011a). Moreover, IFN-γ-deficient, virus-specific T cells were more pathological than their IFN-γ-sufficient counterparts (Wiley et al. 2001). Antibody neutralization of IFN-γ in vivo affected influenza virus induced humoral and cellular immune responses in the lung (Baumgarth and Kelso 1996). Conversely, several studies reported that IFN-γ-deficient mice have negligible defects in virus clearance or generating efficient immune responses (Bot et al. 1998; Nguyen et al. 2000; Price et al. 2000). These studies suggest that spatial and temporal activity of IFN-γ production and signaling likely play key roles in controlling influenza virus infection and the magnitude of the immune response.

In addition to type I and II interferons, type III interferon, λ-interferon, has been detected in both respiratory epithelial cell cultures as well as mouse lung following influenza virus infection (Crotta et al. 2013; Jewell et al. 2010). Interestingly, λ-interferon did not require type I interferon for its induction and appeared to be sufficient to protect mice in the absence of type 1 interferon signaling during influenza virus challenge (Jewell et al. 2010). Administration of λ-interferon prior to influenza virus infection protected type 1 Interferon receptor knockout mice from infection. However, deletion of IL-28Rα, the receptor that recognizes λ-interferon, rendered mice only slightly more susceptible to influenza virus infection (Mordstein et al. 2008). Thus, it appears that Interferon-λ signaling following influenza virus challenge contributes to antiviral protection similar to type I interferon signaling.

2.2 Interleukin-1 (IL-1) and Tumor Necrosis Factor Alpha (TNF-α)

In addition to endosome (TLR3, 7) and cytosolic (RIG-I) sensors, influenza virus infected cells can activate the NLRP3 inflammasome (Ichinohe et al. 2009, 2010). The end result of inflammasome activation is the cleavage of pro-IL-1β and pro-IL-18 to active proteins. In turn, secreted IL-1β can signal through the IL-1R to induce inflammatory gene production through MyD88 signaling. Signaling through IL-1R has been demonstrated to contribute to both host protection and immune pathology following influenza virus infection. One group found that while IL-1R$^{-/-}$ mice displayed reduced lung inflammatory pathology with reduced neutrophil recruitment, IL-1R$^{-/-}$ mice also displayed reduced anti-influenza virus IgM antibody, along with delayed viral clearance and increased mortality (Schmitz et al. 2005). In contrast, a separate study demonstrated delayed mortality in IL-1R$^{-/-}$ mice following infection with H5N1 influenza virus (Perrone et al. 2010). In fact, elevated levels of IL-1β drive proinflammatory responses in patients with acute respiratory distress syndrome (Pugin et al. 1996). Elevated levels of TNF-α have also been linked to morbidity and mortality following highly pathogenic influenza virus infection in humans and animal models (Szretter et al. 2007). Interestingly, anti-TNF-α antibody therapy in mice resulted in reduced recruitment of inflammatory cells, T cell cytokine production, and morbidity in a mouse model of influenza virus infection (Hussell et al. 2001). Conversely, no difference in disease severity or mortality was observed in TNFR$^{-/-}$ mice following H5N1 infection (Salomon et al. 2007). Interestingly, mice lacking both IL-1R and TNFR displayed reduced morbidity, significantly delayed mortality, suppressed cytokine/chemokine production and reduced numbers of neutrophils and macrophages in the lung compared to wild-type mice (Perrone et al. 2010). Whether the disparate results between these two studies are due to the different viral strains used (H1N1/PR8 versus H5N1), differences in the method of depletion (anti-TNF antibody versus congenital TNFR knock out), or redundancy between the TNFR and IL-1R signaling pathways is still unclear.

2.3 Interleukin-6 (IL-6)

Elevated levels of IL-6 were found in human serum from patients infected with H5N1 and H1N1/2009 infections. Moreover, levels of IL-6 correlate directly with symptom formation in human influenza virus infection (Kaiser et al. 2001; Van Reeth 2000). Infection of macaques with the H1N1/1918/1919 pandemic influenza virus generated increased levels of IL-6 in the serum, suggestive of an aberrant inflammatory response (Kobasa et al. 2007). Despite the strong correlation of IL-6 levels and influenza pathogenesis, genetic depletion of IL-6 did not alter mortality following experimental infection of mice with H5N1 infection (Salomon et al. 2007), suggesting IL-6 may not be causal for influenza virus immune pathogenesis. On the other hand, IL-6 signaling was required to survive sublethal influenza virus infection in a mouse model (Dienz et al. 2012). In this study, the absence of IL-6 signaling led to increased lung pathology and viral titers, however, resulted in significant decreases in neutrophils in the lung, which was shown to be attributable to neutrophil death. Signaling through the IL-6 receptor is also essential for CD4 T follicular helper cell generation, B cell and antibody responses, which may explain the inability of IL-6 deficient mice to control influenza viral titers in the lung. The immune stimulatory antiviral properties of IL-6 may also explain why IL-6 deficient mice succumbed at a similar rate following H5N1 infection (Salomon et al. 2007). Alternatively, the different viral strains used in the above studies could explain the disparate clinical outcomes in mice deficient in IL-6 signaling. Nevertheless, fine-tuning will likely be required during inhibition of IL-6 signaling following influenza virus infection to allow for a sufficient immune response to control virus replication.

2.4 Chemokines

In addition to cytokines, multiple chemotactic molecules are induced following influenza virus infection in humans and animal models. In fact, production of several chemokines, both locally and systemically, correlate with influenza virus pathogenesis (de Jong et al. 2006; Kobasa et al. 2007; Van Reeth 2000). Elevated levels of MCP-1 (CCL2) and IP-10 (CXCL10) were found in the serum of patients infected with H5N1 compared to patients with less virulent strains (de Jong et al. 2006; Peiris et al. 2004). Moreover, elevated levels of RANTES (CCL5) mRNA were detected in human primary macrophages following infection with H5N1 as compared to H1N1 or H3N2 infection (Cheung et al. 2002). Influenza virus infected monocytes also express MIP-1α (Sprenger et al. 1996). While there is a clear correlation between increased production of the above chemokines during lethal influenza virus infection and pathology, a causal relationship between individual chemokines and pathogenesis has been difficult to prove. Infection of CCR2 and CCR5-deficient animals with mouse adapted PR8 H1N1 influenza virus yielded opposing results. CCR5 deficient mice developed a severe pro-inflammatory response, pulmonary cell damage, and decreased survival despite normal control of virus replication (Dawson et al. 2000). In contrast to worse pathology observed in CCR5$^{-/-}$ mice following influenza virus infection, CCR2-deficient mice displayed reduced pulmonary innate immune cell infiltration, decreased pulmonary damage, and increased survival. Interestingly, despite reduced pulmonary immune pathology, influenza virus loads were elevated in CCR2$^{-/-}$ mice (Dawson et al. 2000). Based on the above studies, one might assume that neutralization or deletion of CCL2 (or CCR2) during infection with human pathogenic influenza virus strains would result in a favorable clinical outcome. However, it was later determined that CCL2$^{-/-}$ mice succumbed to H5N1 infection at a similar rate and frequency as CCL2$^{+/+}$ control mice (Salomon et al. 2007). Again, the discrepancy could be due to the differences in the virus strains used or that other non-CCL2 chemokines that signal through CCR2 are responsible for immune pathology. However, neutralization of CCR2 signaling with antibody, chemotherapeutic, or genetic deletion in animal models has not been tested following infection with H5N1 or other highly pathogenic influenza virus strains. In light of the increased pathology in $CCR5^{-/-}$ mice, it was demonstrated that CXCR3-deficiency (CXCR3 is a receptor for CXCL10) blunted lung pathology and cytokine levels and ultimately restored survival in $CCR5^{-/-}$ mice (Fadel et al. 2008), suggesting that signaling through CXCR3 in the absence of CCR5 may be detrimental during influenza virus infection. Moreover, blockade of CXCR3 with the drug AMG487 reduced symptom formation and delayed mortality in H5N1 infected ferrets (Cameron et al. 2008).

2.5 Negative Regulatory Cytokines, Interleukin-10 (IL-10), and Tumor Growth Factor-Beta (TGF-β)

In addition to initiating immune responses, the host immune system also utilizes multiple anti-inflammatory cytokines to prevent detrimental immune pathology. One major negative immune regulator, IL-10, is a central factor for regulating immune responses to viruses, bacteria, and parasitic infections (Couper et al. 2008). During human pathogenic influenza virus infection, elevated IL-10 levels are found in severely ill patients (de Jong et al. 2006). However, upregulation of IL-10 in these patients was likely a reactionary response to the excessive inflammation generated. One study reported that blockade of IL-10 signaling using an IL-10R neutralizing antibody following sublethal infection of mice resulted in exacerbated morbidity and mortality. The source of the IL-10 was determined to be effector CD8 T cells infiltrating the lung tissue (Sun et al. 2009). In a separate study, IL-10-deficient mice were protected from death following infection with a lethal dose of influenza virus. However, in this model the source of IL-10 was lung effector CD4 T cells (McKinstry et al. 2009). Moreover, a significant increase in the T helper 17 cell subset was detected in $IL\text{-}10^{-/-}$ mice following lethal influenza virus infection (McKinstry et al. 2009).

The immune regulatory role of Transforming Growth Factor Beta (TGF-β) has been extensively studied (Li et al. 2006). The activity of TGF-β has been reported to increase following influenza virus infection in mice. In fact, the influenza virus neuraminidase (NA) protein was demonstrated to convert inactive TGF-β into its active form (Schultz-Cherry and Hinshaw 1996). Interestingly, it was also discovered that highly pathogenic strains of H5N1 influenza virus fail to activate TGF-β (Carlson et al. 2010). Thus, one might anticipate that TGF-β activation may be essential for host protection during lethal H5N1 infection. In support of that hypothesis, it was determined that exogenous administration of active TGF-β using an adenovirus vector resulted in reduced viral loads and delayed mortality following lethal H5N1 infection in mice (Carlson et al. 2010). Conversely, neutralization of TGF-β produced higher mortality rates in mice infected with non-lethal doses of influenza virus, suggesting that active TGF-β can serve as a protective factor (Carlson et al. 2010). Despite these interesting results, the degree and mechanisms by which TGF-β regulates pathological immune responses or interferes with virus replication during human pathogenic influenza virus infection requires further studies and is likely to be a fruitful area of investigation. Moreover, a better understanding of these and other negative immune regulatory molecules may lead to treatments that blunt immune pathology following pathogenic influenza virus infection in humans.

3 The Role of Innate Immune Cells in Pathogenesis Versus Protection

3.1 Macrophages/Monocytes

Experimental infection with H5N1 and 1918 H1N1 influenza viruses results in recruitment of macrophages/monocytic cells into infected lungs. Recruited monocytic cells can serve as reservoirs for influenza virus replication early following infection (Pang et al. 2013) and can be protected from infection via type 1 interferon signaling (Hermesh et al. 2010). Further, this infiltration may contribute to lung pathology and correlates directly with morbidity and mortality. In addition to infiltrating macrophages and monocytes, lung resident alveolar macrophages (AMs) have been demonstrated to play a role in the control of influenza virus clearance (Tumpey et al. 2005). In fact, administration of clodronate containing liposomes prior to infection with influenza viruses containing genes from the 1918–1919 H1N1 pandemic isolate reduced cytokine/chemokine production, however, also led to increased mortality. Moreover, depletion of AMs prior to sublethal influenza virus infection using clondronate liposomes resulted in uncontrolled viral titers and increased mortality despite reduced cytokine and chemokine expression (Tate et al. 2010). In contrast, AM depletion using clodronate liposomes during lethal PR8 infection did not alter the severity of disease or mortality (Tate et al. 2010). These contrasting results highlight the importance of the infectious dose of virus used and the outcome of immune cell depletion. Moreover, it is important to point out that clodronate liposome administration likely eliminates additional non-AM cell populations in the lungs, and a more extensive analysis of the populations depleted in these studies would be beneficial for interpretation. Further, the selective depletion of specific monocyte populations following influenza virus challenge has not been performed to date.

3.2 Neutrophils

Pathology following infection with highly virulent strains of human pathogenic influenza virus correlates with elevated neutrophil recruitment into lung tissue (Perrone et al. 2008). Moreover, the neutrophil responsive chemokine, IL-8, is elevated in patients displaying severe disease during H5N1 infection compared to infection with seasonal strains (de Jong et al. 2006). However, upon closer review of the literature, both protective and pathogenic roles for neutrophils have been reported following influenza virus infection. Complete depletion of neutrophils using antibody methods increased morbidity and mortality that was accompanied by decreased control of virus replication following infection with various strains of influenza virus (Brandes et al. 2013; Tumpey et al. 2005). Increased neutrophil numbers were detected in influenza virus infected $CCR2^{-/-}$ mice, correlating with reduced lung pathology and survival, despite slightly elevated viral loads (Dawson et al. 2000). Interestingly, a recent report demonstrated that attenuation, not depletion, of the neutrophil response correlated with improved survival following infection of mice with the PR8 strain of influenza virus (Brandes et al. 2013). This latter report suggests that too many or too few neutrophils can result in negative pathological outcomes either through exacerbated lung immune pathology or reduced virus control. Collectively, the above studies suggest that there may be a "sweet spot" in the numbers of neutrophils required to allow for the optimal control of both virus replication and immune pathology following influenza virus infection. In light of the above work, a more detailed understanding of the exact mechanisms of neutrophil-mediated protection and pathology will be crucial to designing therapies to quell lung immune pathology while preserving virus control.

3.3 Dendritic Cells

During respiratory virus infection, lung resident dendritic cells (DCs) play important roles in priming naïve T cells in the lung draining mediastinal lymph nodes. Several different subpopulations of these DCs have been identified by phenotypic flow cytometry analysis, with different populations displaying varying abilities to prime virus-specific T cells (Lambrecht and Hammad 2012). This aspect of influenza immune biology will be discussed in more detail in a separate chapter in this volume. Our focus here will be to discuss what is known about the pathogenic roles of DCs during the innate immune response of influenza virus infection. Several studies have linked DC responses with the immune pathology observed following influenza virus infection. Accumulation of $CCR2^{+}$ monocyte derived DCs in the lung correlates with increased lung pathology, morbidity, and mortality. Importantly, reduced numbers of $CCR2^{+/+}$ monocyte derived DCs are found in the lung of $CCR2^{-/-}$ mice following influenza challenge, and $CCR2^{-/-}$

mice display reduced morbidity and less mortality (Dawson et al. 2000). A similar study reported that TNF-α and Nitric Oxide Producing DC (TipDC) are found in higher numbers in the lung following infection with highly pathogenic compared to less pathogenic influenza virus strains. Moreover, TipDC recruitment was completely abolished in $CCR2^{-/-}$ mice following PR8 influenza virus infection (Aldridge et al. 2009). Despite reduced TipDC numbers in the lungs in $CCR2^{-/-}$ mice, no differences in morbidity or mortality were observed. The authors further demonstrated that TipDCs were essential for priming virus-specific CD8 T cell responses and conclude that complete depletion of TipDCs in their model may prevent the control of influenza virus replication. Interestingly, using the peroxisome proliferator-activated receptor-γ (PPAR-γ) agonist Pioglitazone prior to influenza virus infection reduced TipDCs, MCP-1, and MCP-3 chemokine production in the lungs, promoting increased survival following influenza virus infection (Aldridge et al. 2009). Collectively, the above studies suggest that a fine balance between protection and pathology exists upon depletion of DC populations during influenza virus infection. Therapeutic modulation of influenza virus induced immune pathology will likely require effective blunting without ablation of specific pulmonary DC subsets.

4 Identifying Therapeutic Interventions to Blunt Immune Pathology

Overabundant innate immune responses correlate with increased morbidity and mortality during infection with multiple pathogenic respiratory viruses (Kobasa et al. 2007; Macneil et al. 2011; Thiel and Weber 2008). In fact, cytokine storm during influenza virus infection is a prospective predictor of morbidity and mortality in humans (de Jong et al. 2006). Despite a strong correlation with pathogenesis, a direct causal link between innate immune responses, morbidity, and mortality has been difficult to prove. While cytokines and chemokines are produced at elevated levels during highly pathogenic compared to less pathogenic human influenza virus infection, inhibition of any single inflammatory mediator only modestly improved morbidity and delayed mortality in animal models (Cameron et al. 2008; Salomon et al. 2007; Salomon and Webster 2009; Szretter et al. 2007). These results indicate that isolated neutralization of single immune signaling molecules is insufficient to curb the resultant immune pathology following highly pathogenic influenza virus infection. However, global immune suppressive strategies such as corticosteroids have proven either ineffective or only modestly altered disease course in humans or animal models (Brun-Buisson et al. 2011; Tisoncik et al. 2012). One critical hurdle to generating effective treatments to curb influenza virus mediated immune pathology is a more detailed understanding of the cellular signaling pathways that elicit cytokine storm and potentiate lung pathology.

The balance between influenza virus immune control and pathology is on a knife's edge; too much immune modulation results in the loss of virus control and too little can prove ineffective to blunt immune pathology. One must remain in the "goldilocks zone" for the best efficacy. Perhaps it is best to discuss therapies that have proven effective in blunting immune pathology while simultaneously sparing control of influenza virus replication with the hope of gaining insight into effective immune modulatory strategies to curb pathogenesis. Over the past 5 years, several studies have emerged demonstrating efficacious immune modulation of influenza virus replication and immunopathology. One of the more exciting areas of research that has recently developed is the characterization of lipid species following influenza virus infection and how they contribute to pathogenicity or protection. In fact, the majority of effective immune modulatory therapies that suppress morbidity and mortality following influenza virus infection have targeted various pathways that mediate lipid production or signaling. Performing lipidomic profiling following influenza virus infection using viruses with varying pathogenicity, one group identified lipid species that predominated during the pathogenic phase of infection and others that were associated with the resolution phase. Specifically, the authors found 5-Lipoxygenase metabolites in pathogenic influenza virus infection while 12/15-lipoxygenase metabolites were found in less pathogenic influenza infection (Tam et al. 2013). The generation of the omega-3 polyunsaturated fatty acid-derived lipid mediator, Protectin D1, was determined to inhibit influenza virus replication and result in reduced morbidity and mortality following infection (Morita et al. 2013). Another group identified that the oxidized phospholipid OxPAPC (OxPL) was essential for acute lung injury (ALI) following administration of inactivated H5N1 influenza virus to lungs (Imai et al. 2008). Interestingly, OxPL promoted lung injury and cytokine production by lung macrophages, which was dependent on TLR4-TRIF signaling. Moreover, TLR4- or TRIF-deficiency protected mice from ALI following H5N1 stimulation. Complimentary studies confirmed and extended this work, demonstrating that $TLR4^{-/-}$ mice are less susceptible to mortality following infection with a lethal dose of the PR8 strain of influenza virus (Nhu et al. 2012). Moreover, both prophylactic and therapeutic administration of a TLR4 antagonist, Eritoran, protected mice from lethal infection with either PR8 or the A/California/07/2009 H1N1 virus strain (Shirey et al. 2013). Importantly, Eritoran treatment resulted in reduced levels of oxidized phospholipids, suppressed cytokine/chemokine gene expression and ameliorated lung pathology (Shirey et al. 2013). While early viral titers were comparable between control and Eritoran treated mice infected with influenza virus, viral loads were reduced on day 7 postinfection in Eritoran treated mice compared to controls. Despite significant immune modulatory effects, Eritoran displayed no direct antiviral activities. The above reports indicate that a better understanding of pathogenic lipid species following influenza virus infection may lead to superior therapeutic modalities to blunt disease pathogenesis.

The cyclooxygenase enzymes (COX-1 and 2) convert arachidonic acid into prostaglandins and can control various inflammatory processes. The roles these enzymes play in the outcome of influenza virus pathology have been addressed.

Deletion or pharmacological inhibition of the COX-1 enzyme was detrimental during influenza virus infection, resulting in enhanced morbidity, mortality, and enhanced cytokine/chemokine production. In contrast, COX-2 deficiency or pharmacological inhibition ameliorated pathology, suppressed inflammation and improved survival despite elevated viral loads (Carey et al. 2005, 2010). Notably, coadministration of the COX-2 inhibitor celecoxib and the antiviral drug zanamivir reduced mortality in mice infected with pathogenic H5N1 virus (Zheng et al. 2008). Thus, inhibiting COX-2 activity can be beneficial during influenza virus infection in the presence of antiviral therapies.

Sphingosine-1-Phosphate (S1P) is a lipid metabolite synthesized from intracellular ceramide precursors to sphingosine. Sphingosine is subsequently phosphorylated by sphingosine kinase 1 and 2 (Sphk) to bioactive S1P (Chalfant and Spiegel 2005). The levels of bioactive S1P are stringently regulated through the actions of S1P lyases and phosphatases which degrade and dephosphorylate S1P, respectively. Highest levels of S1P are found in the blood and lymph with significantly lower levels maintained in peripheral tissues (Cyster 2005). S1P binds and signals through five G-protein coupled receptors denoted S1PR1–5. The expression of S1P receptors is heterogeneous, being found on various cell types of both hematopoietic and nonhematopoietic lineages and regulation of S1P signaling is mediated primarily through the expression pattern of the five receptors and stringent regulations of S1P levels (Im 2010). The diverse cellular functions associated with S1P receptor signaling is mediated through coupling to multiple heterotrimeric G-proteins adding an additional level of regulation. Binding through these five receptors is known to modulate multiple cellular functions including: cell adhesion, migration, survival, proliferation, endocytosis, barrier function, and cytokine production (Rivera et al. 2008). Since the initial discovery that the immunomodulatory agent, FTY720, induced lymphopenia, investigators sought to understand how S1P signaling affects immune cell function. To this end, genetically altered mice and selective agonists/antagonists have been developed to probe how S1P signaling on different S1P receptors alters immune cell responses (Marsolais and Rosen 2009; Rosen et al. 2008). FTY720 and AAL-R are prodrug promiscuous S1P receptor agonists and once phosphorylated in vivo by SphK-2, bind and signal through S1P1, 3, 4, and 5R. Both FTY720 and AAL-R have been used extensively to characterize the effects of S1P signaling in vivo and have been shown to alter the outcome of autoimmune disease, toxic shock syndrome, and viral infection (Niessen et al. 2008; Oldstone 2013). In addition, several S1P receptor selective agonists have been developed to probe the cellular functions of S1P-receptor signaling. For instance, S1P1R selective agonists (CYM5442, SEW2781 and AUY954) (Gonzalez-Cabrera et al. 2008; Rosen and Liao 2003) and antagonists (W146 and Ex26) (Cahalan et al. 2013; Gonzalez-Cabrera et al. 2008) have been synthesized and have provided insights into how S1P1R signaling affects lymphocyte trafficking and endothelial cell barrier functions (Rosen and Liao 2003; Shea et al. 2010). More recently, an S1P1R-eGFP knock-in mouse has been created, allowing for fluorescent and biochemical detection of functional S1P1R expression (Cahalan et al. 2011). Further, small molecule probes to S1P3 and S1P4 have been developed and are being used to probe the functions of these receptors in modulating DC activation and in turn pathological T cell responses. Most importantly, FTY720 has been approved for use in humans to treat Multiple Sclerosis (MS) and several S1P1R-selective agonists are in phase 2/3 clinical trials for MS and Colitis. Thus, potential of S1P receptor signaling modulation to modulate immune pathology during influenza virus infection wielded great promise.

Studies using the promiscuous S1P receptor agonist, AAL-R, demonstrated significant reductions in the numbers of macrophages and neutrophils in the lung early following infection with a mouse-adapted strain (WSN) (Marsolais et al. 2009). In addition, activation of lung infiltrating macrophage and NK cells, as measured by CD69 expression, was also significantly attenuated by AAL-R treatment following infection with a human virulent strain (pandemic H1N1 2009) of influenza virus (Walsh et al. 2011). Moreover, early administration of AAL-R resulted in significant reductions of multiple proinflammatory cytokines and chemokines following infection with either WSN or human pandemic H1N1 2009 influenza virus (Marsolais et al. 2009; Walsh et al. 2011). Further, AAL-R-mediated reduction of early innate immune cell recruitment and cytokine/chemokine production correlated directly with reduced lung pathology and improved survival during H1N1 2009 influenza virus infection. While AAL-R clearly inhibited innate immune responses, significant inhibition of activated T cell recruitment into the lung at various times postinfection was also observed in both mouse adapted (Marsolais et al. 2008) and human pathogenic strains of influenza virus (Walsh et al. 2011). Thus, whether AAL-R-mediated survival was due to inhibition of innate or adaptive immune responses could not be determined from these studies. The above results were extended using genetic and chemical tools to probe functions of the S1P1 receptor (S1P1 GFP knock-in transgenic mice, S1P1 receptor agonists and antagonists) revealing that pulmonary endothelial cells are major modulators of innate immune cell recruitment and cytokine/chemokine responses early following influenza virus infection (Teijaro et al. 2011b). While $S1P_1R$ is expressed on endothelial cells and lymphocytes within lung tissue, an $S1P_1R$-selective agonist suppresses cytokines and innate immune cell recruitment in wild-type and lymphocyte-deficient mice, identifying pulmonary endothelial cells as central players in promoting cytokine storm (Teijaro et al. 2011b). Immune cell infiltration and cytokine production were found to be distinct events, both orchestrated by signaling through the $S1P_1R$ located on endothelial cells (Teijaro et al. 2011b). Furthermore, suppression of early innate immune responses through $S1P_1R$ signaling results in reduced mortality during infection with human pathogenic strains (H1N1 swine) of influenza virus without compromising the host's ability to mount a sufficiently effective antiviral immune response to control infection in both mouse and ferret models (Teijaro et al. 2011b, 2014a). Importantly, no differences were observed in T cell functionality or total numbers in the lung during influenza virus infection following $S1P_1R$ agonist treatment (Marsolais et al. 2008), suggesting that the protective effect likely occurred primarily through suppression of early innate immune responses. We extended these findings showing that $S1P_1R$ agonist treatment suppresses global cytokine amplification. Importantly, $S1P_1R$ agonist treatment blunted cytokine/chemokine production and innate immune cell recruitment in the lung independently of endosomal and cytosolic innate sensing pathways (Teijaro et al. 2014b). Further, $S1P_1R$ signaling suppression of cytokine amplification was independent of multiple innate signaling adaptor pathways, indicating common pathway inhibition of cytokine storm is likely essential for protection. Moreover, the MyD88 adaptor molecule was determined to be responsible for the majority of cytokine amplification observed following influenza virus challenge (Teijaro et al. 2014b). Collectively, our results suggest that blunting global cytokine and chemokine production and innate immune cell recruitment is likely required for effective host protection from excessive immunopathology. Collectively, the observations that host-generated lipids and lipid signaling pathways can promote or inhibit aberrant immune responses as well as suppress virus replication reveal new targets that may ultimately be utilized to ameliorate disease following pathogenic influenza virus infection.

5 Future Perspectives

Current research is illuminating the cellular and molecular contributions of immunopathology caused by highly virulent influenza viruses that lead to disease. New therapies should focus on blocking inflammation in conjunction with antiviral therapy to reduce morbidity and mortality following infection. Moreover, it is clear from studies performed recently that global blunting, not ablation, of inflammatory mediators will likely be required to ameliorate disease following highly pathogenic influenza virus infections. Thus, future studies should focus on the signaling pathways necessary for cytokine amplification and seek out ways to globally dampen inflammatory immune responses generated through these pathways. Toward this end, it will be essential to understand in greater detail the mechanisms by which the lipid signaling modulators described above improve the outcome during pathogenic influenza virus infection. Additionally, poor outcome during pathogenic influenza virus infection may be predictable by identifying mutations in genetic loci that alter the production of these lipid species.

Despite encouraging reports that differential lipid signaling can affect the outcome of influenza virus infection, more work is necessary to create a thorough understanding of how different host-generated lipids modulate influenza virus generated pathological immune responses. Blockade or deletion of TLR4 signaling significantly improves the clinical outcome of influenza virus infection in mice. Understanding the pulmonary cells that produce oxidized phospholipid species that target TLR4 will be essential. Moreover, the cell types that require TLR4 signaling to amplify cytokine production, innate immune cell recruitment, and the resulting morbidity and mortality will also be informative. The fact that Eritoran is already FDA approved may expedite its use during influenza virus infection in humans. Further investigation into the cellular and molecular sources of these lipids may lead to novel interventions to relieve immune pathology. The detection of 5-Lipoxygenase metabolites in pathogenic influenza virus infection while 12/15-lipoxygenase or docosahexaenoic acid derived metabolites in less pathogenic influenza infection suggests that some lipid species can indicate resolution of infection or exert antiviral protective effects. Again, the sources of these lipids and how they mediate their protective or pathological effects will be important directions for future research. Whether similar lipid profiles are also observed in human pathogenic influenza virus infection would significantly buttress this area of research.

The identification that S1P signaling dampens influenza virus immune pathology provides insights and tools to dissect influenza virus pathogenesis. S1P receptor signaling inhibits inflammation during both the innate and adaptive immune responses to influenza virus infection. Specific targeting of distinct cell populations as well as selective S1P receptors may differentially dampen innate and adaptive inflammatory responses and thus will be important to explore. Further research will focus on pinpointing the S1P receptors and pulmonary cell subsets responsible for blunting innate and adaptive immune responses during influenza virus infection. To this end, more potent receptor selective drugs and knock-in and knock-out mouse models can be used as tools to further understand the mechanisms and signaling pathways involved during the inflammatory response. Moreover, the development and application of potent, selective agonists will likely decrease the potential of adverse side-effects through more precise targeting of specific receptors, modulating distinct immune functions. Additionally, human susceptibilities to inflammatory disease may correlate directly with differential regulation and/or signaling of the S1P receptor cascade. Modulation of inflammation utilizing S1P receptor signaling may be a general phenomenon that occurs in multiple respiratory viral associated maladies and manipulation of this pathway may provide broad anti-inflammatory therapeutic efficacy during multiple respiratory virus infections.

References

Ahmed R, Oldstone MB, Palese P (2007) Protective immunity and susceptibility to infectious diseases: lessons from the 1918 influenza pandemic. Nat Immunol 8:1188–1193

Aldridge JR Jr, Moseley CE, Boltz DA, Negovetich NJ, Reynolds C, Franks J, Brown SA, Doherty PC, Webster RG, Thomas PG (2009) TNF/iNOS-producing dendritic cells are the necessary evil of lethal influenza virus infection. Proc Nat Acad Sci U.S.A 106:5306–5311

Arankalle VA, Lole KS, Arya RP, Tripathy AS, Ramdasi AY, Chadha MS, Sangle SA, Kadam DB (2010) Role of host immune response and viral load in the differential outcome of pandemic H1N1 (2009) influenza virus infection in Indian patients. PLoS ONE 5(10):e13099

Baumgarth N, Kelso A (1996) In vivo blockade of gamma interferon affects the influenza virus-induced humoral and the local cellular immune response in lung tissue. J Virol 70:4411–4418

Bot A, Bot S, Bona CA (1998) Protective role of gamma interferon during the recall response to influenza virus. J Virol 72:6637–6645

Brandes M, Klauschen F, Kuchen S, Germain RN (2013) A systems analysis identifies a feedforward inflammatory circuit leading to lethal influenza infection. Cell 154:197–212
Brun-Buisson C, Richard JC, Mercat A, Thiebaut AC, Brochard L, REVA-SRLF A/H1N1v 2009 Registry Group (2011) Early corticosteroids in severe influenza A/H1N1 pneumonia and acute respiratory distress syndrome. Am J Respir Crit Care Med 183:1200–1206
Cahalan SM, Gonzalez-Cabrera PJ, Nguyen N, Guerrero M, Cisar EA, Leaf NB, Brown SJ, Roberts E, Rosen H (2013) Sphingosine 1-phosphate receptor 1 (S1P(1)) upregulation and amelioration of experimental autoimmune encephalomyelitis by an S1P(1) antagonist. Mol Pharmacol 83:316–321
Cahalan SM, Gonzalez-Cabrera PJ, Sarkisyan G, Nguyen N, Schaeffer MT, Huang L, Yeager A, Clemons B, Scott F, Rosen H (2011) Actions of a picomolar short-acting S1P(1) agonist in S1P(1)-eGFP knock-in mice. Nat Chem Biol 7:254–256
Cameron CM, Cameron MJ, Bermejo-Martin JF, Ran L, Xu L, Turner PV, Ran R, Danesh A, Fang Y, Chan PK et al (2008) Gene expression analysis of host innate immune responses during lethal H5N1 infection in ferrets. J Virol 82:11308–11317
Carey MA, Bradbury JA, Rebolloso YD, Graves JP, Zeldin DC, Germolec DR (2010) Pharmacologic inhibition of COX-1 and COX-2 in influenza A viral infection in mice. PLoS ONE 5:e11610
Carey MA, Bradbury JA, Seubert JM, Langenbach R, Zeldin DC, Germolec DR (2005) Contrasting effects of cyclooxygenase-1 (COX-1) and COX-2 deficiency on the host response to influenza A viral infection. J Immunol 175:6878–6884
Carlson CM, Turpin EA, Moser LA, O'Brien KB, Cline TD, Jones JC, Tumpey TM, Katz JM, Kelley LA, Gauldie J et al (2010) Transforming growth factor-beta: activation by neuraminidase and role in highly pathogenic H5N1 influenza pathogenesis. PLoS Pathog 6:e1001136
Chalfant CE, Spiegel S (2005) Sphingosine 1-phosphate and ceramide 1-phosphate: expanding roles in cell signaling. J Cell Sci 118:4605–4612
Cheung CY, Poon LL, Lau AS, Luk W, Lau YL, Shortridge KF, Gordon S, Guan Y, Peiris JS (2002) Induction of proinflammatory cytokines in human macrophages by influenza A (H5N1) viruses: a mechanism for the unusual severity of human disease? Lancet 360:1831–1837
Cilloniz C, Shinya K, Peng X, Korth MJ, Proll SC, Aicher LD, Carter VS, Chang JH, Kobasa D, Feldmann F et al (2009) Lethal influenza virus infection in macaques is associated with early dysregulation of inflammatory related genes. PLoS Pathog 5:e1000604
Couper KN, Blount DG, Riley EM (2008) IL-10: the master regulator of immunity to infection. J Immunol 180:5771–5777
Crotta S, Davidson S, Mahlakoiv T, Desmet CJ, Buckwalter MR, Albert ML, Staeheli P, Wack A (2013) Type I and type III interferons drive redundant amplification loops to induce a transcriptional signature in influenza-infected airway epithelia. PLoS Pathog 9:e1003773
Cyster JG (2005) Chemokines, sphingosine-1-phosphate, and cell migration in secondary lymphoid organs. Ann Rev Immunol 23:127–159
Dawson TC, Beck MA, Kuziel WA, Henderson F, Maeda N (2000) Contrasting effects of CCR5 and CCR2 deficiency in the pulmonary inflammatory response to influenza A virus. Am J Pathol 156:1951–1959
de Jong MD, Simmons CP, Thanh TT, Hien VM, Smith GJ, Chau TN, Hoang DM, Chau NV, Khanh TH, Dong VC et al (2006) Fatal outcome of human influenza A (H5N1) is associated with high viral load and hypercytokinemia. Nat Med 12:1203–1207
Dienz O, Rud JG, Eaton SM, Lanthier PA, Burg E, Drew A, Bunn J, Suratt BT, Haynes L, Rincon M (2012) Essential role of IL-6 in protection against H1N1 influenza virus by promoting neutrophil survival in the lung. Mucosal Immunol 5:258–266
Fadel SA, Bromley SK, Medoff BD, Luster AD (2008) CXCR3-deficiency protects influenza-infected CCR5-deficient mice from mortality. Eur J Immunol 38:3376–3387
Garcia-Sastre A (2010) Influenza virus receptor specificity: disease and transmission. Am J Pathol 176:1584–1585

Garcia-Sastre A, Biron CA (2006) Type 1 interferons and the virus-host relationship: a lesson in detente. Science 312:879–882

Garcia-Sastre A, Egorov A, Matassov D, Brandt S, Levy DE, Durbin JE, Palese P, Muster T (1998) Influenza A virus lacking the NS1 gene replicates in interferon-deficient systems. Virology 252:324–330

Gonzalez-Cabrera PJ, Jo E, Sanna MG, Brown S, Leaf N, Marsolais D, Schaeffer MT, Chapman J, Cameron M, Guerrero M et al (2008) Full pharmacological efficacy of a novel S1P1 agonist that does not require S1P-like headgroup interactions. Mol Pharmacol 74:1308–1318

Hale BG, Randall RE, Ortin J, Jackson D (2008) The multifunctional NS1 protein of influenza A viruses. J Gen Virol 89:2359–2376

Hayden FG, Fritz R, Lobo MC, Alvord W, Strober W, Straus SE (1998) Local and systemic cytokine responses during experimental human influenza A virus infection. Relation to symptom formation and host defense. J Clin Invest 101:643–649

Hermesh T, Moltedo B, Moran TM, Lopez CB (2010) Antiviral instruction of bone marrow leukocytes during respiratory viral infections. Cell Host Microbe 7:343–353

Hussell T, Pennycook A, Openshaw PJ (2001) Inhibition of tumor necrosis factor reduces the severity of virus-specific lung immunopathology. Eur J Immunol 31:2566–2573

Ichinohe T, Lee HK, Ogura Y, Flavell R, Iwasaki A (2009) Inflammasome recognition of influenza virus is essential for adaptive immune responses. J Exp Med 206:79–87

Ichinohe T, Pang IK, Iwasaki A (2010) Influenza virus activates inflammasomes via its intracellular M2 ion channel. Nat Immunol 11:404–410

Im DS (2010) Pharmacological tools for lysophospholipid GPCRs: development of agonists and antagonists for LPA and S1P receptors. Acta Pharmacol Sin 31:1213–1222

Imai Y, Kuba K, Neely GG, Yaghubian-Malhami R, Perkmann T, van Loo G, Ermolaeva M, Veldhuizen R, Leung YH, Wang H et al (2008) Identification of oxidative stress and Toll-like receptor 4 signaling as a key pathway of acute lung injury. Cell 133:235–249

Jewell NA, Cline T, Mertz SE, Smirnov SV, Flano E, Schindler C, Grieves JL, Durbin RK, Kotenko SV, Durbin JE (2010) Lambda interferon is the predominant interferon induced by influenza A virus infection in vivo. J Virol 84:11515–11522

Jiao P, Tian G, Li Y, Deng G, Jiang Y, Liu C, Liu W, Bu Z, Kawaoka Y, Chen H (2008) A single amino acid substitution in the NS1 protein changes the pathogenicity of H5N1 avian influenza viruses in mice. J Virol 82:1146–1154

Kaiser L, Fritz RS, Straus SE, Gubareva L, Hayden FG (2001) Symptom pathogenesis during acute influenza: interleukin-6 and other cytokine responses. J Med Virol 64:262–268

Khoufache K, Berri F, Nacken W, Vogel AB, Delenne M, Camerer E, Coughlin SR, Carmeliet P, Lina B, Rimmelzwaan GF et al (2013) PAR1 contributes to influenza A virus pathogenicity in mice. J Clin Invest 123:206–214

Khoufache K, LeBouder F, Morello E, Laurent F, Riffault S, Andrade-Gordon P, Boullier S, Rousset P, Vergnolle N, Riteau B (2009) Protective role for protease-activated receptor-2 against influenza virus pathogenesis via an IFN-gamma-dependent pathway. J Immunol 182:7795–7802

Kobasa D, Jones SM, Shinya K, Kash JC, Copps J, Ebihara H, Hatta Y, Kim JH, Halfmann P, Hatta M et al (2007) Aberrant innate immune response in lethal infection of macaques with the 1918 influenza virus. Nature 445:319–323

Kochs G, Garcia-Sastre A, Martinez-Sobrido L (2007) Multiple anti-interferon actions of the influenza A virus NS1 protein. J Virol 81:7011–7021

La Gruta NL, Kedzierska K, Stambas J, Doherty PC (2007) A question of self-preservation: immunopathology in influenza virus infection. Immunol Cell Biol 85:85–92

Lambrecht BN, Hammad H (2012) Lung dendritic cells in respiratory viral infection and asthma: from protection to immunopathology. Ann Rev Immunol 30:243–270

Li MO, Wan YY, Sanjabi S, Robertson AK, Flavell RA (2006) Transforming growth factor-beta regulation of immune responses. Ann Rev Immunol 24:99–146

Macneil A, Nichol ST, Spiropoulou CF (2011) Hantavirus pulmonary syndrome. Virus Res 162:138–147

Maelfait J, Roose K, Bogaert P, Sze M, Saelens X, Pasparakis M, Carpentier I, van Loo G, Beyaert R (2012) A20 (Tnfaip3) deficiency in myeloid cells protects against influenza A virus infection. PLoS Pathog 8:e1002570

Marsolais D, Hahm B, Edelmann KH, Walsh KB, Guerrero M, Hatta Y, Kawaoka Y, Roberts E, Oldstone MB, Rosen H (2008) Local not systemic modulation of dendritic cell S1P receptors in lung blunts virus-specific immune responses to influenza. Mol Pharmacol 74:896–903

Marsolais D, Hahm B, Walsh KB, Edelmann KH, McGavern D, Hatta Y, Kawaoka Y, Rosen H, Oldstone MB (2009) A critical role for the sphingosine analog AAL-R in dampening the cytokine response during influenza virus infection. Proc Nat Acad Sci U.S.A. 106:1560–1565

Marsolais D, Rosen H (2009) Chemical modulators of sphingosine-1-phosphate receptors as barrier-oriented therapeutic molecules. Nat Rev Drug Discov 8:297–307

McKinstry KK, Strutt TM, Buck A, Curtis JD, Dibble JP, Huston G, Tighe M, Hamada H, Sell S, Dutton RW et al (2009) IL-10 deficiency unleashes an influenza-specific Th17 response and enhances survival against high-dose challenge. J Immunol 182:7353–7363

McKinstry KK, Strutt TM, Kuang Y, Brown DM, Sell S, Dutton RW, Swain SL (2012) Memory CD4+ T cells protect against influenza through multiple synergizing mechanisms. J Clin Invest 122:2847–2856

Morita M, Kuba K, Ichikawa A, Nakayama M, Katahira J, Iwamoto R, Watanebe T, Sakabe S, Daidoji T, Nakamura S et al (2013) The lipid mediator protectin D1 inhibits influenza virus replication and improves severe influenza. Cell 153:112–125

Mahlakõiv T, Ritz D, Mordstein M, DeDiego ML, Enjuanes L, Müller MA, Drosten C, Staeheli P et al (2012) Combined action of type I and type III interferon restricts initial replication of severe acute respiratory syndrome coronavirus in the lung but fails to inhibit systemic virus spread. J Gen Virol 2601-2605 doi:10.1099/vir.0.046284-0

Nguyen HH, van Ginkel FW, Vu HL, Novak MJ, McGhee JR, Mestecky J (2000) Gamma interferon is not required for mucosal cytotoxic T-lymphocyte responses or heterosubtypic immunity to influenza A virus infection in mice. J Virol 74:5495–5501

Nhu QM, Shirey K, Teijaro JR, Farber DL, Netzel-Arnett S, Antalis TM, Fasano A, Vogel SN (2010) Novel signaling interactions between proteinase-activated receptor 2 and toll-like receptors in vitro and in vivo. Mucosal Immunol 3:29–39

Nhu QM, Shirey KA, Pennini ME, Stiltz J, Vogel SN (2012) Proteinase-activated receptor 2 activation promotes an anti-inflammatory and alternatively activated phenotype in LPS-stimulated murine macrophages. Innate Immun 18:193–203

Niessen F, Schaffner F, Furlan-Freguia C, Pawlinski R, Bhattacharjee G, Chun J, Derian CK, Andrade-Gordon P, Rosen H, Ruf W (2008) Dendritic cell PAR1-S1P3 signalling couples coagulation and inflammation. Nature 452:654–658

Oldstone MB (2013) Lessons learned and concepts formed from study of the pathogenesis of the two negative-strand viruses lymphocytic choriomeningitis and influenza. Proc Nat Acad Sci U.S.A 110:4180–4183

Openshaw PJ, Dunning J (2010) Influenza vaccination: lessons learned from the pandemic (H1N1) 2009 influenza outbreak. Mucosal Immunol 3:422–424

Pang IK, Pillai PS, Iwasaki A (2013) Efficient influenza A virus replication in the respiratory tract requires signals from TLR7 and RIG-I. Proc Nat Acad Sci U.S.A 110:13910–13915

Peiris JS, Yu WC, Leung CW, Cheung CY, Ng WF, Nicholls JM, Ng TK, Chan KH, Lai ST, Lim WL et al (2004) Re-emergence of fatal human influenza A subtype H5N1 disease. Lancet 363:617–619

Perrone LA, Plowden JK, Garcia-Sastre A, Katz JM, Tumpey TM (2008) H5N1 and 1918 pandemic influenza virus infection results in early and excessive infiltration of macrophages and neutrophils in the lungs of mice. PLoS Pathog 4:e1000115

Perrone LA, Szretter KJ, Katz JM, Mizgerd JP, Tumpey TM (2010) Mice lacking both TNF and IL-1 receptors exhibit reduced lung inflammation and delay in onset of death following infection with a highly virulent H5N1 virus. J Infect Dis 202:1161–1170

Price GE, Gaszewska-Mastarlarz A, Moskophidis D (2000) The role of alpha/beta and gamma interferons in development of immunity to influenza A virus in mice. J Virol 74:3996–4003

Pugin J, Ricou B, Steinberg KP, Suter PM, Martin TR (1996) Proinflammatory activity in bronchoalveolar lavage fluids from patients with ARDS, a prominent role for interleukin-1. Am J Respir Crit Care Med 153:1850–1856

Rivera J, Proia RL, Olivera A (2008) The alliance of sphingosine-1-phosphate and its receptors in immunity. Nat Rev Immunol 8:753–763

Rosen H, Gonzalez-Cabrera P, Marsolais D, Cahalan S, Don AS, Sanna MG (2008) Modulating tone: the overture of S1P receptor immunotherapeutics. Immunol Rev 223:221–235

Rosen H, Liao J (2003) Sphingosine 1-phosphate pathway therapeutics: a lipid ligand-receptor paradigm. Curr Opin Chem Biol 7:461–468

Salomon R, Hoffmann E, Webster RG (2007) Inhibition of the cytokine response does not protect against lethal H5N1 influenza infection. Proc Nat Acad Sci U.S.A 104:12479–12481

Salomon R, Webster RG (2009) The influenza virus enigma. Cell 136:402–410

Schmitz N, Kurrer M, Bachmann MF, Kopf M (2005) Interleukin-1 is responsible for acute lung immunopathology but increases survival of respiratory influenza virus infection. J Virol 79:6441–6448

Schultz-Cherry S, Hinshaw VS (1996) Influenza virus neuraminidase activates latent transforming growth factor beta. J Virol 70:8624–8629

Seo SU, Kwon HJ, Ko HJ, Byun YH, Seong BL, Uematsu S, Akira S, Kweon MN (2011) Type I interferon signaling regulates Ly6C(hi) monocytes and neutrophils during acute viral pneumonia in mice. PLoS Pathog 7:e1001304

Shea BS, Brooks SF, Fontaine BA, Chun J, Luster AD, Tager AM (2010) Prolonged exposure to sphingosine 1-phosphate receptor-1 agonists exacerbates vascular leak, fibrosis, and mortality after lung injury. Am J Respir Cell Mol Biol 43:662–673

Shirey KA, Lai W, Scott AJ, Lipsky M, Mistry P, Pletneva LM, Karp CL, McAlees J, Gioannini TL, Weiss J et al (2013) The TLR4 antagonist Eritoran protects mice from lethal influenza infection. Nature 497:498–502

Sprenger H, Meyer RG, Kaufmann A, Bussfeld D, Rischkowsky E, Gemsa D (1996) Selective induction of monocyte and not neutrophil-attracting chemokines after influenza A virus infection. J Exp Med 184:1191–1196

Strutt TM, McKinstry KK, Dibble JP, Winchell C, Kuang Y, Curtis JD, Huston G, Dutton RW, Swain SL (2010) Memory CD4+ T cells induce innate responses independently of pathogen. Nat Med 16: 558–564 (1p following 564)

Sun J, Madan R, Karp CL, Braciale TJ (2009) Effector T cells control lung inflammation during acute influenza virus infection by producing IL-10. Nat Med 15:277–284

Szretter KJ, Gangappa S, Lu X, Smith C, Shieh WJ, Zaki SR, Sambhara S, Tumpey TM, Katz JM (2007) Role of host cytokine responses in the pathogenesis of avian H5N1 influenza viruses in mice. J Virol 81:2736–2744

Tam VC, Quehenberger O, Oshansky CM, Suen R, Armando AM, Treuting PM, Thomas PG, Dennis EA, Aderem A (2013) Lipidomic profiling of influenza infection identifies mediators that induce and resolve inflammation. Cell 154:213–227

Tate MD, Pickett DL, van Rooijen N, Brooks AG, Reading PC (2010) Critical role of airway macrophages in modulating disease severity during influenza virus infection of mice. J Virol 84:7569–7580

Teijaro JR, Turner D, Pham Q, Wherry EJ, Lefrancois L, Farber DL (2011a) Cutting edge: tissue-retentive lung memory CD4 T cells mediate optimal protection to respiratory virus infection. J Immunol 187:5510–5514

Teijaro JR, Verhoeven D, Page CA, Turner D, Farber DL (2010) Memory CD4 T cells direct protective responses to influenza virus in the lungs through helper-independent mechanisms. J Virol 84:9217–9226

Teijaro JR, Walsh KB, Cahalan S, Fremgen DM, Roberts E, Scott F, Martinborough E, Peach R, Oldstone MB, Rosen H (2011b) Endothelial cells are central orchestrators of cytokine amplification during influenza virus infection. Cell 146:980–991

Teijaro JR, Walsh KB, Long JP, Tordoff KP, Stark GV, Eisfeld AJ, Kawaoka Y, Rosen H, Oldstone MB (2014a) Protection of ferrets from pulmonary injury due to H1N1 2009 influenza virus infection: immunopathology tractable by sphingosine-1-phosphate 1 receptor agonist therapy. Virology 452–453:152–157

Teijaro JR, Walsh KB, Rice S, Rosen H, Oldstone MB (2014) Mapping the innate signaling cascade essential for cytokine storm during influenza virus infection. Proc Nat Acad Sci U.S.A 111(10):3799–3804

Thiel V, Weber F (2008) Interferon and cytokine responses to SARS-coronavirus infection. Cytokine Growth Factor Rev 19:121–132

Tisoncik JR, Korth MJ, Simmons CP, Farrar J, Martin TR, Katze MG (2012) Into the eye of the cytokine storm. Microbiol Mol Biol Rev (MMBR) 76:16–32

Tscherne DM, Garcia-Sastre A (2011) Virulence determinants of pandemic influenza viruses. J Clin Invest 121:6–13

Tumpey TM, Garcia-Sastre A, Taubenberger JK, Palese P, Swayne DE, Pantin-Jackwood MJ, Schultz-Cherry S, Solorzano A, van Rooijen N, Katz JM et al (2005) Pathogenicity of influenza viruses with genes from the 1918 pandemic virus: functional roles of alveolar macrophages and neutrophils in limiting virus replication and mortality in mice. J Virol 79:14933–14944

Van Reeth K (2000) Cytokines in the pathogenesis of influenza. Vet Microbiol 74:109–116

Walsh KB, Teijaro JR, Wilker PR, Jatzek A, Fremgen DM, Das SC, Watanabe T, Hatta M, Shinya K, Suresh M et al (2011) Suppression of cytokine storm with a sphingosine analog provides protection against pathogenic influenza virus. Proc Nat Acad Sci U.S.A 108:12018–12023

Weiss ID, Wald O, Wald H, Beider K, Abraham M, Galun E, Nagler A, Peled A (2010) IFN-gamma treatment at early stages of influenza virus infection protects mice from death in a NK cell-dependent manner. J Interferon Cytokine Res (the official journal of the International Society for Interferon and Cytokine Research) 30:439–449

Wiley JA, Cerwenka A, Harkema JR, Dutton RW, Harmsen AG (2001) Production of interferon-gamma by influenza hemagglutinin-specific CD8 effector T cells influences the development of pulmonary immunopathology. Am J Pathol 158:119–130

Zheng BJ, Chan KW, Lin YP, Zhao GY, Chan C, Zhang HJ, Chen HL, Wong SS, Lau SK, Woo PC et al (2008) Delayed antiviral plus immunomodulator treatment still reduces mortality in mice infected by high inoculum of influenza A/H5N1 virus. Proc Nat Acad Sci U.S.A 105:8091–8096

Innate Immune Sensing and Response to Influenza

Bali Pulendran and Mohan S. Maddur

Abstract Influenza viruses pose a substantial threat to human and animal health worldwide. Recent studies in mouse models have revealed an indispensable role for the innate immune system in defense against influenza virus. Recognition of the virus by innate immune receptors in a multitude of cell types activates intricate signaling networks, functioning to restrict viral replication. Downstream effector mechanisms include activation of innate immune cells and, induction and regulation of adaptive immunity. However, uncontrolled innate responses are associated with exaggerated disease, especially in pandemic influenza virus infection. Despite advances in the understanding of innate response to influenza in the mouse model, there is a large knowledge gap in humans, particularly in immunocompromised groups such as infants and the elderly. We propose here, the need for further studies in humans to decipher the role of innate immunity to influenza virus, particularly at the site of infection. These studies will complement the existing work in mice and facilitate the quest to design improved vaccines and therapeutic strategies against influenza.

Contents

B. Pulendran (✉) · M.S. Maddur
Emory Vaccine Center, Yerkes National Primate Research Center, Emory University, 954 Gatewood Road, Atlanta, GA 30329, USA
e-mail: bpulend@emory.edu

Current Topics in Microbiology and Immunology (2015) 386: 23–71
DOI: 10.1007/82_2014_405

Published Online: 31 July 2014

1 Introduction

Influenza viruses pose a substantial threat to human and animal health worldwide. Based on the antigenic specificity of their envelope proteins, influenza viruses are classified into three distinct types: A, B, and C. Influenza A virus is the major type that circulates in humans, birds, horses, dogs, and pigs. Influenza virus has a negative sense, single-stranded RNA genome composed of eight segments, which encode up to 13 proteins (Wright et al. 2013). Influenza A virus is further classified into different subtypes based on the antigenic properties of two glycoproteins, the hemagglutinin (HA) and neuraminidase (NA). Influenza virus causes annual epidemics that result in millions of human infections due to the emergence of virus strains arising from high frequency of point mutations (antigenic drift). Furthermore, it also has high potential to cause pandemics, owing to the generation of novel subtypes, especially in animal reservoirs, following the gene reassortments between different influenza viruses (antigenic shift) (Medina and Garcia-Sastre 2011; Tscherne and Garcia-Sastre 2011). Such new variants of influenza virus possess an array of strategies to disarm the host immune system, and enable productive invasion of host cells.

Influenza virus infection in humans can result in a wide range of disease symptoms, from an asymptomatic infection to a severe form of febrile respiratory disease. (Taubenberger and Morens 2008). These acute symptoms may last for 7–10 days, but in most cases influenza virus infection is self-limiting due to the induction of protective immune response (Valkenburg et al. 2011). Enhanced disease severity associated with high mortality is very common in infants, but also in the elderly and in immunocompromised populations (Taubenberger and Morens 2008). Therefore, a key challenge is learning how to induce protective immunity in populations at the extremes of age and in immune compromised subjects. This in turn requires a much deeper understanding of the nature of the innate and adaptive immune systems in these populations.

Although virus is restricted to the respiratory tract and cleared efficiently in most cases, acute fatal infections are associated with systemic spread of virus, particularly in pandemic influenza virus infections (Taubenberger and Morens 2008; Tse et al. 2011). In the United States, more than 36,000 deaths and 200,000 hospitalizations with a total health care cost of $10 billion are associated with influenza infections every year (Mao et al. 2012; Molinari et al. 2007; Taubenberger and Morens 2008). Because of the potentially devastating consequences of influenza pandemics and epidemics, several control measures, such as annual vaccination with either inactivated (IIV) or live attenuated (LAIV) influenza vaccines, are used to prevent the likelihood of future outbreaks. These vaccines incorporate the circulating strains of influenza A/H1, A/H3, and B types, which are expected to emerge in the upcoming season, based on epidemiological data obtained from around the globe (Centers for Disease Control and Prevention 2011). Immunization with influenza vaccines, similar to virus infection, primarily induces virus-specific antibody responses, in the blood as well as the local respiratory tissues (Clements et al. 1986). Although vaccination induce a protective B cell memory response, the numbers of antibody secreting cells wane rapidly over time (Sasaki et al. 2007), leading to reduced antibody titers, which may not be sufficient to prevent virus infection (Castilla et al. 2013; Song et al. 2010). In addition, the potential for emergence of new strains and particularly novel subtypes of influenza virus against which there is no immunological memory in the population, poses major threats to human health.

Based on extensive studies in mouse models and influenza-infected patients, it is becoming clear that the innate immune response is critical for virus control and plays a key role in the induction and regulation of adaptive immune responses. Paradoxically, evidence is also emerging that an exaggerated innate immune response can lead to enhanced pathophysiology including influenza-induced acute respiratory distress syndrome (ARDS) in individuals with secondary complications such as chronic respiratory or cardiac illness, or diabetes. In this review, we discuss recent advances in our understanding of innate immunity to influenza virus, with particular emphasis on the different subsets of innate immune cells involved, the nature of the innate receptors that sense the virus, and the antiviral effector molecules. Furthermore, we highlight the contrasting roles played by the innate immune system in mediating protective antiviral immunity to influenza, versus enhanced pathophysiology and disease severity. Most of these insights have resulted from the mechanistic studies in animal models, in which specific subsets of cells or specific receptors have been ablated using gene targeting. However, the extent to which such insights can be translated into the human model is poorly understood. Thus, we review the knowledge gap about the roles of the various subsets of antigen (Ag) presenting cells and other subpopulations of innate immune cells during influenza infection in humans. We emphasize here, the paramount need for future studies deciphering the role of innate immune response to influenza virus at the site of infection in humans. We believe that these studies will facilitate better understanding of the mechanisms that mediate pathogenesis of disease, and in designing improved vaccine and therapeutic strategies against influenza.

2 Innate Immunity to Influenza Virus

Influenza virus primarily targets the respiratory epithelial cells after breaking through the first innate barrier, the mucous layer. In the majority of individuals infected with the seasonal influenza virus, the virus replication is restricted to the upper respiratory tract (nose, pharynx, and larynx). However, in some cases, the virus can also reach the lower respiratory tract (trachea, bronchi, and lung alveoli) in infections with pandemic strains, especially in children and the elderly. Avian influenza virus, such as H5N1 and H7N9, can even reach the blood circulation to infect cells in distant tissues (Taubenberger and Morens 2008; Tse et al. 2011). Attachment to cells via virus-binding receptors enables endocytic uptake resulting in recognition of the virus through innate receptors, which trigger intricate signaling networks to produce antiviral effector molecules that are capable of conferring the protective immunity.

3 Cells of the Innate Immune System Involved in Immunity to Influenza

3.1 Respiratory Epithelial Cells

It has been demonstrated in fatal human cases as well as in mouse model that the epithelial cells of alveoli (type I and II pneumocytes), trachea, bronchi, nose, pharynx and larynx, and sub mucosal glands are infected by influenza virus (Manicassamy et al. 2010; Nakajima et al. 2012, 2013; Pan et al. 2013). Influenza virus causes productive infection of these epithelial cells resulting in the release of large numbers of infectious virus progeny. Notably, the temperature of nose and pharynx is 30–34 °C, which is relatively lower than the tracheal and internal body temperature (36–37 °C). Human influenza viruses, but not avian viruses, can replicate efficiently at this lower temperature of upper respiratory tract, similar to that at 37 °C (Boonnak et al. 2012; Pelletier et al. 2011). Although different innate immune cells are found in nasal and pharyngeal cavity, the functional features of innate immunity against pathogens at this lower temperature is not known.

In vitro, primary human type II alveolar cells produced type III IFNs in response to human seasonal influenza virus (Wang et al. 2009), whereas differentiated/polarized human bronchial epithelial cells upregulated the expression of type I IFNs upon infection with human influenza virus, but not avian H5N1 influenza virus (Chan et al. 2010; Gerlach et al. 2013; Hsu et al. 2012; Zeng et al. 2007). These findings are consistent with the idea that the activation of type I IFN response in respiratory epithelial cells is crucial for limiting the initial viral infection, since the impaired type I IFN production by H5N1 virus is associated with severe virulence.

In addition to the initial IFN-mediated antiviral response, epithelial cells secrete various cytokines and chemokines such as IL-6, TNF-α, IL-8/CXCL8, CXCL10, CCL2, CCL5 (Chan et al. 2005, 2009; Vareille et al. 2011; Wang et al. 2011; Yu et al. 2011). Furthermore, influenza virus-infected epithelial cells trigger recruitment of an array of innate immune cells, which participate in the protective immune response (Table 1). Interestingly, a recent study in mice showed that expression of GM-CSF by influenza virus-infected alveolar epithelium is essential for effective viral clearance mediated by $CD103^+$ DC-induced $CD8^+$ T cells (Unkel et al. 2012).

3.2 *Neutrophils*

Neutrophils arrive very early at the site of infection, and together with the tissue-resident macrophages are among the first line of cellular defense against pathogens. Although influenza viruses are phagocytized by neutrophils in humans and mice (Brandes et al. 2013), neutrophils are not permissible for productive infection in vitro (Tate et al. 2011). Neutrophils are shown to be important for controlling replication and spread of influenza virus in mouse models (Fujisawa 2001). Lethal dose infection of mice depleted of neutrophils results in increased virus titers in the lungs and in extrapulmonary sites with increased mortality (Tate et al. 2008, 2009, 2011; Tumpey et al. 2005) (Table 1). Consistent with this, in an in vitro culture of human bronchoalveolar lavage fluid (BALF), addition of neutrophils, particularly activated neutrophils, resulted in significantly greater clearance of influenza virus (White et al. 2007). As phagocytic cells, neutrophils can uptake influenza virus-infected apoptotic cells in the lungs to augment clearance of virus (Hashimoto et al. 2007; Watanabe et al. 2005). Despite neutrophils being important participants in the antiviral response in mouse models, the phenotype and functional relevance of large number of neutrophils that accumulate at the site of infection in influenza virus-infected patients, and their mechanisms of anti viral immunity, are poorly understood.

3.3 Macrophages (MΦ)

These include both tissue-resident alveolar macrophages (aMΦ) as well as recently recruited MΦ derived from circulating monocytes (moMΦ) (Table 1). In mouse models, during the course of influenza virus infection, aMΦ are outnumbered by the migrant monocytes, which differentiate into MΦ with an activated phenotype (Herold et al. 2008). Because of their efficient phagocytic capacity, like neutrophils MΦ are critical for clearance of virus-infected and apoptotic cells (Hashimoto et al. 2007; Hoeve et al. 2012; Watanabe et al. 2005). In the absence of MΦ, influenza virus replication is enhanced, leading to greater disease severity and mortality, in mice and pigs (Ito et al. 2011; Kim et al. 2008, 2013; Tate et al. 2010; Tumpey et al. 2005). In humans, most of the studies were done employing in vitro culture of aMΦ obtained from BALF or lung specimens and blood monocyte-derived MΦ (moMΦ). Compared to moMΦ, aMΦ are considered to be resistant to productive infection with the seasonal human influenza virus strains in vitro. Consistent with this, influenza virus replication and induction of proinflammatory cytokine responses were much poorer in aMΦ when compared with moMΦ (van Riel et al. 2011). In the case of avian influenza, however, the virus is able to productively infect both moMΦ and aMΦ (reviewed in Short et al. 2012). Notably, highly pathogenic H5N1 viruses are found to induce more potent proinflammatory cytokine responses, and IFN production than seasonal human viruses (Cheung et al. 2002; Geiler et al. 2011; Lee et al. 2009; Perrone et al. 2008; Yu et al. 2011; Zhou et al. 2006). Moreover, aMΦ are believed to be the main producers of type I IFN, since they are shown to produce significantly more type I IFNs than DCs during influenza virus infection (Helft et al. 2012). Thus, MΦ appear to play critical role in the early innate response to influenza virus infection.

3.4 Monocytes

There are three monocyte subsets identified in the blood, which includes classical monocytes ($CD14^{++}CD16^{-}$ in humans), intermediate monocytes ($CD14^{++}CD16^{+}$ in humans), and the so-called patrolling monocytes ($CD14^{lo}CD16^{++}$ in humans) (Cros et al. 2010; Ziegler-Heitbrock et al. 2010) (Table 1).

Increased number of monocytes are found in the nasal mucosae, the first site of infection (Gill et al. 2005, 2008; Oshansky et al. 2013) as well as in the peripheral blood of influenza virus-infected patients (Giamarellos-Bourboulis et al. 2009; Gill et al. 2005, 2008; McClain et al. 2013; Oshansky et al. 2013). Interestingly, in influenza virus-infected mice, type I IFN-signaling was found to augment the differentiation of stem cells into CCL2-producing monocytes, which mediate the recruitment of additional monocytes (Brandes et al. 2013; Seo et al. 2011). Consistent with this, influenza virus infection of human monocytes induces the release of CCL2 and CXCL10 (Hoeve et al. 2012; Maddur and Pulendran, unpublished data),

Table 1 Cells of the innate immune system involved in immunity to influenza

Cell type	Phenotype markers		Virus binding receptors	Virus sensing receptors	Innate response	Degree of productive infection	Outcome in cell-depleted mice		
	Mice	Humans					Virus load	Disease	References
Respiratory epithelial cells			SAα2,6-absent in mice						
Upper tract	$CD45^{-}$	$CD45^{-}$	SAα2,6 > SAα2,3	TLR3, TLR7, RIG-1, NLRP3	IFNs (low), IL-1β, IL-6, TNFα, IL-8, CCL2, CCL5	++++	NA	NA	NA
Lower tract	$CD45^{-}$	$CD45^{-}$	SAα2,3 > SAα2,6			++++			
Neutrophils									
$CD11c^{-}MHCII^{-}CD11b^{hi}$	$LyC6^{int}$ $Ly6G^{hi}$	$CD16^{hi}$			IL-1β,				Tumpey et al. 2005*
	Siglec-F^{-}	$CD15^{+}$	SAα2,6 > SAα2,3	TLR7, NLRP3?	TNFα,	–	↑	↑	Tate et al. 2008, 2011**
		$CD33^{+}$			IL-8, CXCL2				Brandes et al. 2013**
Macrophages	F4/80^{+}	$CD68^{+}$							
Alveolar	$MHCII^{int}$	$CD14^{-}$	SAα2,6 > SAα2,3	TLR3	IFNs (low), IL-1β,				Tumpey et al. 2005*
$AF^{hi}CD11b^{lo}CD11c^{hi}$	Siglec-F^{hi}	$CD163^{+}$	DC-SIGN, MMR,	RIG-I	IL-6, CCL2,	±	↑	↑	Tate et al. 2010**
	$CD64^{+}$	$CD36^{+}$		NLRP3	CCL5				
Monocyte-derived	$MHCII^{-}$	$CD14^{+}$	SAα2,6 > SAα2,3	TLR3	IL-1β,				Lin et al. 2008**
$CD11b^{hi}CD11c^{lo}$	$CD64^{+/-}$	$CD163^{+}$	DC-SIGN, MMR,	TLR8	IL-6, IL-10,	+++	NC	↓	Lin et al. 2011**
	$Ly6C^{+}$	$CD169^{+}$	MGL	RIG-I, NLRP3	CCL2, CCL5				

(continued)

Table 1 (continued)

Cell type	Phenotype markers		Virus binding receptors	Virus sensing receptors	Innate response	Degree of productive infection	Outcome in cell-depleted mice		
	Mice	Humans					Virus load	Disease	References
Monocytes	MHCII– CD115^{+}	HLA–DR^{+} CD11c^{+}							
Classical	Ly6C^{hi} CD43^{lo}	CD14^{hi} CD16^{-}		TLR7/8	IL-1β				
		CD11b^{hi}	SAα2,6 > SAα2,3	RIG-I	TNFα	+++	NC	↓	Lin et al. 2008**
	CCR2^{hi}	CCR2^{hi}		NLRP3	IL-6				Lin et al. 2011**
	CX3CR1^{lo}	CX3CR1^{lo}			CCL2, CXCL10				
Intermediate	LY6C^{hi} CD43^{hi}	CD14^{hi} CD16^{+}		TLR7/8					
		CD11b^{hi}	SAα2,6 > SAα2,3	RIG-I	ND	+++	ND	ND	NA
		CCR2^{lo}		NLRP3					
		CX3CR1^{hi}							
Non-classical/patrolling	LY6C^{lo} CD43^{hi}	CD14^{lo} CD16^{hi}		TLR7/8					
		CD11b^{lo}	SAα2,6 > SAα2,3	RIG-I	ND	+++	ND	ND	NA
	CX3CR^{hi}	CX3CR^{hi}		NLRP3					
	CCR2^{lo}	CCR2^{lo}							

(continued)

Table 1 (continued)

Cell type	Phenotype markers		Virus binding receptors	Virus sensing receptors	Innate response	Degree of productive infection	Outcome in cell-depleted mice		
	Mice	Humans					Virus load	Disease	References
Dentritic cells (DCs)	$MHCII^{hi}$	$HLA\text{-}DR^{hi}$							
$CD11b^{hi}$ $CD103^{-}$	$SIRP\alpha^{+}$	$SIRP\alpha^{+}$	$SA\alpha2,6 > SA\alpha2,3$		IFN-α (low)				
$CD11c^{hi}$ cDCs	$CX3CR1^{int}$	$CD11b^{lo}$		TLR3	IL-6				McGill et al. 2008*
	CD64–	$Langerin^{+/-}$		RIG-1	IL-12	+++	↑	↑	GeurtsvanKessel et al. 2008*
$CD1c^{+}$ $CD11c^{hi}$ mDC1	$Langerin^{-}$	$CD1a^{+}$	MMR (mDC1)	TLR4	TNFα				
	$CD24^{lo}$				CXCL10				
$CD103^{+}$ $CD11b^{lo}$	$Langerin^{+}$	$Langerin^{-}$							
$CD11c^{hi}$ cDCs	$XCR1^{+}$	$SIRP\alpha^{-}$		TLR3					GeurtsvanKessel et al. 2008*
	$CLEC9a^{+}$	$XCR1^{+}$	$SA\alpha2,6 > SA\alpha2,3$	RIG-I	IL-6	++	↑	↑	
$CD141^{hi}$ $CD11c^{lo}$ mDC2	$CD64^{-}$	$CLEC9a^{+}$		TLR4	TNFα				Unkel et al. 2012*
	$CD24^{hi}$	$CD11b^{lo}$							
Monocyte-derived DCs	$CD64^{+}$	$CD1a^{+}$	$SA\alpha2,6 > SA\alpha2,3$	TLR3					
$Ly6C^{hi/lo}$ $CD11b^{+}$ $CD11c^{+}$	$Mar\text{-}1^{+}$	$DC\text{-}SIGN^{hi}$	DC-SIGN	RIG-I	IL-6	+++	NC	↓	Lin et al. 2008**
	$SIRP\alpha^{+}$	$CD1c^{hi}$	MMR	NLRP3	IL-12				Lin et al. 2011**
$DC\text{-}SIGN^{hi}$ $CD11b^{+}$ $CD11c^{+}$	$CX3CR1^{int}$	$CD14^{-}$	MGL	TLR4	TNFα				
$CD11c^{lo}$ Plasmacytoid DCs (pDCs)	$MHCII^{lo}$	$HLA\text{-}DR^{+}$							
	$CD11b^{-}$	$CD123^{hi}$	$SA\alpha2,6 > SA\alpha2,3$	TLR7	IFN-α (high)	+	↑	↑	Kaminski et al. 2012**
	$LyC6^{+}$ $mPDCA\text{-}1^{+}$	$CD11b^{-}$			IL-6				

(continued)

Table 1 (continued)

Cell type	Phenotype markers		Virus binding receptors	Virus sensing receptors	Innate response	Degree of productive infection	Outcome in cell-depleted mice		
	Mice	Humans					Virus load	Disease	References
		$CD302^+$			TNFα				
Natural killer cells ($CD3^-$)	NK1.1	$CD56^{hi/lo/-}$			IFN-γ				
	$CD49b^+$	$CD16^{+/-}$	SAα2,6 = SAα2,3	NKp46	Granzyme B	++	↑	↑	Gazit et al. 2006*
	$CD11b^+$	$KIR^{+/-}$		NKG2D	Perforin				
	$CD27^+$								
Natural killer T (NKT) cells ($CD3^+$)	NK1.1	CD56+	ND	ND	IFN-γ, IL-22	ND	↑	↑	de Santo et al. 2008**
Innate lymphoid cells (ILCs)									
ILC2	$CD25^+$	$CD25^{lo}$			Amphiregulin				
	$CD90^+$	$CD117^{+/-}$	ND	ND	IL-13	ND	ND	↑	Monticelli et al. 2011*
	$CD127^+$	$CD127^+$			IL-5				

cDCs Conventional DCs (Mice)
mDCs Myeloid DCs (Humans)
SAα2,6 Sialic acid with α2,6 linkage to galatose
SAα2,3 Sialic acid with α2,3 linkage to galatose
NA Not applicable
NC Not changed
ND Not determined
* Sublethal low dose infection
** Lethal high dose infection

but inhibits the responsiveness to chemokines, such as CCL2, CCL3, CCL4, and CCL5 by downregulation of their respective chemokine receptors (Salentin et al. 2003), presumably to retain these cells at the site of infection.

As discussed earlier, in addition to transformation to moMΦ, monocytes that migrate to influenza virus-infected tissues can also differentiate into monocyte-derived dendritic cells (moDCs) (Cao et al. 2012; Lin et al. 2008; Unkel et al. 2012). In vitro studies have shown that productive influenza virus infection of human monocytes induces secretion of TNF-α and GM-CSF, and triggers rapid transformation into cells with phenotypic features of DCs (Cao et al. 2012; Hou et al. 2012; Qu et al. 2003). In contrast, we found that infection of monocytes with influenza virus did not induce activation and TNF-α secretion, but merely induces the loss of CD14 resulting in DC-like phenotype ($CD11c^{+}CD14^{-}$). Despite the phenotypic similarity to DCs, these $CD14^{-}$ cells lack the functional properties of DCs (Maddur and Pulendran unpublished data). Mice with reduced numbers of monocytes at the site of infection, such as $CCR2^{-/-}$ mice or mice treated with a CCR2 antagonist did not show increased viral loads, raising the question of the direct role of monocytes in virus clearance (Lin et al. 2008, 2011). Furthermore, the relevance of these findings of mouse models and in vitro studies to influenza human patients is not clear and is worth investigating for understanding the role of monocytes in influenza.

3.5 Dendritic Cells (DCs)

DCs are rare but widely distributed throughout the body, and function as key orchestrators of the immune response (Banchereau and Steinman 1998; Manicassamy and Pulendran 2011; Pulendran et al. 2010b; Steinman and Banchereau 2007).

3.5.1 DC Subsets

In mice, DCs can be broadly classified as $CD11c^{hi}$ conventional DCs (cDCs) and $CD11c^{lo}$ $B220^{+}$ plasmacytoid DCs (pDCs). In the steady-state respiratory tract, the epithelial layer of conducting airways is lined by $CD103^{+}CD11b^{lo}$ cDCs (langerin^{+}), which extends their long dendrites into the airway lumen. The lamina propria, which is beneath the epithelial layer, contains $CD103^{-}CD11b^{hi}$ cDCs (langerin^{-}) as well as $CD11c^{lo}$ pDCs. Further, all the three DC subsets are found in the alveolar septa of lung parenchyma. Under inflammatory conditions, additional $CD11c^{lo}CD11b^{+}Ly6C^{+}$ moDCs are recruited to the conducting airways and lung parenchyma (Guilliams et al. 2013; Helft et al. 2010; Lambrecht and Hammad 2009, 2012). Of note, in the lungs, MΦ subsets, which are $CD11c^{hi}$, must be distinguished from cDCs based on other markers (Table 1). The respiratory tract draining lymphoid tissues contain resident DC subsets such as, $CD8\alpha^{+}$ cDCs, and $CD11b^{+}$ cDCs as well as $CD11c^{lo}$ pDCs, in addition to migratory DCs (Haniffa et al. 2013; Helft et al. 2010).

In influenza virus-infected mice, there is an increased accumulation of $CD103^{-}CD11b^{hi}$ cDCs as well as $CD103^{+}CD11b^{lo}$ cDCs in the trachea and lung interstitial tissue, with a transient increase in $CD11c^{lo}$ pDCs, all of which display an activated phenotype (GeurtsvanKessel et al. 2008; Ho et al. 2011; McGill et al. 2008). In addition, $CD11c^{lo}CD11b^{+}Ly6C^{+}$ moDCs also infiltrate the lungs in high number (Guilliams et al. 2013; Lin et al. 2008, 2011). pDCs are considered to be less susceptible to influenza virus infection, compared to the highest susceptibility of $CD103^{+}$ cDCs and $CD11b^{+}Ly6C^{+}$ moDCs, and that of intermediate susceptibility of $CD11b^{hi}$ cDCs (Hao et al. 2008; Hargadon et al. 2011). Of relevance, murine DCs are considered to be less susceptible to productive influenza virus infection than human DCs in vitro (Hartmann et al. 2013; Ioannidis et al. 2012).

In addition to secretion of inflammatory cytokines and chemokines, DCs efficiently migrated to the regional mediastinal LN (MLN) and induce protective adaptive immune responses to augment viral clearance (see later sections) (GeurtsvanKessel et al. 2008; Helft et al. 2012; Ho et al. 2011; Kim and Braciale 2009; McGill et al. 2008; Unkel et al. 2012). Consistent with these findings, an effective reduction in influenza virus replication in the lungs and enhanced survival of infected mice was observed following adoptive transfer of $CD11c^{hi}$ cDCs 1 day before infection (GeurtsvanKessel et al. 2008) or influenza virus-activated bone marrow-derived DCs (BMDCs) 1 day after infection (Boonnak et al. 2013). Conversely, removal or loss of pDCs and/or migratory cDCs in mice prior to influenza virus infection resulted in higher viral load in the lungs with increased mortality, supporting the contribution of DCs in viral control (GeurtsvanKessel et al. 2008; Kaminski et al. 2012; McGill et al. 2008).

In humans, similar to mice, two lineages of DCs are identified, which include $CD11c^{+}CD123^{lo}$ myeloid DCs (mDCs) and $CD11c^{-}CD123^{hi}$ pDCs. The respiratory tract has both mDCs and pDCs. Further, $CD1c^{+}$ mDC1 ($CD1a^{+}langerin^{-/+}$), which resemble Langerhans cells and $CD141^{+}$ mDC2 ($CD1a^{-}langerin^{-}$) subsets of mDCs identified in the human lungs are proposed to correspond to $CD103^{-}CD11b^{hi}$ cDC and $CD103^{+}CD11b^{lo}langerin^{+}$ cDC subsets in mice, respectively (Haniffa et al. 2012; Yu et al. 2013) (Table 1). The draining lymphoid tissue contains pDCs and $CD1c^{+}$ mDC1 as well as $CD141^{+}$ mDC2 (Segura et al. 2012).

Studies have observed an increased number of mDCs and pDCs in the nasal mucosa, but a decreased number in the peripheral blood of influenza virus-infected patients (Gill et al. 2005, 2008; Huang et al. 2013), supporting the recruitment of circulating DCs to the site of infection. Furthermore, influenza virus infection induced activation of human DC subsets including $CD1c^{+}$ mDC1, pDC and moDCs characterized by upregulation of expression of HLA-DR, HLA-ABC, CD80, CD86, CD40, and CCR7 (Fonteneau et al. 2003; Larsson et al. 2000; le Nouen et al. 2011; Osterlund et al. 2005; Piqueras et al. 2006; Smed-Sorensen et al. 2012). Interestingly, although enhanced production of IL-6, IL-8, and CCL2 was observed in pandemic H1N1 2009 influenza virus-infected patients (Lee et al. 2011), in vitro virus infection failed to enhance cytokine secretion in human moDCs (Osterlund et al. 2010). Consistent with this, influenza virus infection of moDCs failed to induce maturation and production of IFN-α, TNF-α, and IL-6, due to the suppressive effects of NS1 protein (Fernandez-Sesma et al. 2006). Notably, exposure to type I IFNs prior to influenza virus infection was found to enhance the activation and cytokine secretion of mDCs and pDCs, by partially overcoming the inhibition by IFN antagonist NS1 protein of influenza virus (Fernandez-Sesma et al. 2006; Phipps-Yonas et al. 2008).

3.6 Natural Killer (NK) Cells

NK cells possess unique natural cytotoxicity receptors (NCRs) such as NCR1 in mice, and NKp30, NKp44, and NKp46 in humans, involved in recognition of viral- and tumor-associated molecules and activation of NK cells (Jost and Altfeld 2013). Influenza virus productively infects human NK cells in vitro (Mao et al. 2009, 2010) as well as mice NK cells in vivo (Guo et al. 2009). In mouse models of influenza virus infection, there is a substantial increase in the population of activated NK cells expressing CD107a and IFN-γ in the lungs, which can lyse influenza virus-infected cells through granzyme B and perforin, and contribute to the virus control (Ge et al. 2012; He et al. 2004; Hwang et al. 2012; Verbist et al. 2012). Accordingly, NK cell–depletion (Ge et al. 2012) or defects in NK cell activity (Gazit et al. 2006) resulted in delayed virus clearance from the lungs with worsen disease in mouse models of sublethal influenza virus infection.

Consistent with this, in humans, NKp46 and NKG2D-mediated recognition of HA on influenza virus-infected cells induced NK cell-mediated cytolysis of target cells (Draghi et al. 2007; Mandelboim et al. 2001). However, in contrast to these in vitro findings, virus infection was associated with transient deficiency of circulating NK cells, particularly CD56^{+++} NK cells, and downregulation of NK cell activity, especially with pandemic H1N1 2009 influenza patients (Denney et al. 2010; Fox et al. 2012; Guo et al. 2011; Heltzer et al. 2009). It is not clear whether the reduced number of NK cells in peripheral blood is a reflection of augmented recruitment of NK cells to the site of infection, the respiratory tract. However, the fatal cases of influenza virus infections showed reduced number or absence of NK cells in lung inflammatory infiltrate (Denney et al. 2010; Welliver et al. 2007). Consistent with this, studies have found that influenza virus-infection of NK cells inhibits their functions of cytotoxicity and cytokine and chemokine secretion in humans (Mao et al. 2010) as well as in mice (Guo et al. 2009).

3.7 Natural Killer T (NKT) Cells

These are a heterogeneous group of T cells that share properties of both T cells and natural killer (NK) cells. Many of these cells recognize the non-polymorphic CD1d molecule, an Ag-presenting molecule that binds self- and foreign lipids and glycolipids (reviewed in Bendelac et al. 2007).

In mice, influenza virus-activated invariant NKT cells were found to reduce viral load and the immune-pathology during lethal influenza virus infection by different mechanisms mediated by IFN-γ and IL-22 (Kok et al. 2012; Paget et al. 2011). Interestingly, in influenza virus-infected mice as well as in humans, activated iNKT cells were found to diminish the immunosuppressive effect of influenza virus-induced myeloid-derived suppressor cells (MDSCs) through CD1d- and CD40-mediated interactions (de Santo et al. 2008). Despite these striking observation, the role of NKT cells in humans, particularly at the site of infection is unexplored.

3.8 Innate Lymphoid Cells (ILCs)

In mice as well as in humans, ILCs include three groups of cells, (1) IFN-γ-producing NK cells and ILC1, (2) IL-4/IL-5/IL-13-producing ILC2, and (3) IL-17/IL-22-producing ILC3 and LTi (lymphoid tissue-induce) cells (Spits et al. 2013). Recent studies have revealed the diverse role of ILC2 in influenza virus infection. In mice lacking T cells and B cells, ILC2 cells were found to accumulate in the lungs following sublethal influenza virus infection, and were critical for sustaining lung epithelial barrier and remodeling of respiratory tissue through secretion of amphiregulin (Monticelli et al. 2011). In contrast, sublethal influenza virus infection triggered airway hyper-reactivity (AHR) is shown to be mediated by IL-5 and IL-13–producing ILC2 (natural helper cells) that are activated by IL-33 secreted by aMΦ and NKT cells (Chang et al. 2011; Gorski et al. 2013). The significance of these cells during human influenza needs to be determined.

3.9 Other Innate Immune Cells

In spite of the presence of other innate immune cells like mast cells, eosinophils and basophils in the lungs and airways, the interaction of these cells with influenza virus is not fully explored.

4 Virus Binding Surface Receptors

4.1 Sialic Acid-Containing Receptors

Sialic acid (SA, N-acetylneuraminic acid) is identified as the primary attachment site on the cell surface that interacts with the receptor-binding site within the globular head of HA of influenza viruses (Skehel and Wiley 2000; Wilson and Cox 1990). Following the interaction of virus with SA-containing receptors, entry into the cell might involve clathrin-mediated endocytosis or caveolin and clathrin independent mechanism (de Vries et al. 2011; Lakadamyali et al. 2006).

Sialic acid is added to surface proteins as part of post-translational modification. SA consists of nine carbon sugar frequently attached to underlying terminal galactose residue of glycoproteins or glycolipids of cell surface receptors by either α2,3 (SAα2,3Gal) or α2,6 (SAα2,6Gal) linkage (Wilson and Cox 1990). The SA and its linkage is critical for facilitating influenza virus infection of epithelial and immune cells, since enzymatic switching of SA linkage or removal of cell-surface SA can alter susceptibility or confer resistance to influenza virus infection. It has been observed that human influenza virus strains usually bind SAα2,6Gal, whereas avian influenza virus strains have preference for SAα2,3Gal linkage, (reviewed in Londrigan et al. 2012). Thus, SA is considered to be an important determinant of virus tropism and contributes to viral pathogenesis and induction of immune response.

In the human respiratory tract, using lectins specific for SA linkage, epithelial cells of the nasal mucosa, paranasal sinuses, the pharynx, the trachea, and the bronchi and bronchioles were found to predominantly express SAα2,6Gal, with SAα2,3Gal expression being rare (Shinya et al. 2006). However, the cells of the lower respiratory tract, including non-ciliated cuboidal bronchiolar cells and the type II pneumocytes of alveoli predominantly expressed SAα2,3Gal (Ibricevic et al. 2006; Shinya et al. 2006; Thompson et al. 2006). Although a similar pattern of SAα2,3Gal expression is observed in mouse respiratory tract, SAα2,6Gal is not expressed (Ibricevic et al. 2006) (Table 1). In the human innate immune cells, cell surface expression of SAα2,6Gal is found to be predominant compared to SAα2,3Gal (Corral et al. 1990; Hartshorn et al. 1995; Nicholls et al. 2007; Ramos et al. 2011; Sakabe et al. 2011; Videira et al. 2008) (Table 1).

Despite these observations of differential expression of SA-linkages on cells and its significance in virus attachment, the identity of SA-containing receptors is unexplored. Further, it is also not clear whether virus binding SA-containing receptors trigger intracellular signals for activation and cytokine production in innate cells. However, study using UV-inactivated genetically modified human influenza viruses showed that virus binding to SAα2,3Gal induced higher levels of proinflammatory cytokines and IFN-inducible genes in DCs and MΦ compared to influenza virus with SAα2,6Gal binding specificity (Ramos et al. 2011), suggesting a viral replication-independent induction of innate response. These finding indicate that the binding of SA-containing receptors to HA can induce differential innate antiviral responses. Further, inactivated influenza vaccine (IIV) used in humans is a split vaccine mainly containing HA, and hence, the interaction of IIV with SA-containing receptors is likely to play role in the vaccine-induced immunity. Therefore, deciphering the identity, structure, and functional features (like cytoplasmic signaling network) of SA-containing receptors involved in influenza is warranted.

Although SA is critical for virus binding and tropism, the cells lacking surface SA were found to be permissive to virus entry and infection, although to lesser extent (Thompson et al. 2006). Further, it is believed that SA enhances the binding of influenza virus to cell surface to facilitate the interaction with other receptors required for virus entry (Londrigan et al. 2012). Consistent with this, several cell surface carbohydrate-recognizing receptors are also proposed in binding to sugar residues within the surface glycoproteins of influenza virus to augment virus uptake. They include C-type lectin receptors (CLRs), which are the innate recognition receptors of host (discussed below).

5 Virus Sensing Receptors

Influenza virus is sensed by different pattern-recognition receptors (PRRs). Detection of viral components by PRRs triggers intracellular signaling cascades responsible for secretion of type I IFNs, proinflammatory cytokines, and chemokines, and acquisition of activation status. Recent studies have shown that influenza virus is sensed by PRRs such as, CLRs, Toll-like receptors (TLRs), retinoic acid-inducible gene I (RIG-I)-like receptors (RLRs), and nucleotide oligomerization domain (NOD)-like receptors (NLRs).

5.1 C-Type Lectin Receptors (CLRs)

These are a diverse family of transmembrane proteins that contain one or more carbohydrate recognition domains (CRDs), but do not bind only carbohydrate structures (Geijtenbeek and Gringhuis 2009; Sancho and Reis e Sousa 2012). Interaction between influenza virus and CLRs specific to mannose and galactose, which serve as the receptor for virus attachment and infection of cells, has been observed. These CLRs include (i) macrophage mannose receptor (MMR, CD206, which binds to mannose, fucose, and sulphated sugars), (ii) macrophage galactose-type lectin (MGL, CD301, which binds mainly to terminal GalNAc residues, but also to galactose and Lewis-X structures) and (iii) DC-specific ICAM3-grabbing non-integrin (DC-SIGN, CD209, which binds mannose-rich glycans) (Geijtenbeek and Gringhuis 2009; Sancho and Reis e Sousa 2012).

These CLRs are primarily expressed on monocytes, MΦ, and mDCs (Table 1). They can mediate influenza virus binding to augment the SA-dependent virus up take by cells resulting in enhanced susceptibility to infection. However, these receptors alone do not mediate efficient infection in the absence of SA (Londrigan et al. 2011; Wang et al. 2008). Furthermore, these CLRs, which are known to bind influenza virus lack both activating-ITAM as well as inhibitory-ITIM cytoplasmic signaling motifs, but possess tyrosine motifs involved in endocytosis (Geijtenbeek and Gringhuis 2009; Sancho and Reis e Sousa 2012). Hence, based on the recent findings, it is speculated that virus-bound CLRs can employ the endocytic equipment to direct the captured viral antigenic cargo for processing and cross-presentation to T cells, especially MMR and MGL (Sancho and Reis e Sousa 2012). Furthermore, despite being unable to induce myeloid cell activation by themselves, these CLRs, particularly DC-SIGN, are found to modulate the outcome of signaling by other PRRs (Geijtenbeek and Gringhuis 2009; Sancho and Reis e Sousa 2012). It is therefore important to determine the effect of binding of influenza virus to these CLRs on the activation and function of myeloid cells induced by other PRRs, and also the ensuing $CD8^+$ T cell immune response.

5.2 Toll-Like Receptors (TLRs)

TLRs have emerged as key sensors of innate immunity to viruses recognizing their PAMPs. TLR2 and TLR4 on cell surface detect the envelope glyco/lipoproteins and that of intracellular/endosomal TLR3, TLR7, TLR8, and TLR9 sense viral nucleic acids (Finberg et al. 2007; Kawai and Akira 2011).

All TLRs recruit a specific set of adaptor molecules that harbor TIR (Toll-IL-1 receptor) domain, such as MyD88, TIRAP, TRIF, or TRAM, a combination of which decides the response to ligand. MyD88 is employed by all TLRs, except TLR3, which uses TRIF. Whereas TLR4 can utilize TIRAP or TRAM to recruit MyD88 or TRIF, TLR2 uses TIRAP to recruit MyD88. Further, MyD88-dependent and TRIF-dependent signaling pathways activate NF-kB, interferon regulatory factor7 (IRF7) or IRF3 through IRAKs, TRAF6, TAK1, and IKK complex, resulting in induction of antiviral status and secretion of cytokines. Interestingly, TLRs cooperate with other PRRs like NLRs and RLRs to induce innate immunity to pathogens including influenza (reviewed in Kawai and Akira 2011) (Fig. 1). Studies have shown that influenza virus is recognized by different TLRs, such as TLR7/8 that bind ssRNA and TLR3, which senses the dsRNA in the endosomes. In addition, TLR4 can detect the damage-associated molecular patterns (DAMPs) released from virus-infected cells (Table 2).

5.2.1 TLR3

Although absent in pDCs, monocytes, and neutrophils, low levels of TLR3 is expressed in MΦ, mDCs, moDCs (Kadowaki et al. 2001) and primary respiratory epithelial cells of mice (le Goffic et al. 2006) and humans (Guillot et al. 2005; Ioannidis et al. 2013) (Table 1). It is important to note that due to the action of RNA helicase DDX39B, dsRNA is not generated during replication of influenza virus (Pichlmair et al. 2006; Wisskirchen et al. 2011). It is therefore important to determine whether TLR3 plays a significant role in antiviral immunity during influenza virus infections and to identify the ligands for TLR3 within the influenza-infected cells.

Pretreatment of human moDCs with TLR3 ligand (poly I:C) conferred resistance to infection with H5N1 influenza virus (Thitithanyanont et al. 2007). Consistent with this, intranasal pretreatment of mice with poly I:C provided high level of protection against lethal challenge with influenza virus (Wong et al. 2009).

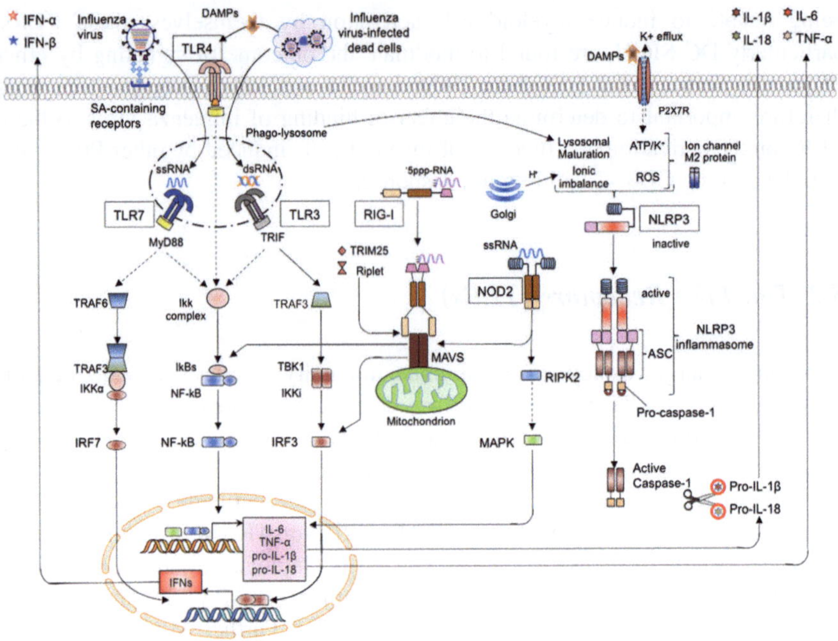

Fig. 1 Recognition of influenza virus infection by pattern-recognition receptors. Activation of TLRs upon detection of viral RNA (TLR3 and TLR7/8) or binding of death-associated molecular patterns (DAMPS; TLR4) recruits adaptor molecules (MyD88 and TRIF) triggering distinct signaling pathways that activates nuclear translocation of transcription factors (IRF3/7 and NF-kB) to induce production of type I interferons (I IFNs) and inflammatory cytokines (IL-6, TNF and pro-IL-1β and -IL-18). Recognition of 5'ppp-RNA by RIG-I activates recruitment of MAVS on mitochondrion, which in turn induces the production of cytokines through IRF3/IRF7. Of the NLRs, NOD2 detects ssRNA to activate translocation of MAPK and IRF3/IRF7 by recruiting adaptor molecules, RIPK2 and MAVS, respectively, to induce cytokine production. Activation of NLRP3 mediated by diverse stimuli, dependent on ionic channel M2 protein of influenza virus, recruits ASC (apoptosis-associated speck-like protein containing a caspase recruitment domain), which in turn interact with pro-caspase-1 to form NLRP3 inflammasome. Autoactivation of caspase-1 cleaves pro-IL-1β/IL-18 to mature IL-1β/IL-18 for their secretion

Furthermore, lethal dose influenza virus-infected mice showed TLR3-mediated enhancement of inflammatory reaction and CD8+ T cell response, associated with augmented viral clearance, compared to TLR3−/− mice (le Goffic et al. 2006) (Table 2). However, TLR3−/− mice survived longer than control mice (le Goffic et al. 2006), suggesting that TLR3-triggered innate response inhibits viral spread, but the ensuing adaptive immunity is detrimental to the host.

5.2.2 TLR7/8

In humans, the highest levels of TLR7 is expressed in pDCs (Kadowaki et al. 2001), whereas mDC1, mDC2, LCs, and NK cells lack TLR7 (Kadowaki et al. 2001;

Table 2 Innate receptors involved in immunity to influenza

Innate receptors	Virus derived or induced ligands	Source of ligand	Virus dose	Outcome of infection or vaccination in knock-out mice			References
				Virus load	Mortality	Control of adaptive immunity	
Toll-like receptor (TLR)							
TLR3	dsRNA?	Uptake of dead-infected cells	LD	↑ (9 days)	↓	Reduced $CD8^+$ T cells	le Goffic et al. 2006
			SLD	ND	ND	Normal $CD8^+$ T cell, $CD4^+$ T cell and antibody response	Seo et al. 2010; Koyama et al. 2007
			Vaccine	–	–	ND	–
TLR7	ssRNA	Live or inactivated virus	LD	NC/↑	NC/↑	Reduced virus-specific antibody response	Jeisy-Scott et al. 2012
			SLD	NC	NC	Reduced $CD4^+$ T cell and antibody response	Seo et al. 2010; Pang et al. 2013a, b
			Vaccine	–	–	Reduced $CD4^+$ T cell and antibody response	Koyama et al. 2007, 2010
TLR4	DAMPs-S100A9	Released from virus-infected cells	LD	↓	↓	ND	Shirey et al. 2013; Tsai et al. 2014
			SLD	ND	ND	ND	–
			Vaccine	–	–	ND	–
RIG-1-Like receptor (RLR)							
RIG-I	5ppp RNA with panhandle structure	Generated by viral replication	LD	↑	↑	ND	Pang et al. 2013a, b
			SLD	NC	NC	Normal $CD8^+$ T cell, $CD4^+$ T cell and antibody response	Koyama et al. 2007
			Vaccine	–	–	Normal $CD4^+$ T cell and antibody response	Koyama et al. 2007, 2010

(continued)

Table 2 (continued)

Innate receptors	Virus derived or induced ligands	Source of ligand	Virus dose	Outcome of infection or vaccination in knock-out mice			References
				Virus load	Mortality	Control of adaptive immunity	
NOD-Like receptor (NLR)							
NLRP3-ASC-Caspase-1 Inflammasome	M2 protein PB1-F2	Viral replication triggered signals (cellular damage)	LD	NC	↑	Reduced $CD8^+$ T cell, $CD4^+$ T cell and Mucosal IgA response	Ichinohe et al. 2009; Thomas et al. 2009; Allen et al. 2009
			SLD	↑ (8 days)	↑	Reduced/Normal $CD8^+$ T cell, $CD4^+$ T cell and B cell response	Ichinohe et al. 2009; Pang et al. 2013a, b; Thomas et al. 2009
			Vaccine	–	–	ND	–
NOD2	ssRNA	Generated by viral replication	LD	↑	↑	Reduced $CD8^+$ T cell response	Sabbah et al. 2009; Lupfer et al. 2014
			SLD	ND	ND	ND	–
			Vaccine	–	–	ND	–
NLRX1	PB1-F2	Generated by viral replication	LD	↑	NC	ND	Jaworska et al. 2014
			SLD	ND	ND	ND	–
			Vaccine	–	–	ND	–

LD Lethal high dose infection
SLD Sublethal low dose infection
Vaccine Inactivated whole virus vaccine
NC Not changed
ND Not determined

Merad et al. 2013). However, TLR8 is expressed at low levels by moMΦ (Hui et al. 2011) and mDCs, but not pDCs (Kadowaki et al. 2001). In mice, CD8α^+ cDCs lack TLR7, but express TLR3, whereas CD8α^- cDCs, pDCs, and BMDCs (Edwards et al. 2003), and also BMMΦ (Kawai and Akira 2011) express TLR7 (Table 1).

In response to live or inactivated influenza virus in vitro, pDCs produced high levels of IFN-α, and also inflammatory cytokines in a TLR7-and MyD88-dependent manner through recognition of viral ssRNA (Diebold et al. 2004; Koyama et al. 2007; Lund et al. 2004) (Fig. 1). TLR7-mediated sensing of inactivated-influenza virus by pDCs is required to confer protective primary adaptive immune response in mice (Geeraedts et al. 2008; Koyama et al. 2007, 2010). In contrast, cytokine production in the lungs following live influenza virus infection did not require TLR7-signaling in pDCs (Koyama et al. 2010). Despite the uncontrolled viral load and mortality observed in TLR7/MyD88-deficit mice infected with lethal dose of influenza virus in a previous study (Seo et al. 2010), the lack of TLR7 did not markedly alter the viral load, disease pathology and inflammatory cytokine response in following lethal dose (Jeisy-Scott et al. 2011) or sublethal dose (Pang et al. 2013b). Consistent with this finding, TLR7-induced type I IFN in pDCs was dispensable for induction of protective response to influenza virus in mice vaccinated with live-virus vaccine (Koyama et al. 2010). Furthermore, IFN-α secretion by murine mDC/BMDCs in response to influenza virus is found to be dependent on live virus replication, but not on TLR7/MyD88- signaling (Barchet et al. 2005; Koyama et al. 2007). Nevertheless, in murine BMDCs, TLR7-signaling was required for the induction of pro-IL-1β and secretion of mature IL-1β after influenza virus infection (Ichinohe et al. 2010). These results suggest a cell-specific role of TLR7 in the induction of innate immune response to influenza virus infection as well as vaccination.

5.2.3 TLR4

TLR4 is expressed mainly on myeloid cells including, neutrophils, monocytes, mDCs, moDCs, and MΦ (Table 2). Although the ligand for TLR4 in influenza virus is not known, a DAMP molecule, S100A9 released in influenza virus-infected lungs was found to trigger TLR4-MyD88-signaling pathway in MΦ to induce exaggerating proinflammatory response, cell-death, and virus pathogenesis following lethal infection (Tsai et al. 2014) (Fig. 1). Furthermore, similar to TLR4 deficient mice (Nhu et al. 2010), treatment of mice with a TLR4 antagonist, Eritoran, was found to protect from lethal influenza infection by alleviating lung pathology, clinical symptoms, cytokine, and oxidized phospholipid expression, as well as by controlling viral loads, a process dependent on CD14 and TLR2 expression (Shirey et al. 2013). Activation of TLR4-signaling during influenza infection seems to induce an exaggerated inflammatory response.

5.3 RIG-I-Like Receptors (RLRs)

These are the RNA-sensing PRRs expressed in the cytosol of majority of the mammalian cells. RLRs represent a family of RNA helicases, which includes three members, RIG-I, melanoma differentiation-associated gene 5 (MDA5), and laboratory of genetics and physiology-2 (LGP-2) (Takeuchi and Akira 2009). In addition to the RNA helicase domain, RIG-I and MDA5 contain two N-terminal caspase recruitment domains (CARDs), whereas LGP2 lacks a CARD component, and functions as a negative regulator of RIG-I/MDA5-signaling (Loo and Gale 2011). RIG-I recognizes RNA containing 5'-triphosphate with panhandle-like secondary structures, whereas MDA5 preferentially senses long dsRNA (>2 kb) (Takeuchi and Akira 2009). RLRs signal through a common adaptor IFN-β promoter stimulator-1 (IPS-1), also known as mitochondrial antiviral signaling (MAVS) leading to phosphorylation of IRF7/3 and NF-kB , which in turn induce type I IFNs, and proinflammatory cytokines and chemokines, respectively (Loo and Gale 2011). The recruitment of the adaptor MAVS is dependent on E3-ligase tripartite motif containing 25 (TRIM25)- and Riplet-dependent ubiquitination of RIG-I (Loo and Gale 2011). Under steady state, RLR is expressed at low levels, but is greatly increased in response to IFN and after virus infection (Loo and Gale 2011) (Fig. 1).

In influenza virus-infected cells, RIG-I is the RLR that senses the virus in cytosol by recognizing the 5'-triphosphate -RNA sequence motifs along RNA containing some dsRNA part (panhandle), which is generated by active viral replication within the cells (Kato et al. 2006; Pichlmair et al. 2006; Rehwinkel et al. 2010). Of note, a recent study revealed that influenza virus lacking NS1 induces antiviral stress granules that contain viral RNA together with RIG-I and antiviral proteins including protein kinase R (PKR). These antiviral stress granules are shown to serve as the site of 5'ppp RNA-induced activation of RIG-I-signaling (Onomoto et al. 2012). Consistent with this, influenza virus infection boosted an early transient expression and activation of RIG-I in respiratory epithelial cells (Crotta et al. 2013; le Goffic et al. 2007), MΦ (Ohman et al. 2009; Wang et al. 2012), BMDCs (Koyama et al. 2007) and mast cells (Graham et al. 2013). Although dispensable for viral control following sublethal dose, signaling from RIG-I and TLR7 was required for survival and restricting the virus growth after lethal dose influenza infection in mice (Koyama et al. 2007; Pang et al. 2013b). Furthermore, expression on RIG-I and MDA5 were enhanced in peripheral blood cells (Lee et al. 2013) and patients who exhibit a polymorphism resulting in the expression of a nonfunctional variant of RIG-I were severely attenuated in antiviral responses against influenza virus (Pothlichet et al. 2009). These findings support an important role for the RIG-I-mediated responses in restraining the influenza virus.

5.4 NOD-Like Receptors (NLRs)

The NLR family comprises more than 20 receptors that are expressed intracellularly in the cytosol, and respond to various PAMPs to trigger inflammatory response. NLRs can trigger several signaling pathways including MAPK, NF-kB, and MAVS-IRF3 to induce production of IL-6, TNF-α, pro- IL-1β/IL-18, and also type I IFNs, respectively (Kanneganti 2010) (Fig. 1). Importantly, some of the NLRs can recruit the adaptor ASC (apoptosis-associated speck-like protein containing a CARD), which in turn interact with the pro-caspase-1 to form the "inflammasome" (Franchi et al. 2009). Assembly of inflammasome leads to autoactivation of caspase-1, which cleaves pro-IL-1β/IL-18 to mature IL-1β/IL-18 for secretion (Yu and Finlay 2008) (Fig. 1).

Studies have shown that NLRP3 (NLR family PYD-containing protein 3/Cryopyrin), NLRC2 (NLR family CARD-containing protein 2), and NLRX1 are the NLRs responding to influenza virus (Kanneganti 2010). Whereas NLRP3 inflammasome induces the secretion of mature IL-1β/IL-18, NLRC2/NOD2, and NLRX1 signals the production of type I IFNs in response to influenza virus.

Influenza virus-induced NLRP3-mediated IL-1β and IL-18 production involve two steps that include, enhancing the transcription of genes encoding pro-IL- 1β and pro-IL-18 and NLRP3 (signal 1) and activating NLRP3 inflammasome (signal 2). Signal 1 is initiated by the detection of viral RNA by TLR7, which activates NF-kB. Although initial studies showed that NLRP3 detects influenza virus via recognition of viral RNA (Allen et al. 2009; Thomas et al. 2009), it is now clear that many sources contribute to signal 2 either in combination or alone, and all depend on the newly synthesized viral M2 protein. These include, (i) ionic imbalance of the trans-Golgi pH, (ii) potassium efflux through the P2X7 receptor, an ATP-gated cation channel, (iii) lysosomal maturation and release of cathepsin B and (iv) cellular reactive oxygen species (Ichinohe et al. 2010; Lietzen et al. 2011) (Fig. 1). Recently, influenza virus virulence protein polymerase basic protein 1-frame 2 (PB1-F2) alone in aggregated form was found to be sufficient to activate NLRP3 inflammasome-induced IL-1β (McAuley et al. 2013). In addition, recent evidences support the role of commensal microbiota derived PAMPs as signal 1 for NLRP3 inflammasome activation (Ichinohe et al. 2011). Despite these findings, the specific PAMP in influenza virus interacting with NLRP3 is not yet known. Apart from the cleavage of pro-IL-1β and pro-IL-18, NLRP3-inflammasome activation also results in the initiation of a proinflammatory form of cell death known as pyroptosis (Schroder and Tschopp 2010).

Studies have shown that live influenza virus infection induces the expression and activation of NLRP3 inflammasome components (NLRP3, ASC, and Caspase-1) to mediate IL-1β and IL-18 production in different cell types in vitro; such as mice BMDCs and BMMΦ, human MΦ, nasal airway epithelial cell line and monocytic cell line THP-1 (Allen et al. 2009; Ichinohe et al. 2009; Kanneganti et al. 2006; Thomas et al. 2009). Accordingly, mice lacking any of the NLRP3 inflammasome components did not produce IL-1β and IL-18 following the high-lethal dose influenza virus infection (Allen et al. 2009; Thomas et al. 2009). Furthermore, NLRP3-deficient mice showed a reduced protective inflammation including the suppressed accumulation of neutrophils and monocytes to the lungs and airways upon influenza virus infection, which resulted in higher mortality (Allen et al. 2009; Thomas et al. 2009). Strikingly, NLRP3-deficient mice showed collagen deposits in lungs suggesting the delayed resolution of lung injury due to the absence of pro-fibrotic role of IL-1β (Thomas et al. 2009). Notably, the inflammasome complex was found to be dispensable for early clearance (up to 6 days) of the virus (Thomas et al. 2009), but was essential for reducing the viral load in later stage of infection (Allen et al. 2009; Ichinohe et al. 2009). These findings suggested that NLRP3-inflammasome induced inflammatory response, rather than direct viral control, mediates the protective immunity to influenza virus infection, possibly via adaptive immune responses.

NLRC2 (or NOD2) is believed to recognize the viral genomic ssRNA to recruit MAVS adaptor protein to activate IRF3-mediated type I IFN production in DCs and MΦ in response to influenza virus (Fig. 1). In agreement, NOD2-deficient mice showed decreased type I IFNs and DC activation, and exhibited enhanced susceptibility to lethal dose virus-induced pathogenesis (Lupfer et al. 2014; Sabbah et al. 2009). Further, NLRX1, NLR located in mitochondria, binds to viral protein PB1-F2. NLRX-signaling prevents virus-induced MΦ apoptosis and promotes both MΦ survival as well as type I IFN signaling in mice infection with lethal dose (Jaworska et al. 2014). On contrary, NOD2 and NLRX1 are found to negatively regulate the NLRP3 and RIG-induced inflammatory response to lethal dose influenza virus, respectively, and control the immunopathology (Allen et al. 2011; Lupfer et al. 2013). Together, these findings suggest that NLRs execute differential role in response to influenza virus infection to obtain a balanced innate immunity.

6 Effector Molecules of Innate Immunity

6.1 *Cytokines and Chemokines*

These mainly activate and attract various immune cells to the site of infection. Type I IFNs are the principal antiviral effectors to inhibit viral replication, and also promote greater activation of innate immune cells, particularly DCs, to facilitate the induction of adaptive immunity.

6.2 *Soluble Innate Mediators*

These function mainly by direct interaction with the virus outside the cells, resulting in either inhibition of viral binding to target cells, or in disruption of viral membranes (reviewed in Tripathi et al. 2013). Some of these soluble innate mediators, such as mucins, surfactant protein A (SP-A), glycoprotein-340, pentraxins, ficolins- inhibit the attachment of influenza virus to cells by presenting SA to the viral HA. Whereas other mediators, such as SP-D, mannose binding lectin (MBL), H-ficolins possess a lectin activity, and can interact with glycans on viral HA to form aggregate, which prevents the binding of virus to cells. In addition, there are antimicrobial peptides, such as α-defensins (human neutrophil peptides) and β-defensins, which cause viral aggregates, and also LL-37 that causes disruption of viral membrane. Furthermore, complement proteins activated by either soluble innate mediator, MBL, or natural IgM are also shown to exert beneficial role in influenza virus infection (Tripathi et al. 2013).

6.3 Intrinsic Antiviral Factors

These factors directly interact with the virus inside host cells to restrict the entry, replication, and assembly of virus, thereby rendering the cells nonpermissive to virus. This form of immunity to virus is referred as intrinsic antiviral immunity (Yan and Chen 2012). These factors are preexistent, but can be further enhanced by viral infection and type I IFNs, the principal mediator of antiviral innate response.

Type I IFNs activate the JAK/STAT pathway upon binding to its receptor, IFNAR. In addition to upregulating the innate recognition receptors (discussed earlier), IFNAR-signaling results in transcriptional upregulation of interferon-stimulated genes (ISGs), which in turn restrict the viral replication.

6.3.1 Mx

The myxovirus resistance gene, or *Mx*, was the first ISG found to restrict influenza virus replication. The human MxA and MxB, and the murine Mx2 are cytoplasmic proteins, whereas the murine Mx1 is localized within the nucleus (Haller et al. 2009). In mice, Mx1 inhibits the influenza virus infection, but Mx2 does not. In humans, MxA inhibits influenza as well as other viruses, but MxB has no effect on influenza infection. Mx proteins are reported to interact with viral NP and RNA helicases involved in the transport of viral RNA to the nucleus, which is the site of viral transcription and replication, resulting in the inhibition of viral growth (von der Malsburg et al. 2011). Different strains of influenza virus vary in their sensitivity to these proteins (Zimmermann et al. 2011). Of note, since most of the inbred mice strains are devoid of functional Mx proteins, the extrapolation of mouse data to humans has to be done with extreme caution.

6.3.2 Protein Kinase R (PKR)

It is an IFN inducible protein kinase that becomes activated upon binding to dsRNA in cytosol. In case of influenza virus, this is shown to be mediated by the panhandle secondary structure formed by 5’ppp end of RNA (Dauber et al. 2009).

While there have been multiple substrates identified for PKR, most of the antiviral activity of PKR is due to phosphorylation of eIF2α, which results in a general translational block, limiting viral replication (Pindel and Sadler 2011). NS1 of influenza A virus inhibits the activity of PKR (Li et al. 2006), and PKR-KO mice are highly susceptible to infection with NS1 defective influenza A virus (Bergmann et al. 2000), highlighting the contribution of PKR in restricting influenza virus replication. In addition to its role in inhibiting the translation of viral RNA, PKR activation also initiates signal transduction via NF-kB leading to cell growth arrest and autophagy, which result in an enhanced anti-viral immunity (Sadler and Williams 2008).

6.3.3 OAS/RNAseL

OAS (oligoadenylate synthetase) and RNase L is one of the first interferon-induced antiviral pathways discovered. Similar to PKR, OAS requires binding to dsRNA for activation of its enzymatic activity in cytosol. Upon activation, OAS generates 2'–5' oligoadenylates that act as a cofactor for a latent cytoplasmic RNAse, RNAseL. Activated RNAseL cleaves viral and cellular RNA stopping the viral replication (Chakrabarti et al. 2011).

6.3.4 ISG15

ISG15 is a 17kDa protein present in cytosol that has structural resemblance to two covalently linked ubiquitins. Like ubiquitin, ISG15 is conjugated to proteins through lysine residues. While the outcome of ISGylation are still unclear, ISG15-KO mice are more prone to infection by several viruses, including influenza A and B viruses, supporting the antiviral activity of this molecule (Lenschow et al. 2007). Importantly, NS1 protein of influenza A virus was shown to be conjugated by ISG15 resulting in the inhibition of NS1 function, and is believed to restrict the influenza virus replication (reviewed in Garcia-Sastre 2011).

6.3.5 Viperin and Tetherin

These are the recently discovered ISGs expressed on cell surface that exhibit the ability to inhibit influenza virus infection. Viperin is localized in the endoplasmic reticulum. It interferes with the enzymatic process of membrane fluidity and membrane microdomains to inhibit the efficient budding of influenza virus from infected cells (Wang et al. 2007). Tetherin (also known as BST2), like viperin, also restricts viral budding. By retaining newly assembled virions attached to the plasma membrane, tetherin restricts the formation of influenza virus like particles (reviewed in Garcia-Sastre 2011).

6.3.6 IFITM and IFIT

IFITM (IFN-inducible transmembrane protein) are ISGs that restrict viral entry (Brass et al. 2009; Everitt et al. 2012). IFITM3 has been identified as an important host restriction factor for influenza virus. IFITM3 proteins block infection early during cytosolic entry of viruses that utilize the endosomal pathway (Feeley et al. 2011), suggesting that they affect the function of viral proteins involved in viral fusion in the endosome (Garcia-Sastre 2011). Infection of IFITM3 deficient mice with low virulence influenza A virus resulted in a severe form of disease, similar to that caused by high virulence virus (Brass et al. 2009; Everitt et al. 2012). Interestingly, avian cells do not seem to express a homolog to IFITM3, which raises the possibility that IFITM proteins might influence viral tropism (reviewed in Yan and Chen 2012).

The IFIT family (interferon-induced proteins with tetratricopeptide repeats) includes four members, IFIT1, 2, 3, and 5, which are the cytoplasmic proteins that recognize viral RNA with 5'triphosphate or without 2'-O-methylation. IFIT1 is found to inhibit cellular translation by binding to the eIF3 initiation factor to suppress the viral translation and replication (Yan and Chen 2012).

7 Innate Control of Adaptive Immunity to Influenza

7.1 Innate Immune Cells

At the cellular level, innate immune cells, particularly DCs, which sense the viral invasion through unique innate receptors, are also endowed with the ability to prime adaptive immune cells, such as T cells and B cells, to induce a virus-specific long-lasting immunity (Braciale et al. 2012; Iwasaki and Medzhitov 2010; Manicassamy and Pulendran 2009, 2011; Pulendran et al. 2010b).

7.1.1 DCs

DCs are well known for their critical role in the initiation of Ag-specific response owing to their ability to uptake and process Ags, and to migrate to the lymphoid tissues for presentation to naïve Ag-specific T cells. Furthermore, DCs in airways are believed to derive viral Ag for presentation via two unique ways, endogenous Ag following direct infection or exogenous Ag by uptake of infected dead cells.

Extensive studies have shown that respiratory DC subsets, such as $CD103^{+}CD11b^{lo}$cDCs and $CD11b^{hi}CD103^{-}$ cDCs acquire a mature phenotype in the presence of type I IFNs and migrate to the regional LN in CCR7-dependent manner (Fig. 2). Among the DCs in LN, respiratory $CD103^{+}CD11b^{lo}$ cDCs are found to be the only DCs that prime virus-specific naïve $CD8^{+}$ T cells in the LN to differentiate into effector cells (GeurtsvanKessel et al. 2008; Helft et al. 2012;

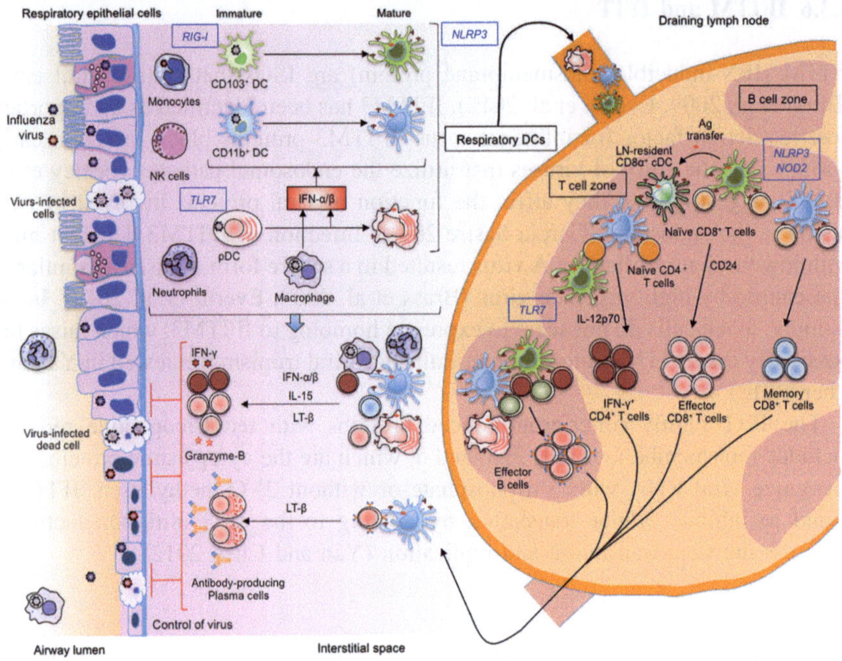

Fig. 2 Innate control of adaptive immunity to influenza. Innate immune cells, particularly dendritic cells (DCs) in the respiratory tissues acquire antigens either through direct infection or by uptake of influenza-infected dead cells and undergo maturation process triggered by TLR7 or RIG-I-signaling, under the influence of type I IFNs produced by macrophages and pDCs. Respiratory DC subsets (CD103$^+$ cDCs, CD11b$^+$ cDCs and pDCs) migrate to the draining lymph node (LN), where they can transfer influenza antigens (Ag) to LN-resident CD8α$^+$ cDC. In the LN, respiratory CD103$^+$ cDCs together with CD8α$^+$ cDCs stimulate the naïve CD8$^+$ T cells to proliferate and differentiate into cytotoxic effector CD8$^+$ T cells, in a CD24-dependent manner. On the other hand, CD11b$^+$ cDCs drive the activation of CD8$^+$ T cells, mainly effector T cells at later stage of infection, to induce memory CD8$^+$ T cells. Interaction of naïve CD4$^+$ T cells with cDCs generates IFN-γ-producing Th1 cells, which in turn facilitates the differentiation of effector B cells in a TLR7-dependent manner. These effector cells migrate from LN to respiratory tissues, where they have second interaction with Ag-bearing innate immune cells to undergo further activation and differentiation to terminal effector cells that secrete effector molecules to control virus spread

Ho et al. 2011; Kim and Braciale 2009; Kim et al. 2014; Unkel et al. 2012). This is because, type I IFN-dependent antiviral status of CD103$^+$CD11b^{lo} cDCs restrains their productive infection, and they preferentially uptake influenza virus-infected apoptotic cells in the lungs (Desch et al. 2011; Helft et al. 2012). This results in an influx of high number of activated CD103$^+$CD11b^{lo}cDCs that carry viral Ags into LN for cross-priming of virus-specific CD8$^+$ T cells, early during the infection (Albert et al. 1998; Desch et al. 2011; Helft et al. 2012; Ho et al. 2011) (Fig. 2).

On the contrary, CD11b^{hi}CD103$^-$ cDCs, which is the major migratory DC subset in LN at the peak of infection, are found to drive the generation of central memory CD8$^+$T cells (Kim et al. 2014) (Fig. 2). The differential function of cDC subsets is attributed to an enhanced expression of CD24 on $CD103^+CD11b^{lo}$cDCs, which regulate $CD8^+$ T cell activation through HMGB1-mediated engagement of T cell RAGE (Kim et al. 2014). Although $CD11c^{lo}$ pDCs and $CD11b^+Ly6C^+$ moDCs migrate to the LN in high number, and are shown to carry viral Ags, they were inefficient in activating naïve $CD8^+$T cells, compared to $CD103^+$ cDCs and $CD11b^{hi}$ cDCs (Ballesteros-Tato et al. 2010; GeurtsvanKessel et al. 2008; Kim and Braciale 2009).

In addition to migratory respiratory DCs, some studies suggested that LN-resident $CD8\alpha^+$ cDCs are also able to activate naïve $CD8^+$ T cells by cross-presentation of Ag acquired from migratory DCs (Belz et al. 2007; Waithman et al. 2013). Notably, together with neutrophils and MΦ (Hufford et al. 2012; Kohlmeier et al. 2010; Tate et al. 2012), respiratory DCs at the site of infection were essential for the survival of effector T cells in Ag (cross-) presentation, IL-15 trans-presentation- and lymphotoxin (LT) β-dependent manner (McGill et al. 2008, 2010) (Fig. 2). Thus, the non-redundant role of DC subsets facilitates rapid generation and maintenance of the effector T cells needed to clear acute infection, followed by slower development of the cells needed for sustained memory.

Furthermore, both $CD103^+CD11b^{lo}$ cDCs and $CD11b^{hi}CD103^-$ cDCs are found to efficiently activate naïve virus-specific $CD4^+$ T cells in the LN (Fig. 2), compared to other migratory DC subsets, in mice exposed to infectious as well as inactivated influenza virus (GeurtsvanKessel et al. 2008; Kim and Braciale 2009). However, blood monocyte-derived moDC recruited to LN are reported to stimulate IL-12p70-mediated Th1 response in mice (Nakano et al. 2009). Recent studies in influenza-infected mice (Leon et al. 2014) and influenza-vaccinated humans (Bentebibel et al. 2013) showed that follicular $CD4^+$ T (Tfh) cells are present in LN and circulation, respectively, and are essential for germinal center (GC) reactions and antibody production. Notably, pDCs were found to be essential for enhancement of virus-specific primary antibody response following influenza infection (GeurtsvanKessel et al. 2008; McGill et al. 2008) and vaccination (Koyama et al. 2010). Further, $CD11c^{hi}$ cDCs in the lungs were crucial for maintenance of GC reactions in tertiary lymphoid structures, and to sustain virus-specific antibodies (GeurtsvanKessel et al. 2009). Despite these observations, the role of DC subsets in the generation of Tfh cells and primary antibody response is not clearly known.

In humans, consistent with the high susceptibility to productive infection in vitro, influenza virus-exposed mDCs were impaired in Ag (cross-) presentation to $CD8^+$ T cells (Smed-Sorensen et al. 2012) and $CD4^+$ T cells (Fernandez-Sesma et al. 2006). However, mDCs exposed to inactivated virus or infected dead cells were highly efficient in Ag (cross-) presentation to activate $CD8^+$ T cells (Smed-Sorensen et al. 2012). Furthermore, when LAIV was administered to humanized mice, the lung-resident $CD1c^+$ mDC1, but not $CD141^+$ mDC2, are found to drive the expansion of influenza virus-specific CD103-expressing mucosal $CD8^+$ T cells through membrane-bound TGF-β-dependent mechanisms (Yu et al. 2013).

Recent studies showed that pDCs are less efficient than mDCs, in both cross- as well as direct presentation of influenza Ag to T cells in vitro (Lui et al. 2009; Smed-Sorensen et al. 2012). Strikingly, influenza virus-activated pDCs were able to induce a strong Th1 polarization through synergistic effect of IL-12 and type I IFNs (Cella et al. 2000). Furthermore, influenza virus triggered secretion of type I IFNs and IL-6 from pDCs induced differentiation of plasma cells and virus-specific antibody production from B cells activated by T cells (Jego et al. 2003). These findings indicate that human mDCs are likely important for the induction of $CD8^+$ T cell response and that of pDCs in $CD4^+$ T cell-dependent virus-specific antibody response.

Despite these studies in mouse models and in vitro human studies on how influenza virus-exposed mDCs and pDCs influence different aspects of adaptive immunity; the phenotype, activation status and functional role of DC subsets in influenza virus-infected patients, particularly at the site of infection, is not known.

7.2 Virus Sensing Receptors

7.2.1 TLRs and RLRs

Although a previous study implicated TLR3 in the enhancement of $CD8^+$ T cell response in lethal dose influenza virus-infected mice (le Goffic et al. 2006), later studies found that TLR3 and its associated adapter molecule, TRIF, do not play a significant role in the development of influenza virus-specific $CD4^+$ or $CD8^+$ T cell or B cell responses following sublethal infection (Heer et al. 2007; Koyama et al. 2007; Seo et al. 2010) (Table 2). Surprisingly, TLR7/MyD88 and RIG-I-signaling are also found to play negligible roles in $CD8^+$ T cell activation and effector functions in sublethal dose influenza virus-infected mice (Heer et al. 2007; Koyama et al. 2007; Pang et al. 2013a). However, $CD4^+$ T cell response, the number of antibody-secreting cells in secondary lymphoid organs, and the production of virus-specific antibodies following sublethal intranasal infection were dependent on TLR7 signaling, but not RIG-I signaling (Jeisy-Scott et al. 2012; Koyama et al. 2007). Furthermore, TLR7-signaling in pDCs, was essential for protective antibody response induced by virion RNA-containing split vaccine (Jeisy-Scott et al. 2012) and inactivated whole virus vaccine (Koyama et al. 2007, 2010) (Table 2). Here, along with stimulation of TLRs on B cells, TLR7-mediated induction of type I IFNs in pDCs was found to be critical for T cell-dependent antibody response following infection and vaccination (Heer et al. 2007; Koyama et al. 2010). Based on these findings, it appears that TLRs rather than RLRs contribute to the induction of effective T cell-dependent antibody response to influenza virus, whereas TLR-independent and RLR-independent mechanisms might exist with regards to $CD8^+$ T cell responses. In this context, our recent study showed that activation of induced general control nonderepressible 2 kinase (GCN2) in DCs by the yellow fever vaccine (YF-17D) is crucial for generation of $CD8^+$ T cell response through autophagy and enhanced Ag presentation (Ravindran et al. 2014). Interestingly, induction of $CD8^+$ T cell responses to the LAIV was also dependent on GCN2 (Ravindran et al. 2014).

7.2.2 NLRs and Caspase-1

Mice deficient of caspase-1, ASC, and NLRP3, which lacked IL-1β and that of IL-1R-deficient mice showed a failure in the activation of virus-specific IFN-γ-secreting CD4$^+$ and CD8$^+$ T cells, and to generate nasal IgA and serum IgG response following sublethal dose of influenza virus infection (Ichinohe et al. 2009; Pang et al. 2013a) (Table 2). Furthermore, microbiota-mediated NLRP3-inflammasome-caspase-1 activation-induced IL-1β is believed to be essential for activation and migration of DCs from the lungs to the LN for T cell priming during sublethal dose influenza virus infection in mice (Ichinohe et al. 2011). Supporting these previous findings, a recent study showed that signaling through the IL-1R (by IL-1β/IL-1α) in uninfected DCs carrying viral Ag was required and sufficient for productive priming of CD8$^+$ T cells, but signaling through TLR7 and RIG-I was dispensable (Pang et al. 2013a). In contrast, a previous study found that antibody production, as well as the influenza virus-specific CD8$^+$ T cell number in the BAL, of both Nlrp3 and caspase-1-deficient mice was similar to wild type mice infected with sublethal dose of influenza virus between 7 and 11 days of infection (Thomas et al. 2009) (Table 2). While several studies favored the role of influenza virus-triggered caspase-1 activation in CD8$^+$ T cell response, further studies are needed to clarify these findings. A recent study revealed that NOD2-deficiency causes reduced generation of virus-specific CD8$^+$ T cell response following lethal infection in mice (Lupfer et al. 2014) (Table 2).

In summary, despite a unique indispensable role of innate immune system in antiviral immunity, cooperation with CD8$^+$ T cell and CD4$^+$ T cell-dependent virus-neutralizing antibody response, is essential for protection, especially heterosubtypic influenza virus immunity.

8 Pathogenic Role of Innate Immunity to Influenza Virus Infection

A major form of innate immune-mediated pathology following influenza virus infection is viral pneumonia, which leads to ARDS resulting in multiorgan failure and a high mortality rate (Short et al. 2014). In addition to virus-induced cell injury, ARDS is attributed to hyperactivation of innate immune cells, such as neutrophils, monocytes, and NK cells. These cells induce excessive inflammatory responses involving reactive oxygen species, TNF-related apoptosis-inducing ligand (TRAIL), inducible nitric oxide synthase (iNOS2) and proinflammatory cytokines (Herold et al. 2008; Hogner et al. 2013; Lin et al. 2008; Short et al. 2014).

Increased accumulation of innate cells through a chemokine-mediated feed-forward loop is observed in the lung lesions of high dose lethal infection associated with poor innate control of influenza virus (Aldridge et al. 2009; Brandes et al. 2013; Lin et al. 2008; Narasaraju et al. 2011; Seo et al. 2011). Consistent with this, interfering with the massive infiltration of these innate cells through chemokine antagonism (CCR2 for monocytes) or partial cell depletion (Aldridge et al. 2009; Brandes et al. 2013; Lin et al. 2011) was found to alleviate the immune-mediated pathology.

9 Systems Vaccinology of Influenza Vaccines

System vaccinology employs a number of high-throughput technologies like DNA microarrays, protein arrays, deep sequencing, and mass spectrometry to generate system-wide unbiased molecular measurements to reconstruct the events in an immune response (Pulendran et al. 2010a). Over the last few years, several studies have used systems biology approaches to obtain a global picture of the immune responses to vaccination, and to identify molecular signatures that can be used to predict vaccine immunity in humans, and also to understand the mechanisms involved in the vaccine-induced immunity (Li et al. 2013, 2014; Nakaya et al. 2011, 2012; Pulendran 2009; Pulendran et al. 2010a; Querec et al. 2009; Ravindran et al. 2014; Tsang et al. 2014).

A comparative study of immune response to trivalent inactivated influenza vaccine (TIV) and live attenuated influenza vaccine (LAIV) using systems biology approach revealed salient common as well as contrasting features between them. While LAIV induced the expression of several interferon-related genes, which are similar to live viral vaccines, the TIV induced a signature composed of genes highly expressed in plasma B cells (Nakaya et al. 2011). For TIV, of the 44 genes identified to accurately predict the outcome of immunization as either high or low antibody titers, one gene-CAMKIV- had no known function in regulating immunity, but was negatively correlated with antibody titers. Consistent with this, CAMKIV-deficit mice developed high antibody titers after vaccination (Nakaya et al. 2011). Furthermore, the expression of TLR5 few days after TIV administration highly correlated with the antibody titers 4 weeks post vaccination. However, TIV did not activate TLR5 signaling per se (Jason and Pulendran unpublished data). TLR5 is sensor of bacterial flagellin, which could be derived from commensal flora. In this context, perturbation of gut microbiota was found to influence the host immune response involved in the clearance of virus from lungs in influenza infected mice (Ichinohe et al. 2011). Consistent with this, our preliminary results support the significant influence of intestinal flora on TIV-induced antibody response in mouse model (Jason and Pulendran unpublished data).

In addition, studies are also being performed in influenza virus-infected patients and animal models for better understanding of the disease pathogenesis that might help in efficient control (Huang et al. 2011; Korth et al. 2013; Woods et al. 2013; Zaslavsky et al. 2013). A temporal pattern of host molecular responses was identified by systems biology approach in the peripheral blood of influenza virus-infected human volunteers, which differentiated symptomatic from asymptomatic infections of influenza virus strains (Huang et al. 2011; Woods et al. 2013).

Further, while symptomatic patients showed multiple PRR-mediated antiviral and inflammatory responses, asymptomatic individuals revealed a highly regulated antiviral responses together with enhanced cell-mediated and antioxidant responses (Huang et al. 2011; Woods et al. 2013). Similarly, differential induction of inflammatory gene expression is observed in the mouse lungs following infection with influenza virus causing mild or severe respiratory disease, which is largely accounted by neutrophils (Brandes et al. 2013; Kash et al. 2006; Korth et al. 2013). Furthermore, by integrating the large-scale lipid measurements with targeted gene expression, a recent study in influenza mouse model and human patients showed that 5-lipoxygenase metabolites correlate with the pathogenic phase of the infection, whereas 12/15-lipoxygenase metabolites associate with the resolution phase (Tam et al. 2013).

10 Conclusions and Perspectives

In this review, we summarized our current knowledge of the innate immune responses to influenza. At the cellular level, respiratory epithelial cells being the primary target support the viral replication to release progeny viruses; but together with DCs and MΦ, trigger trafficking of increased number of immune cells to the site of infection. Uptake of influenza virus mainly through the SA-containing receptors and recognition of viral components by the innate receptors trigger activation and upregulation of antiviral program in respiratory epithelial as well as immune cells recruited to the airways. Antiviral innate response mainly includes type I and III IFNs and the IFN-stimulated genes, in addition to various inflammatory cytokines and chemokines. Although innate immunity seems to achieve the protective viral clearance in concert with adaptive immune response, damaging role of innate immunity in the pathogenesis of influenza is also emerging with the recent studies. Of note, variation in the amplitude of innate immune response has been linked to both virus dose and strains as well as host factors.

There is an impressive amount of knowledge emerging on innate immunity to influenza virus from experimental studies in mice. However, there is a paucity of knowledge about the mechanisms that mediate innate and adaptive immunity to influenza in humans, particularly among those populations that show enhanced morbidity and mortality to infection, such as the infants and the elderly. Thus, there is an imperative to study innate immunity in humans using cutting edge tools like systems biology, in order to acquire a deeper understanding for devising rational prophylactic and therapeutic strategies for the control of influenza.

Acknowledgments This work was supported by grants from the U.S. National Institutes of Health (grants HHSN272201400004C, N01 AI50019, and N01 AI50025, R37 DK057665, R37 AI048638, U19 AI090023, U19 AI057266, U54 AI057157, U54 AI057160).

References

Albert ML, Sauter B, Bhardwaj N (1998) Dendritic cells acquire antigen from apoptotic cells and induce class I-restricted CTLs. Nature 392:86–89. doi:10.1038/32183

Aldridge JR Jr, Moseley CE, Boltz DA, Negovetich NJ, Reynolds C, Franks J, Brown SA, Doherty PC, Webster RG, Thomas PG (2009) TNF/iNOS-producing dendritic cells are the necessary evil of lethal influenza virus infection. Proc Nat Acad Sci U.S.A 106:5306–5311. doi:10.1073/pnas.0900655106

Allen IC, Moore CB, Schneider M, Lei Y, Davis BK, Scull MA, Gris D, Roney KE, Zimmermann AG, Bowzard JB, Ranjan P, Monroe KM, Pickles RJ, Sambhara S, Ting JP (2011) NLRX1 protein attenuates inflammatory responses to infection by interfering with the RIG-I-MAVS and TRAF6-NF-kappaB signaling pathways. Immunity 34:854–865. doi:10.1016/j.immuni.2011.03.026 S1074-7613(11)00226-3 [PII]

Allen IC, Scull MA, Moore CB, Holl EK, McElvania-TeKippe E, Taxman DJ, Guthrie EH, Pickles RJ, Ting JP (2009) The NLRP3 inflammasome mediates in vivo innate immunity to influenza A virus through recognition of viral RNA. Immunity 30:556–565. doi:10.1016/j.immuni.2009.02.005

Ballesteros-Tato A, Leon B, Lund FE, Randall TD (2010) Temporal changes in dendritic cell subsets, cross-priming and costimulation via CD70 control CD8(+) T cell responses to influenza. Nat Immunol 11:216–224. doi:10.1038/ni.1838

Banchereau J, Steinman RM (1998) Dendritic cells and the control of immunity. Nature 392:245–252. doi:10.1038/32588

Barchet W, Krug A, Cella M, Newby C, Fischer JA, Dzionek A, Pekosz A, Colonna M (2005) Dendritic cells respond to influenza virus through TLR7- and PKR-independent pathways. Eur J Immunol 35:236–242. doi:10.1002/eji.200425583

Belz GT, Bedoui S, Kupresanin F, Carbone FR, Heath WR (2007) Minimal activation of memory CD8+ T cell by tissue-derived dendritic cells favors the stimulation of naive CD8+ T cells. Nat Immunol 8:1060–1066. doi:10.1038/ni1505

Bendelac A, Savage PB, Teyton L (2007) The biology of NKT cells. Ann Rev Immunol 25:297–336. doi:10.1146/annurev.immunol.25.022106.141711

Bentebibel SE, Lopez S, Obermoser G, Schmitt N, Mueller C, Harrod C, Flano E, Mejias A, Albrecht RA, Blankenship D, Xu H, Pascual V, Banchereau J, Garcia-Sastre A, Palucka AK, Ramilo O, Ueno H (2013) Induction of ICOS+CXCR3+CXCR5+ TH cells correlates with antibody responses to influenza vaccination. Sci Transl Med 5:176ra32. doi: 10.1126/scitranslmed.3005191 5/176/176ra32 [PII]

Bergmann M, Garcia-Sastre A, Carnero E, Pehamberger H, Wolff K, Palese P, Muster T (2000) Influenza virus NS1 protein counteracts PKR-mediated inhibition of replication. J Virol 74:6203–6206

Boonnak K, Paskel M, Matsuoka Y, Vogel L, Subbarao K (2012) Evaluation of replication, immunogenicity and protective efficacy of a live attenuated cold-adapted pandemic H1N1 influenza virus vaccine in non-human primates. Vaccine 30:5603–5610. doi:10.1016/j.vaccine.2012.06.088

Boonnak K, Vogel L, Orandle M, Zimmerman D, Talor E, Subbarao K (2013) Antigen-activated dendritic cells ameliorate influenza A infections. J Clin Invest 123:2850–2861. doi:10.1172/JCI67550

Braciale TJ, Sun J, Kim TS (2012) Regulating the adaptive immune response to respiratory virus infection. Nat Rev Immunol 12:295–305. doi:10.1038/nri3166

Brandes M, Klauschen F, Kuchen S, Germain RN (2013) A systems analysis identifies a feedforward inflammatory circuit leading to lethal influenza infection. Cell 154:197–212. doi:10.1016/j.cell.2013.06.013

Brass AL, Huang IC, Benita Y, John SP, Krishnan MN, Feeley EM, Ryan BJ, Weyer JL, van der Weyden L, Fikrig E, Adams DJ, Xavier RJ, Farzan M, Elledge SJ (2009) The IFITM proteins mediate cellular resistance to influenza A H1N1 virus, West Nile virus, and dengue virus. Cell 139:1243–1254. doi:10.1016/j.cell.2009.12.017

Cao W, Taylor AK, Biber RE, Davis WG, Kim JH, Reber AJ, Chirkova T, de la Cruz JA, Pandey A, Ranjan P, Katz JM, Gangappa S, Sambhara S (2012) Rapid differentiation of monocytes into type I IFN-producing myeloid dendritic cells as an antiviral strategy against influenza virus infection. J Immunol 189:2257–2265. doi:10.4049/jimmunol.1200168

Castilla J, Martinez-Baz I, Martinez-Artola V, Reina G, Pozo F, Garcia Cenoz M, Guevara M, Moran J, Irisarri F, Arriazu M, Albeniz E, Ezpeleta C, Barricarte A (2013) Decline in influenza vaccine effectiveness with time after vaccination, Navarre, Spain, season 2011/12. Euro Surveill 18:1–8. http://www.eurosurveillance.org/ViewArticle.aspx?ArticleId=20388

Cella M, Facchetti F, Lanzavecchia A, Colonna M (2000) Plasmacytoid dendritic cells activated by influenza virus and CD40L drive a potent TH1 polarization. Nat Immunol 1:305–310. doi:10.1038/79747

Centers for Disease Control and Prevention US (2011) Prevention and control of influenza with vaccines: recommendations of the Advisory Committee on Immunization Practices (ACIP), 2011. MMWR, vol 60, US Centers for Disease Control and Prevention, pp 1128–1132

Chakrabarti A, Jha BK, Silverman RH (2011) New insights into the role of RNase L in innate immunity. J Interferon Cytokine Res 31:49–57. doi:10.1089/jir.2010.0120

Chan MC, Chan RW, Yu WC, Ho CC, Chui WH, Lo CK, Yuen KM, Guan YI, Nicholls JM, Peiris JS (2009) Influenza H5N1 virus infection of polarized human alveolar epithelial cells and lung microvascular endothelial cells. Respir Res 10:102. doi:10.1186/1465-9921-10-102

Chan MC, Cheung CY, Chui WH, Tsao SW, Nicholls JM, Chan YO, Chan RW, Long HT, Poon LL, Guan Y, Peiris JS (2005) Proinflammatory cytokine responses induced by influenza A (H5N1) viruses in primary human alveolar and bronchial epithelial cells. Respir Res 6:135. doi:10.1186/1465-9921-6-135

Chan RW, Yuen KM, Yu WC, Ho CC, Nicholls JM, Peiris JS, Chan MC (2010) Influenza H5N1 and H1N1 virus replication and innate immune responses in bronchial epithelial cells are influenced by the state of differentiation. PLoS ONE 5:e8713. doi:10.1371/journal.pone.0008713

Chang YJ, Kim HY, Albacker LA, Baumgarth N, McKenzie AN, Smith DE, Dekruyff RH, Umetsu DT (2011) Innate lymphoid cells mediate influenza-induced airway hyper-reactivity independently of adaptive immunity. Nat Immunol 12:631–638. doi:10.1038/ni.2045

Cheung CY, Poon LL, Lau AS, Luk W, Lau YL, Shortridge KF, Gordon S, Guan Y, Peiris JS (2002) Induction of proinflammatory cytokines in human macrophages by influenza A (H5N1) viruses: a mechanism for the unusual severity of human disease? Lancet 360:1831–1837. doi:10.1016/S0140-6736(02)11772-7 S0140673602117727 [PII]

Clements ML, Betts RF, Tierney EL, Murphy BR (1986) Serum and nasal wash antibodies associated with resistance to experimental challenge with influenza A wild-type virus. J Clin Microbiol 24:157–160

Corral L, Singer MS, Macher BA, Rosen SD (1990) Requirement for sialic acid on neutrophils in a GMP-140 (PADGEM) mediated adhesive interaction with activated platelets. Biochem Biophys Res Commun 172:1349–1356

Cros J, Cagnard N, Woollard K, Patey N, Zhang SY, Senechal B, Puel A, Biswas SK, Moshous D, Picard C, Jais JP, D'Cruz D, Casanova JL, Trouillet C, Geissmann F (2010) Human CD14dim monocytes patrol and sense nucleic acids and viruses via TLR7 and TLR8 receptors. Immunity 33:375–386. doi:10.1016/j.immuni.2010.08.012 S1074-7613(10)00317-1 [PII]

Crotta S, Davidson S, Mahlakoiv T, Desmet CJ, Buckwalter MR, Albert ML, Staeheli P, Wack A (2013) Type I and type III interferons drive redundant amplification loops to induce a transcriptional signature in influenza-infected airway epithelia. PLoS Pathog 9:e1003773. doi:10.1371/journal.ppat.1003773

Dauber B, Martinez-Sobrido L, Schneider J, Hai R, Waibler Z, Kalinke U, Garcia-Sastre A, Wolff T (2009) Influenza B virus ribonucleoprotein is a potent activator of the antiviral kinase PKR. PLoS Pathog 5:e1000473. doi:10.1371/journal.ppat.1000473

de Santo C, Salio M, Masri SH, Lee LY, Dong T, Speak AO, Porubsky S, Booth S, Veerapen N, Besra GS, Grone HJ, Platt FM, Zambon M, Cerundolo V (2008) Invariant NKT cells reduce the immunosuppressive activity of influenza A virus-induced myeloid-derived suppressor cells in mice and humans. J Clin Invest 118:4036–4048. doi:10.1172/JCI36264

de Vries E, Tscherne DM, Wienholts MJ, Cobos-Jimenez V, Scholte F, Garcia-Sastre A, Rottier PJ, de Haan CA (2011) Dissection of the influenza A virus endocytic routes reveals macropinocytosis as an alternative entry pathway. PLoS Pathog 7:e1001329. doi:10.1371/journal.ppat.1001329

Denney L, Aitken C, Li CK, Wilson-Davies E, Kok WL, Clelland C, Rooney K, Young D, Dong T, McMichael AJ, Carman WF, Ho LP (2010) Reduction of natural killer but not effector CD8 T lymphocytes in three consecutive cases of severe/lethal H1N1/09 influenza A virus infection. PLoS ONE 5:e10675. doi:10.1371/journal.pone.0010675

Desch AN, Randolph GJ, Murphy K, Gautier EL, Kedl RM, Lahoud MH, Caminschi I, Shortman K, Henson PM, Jakubzick CV (2011) CD103+ pulmonary dendritic cells preferentially acquire and present apoptotic cell-associated antigen. J Exp Med 208:1789–1797. doi:10.1084/jem.20110538

Diebold SS, Kaisho T, Hemmi H, Akira S, Reis e Sousa C (2004) Innate antiviral responses by means of TLR7-mediated recognition of single-stranded RNA. Science 303:1529–1531. doi:10.1126/science.1093616

Draghi M, Pashine A, Sanjanwala B, Gendzekhadze K, Cantoni C, Cosman D, Moretta A, Valiante NM, Parham P (2007) NKp46 and NKG2D recognition of infected dendritic cells is necessary for NK cell activation in the human response to influenza infection. J Immunol 178:2688–2698

Edwards AD, Diebold SS, Slack EM, Tomizawa H, Hemmi H, Kaisho T, Akira S, Reis e Sousa C (2003) Toll-like receptor expression in murine DC subsets: lack of TLR7 expression by CD8 alpha+ DC correlates with unresponsiveness to imidazoquinolines. Eur J Immunol 33:827–833. doi:10.1002/eji.200323797

Everitt AR, Clare S, Pertel T, John SP, Wash RS, Smith SE, Chin CR, Feeley EM, Sims JS, Adams DJ, Wise HM, Kane L, Goulding D, Digard P, Anttila V, Baillie JK, Walsh TS, Hume DA, Palotie A, Xue Y, Colonna V, Tyler-Smith C, Dunning J, Gordon SB, Smyth RL, Openshaw PJ, Dougan G, Brass AL, Kellam P (2012) IFITM3 restricts the morbidity and mortality associated with influenza. Nature 484:519–523. doi:10.1038/nature10921

Feeley EM, Sims JS, John SP, Chin CR, Pertel T, Chen LM, Gaiha GD, Ryan BJ, Donis RO, Elledge SJ, Brass AL (2011) IFITM3 inhibits influenza A virus infection by preventing cytosolic entry. PLoS Pathog 7:e1002337. doi:10.1371/journal.ppat.1002337

Fernandez-Sesma A, Marukian S, Ebersole BJ, Kaminski D, Park MS, Yuen T, Sealfon SC, Garcia-Sastre A, Moran TM (2006) Influenza virus evades innate and adaptive immunity via the NS1 protein. J Virol 80:6295–6304. doi:10.1128/JVI.02381-05

Finberg RW, Wang JP, Kurt-Jones EA (2007) Toll like receptors and viruses. Rev Med Virol 17:35–43. doi:10.1002/rmv.525

Fonteneau JF, Gilliet M, Larsson M, Dasilva I, Munz C, Liu YJ, Bhardwaj N (2003) Activation of influenza virus-specific CD4+ and CD8+ T cells: a new role for plasmacytoid dendritic cells in adaptive immunity. Blood 101:3520–3526. doi:10.1182/blood-2002-10-3063-10-3063

Fox A, Le NM, Horby P, van Doorn HR, Nguyen VT, Nguyen HH, Nguyen TC, Vu DP, Nguyen MH, Diep NT, Bich VT, Huong HT, Taylor WR, Farrar J, Wertheim H, Nguyen VK (2012) Severe pandemic H1N1 2009 infection is associated with transient NK and T deficiency and aberrant CD8 responses. PLoS ONE 7:e31535. doi:10.1371/journal.pone.0031535

Franchi L, Eigenbrod T, Munoz-Planillo R, Nunez G (2009) The inflammasome: a caspase-1-activation platform that regulates immune responses and disease pathogenesis. Nat Immunol 10:241–247. doi:10.1038/ni.1703

Fujisawa H (2001) Inhibitory role of neutrophils on influenza virus multiplication in the lungs of mice. Microbiol Immunol 45:679–688

Garcia-Sastre A (2011) Induction and evasion of type I interferon responses by influenza viruses. Virus Res 162:12–18. doi:10.1016/j.virusres.2011.10.017 S0168-1702(11)00411-4 [PII]

Gazit R, Gruda R, Elboim M, Arnon TI, Katz G, Achdout H, Hanna J, Qimron U, Landau G, Greenbaum E, Zakay-Rones Z, Porgador A, Mandelboim O (2006) Lethal influenza infection in the absence of the natural killer cell receptor gene Ncr1. Nat Immunol 7:517–523. doi:10.1038/ni1322

Ge MQ, Ho AW, Tang Y, Wong KH, Chua BY, Gasser S, Kemeny DM (2012) NK cells regulate CD8+ T cell priming and dendritic cell migration during influenza A infection by IFN-gamma and perforin-dependent mechanisms. J Immunol 189:2099–2109. doi:10.4049/jimmunol.1103474

Geeraedts F, Goutagny N, Hornung V, Severa M, de Haan A, Pool J, Wilschut J, Fitzgerald KA, Huckriede A (2008) Superior immunogenicity of inactivated whole virus H5N1 influenza vaccine is primarily controlled by toll-like receptor signalling. PLoS Pathog 4:e1000138. doi:10.1371/journal.ppat.1000138

Geijtenbeek TB, Gringhuis SI (2009) Signalling through C-type lectin receptors: shaping immune responses. Nat Rev Immunol 9:465–479. doi:10.1038/nri2569

Geiler J, Michaelis M, Sithisarn P, Cinatl J Jr (2011) Comparison of pro-inflammatory cytokine expression and cellular signal transduction in human macrophages infected with different influenza A viruses. Med Microbiol Immunol 200:53–60. doi:10.1007/s00430-010-0173-y

Gerlach RL, Camp JV, Chu YK, Jonsson CB (2013) Early host responses of seasonal and pandemic influenza a viruses in primary well-differentiated human lung epithelial cells. PLoS ONE 8:e78912. doi:10.1371/journal.pone.0078912 PONE-D-13-28042s [PII]

GeurtsvanKessel CH, Willart MA, Bergen IM, van Rijt LS, Muskens F, Elewaut D, Osterhaus AD, Hendriks R, Rimmelzwaan GF, Lambrecht BN (2009) Dendritic cells are crucial for maintenance of tertiary lymphoid structures in the lung of influenza virus-infected mice. J Exp Med 206:2339–2349. doi:10.1084/jem.20090410

GeurtsvanKessel CH, Willart MA, van Rijt LS, Muskens F, Kool M, Baas C, Thielemans K, Bennett C, Clausen BE, Hoogsteden HC, Osterhaus AD, Rimmelzwaan GF, Lambrecht BN (2008) Clearance of influenza virus from the lung depends on migratory langerin+CD11b− but not plasmacytoid dendritic cells. J Exp Med 205:1621–1634. doi:10.1084/jem.20071365jem.20071365

Giamarellos-Bourboulis EJ, Raftogiannis M, Antonopoulou A, Baziaka F, Koutoukas P, Savva A, Kanni T, Georgitsi M, Pistiki A, Tsaganos T, Pelekanos N, Athanassia S, Galani L, Giannitsioti E, Kavatha D, Kontopidou F, Mouktaroudi M, Poulakou G, Sakka V, Panagopoulos P, Papadopoulos A, Kanellakopoulou K, Giamarellou H (2009) Effect of the novel influenza A (H1N1) virus in the human immune system. PLoS ONE 4:e8393. doi:10.1371/journal.pone.0008393

Gill MA, Long K, Kwon T, Muniz L, Mejias A, Connolly J, Roy L, Banchereau J, Ramilo O (2008) Differential recruitment of dendritic cells and monocytes to respiratory mucosal sites in children with influenza virus or respiratory syncytial virus infection. J Infect Dis 198:1667–1676. doi:10.1086/593018

Gill MA, Palucka AK, Barton T, Ghaffar F, Jafri H, Banchereau J, Ramilo O (2005) Mobilization of plasmacytoid and myeloid dendritic cells to mucosal sites in children with respiratory syncytial virus and other viral respiratory infections. J Infect Dis 191:1105–1115. doi:10.1086/428589 JID33373 [PII]

Gorski SA, Hahn YS, Braciale TJ (2013) Group 2 innate lymphoid cell production of IL-5 is regulated by NKT cells during influenza virus infection. PLoS Pathog 9:e1003615. doi:10.1371/journal.ppat.1003615

Graham AC, Hilmer KM, Zickovich JM, Obar JJ (2013) Inflammatory response of mast cells during influenza A virus infection is mediated by active infection and RIG-I signaling. J Immunol 190:4676–4684. doi:10.4049/jimmunol.1202096

Guilliams M, Lambrecht BN, Hammad H (2013) Division of labor between lung dendritic cells and macrophages in the defense against pulmonary infections. Mucosal Immunol 6:464–473. doi:10.1038/mi.2013.14

Guillot L, le Goffic R, Bloch S, Escriou N, Akira S, Chignard M, Si-Tahar M (2005) Involvement of toll-like receptor 3 in the immune response of lung epithelial cells to double-stranded RNA and influenza A virus. J Biol Chem 280:5571–5580. doi:10.1074/jbc.M410592200

Guo H, Kumar P, Moran TM, Garcia-Sastre A, Zhou Y, Malarkannan S (2009) The functional impairment of natural killer cells during influenza virus infection. Immunol Cell Biol 87:579–589. doi:10.1038/icb.2009.60

Guo X, Chen Y, Li X, Kong H, Yang S, Ye B, Cui D, Wu W, Li L (2011) Dynamic variations in the peripheral blood lymphocyte subgroups of patients with 2009 pandemic H1N1 swine-origin influenza A virus infection. Virol J 8:215. doi:10.1186/1743-422X-8-215

Haller O, Staeheli P, Kochs G (2009) Protective role of interferon-induced Mx GTPases against influenza viruses. Rev Sci Tech 28:219–231

Haniffa M, Collin M, Ginhoux F (2013) Ontogeny and functional specialization of dendritic cells in human and mouse. Adv Immunol 120:1–49. doi:10.1016/B978-0-12-417028-5.00001-6

Haniffa M, Shin A, Bigley V, McGovern N, Teo P, See P, Wasan PS, Wang XN, Malinarich F, Malleret B, Larbi A, Tan P, Zhao H, Poidinger M, Pagan S, Cookson S, Dickinson R, Dimmick I, Jarrett RF, Renia L, Tam J, Song C, Connolly J, Chan JK, Gehring A, Bertoletti A, Collin M, Ginhoux F (2012) Human tissues contain CD141hi cross-presenting dendritic cells with functional homology to mouse CD103+ nonlymphoid dendritic cells. Immunity 37:60–73. doi:10.1016/j.immuni.2012.04.012 S1074-7613(12)00279-8 [PII]

Hao X, Kim TS, Braciale TJ (2008) Differential response of respiratory dendritic cell subsets to influenza virus infection. J Virol 82:4908–4919. doi:10.1128/JVI.02367-07

Hargadon KM, Zhou H, Albrecht RA, Dodd HA, Garcia-Sastre A, Braciale TJ (2011) Major histocompatibility complex class II expression and hemagglutinin subtype influence the infectivity of type A influenza virus for respiratory dendritic cells. J Virol 85:11955–11963. doi:10.1128/JVI.05830-11

Hartmann BM, Li W, Jia J, Patil S, Marjanovic N, Martinez-Romero C, Albrecht RA, Hayot F, Garcia-Sastre A, Wetmur JG, Moran TM, Sealfon SC (2013) Mouse dendritic cell (DC) influenza virus infectivity is much lower than that for human DCs and is hemagglutinin subtype dependent. J Virol 87:1916–1918. doi:10.1128/JVI.02980-12

Hartshorn KL, Liou LS, White MR, Kazhdan MM, Tauber JL, Tauber AI (1995) Neutrophil deactivation by influenza A virus. Role of hemagglutinin binding to specific sialic acid-bearing cellular proteins. J Immunol 154:3952–3960

Hashimoto Y, Moki T, Takizawa T, Shiratsuchi A, Nakanishi Y (2007) Evidence for phagocytosis of influenza virus-infected, apoptotic cells by neutrophils and macrophages in mice. J Immunol 178:2448–2457. doi:10.4049/jimmunol.178.4.2448

He XS, Draghi M, Mahmood K, Holmes TH, Kemble GW, Dekker CL, Arvin AM, Parham P, Greenberg HB (2004) T cell-dependent production of IFN-gamma by NK cells in response to influenza A virus. J Clin Invest 114:1812–1819. doi:10.1172/JCI22797

Heer AK, Shamshiev A, Donda A, Uematsu S, Akira S, Kopf M, Marsland BJ (2007) TLR signaling fine-tunes anti-influenza B cell responses without regulating effector T cell responses. J Immunol 178:2182–2191. doi:10.4049/jimmunol.178.4.2182

Helft J, Ginhoux F, Bogunovic M, Merad M (2010) Origin and functional heterogeneity of non-lymphoid tissue dendritic cells in mice. Immunol Rev 234:55–75. doi:10.1111/j.0105-2896.2009.00885.x

Helft J, Manicassamy B, Guermonprez P, Hashimoto D, Silvin A, Agudo J, Brown BD, Schmolke M, Miller JC, Leboeuf M, Murphy KM, Garcia-Sastre A, Merad M (2012) Cross-presenting CD103+ dendritic cells are protected from influenza virus infection. J Clin Invest 122:4037–4047. doi:10.1172/JCI60659

Heltzer ML, Coffin SE, Maurer K, Bagashev A, Zhang Z, Orange JS, Sullivan KE (2009) Immune dysregulation in severe influenza. J Leukoc Biol 85:1036–1043. doi:10.1189/jlb.1108710

Herold S, Steinmueller M, von Wulffen W, Cakarova L, Pinto R, Pleschka S, Mack M, Kuziel WA, Corazza N, Brunner T, Seeger W, Lohmeyer J (2008) Lung epithelial apoptosis in influenza virus pneumonia: the role of macrophage-expressed TNF-related apoptosis-inducing ligand. J Exp Med 205:3065–3077. doi:10.1084/jem.20080201

Ho AW, Prabhu N, Betts RJ, Ge MQ, Dai X, Hutchinson PE, Lew FC, Wong KL, Hanson BJ, Macary PA, Kemeny DM (2011) Lung CD103+ dendritic cells efficiently transport influenza virus to the lymph node and load viral antigen onto MHC class I for presentation to CD8 T cells. J Immunol 187:6011–6021. doi:10.4049/jimmunol.1100987

Hoeve MA, Nash AA, Jackson D, Randall RE, Dransfield I (2012) Influenza virus A infection of human monocyte and macrophage subpopulations reveals increased susceptibility associated with cell differentiation. PLoS ONE 7:e29443. doi:10.1371/journal.pone.0029443 PONE-D-11-16347 [PII]

Hogner K, Wolff T, Pleschka S, Plog S, Gruber AD, Kalinke U, Walmrath HD, Bodner J, Gattenlohner S, Lewe-Schlosser P, Matrosovich M, Seeger W, Lohmeyer J, Herold S (2013) Macrophage-expressed IFN-beta contributes to apoptotic alveolar epithelial cell injury in severe influenza virus pneumonia. PLoS Pathog 9:e1003188. doi:10.1371/journal.ppat.1003188 PPATHOGENS-D-12-00914

Hou W, Gibbs JS, Lu X, Brooke CB, Roy D, Modlin RL, Bennink JR, Yewdell JW (2012) Viral infection triggers rapid differentiation of human blood monocytes into dendritic cells. Blood 119:3128–3131. doi:10.1182/blood-2011-09-379479

Hsu AC, Parsons K, Barr I, Lowther S, Middleton D, Hansbro PM, Wark PA (2012) Critical role of constitutive type I interferon response in bronchial epithelial cell to influenza infection. PLoS One 7:e32947. doi:10.1371/journal.pone.0032947 PONE-D-11-20761 [PII]

Huang Y, Zaas AK, Rao A, Dobigeon N, Woolf PJ, Veldman T, Oien NC, McClain MT, Varkey JB, Nicholson B, Carin L, Kingsmore S, Woods CW, Ginsburg GS, Hero AO 3rd (2011) Temporal dynamics of host molecular responses differentiate symptomatic and asymptomatic influenza a infection. PLoS Genet 7:e1002234. doi:10.1371/journal.pgen.1002234

Huang Y, Zhu W, Zeng X, Li S, Li X, Lu C (2013) Innate and adaptive immune responses in patients with pandemic influenza A(H1N1)pdm09. Arch Virol 158:2267–2272. doi:10.1007/s00705-013-1692-9

Hufford MM, Richardson G, Zhou H, Manicassamy B, Garcia-Sastre A, Enelow RI, Braciale TJ (2012) Influenza-infected neutrophils within the infected lungs act as antigen presenting cells for anti-viral CD8(+) T cells. PLoS ONE 7:e46581. doi:10.1371/journal.pone.0046581 PONE-D-12-19398 [PII]

Hui KP, Lee SM, Cheung CY, Mao H, Lai AK, Chan RW, Chan MC, Tu W, Guan Y, Lau YL, Peiris JS (2011) H5N1 influenza virus-induced mediators upregulate RIG-I in uninfected cells by paracrine effects contributing to amplified cytokine cascades. J Infect Dis 204:1866–1878. doi:10.1093/infdis/jir665

Hwang I, Scott JM, Kakarla T, Duriancik DM, Choi S, Cho C, Lee T, Park H, French AR, Beli E, Gardner E, Kim S (2012) Activation mechanisms of natural killer cells during influenza virus infection. PLoS ONE 7:e51858. doi:10.1371/journal.pone.0051858 PONE-D-12-23463 [PII]

Ibricevic A, Pekosz A, Walter MJ, Newby C, Battaile JT, Brown EG, Holtzman MJ, Brody SL (2006) Influenza virus receptor specificity and cell tropism in mouse and human airway epithelial cells. J Virol 80:7469–7480. doi:10.1128/JVI.02677-05

Ichinohe T, Lee HK, Ogura Y, Flavell R, Iwasaki A (2009) Inflammasome recognition of influenza virus is essential for adaptive immune responses. J Exp Med 206:79–87. doi:10.1084/jem.20081667

Ichinohe T, Pang IK, Iwasaki A (2010) Influenza virus activates inflammasomes via its intracellular M2 ion channel. Nat Immunol 11:404–410. doi:10.1038/ni.1861

Ichinohe T, Pang IK, Kumamoto Y, Peaper DR, Ho JH, Murray TS, Iwasaki A (2011) Microbiota regulates immune defense against respiratory tract influenza A virus infection. Proc Natl Acad Sci U S A 108:5354–5359. doi:10.1073/pnas.1019378108

Ioannidis I, Ye F, McNally B, Willette M, Flano E (2013) Toll-like receptor expression and induction of type I and type III interferons in primary airway epithelial cells. J Virol 87:3261–3270. doi:10.1128/JVI.01956-12
Ioannidis LJ, Verity EE, Crawford S, Rockman SP, Brown LE (2012) Abortive replication of influenza virus in mouse dendritic cells. J Virol 86:5922–5925. doi:10.1128/JVI.07060-11
Ito T, Allen RM, Carson WFt, Schaller M, Cavassani KA, Hogaboam CM, Lukacs NW, Matsukawa A, Kunkel SL (2011) The critical role of Notch ligand Delta-like 1 in the pathogenesis of influenza A virus (H1N1) infection. PLoS Pathog 7:e1002341. doi:10.1371/journal.ppat.1002341 PPATHOGENS-D-11-00960 [PII]
Iwasaki A, Medzhitov R (2010) Regulation of adaptive immunity by the innate immune system. Science 327:291–295. doi:10.1126/science.1183021
Jaworska J, Coulombe F, Downey J, Tzelepis F, Shalaby K, Tattoli I, Berube J, Rousseau S, Martin JG, Girardin SE, McCullers JA, Divangahi M (2014) NLRX1 prevents mitochondrial induced apoptosis and enhances macrophage antiviral immunity by interacting with influenza virus PB1-F2 protein. Proc Nat Acad Sci U.S.A 111:E2110–E2119. doi:10.1073/pnas.1322118111
Jego G, Palucka AK, Blanck JP, Chalouni C, Pascual V, Banchereau J (2003) Plasmacytoid dendritic cells induce plasma cell differentiation through type I interferon and interleukin 6. Immunity 19:225–234
Jeisy-Scott V, Davis WG, Patel JR, Bowzard JB, Shieh WJ, Zaki SR, Katz JM, Sambhara S (2011) Increased MDSC accumulation and Th2 biased response to influenza A virus infection in the absence of TLR7 in mice. PLoS ONE 6:e25242. doi:10.1371/journal.pone.0025242 PONE-D-11-14981 [PII]
Jeisy-Scott V, Kim JH, Davis WG, Cao W, Katz JM, Sambhara S (2012) TLR7 recognition is dispensable for influenza virus A infection but important for the induction of hemagglutinin-specific antibodies in response to the 2009 pandemic split vaccine in mice. J Virol 86:10988–10998. doi:10.1128/JVI.01064-12
Jost S, Altfeld M (2013) Control of human viral infections by natural killer cells. Annu Rev Immunol 31:163–194. doi:10.1146/annurev-immunol-032712-100001
Kadowaki N, Ho S, Antonenko S, Malefyt RW, Kastelein RA, Bazan F, Liu YJ (2001) Subsets of human dendritic cell precursors express different toll-like receptors and respond to different microbial antigens. J Exp Med 194:863–869
Kaminski MM, Ohnemus A, Cornitescu M, Staeheli P (2012) Plasmacytoid dendritic cells and toll-like receptor 7-dependent signalling promote efficient protection of mice against highly virulent influenza A virus. J Gen Virol 93:555–559. doi:10.1099/vir.0.039065-0
Kanneganti TD (2010) Central roles of NLRs and inflammasomes in viral infection. Nat Rev Immunol 10:688–698. doi:10.1038/nri2851
Kanneganti TD, Body-Malapel M, Amer A, Park JH, Whitfield J, Franchi L, Taraporewala ZF, Miller D, Patton JT, Inohara N, Nunez G (2006) Critical role for Cryopyrin/Nalp3 in activation of caspase-1 in response to viral infection and double-stranded RNA. J Biol Chem 281:36560–36568. doi:10.1074/jbc.M607594200
Kash JC, Tumpey TM, Proll SC, Carter V, Perwitasari O, Thomas MJ, Basler CF, Palese P, Taubenberger JK, Garcia-Sastre A, Swayne DE, Katze MG (2006) Genomic analysis of increased host immune and cell death responses induced by 1918 influenza virus. Nature 443:578–581. doi:10.1038/nature05181
Kato H, Takeuchi O, Sato S, Yoneyama M, Yamamoto M, Matsui K, Uematsu S, Jung A, Kawai T, Ishii KJ, Yamaguchi O, Otsu K, Tsujimura T, Koh CS, Reis e Sousa C, Matsuura Y, Fujita T, Akira S (2006) Differential roles of MDA5 and RIG-I helicases in the recognition of RNA viruses. Nature 441:101–105. doi:10.1038/nature04734
Kawai T, Akira S (2011) Toll-like receptors and their crosstalk with other innate receptors in infection and immunity. Immunity 34:637–650. doi:10.1016/j.immuni.2011.05.006
Kim HM, Kang YM, Ku KB, Park EH, Yum J, Kim JC, Jin SY, Lee JS, Kim HS, Seo SH (2013) The severe pathogenicity of alveolar macrophage-depleted ferrets infected with 2009 pandemic H1N1 influenza virus. Virology 444:394–403. doi:10.1016/j.virol.2013.07.006 S0042-6822(13)00408-X [PII]

Kim HM, Lee YW, Lee KJ, Kim HS, Cho SW, van Rooijen N, Guan Y, Seo SH (2008) Alveolar macrophages are indispensable for controlling influenza viruses in lungs of pigs. J Virol 82:4265–4274. doi:10.1128/JVI.02602-07

Kim TS, Braciale TJ (2009) Respiratory dendritic cell subsets differ in their capacity to support the induction of virus-specific cytotoxic CD8+ T cell responses. PLoS ONE 4:e4204. doi:10.1371/journal.pone.0004204

Kim TS, Gorski SA, Hahn S, Murphy KM, Braciale TJ (2014) Distinct dendritic cell subsets dictate the fate decision between effector and memory CD8(+) T cell differentiation by a CD24-dependent mechanism. Immunity 40:400–413. doi:10.1016/j.immuni.2014.02.004

Kohlmeier JE, Cookenham T, Roberts AD, Miller SC, Woodland DL (2010) Type I interferons regulate cytolytic activity of memory CD8(+) T cells in the lung airways during respiratory virus challenge. Immunity 33:96–105. doi:10.1016/j.immuni.2010.06.016 S1074-7613(10)00242-6 [PII]

Kok WL, Denney L, Benam K, Cole S, Clelland C, McMichael AJ, Ho LP (2012) Pivotal advance: invariant NKT cells reduce accumulation of inflammatory monocytes in the lungs and decrease immune-pathology during severe influenza A virus infection. J Leukoc Biol 91:357–368. doi:10.1189/jlb.0411184

Korth MJ, Tchitchek N, Benecke AG, Katze MG (2013) Systems approaches to influenza-virus host interactions and the pathogenesis of highly virulent and pandemic viruses. Semin Immunol 25:228–239. doi:10.1016/j.smim.2012.11.001

Koyama S, Aoshi T, Tanimoto T, Kumagai Y, Kobiyama K, Tougan T, Sakurai K, Coban C, Horii T, Akira S, Ishii KJ (2010) Plasmacytoid dendritic cells delineate immunogenicity of influenza vaccine subtypes. Sci Transl Med 2:25ra24. doi: 10.1126/scitranslmed.3000759

Koyama S, Ishii KJ, Kumar H, Tanimoto T, Coban C, Uematsu S, Kawai T, Akira S (2007) Differential role of TLR- and RLR-signaling in the immune responses to influenza A virus infection and vaccination. J Immunol 179:4711–4720. doi:10.3410/f.1091005.544378 179/7/4711 [PII]

Lakadamyali M, Rust MJ, Zhuang X (2006) Ligands for clathrin-mediated endocytosis are differentially sorted into distinct populations of early endosomes. Cell 124:997–1009. doi:10.1016/j.cell.2005.12.038 S0092-8674(06)00123-1 [PII]

Lambrecht BN, Hammad H (2009) Biology of lung dendritic cells at the origin of asthma. Immunity 31:412–424. doi:10.1016/j.immuni.2009.08.008

Lambrecht BN, Hammad H (2012) Lung dendritic cells in respiratory viral infection and asthma: from protection to immunopathology. Ann Rev Immunol 30:243–270. doi:10.1146/annurev-immunol-020711-075021

Larsson M, Messmer D, Somersan S, Fonteneau JF, Donahoe SM, Lee M, Dunbar PR, Cerundolo V, Julkunen I, Nixon DF, Bhardwaj N (2000) Requirement of mature dendritic cells for efficient activation of influenza A-specific memory CD8+ T cells. J Immunol 165:1182–1190

le Goffic R, Balloy V, Lagranderie M, Alexopoulou L, Escriou N, Flavell R, Chignard M, Si-Tahar M (2006) Detrimental contribution of the toll-like receptor (TLR)3 to influenza A virus-induced acute pneumonia. PLoS Pathog 2:e53. doi:10.1371/journal.ppat.0020053

le Goffic R, Pothlichet J, Vitour D, Fujita T, Meurs E, Chignard M, Si-Tahar M (2007) Cutting Edge: Influenza A virus activates TLR3-dependent inflammatory and RIG-I-dependent antiviral responses in human lung epithelial cells. J Immunol 178:3368–3372 178/6/3368 [PII]

le Nouen C, Hillyer P, Winter CC, McCarty T, Rabin RL, Collins PL, Buchholz UJ (2011) Low CCR7-mediated migration of human monocyte derived dendritic cells in response to human respiratory syncytial virus and human metapneumovirus. PLoS Pathog 7:e1002105. doi:10.1371/journal.ppat.1002105 PPATHOGENS-D-10-00578 [PII]

Lee N, Wong CK, Chan PK, Chan MC, Wong RY, Lun SW, Ngai KL, Lui GC, Wong BC, Lee SK, Choi KW, Hui DS (2011) Cytokine response patterns in severe pandemic 2009 H1N1 and seasonal influenza among hospitalized adults. PLoS ONE 6:e26050. doi:10.1371/journal.pone.0026050

Lee N, Wong CK, Hui DS, Lee SK, Wong RY, Ngai KL, Chan MC, Chu YJ, Ho AW, Lui GC, Wong BC, Wong SH, Yip SP, Chan PK (2013) Role of human toll-like receptors in naturally occurring influenza A infections. Influenza Other Respir Viruses 7:666–675. doi:10.1111/irv.12109

Lee SM, Gardy JL, Cheung CY, Cheung TK, Hui KP, Ip NY, Guan Y, Hancock RE, Peiris JS (2009) Systems-level comparison of host-responses elicited by avian H5N1 and seasonal H1N1 influenza viruses in primary human macrophages. PLoS ONE 4:e8072. doi:10.1371/journal.pone.0008072

Lenschow DJ, Lai C, Frias-Staheli N, Giannakopoulos NV, Lutz A, Wolff T, Osiak A, Levine B, Schmidt RE, Garcia-Sastre A, Leib DA, Pekosz A, Knobeloch KP, Horak I, Virgin HWt (2007) IFN-stimulated gene 15 functions as a critical antiviral molecule against influenza, herpes, and Sindbis viruses. Proc Nat Acad Sci U.S.A 104:1371–1376. doi:10.1073/pnas.0607038104

Leon B, Bradley JE, Lund FE, Randall TD, Ballesteros-Tato A (2014) FoxP3+ regulatory T cells promote influenza-specific Tfh responses by controlling IL-2 availability. Nat Commun 5:3495. doi:10.1038/ncomms4495

Li S, Min JY, Krug RM, Sen GC (2006) Binding of the influenza A virus NS1 protein to PKR mediates the inhibition of its activation by either PACT or double-stranded RNA. Virology 349:13–21. doi:10.1016/j.virol.2006.01.005 S0042-6822(06)00008-0 [PII]

Li S, Nakaya HI, Kazmin DA, Oh JZ, Pulendran B (2013) Systems biological approaches to measure and understand vaccine immunity in humans. Semin Immunol 25:209–218. doi:10.1016/j.smim.2013.05.003 S1044-5323(13)00032-8 [PII]

Li S, Rouphael N, Duraisingham S, Romero-Steiner S, Presnell S, Davis C, Schmidt DS, Johnson SE, Milton A, Rajam G, Kasturi S, Carlone GM, Quinn C, Chaussabel D, Palucka AK, Mulligan MJ, Ahmed R, Stephens DS, Nakaya HI, Pulendran B (2014) Molecular signatures of antibody responses derived from a systems biology study of five human vaccines. Nat Immunol 15:195–204. doi:10.1038/ni.2789

Lietzen N, Ohman T, Rintahaka J, Julkunen I, Aittokallio T, Matikainen S, Nyman TA (2011) Quantitative subcellular proteome and secretome profiling of influenza A virus-infected human primary macrophages. PLoS Pathog 7:e1001340. doi:10.1371/journal.ppat.1001340 10-PLPA-RA-4245R2 [PII]

Lin KL, Suzuki Y, Nakano H, Ramsburg E, Gunn MD (2008) CCR2+ monocyte-derived dendritic cells and exudate macrophages produce influenza-induced pulmonary immune pathology and mortality. J Immunol 180:2562–2572. doi:10.4049/jimmunol.180.4.2562 180/4/2562 [PII]

Lin KL, Sweeney S, Kang BD, Ramsburg E, Gunn MD (2011) CCR2-antagonist prophylaxis reduces pulmonary immune pathology and markedly improves survival during influenza infection. J Immunol 186:508–515. doi:10.4049/jimmunol.1001002

Londrigan SL, Tate MD, Brooks AG, Reading PC (2012) Cell-surface receptors on macrophages and dendritic cells for attachment and entry of influenza virus. J Leukoc Biol 92:97–106. doi:10.1189/jlb.1011492

Londrigan SL, Turville SG, Tate MD, Deng YM, Brooks AG, Reading PC (2011) N-linked glycosylation facilitates sialic acid-independent attachment and entry of influenza A viruses into cells expressing DC-SIGN or L-SIGN. J Virol 85:2990–3000. doi:10.1128/JVI.01705-10

Loo YM, Gale M Jr (2011) Immune signaling by RIG-I-like receptors. Immunity 34:680–692. doi:10.1016/j.immuni.2011.05.003 S1074-7613(11)00187-7 [PII]

Lui G, Manches O, Angel J, Molens JP, Chaperot L, Plumas J (2009) Plasmacytoid dendritic cells capture and cross-present viral antigens from influenza-virus exposed cells. PLoS ONE 4:e7111. doi:10.1371/journal.pone.0007111

Lund JM, Alexopoulou L, Sato A, Karow M, Adams NC, Gale NW, Iwasaki A, Flavell RA (2004) Recognition of single-stranded RNA viruses by toll-like receptor 7. Proc Nat Acad Sci U.S.A 101:5598–5603. doi:10.1073/pnas.0400937101

Lupfer C, Thomas PG, Anand PK, Vogel P, Milasta S, Martinez J, Huang G, Green M, Kundu M, Chi H, Xavier RJ, Green DR, Lamkanfi M, Dinarello CA, Doherty PC, Kanneganti TD (2013) Receptor interacting protein kinase 2-mediated mitophagy regulates inflammasome activation during virus infection. Nat Immunol 14:480–488. doi:10.1038/ni.2563

Lupfer C, Thomas PG, Kanneganti TD (2014) NOD2 dependent DC activation is necessary for innate immunity and optimal CD8+ T cell responses to influenza A virus infection. J Virol. doi:10.1128/JVI.01110-14
Mandelboim O, Lieberman N, Lev M, Paul L, Arnon TI, Bushkin Y, Davis DM, Strominger JL, Yewdell JW, Porgador A (2001) Recognition of haemagglutinins on virus-infected cells by NKp46 activates lysis by human NK cells. Nature 409:1055–1060. doi:10.1038/35059110
Manicassamy B, Manicassamy S, Belicha-Villanueva A, Pisanelli G, Pulendran B, Garcia-Sastre A (2010) Analysis of in vivo dynamics of influenza virus infection in mice using a GFP reporter virus. Proc Nat Acad Sci U.S.A 107:11531–11536. doi:10.1073/pnas.0914994107
Manicassamy S, Pulendran B (2009) Modulation of adaptive immunity with toll-like receptors. Semin Immunol 21:185–193. doi:10.1016/j.smim.2009.05.005 S1044-5323(09)00048-7 [PII]
Manicassamy S, Pulendran B (2011) Dendritic cell control of tolerogenic responses. Immunol Rev 241:206–227. doi:10.1111/j.1600-065X.2011.01015.x
Mao H, Tu W, Liu Y, Qin G, Zheng J, Chan PL, Lam KT, Peiris JS, Lau YL (2010) Inhibition of human natural killer cell activity by influenza virions and hemagglutinin. J Virol 84:4148–4157. doi:10.1128/JVI.02340-09
Mao H, Tu W, Qin G, Law HK, Sia SF, Chan PL, Liu Y, Lam KT, Zheng J, Peiris M, Lau YL (2009) Influenza virus directly infects human natural killer cells and induces cell apoptosis. J Virol 83:9215–9222. doi:10.1128/JVI.00805-09
Mao L, Yang Y, Qiu Y, Yang Y (2012) Annual economic impacts of seasonal influenza on US counties: spatial heterogeneity and patterns. Int J Health Geogr 11:16. doi:10.1186/1476-072X-11-16
McAuley JL, Tate MD, MacKenzie-Kludas CJ, Pinar A, Zeng W, Stutz A, Latz E, Brown LE, Mansell A (2013) Activation of the NLRP3 inflammasome by IAV virulence protein PB1-F2 contributes to severe pathophysiology and disease. PLoS Pathog 9:e1003392. doi:10.1371/journal.ppat.1003392
McClain MT, Park LP, Nicholson B, Veldman T, Zaas AK, Turner R, Lambkin-Williams R, Gilbert AS, Ginsburg GS, Woods CW (2013) Longitudinal analysis of leukocyte differentials in peripheral blood of patients with acute respiratory viral infections. J Clin Virol 58:689–695. doi:10.1016/j.jcv.2013.09.015 S1386-6532(13)00406-X [PII]
McGill J, van Rooijen N, Legge KL (2008) Protective influenza-specific CD8 T cell responses require interactions with dendritic cells in the lungs. J Exp Med 205:1635–1646. doi:10.1084/jem.20080314
McGill J, van Rooijen N, Legge KL (2010) IL-15 trans-presentation by pulmonary dendritic cells promotes effector CD8 T cell survival during influenza virus infection. J Exp Med 207:521–534. doi:10.1084/jem.20091711
Medina RA, Garcia-Sastre A (2011) Influenza A viruses: new research developments. Nat Rev Microbiol 9:590–603. doi:10.1038/nrmicro2613
Merad M, Sathe P, Helft J, Miller J, Mortha A (2013) The dendritic cell lineage: ontogeny and function of dendritic cells and their subsets in the steady state and the inflamed setting. Ann Rev Immunol 31:563–604. doi:10.1146/annurev-immunol-020711-074950
Molinari NA, Ortega-Sanchez IR, Messonnier ML, Thompson WW, Wortley PM, Weintraub E, Bridges CB (2007) The annual impact of seasonal influenza in the US: measuring disease burden and costs. Vaccine 25:5086–5096. doi:10.1016/j.vaccine.2007.03.046
Monticelli LA, Sonnenberg GF, Abt MC, Alenghat T, Ziegler CG, Doering TA, Angelosanto JM, Laidlaw BJ, Yang CY, Sathaliyawala T, Kubota M, Turner D, Diamond JM, Goldrath AW, Farber DL, Collman RG, Wherry EJ, Artis D (2011) Innate lymphoid cells promote lung-tissue homeostasis after infection with influenza virus. Nat Immunol 12:1045–1054. doi:10.1031/ni.2131
Nakajima N, Sato Y, Katano H, Hasegawa H, Kumasaka T, Hata S, Tanaka S, Amano T, Kasai T, Chong JM, Iizuka T, Nakazato I, Hino Y, Hamamatsu A, Horiguchi H, Tanaka T, Hasegawa A, Kanaya Y, Oku R, Oya T, Sata T (2012) Histopathological and immunohistochemical findings of 20 autopsy cases with 2009 H1N1 virus infection. Mod Pathol 25:1–13. doi:10.1038/modpathol.2011.125

Nakajima N, van Tin N, Sato Y, Thach HN, Katano H, Diep PH, Kumasaka T, Thuy NT, Hasegawa H, San LT, Kawachi S, Liem NT, Suzuki K, Sata T (2013) Pathological study of archival lung tissues from five fatal cases of avian H5N1 influenza in Vietnam. Mod Pathol 26:357–369. doi:10.1038/modpathol.2012.193

Nakano H, Lin KL, Yanagita M, Charbonneau C, Cook DN, Kakiuchi T, Gunn MD (2009) Blood-derived inflammatory dendritic cells in lymph nodes stimulate acute T helper type 1 immune responses. Nat Immunol 10:394–402. doi:10.1038/ni.1707

Nakaya HI, Li S, Pulendran B (2012) Systems vaccinology: learning to compute the behavior of vaccine induced immunity. Wiley Interdiscip Rev Syst Biol Med 4:193–205. doi:10.1002/wsbm.163

Nakaya HI, Wrammert J, Lee EK, Racioppi L, Marie-Kunze S, Haining WN, Means AR, Kasturi SP, Khan N, Li GM, McCausland M, Kanchan V, Kokko KE, Li S, Elbein R, Mehta AK, Aderem A, Subbarao K, Ahmed R, Pulendran B (2011) Systems biology of vaccination for seasonal influenza in humans. Nat Immunol 12:786–795. doi:10.1038/ni.2067

Narasaraju T, Yang E, Samy RP, Ng HH, Poh WP, Liew AA, Phoon MC, van Rooijen N, Chow VT (2011) Excessive neutrophils and neutrophil extracellular traps contribute to acute lung injury of influenza pneumonitis. Am J Pathol 179:199–210. doi:10.1016/j.ajpath.2011.03.013 S0002-9440(11)00329-4 [PII]

Nhu QM, Shirey K, Teijaro JR, Farber DL, Netzel-Arnett S, Antalis TM, Fasano A, Vogel SN (2010) Novel signaling interactions between proteinase-activated receptor 2 and toll-like receptors in vitro and in vivo. Mucosal Immunol 3:29–39. doi:10.1038/mi.2009.120

Nicholls JM, Chan MC, Chan WY, Wong HK, Cheung CY, Kwong DL, Wong MP, Chui WH, Poon LL, Tsao SW, Guan Y, Peiris JS (2007) Tropism of avian influenza A (H5N1) in the upper and lower respiratory tract. Nat Med 13:147–149. doi:10.1038/nm1529

Ohman T, Rintahaka J, Kalkkinen N, Matikainen S, Nyman TA (2009) Actin and RIG-I/MAVS signaling components translocate to mitochondria upon influenza A virus infection of human primary macrophages. J Immunol 182:5682–5692. doi:10.4049/jimmunol.0803093

Onomoto K, Jogi M, Yoo JS, Narita R, Morimoto S, Takemura A, Sambhara S, Kawaguchi A, Osari S, Nagata K, Matsumiya T, Namiki H, Yoneyama M, Fujita T (2012) Critical role of an antiviral stress granule containing RIG-I and PKR in viral detection and innate immunity. PLoS ONE 7:e43031. doi:10.1371/journal.pone.0043031

Oshansky CM, Gartland AJ, Wong SS, Jeevan T, Wang D, Roddam PL, Caniza MA, Hertz T, Devincenzo JP, Webby RJ, Thomas PG (2013) Mucosal immune responses predict clinical outcomes during influenza infection independently of age and viral load. Am J Respir Crit Care Med. doi:10.1164/rccm.201309-1616OC

Osterlund P, Pirhonen J, Ikonen N, Ronkko E, Strengell M, Makela SM, Broman M, Hamming OJ, Hartmann R, Ziegler T, Julkunen I (2010) Pandemic H1N1 2009 influenza A virus induces weak cytokine responses in human macrophages and dendritic cells and is highly sensitive to the antiviral actions of interferons. J Virol 84:1414–1422. doi:10.1128/JVI.01619-09

Osterlund P, Veckman V, Siren J, Klucher KM, Hiscott J, Matikainen S, Julkunen I (2005) Gene expression and antiviral activity of alpha/beta interferons and interleukin-29 in virus-infected human myeloid dendritic cells. J Virol 79:9608–9617. doi:10.1128/JVI.79.15.9608-9617.2005

Paget C, Ivanov S, Fontaine J, Blanc F, Pichavant M, Renneson J, Bialecki E, Pothlichet J, Vendeville C, Barba-Spaeth G, Huerre MR, Faveeuw C, Si-Tahar M, Trottein F (2011) Potential role of invariant NKT cells in the control of pulmonary inflammation and CD8+ T cell response during acute influenza A virus H3N2 pneumonia. J Immunol 186:5590–5602. doi:10.4049/jimmunol.1002348

Pan W, Dong Z, Li F, Meng W, Feng L, Niu X, Li C, Luo Q, Li Z, Sun C, Chen L (2013) Visualizing influenza virus infection in living mice. Nat Commun 4:2369. doi:10.1038/ncomms3369

Pang IK, Ichinohe T, Iwasaki A (2013a) IL-1R signaling in dendritic cells replaces pattern-recognition receptors in promoting CD8(+) T cell responses to influenza A virus. Nat Immunol 14:246–253. doi:10.1038/ni.2514

Pang IK, Pillai PS, Iwasaki A (2013b) Efficient influenza A virus replication in the respiratory tract requires signals from TLR7 and RIG-I. Proc Nat Acad Sci U.S.A 110:13910–13915. doi:10.1073/pnas.1303275110

Pelletier I, Rousset D, Enouf V, Colbere-Garapin F, van der Werf S, Naffakh N (2011) Highly heterogeneous temperature sensitivity of 2009 pandemic influenza A(H1N1) viral isolates, northern France. Euro Surveill 16:1–7. http://www.eurosurveillance.org/ViewArticle.aspx?ArticleId=19999

Perrone LA, Plowden JK, Garcia-Sastre A, Katz JM, Tumpey TM (2008) H5N1 and 1918 pandemic influenza virus infection results in early and excessive infiltration of macrophages and neutrophils in the lungs of mice. PLoS Pathog 4:e1000115. doi:10.1371/journal.ppat.1000115

Phipps-Yonas H, Seto J, Sealfon SC, Moran TM, Fernandez-Sesma A (2008) Interferon-beta pretreatment of conventional and plasmacytoid human dendritic cells enhances their activation by influenza virus. PLoS Pathog 4:e1000193. doi:10.1371/journal.ppat.1000193

Pichlmair A, Schulz O, Tan CP, Naslund TI, Liljestrom P, Weber F, Reis e Sousa C (2006) RIG-I-mediated antiviral responses to single-stranded RNA bearing 5'-phosphates. Science 314:997–1001. doi:10.1126/science.1132998

Pindel A, Sadler A (2011) The role of protein kinase R in the interferon response. J Interferon Cytokine Res 31:59–70. doi:10.1089/jir.2010.0099

Piqueras B, Connolly J, Freitas H, Palucka AK, Banchereau J (2006) Upon viral exposure, myeloid and plasmacytoid dendritic cells produce 3 waves of distinct chemokines to recruit immune effectors. Blood 107:2613–2618. doi:10.1182/blood-2005-07-2965

Pothlichet J, Burtey A, Kubarenko AV, Caignard G, Solhonne B, Tangy F, Ben-Ali M, Quintana-Murci L, Heinzmann A, Chiche JD, Vidalain PO, Weber AN, Chignard M, Si-Tahar M (2009) Study of human RIG-I polymorphisms identifies two variants with an opposite impact on the antiviral immune response. PLoS ONE 4:e7582. doi:10.1371/journal.pone.0007582

Pulendran B (2009) Learning immunology from the yellow fever vaccine: innate immunity to systems vaccinology. Nat Rev Immunol 9:741–747. doi:10.1038/nri2629

Pulendran B, Li S, Nakaya HI (2010a) Systems vaccinology. Immunity 33:516–529. doi:10.1016/j.immuni.2010.10.006 S1074-7613(10)00366-3 [PII]

Pulendran B, Tang H, Manicassamy S (2010b) Programming dendritic cells to induce T(H)2 and tolerogenic responses. Nat Immunol 11:647–655. doi:10.1038/ni.1894

Qu C, Moran TM, Randolph GJ (2003) Autocrine type I IFN and contact with endothelium promote the presentation of influenza A virus by monocyte-derived APC. J Immunol 170:1010–1018

Querec TD, Akondy RS, Lee EK, Cao W, Nakaya HI, Teuwen D, Pirani A, Gernert K, Deng J, Marzolf B, Kennedy K, Wu H, Bennouna S, Oluoch H, Miller J, Vencio RZ, Mulligan M, Aderem A, Ahmed R, Pulendran B (2009) Systems biology approach predicts immunogenicity of the yellow fever vaccine in humans. Nat Immunol 10:116–125. doi:10.1038/ni.1688

Ramos I, Bernal-Rubio D, Durham N, Belicha-Villanueva A, Lowen AC, Steel J, Fernandez-Sesma A (2011) Effects of receptor binding specificity of avian influenza virus on the human innate immune response. J Virol 85:4421–4431. doi:10.1128/JVI.02356-10

Ravindran R, Khan N, Nakaya HI, Li S, Loebbermann J, Maddur MS, Park Y, Jones DP, Chappert P, Davoust J, Weiss DS, Virgin HW, Ron D, Pulendran B (2014) Vaccine activation of the nutrient sensor GCN2 in dendritic cells enhances antigen presentation. Science 343:313–317. doi:10.1126/science.1246829

Rehwinkel J, Tan CP, Goubau D, Schulz O, Pichlmair A, Bier K, Robb N, Vreede F, Barclay W, Fodor E, Reis e Sousa C (2010) RIG-I detects viral genomic RNA during negative-strand RNA virus infection. Cell 140:397–408. doi:10.1016/j.cell.2010.01.020 S0092-8674(10)00021-8 [PII]

Sabbah A, Chang TH, Harnack R, Frohlich V, Tominaga K, Dube PH, Xiang Y, Bose S (2009) Activation of innate immune antiviral responses by Nod2. Nat Immunol 10:1073–1080. doi:10.1038/ni.1782

Sadler AJ, Williams BR (2008) Interferon-inducible antiviral effectors. Nat Rev Immunol 8:559–568. doi:10.1038/nri2314

Sakabe S, Iwatsuki-Horimoto K, Takano R, Nidom CA, Le M, Nagamura-Inoue T, Horimoto T, Yamashita N, Kawaoka Y (2011) Cytokine production by primary human macrophages infected with highly pathogenic H5N1 or pandemic H1N1 2009 influenza viruses. J Gen Virol 92:1428–1434. doi:10.1099/vir.0.030346-0

Salentin R, Gemsa D, Sprenger H, Kaufmann A (2003) Chemokine receptor expression and chemotactic responsiveness of human monocytes after influenza A virus infection. J Leukoc Biol 74:252–259

Sancho D, Reis e Sousa C (2012) Signaling by myeloid C-type lectin receptors in immunity and homeostasis. Annu Rev Immunol 30:491–529. doi:10.1146/annurev-immunol-031210-101352

Sasaki S, Jaimes MC, Holmes TH, Dekker CL, Mahmood K, Kemble GW, Arvin AM, Greenberg HB (2007) Comparison of the influenza virus-specific effector and memory B-cell responses to immunization of children and adults with live attenuated or inactivated influenza virus vaccines. J Virol 81:215–228. doi:10.1128/JVI.01957-06

Schroder K, Tschopp J (2010) The inflammasomes. Cell 140:821–832. doi:10.1016/j.cell.2010.01.040 S0092-8674(10)00075-9 [PII]

Segura E, Valladeau-Guilemond J, Donnadieu MH, Sastre-Garau X, Soumelis V, Amigorena S (2012) Characterization of resident and migratory dendritic cells in human lymph nodes. J Exp Med 209:653–660. doi:10.1084/jem.20111457

Seo SU, Kwon HJ, Ko HJ, Byun YH, Seong BL, Uematsu S, Akira S, Kweon MN (2011) Type I interferon signaling regulates Ly6C(hi) monocytes and neutrophils during acute viral pneumonia in mice. PLoS Pathog 7:e1001304. doi:10.1371/journal.ppat.1001304

Seo SU, Kwon HJ, Song JH, Byun YH, Seong BL, Kawai T, Akira S, Kweon MN (2010) MyD88 signaling is indispensable for primary influenza A virus infection but dispensable for secondary infection. J Virol 84:12713–12722. doi:10.1128/JVI.01675-10

Shinya K, Ebina M, Yamada S, Ono M, Kasai N, Kawaoka Y (2006) Avian flu: influenza virus receptors in the human airway. Nature 440:435–436. doi:10.1038/440435a

Shirey KA, Lai W, Scott AJ, Lipsky M, Mistry P, Pletneva LM, Karp CL, McAlees J, Gioannini TL, Weiss J, Chen WH, Ernst RK, Rossignol DP, Gusovsky F, Blanco JC, Vogel SN (2013) The TLR4 antagonist Eritoran protects mice from lethal influenza infection. Nature 497:498–502. doi:10.1038/nature12118

Short KR, Brooks AG, Reading PC, Londrigan SL (2012) The fate of influenza A virus after infection of human macrophages and dendritic cells. J Gen Virol 93:2315–2325. doi:10.1099/vir.0.045021-0

Short KR, Kroeze EJ, Fouchier RA, Kuiken T (2014) Pathogenesis of influenza-induced acute respiratory distress syndrome. Lancet Infect Dis 14:57–69. doi:10.1016/S1473-3099(13)70286-X S1473-3099(13)70286-X [PII]

Skehel JJ, Wiley DC (2000) Receptor binding and membrane fusion in virus entry: the influenza hemagglutinin. Ann Rev Biochem 69:531–569. doi:10.1146/annurev.biochem.69.1.531

Smed-Sorensen A, Chalouni C, Chatterjee B, Cohn L, Blattmann P, Nakamura N, Delamarre L, Mellman I (2012) Influenza A virus infection of human primary dendritic cells impairs their ability to cross-present antigen to CD8 T cells. PLoS Pathog 8:e1002572. doi:10.1371/journal.ppat.1002572 PPATHOGENS-D-11-01789

Song JY, Cheong HJ, Hwang IS, Choi WS, Jo YM, Park DW, Cho GJ, Hwang TG, Kim WJ (2010) Long-term immunogenicity of influenza vaccine among the elderly: risk factors for poor immune response and persistence. Vaccine 28:3929–3935. doi:10.1016/j.vaccine.2010.03.067

Spits H, Artis D, Colonna M, Diefenbach A, Di Santo JP, Eberl G, Koyasu S, Locksley RM, McKenzie AN, Mebius RE, Powrie F, Vivier E (2013) Innate lymphoid cells—a proposal for uniform nomenclature. Nat Rev Immunol 13:145–149. doi:10.1038/nri3365

Steinman RM, Banchereau J (2007) Taking dendritic cells into medicine. Nature 449:419–426. doi:10.1038/nature06175

Takeuchi O, Akira S (2009) Innate immunity to virus infection. Immunol Rev 227:75–86. doi:10.1111/j.1600-065X.2008.00737.x IMR737 [PII]

Tam VC, Quehenberger O, Oshansky CM, Suen R, Armando AM, Treuting PM, Thomas PG, Dennis EA, Aderem A (2013) Lipidomic profiling of influenza infection identifies mediators that induce and resolve inflammation. Cell 154:213–227. doi:10.1016/j.cell.2013.05.052 S0092-8674(13)00695-8 [PII]

Tate MD, Brooks AG, Reading PC (2008) The role of neutrophils in the upper and lower respiratory tract during influenza virus infection of mice. Respir Res 9:57. doi:10.1186/1465-9921-9-57

Tate MD, Brooks AG, Reading PC, Mintern JD (2012) Neutrophils sustain effective CD8(+) T-cell responses in the respiratory tract following influenza infection. Immunol Cell Biol 90:197–205. doi:10.1038/icb.2011.26

Tate MD, Deng YM, Jones JE, Anderson GP, Brooks AG, Reading PC (2009) Neutrophils ameliorate lung injury and the development of severe disease during influenza infection. J Immunol 183:7441–7450. doi:10.4049/jimmunol.0902497

Tate MD, Ioannidis LJ, Croker B, Brown LE, Brooks AG, Reading PC (2011) The role of neutrophils during mild and severe influenza virus infections of mice. PLoS ONE 6:e17618. doi:10.1371/journal.pone.0017618

Tate MD, Pickett DL, van Rooijen N, Brooks AG, Reading PC (2010) Critical role of airway macrophages in modulating disease severity during influenza virus infection of mice. J Virol 84:7569–7580. doi:10.1128/JVI.00291-10

Taubenberger JK, Morens DM (2008) The pathology of influenza virus infections. Ann Rev Pathol 3:499–522. doi:10.1146/annurev.pathmechdis.3.121806.154316

Thitithanyanont A, Engering A, Ekchariyawat P, Wiboon-ut S, Limsalakpetch A, Yongvanitchit K, Kum-Arb U, Kanchongkittiphon W, Utaisincharoen P, Sirisinha S, Puthavathana P, Fukuda MM, Pichyangkul S (2007) High susceptibility of human dendritic cells to avian influenza H5N1 virus infection and protection by IFN-alpha and TLR ligands. J Immunol 179:5220–5227 179/8/5220 [PII] doi:10.4049/jimmunol.179.8.5220

Thomas PG, Dash P, Aldridge JR Jr, Ellebedy AH, Reynolds C, Funk AJ, Martin WJ, Lamkanfi M, Webby RJ, Boyd KL, Doherty PC, Kanneganti TD (2009) The intracellular sensor NLRP3 mediates key innate and healing responses to influenza A virus via the regulation of caspase-1. Immunity 30:566–575. doi:10.1016/j.immuni.2009.02.006

Thompson CI, Barclay WS, Zambon MC, Pickles RJ (2006) Infection of human airway epithelium by human and avian strains of influenza a virus. J Virol 80:8060–8068. doi:10.1128/JVI.00384-06

Tripathi S, White MR, Hartshorn KL (2013) The amazing innate immune response to influenza A virus infection. Innate Immun. doi:10.1177/1753425913508992

Tsai SY, Segovia JA, Chang TH, Morris IR, Berton MT, Tessier PA, Tardif MR, Cesaro A, Bose S (2014) DAMP molecule S100A9 acts as a molecular pattern to enhance inflammation during influenza A virus infection: role of DDX21-TRIF-TLR4-MyD88 pathway. PLoS Pathog 10:e1003848. doi:10.1371/journal.ppat.1003848 PPATHOGENS-D-13-00524 [PII]

Tsang JS, Schwartzberg PL, Kotliarov Y, Biancotto A, Xie Z, Germain RN, Wang E, Olnes MJ, Narayanan M, Golding H, Moir S, Dickler HB, Perl S, Cheung F (2014) Global analyses of human immune variation reveal baseline predictors of postvaccination responses. Cell 157:499–513. doi:10.1016/j.cell.2014.03.031

Tscherne DM, Garcia-Sastre A (2011) Virulence determinants of pandemic influenza viruses. J Clin Invest 121:6–13. doi:10.1172/JCI44947

Tse H, To KK, Wen X, Chen H, Chan KH, Tsoi HW, Li IW, Yuen KY (2011) Clinical and virological factors associated with viremia in pandemic influenza A/H1N1/2009 virus infection. PLoS ONE 6:e22534. doi:10.1371/journal.pone.0022534

Tumpey TM, Garcia-Sastre A, Taubenberger JK, Palese P, Swayne DE, Pantin-Jackwood MJ, Schultz-Cherry S, Solorzano A, van Rooijen N, Katz JM, Basler CF (2005) Pathogenicity of influenza viruses with genes from the 1918 pandemic virus: functional roles of alveolar macrophages and neutrophils in limiting virus replication and mortality in mice. J Virol 79:14933–14944. doi:10.1128/JVI.79.23.14933-14944.2005

Unkel B, Hoegner K, Clausen BE, Lewe-Schlosser P, Bodner J, Gattenloehner S, Janssen H, Seeger W, Lohmeyer J, Herold S (2012) Alveolar epithelial cells orchestrate DC function in murine viral pneumonia. J Clin Invest 122:3652–3664. doi:10.1172/JCI62139

Valkenburg SA, Rutigliano JA, Ellebedy AH, Doherty PC, Thomas PG, Kedzierska K (2011) Immunity to seasonal and pandemic influenza A viruses. Microbes Infect 13:489–501. doi:10.1016/j.micinf.2011.01.007 S1286-4579(11)00037-2 [PII]

van Riel D, Leijten LM, van der Eerden M, Hoogsteden HC, Boven LA, Lambrecht BN, Osterhaus AD, Kuiken T (2011) Highly pathogenic avian influenza virus H5N1 infects alveolar macrophages without virus production or excessive TNF-alpha induction. PLoS Pathog 7:e1002099. doi:10.1371/journal.ppat.1002099 PPATHOGENS-D-10-00224 [PII]

Vareille M, Kieninger E, Edwards MR, Regamey N (2011) The airway epithelium: soldier in the fight against respiratory viruses. Clin Microbiol Rev 24:210–229. doi:10.1128/CMR.00014-10

Verbist KC, Rose DL, Cole CJ, Field MB, Klonowski KD (2012) IL-15 participates in the respiratory innate immune response to influenza virus infection. PLoS ONE 7:e37539. doi:10.1371/journal.pone.0037539

Videira PA, Amado IF, Crespo HJ, Alguero MC, Dall'Olio F, Cabral MG, Trindade H (2008) Surface alpha 2-3- and alpha 2-6-sialylation of human monocytes and derived dendritic cells and its influence on endocytosis. Glycoconj J 25:259–268. doi:10.1007/s10719-007-9092-6

von der Malsburg A, Abutbul-Ionita I, Haller O, Kochs G, Danino D (2011) Stalk domain of the dynamin-like MxA GTPase protein mediates membrane binding and liposome tubulation via the unstructured L4 loop. J Biol Chem 286:37858–37865. doi:10.1074/jbc.M111.249037

Waithman J, Zanker D, Xiao K, Oveissi S, Wylie B, Ng R, Togel L, Chen W (2013) Resident CD8(+) and migratory CD103(+) dendritic cells control CD8 T cell immunity during acute influenza infection. PLoS ONE 8:e66136. doi:10.1371/journal.pone.0066136 PONE-D-13-05069

Wang J, Nikrad MP, Phang T, Gao B, Alford T, Ito Y, Edeen K, Travanty EA, Kosmider B, Hartshorn K, Mason RJ (2011) Innate immune response to influenza A virus in differentiated human alveolar type II cells. Am J Respir Cell Mol Biol 45:582–591. doi:10.1165/rcmb.2010-0108OC

Wang J, Nikrad MP, Travanty EA, Zhou B, Phang T, Gao B, Alford T, Ito Y, Nahreini P, Hartshorn K, Wentworth D, Dinarello CA, Mason RJ (2012) Innate immune response of human alveolar macrophages during influenza A infection. PLoS ONE 7:e29879. doi:10.1371/journal.pone.0029879 PONE-D-11-13862 [PII]

Wang J, Oberley-Deegan R, Wang S, Nikrad M, Funk CJ, Hartshorn KL, Mason RJ (2009) Differentiated human alveolar type II cells secrete antiviral IL-29 (IFN-lambda 1) in response to influenza A infection. J Immunol 182:1296–1304. doi:10.4049/jimmunol.182.3.1296

Wang SF, Huang JC, Lee YM, Liu SJ, Chan YJ, Chau YP, Chong P, Chen YM (2008) DC-SIGN mediates avian H5N1 influenza virus infection in cis and in trans. Biochem Biophys Res Commun 373:561–566. doi:10.1016/j.bbrc.2008.06.078

Wang X, Hinson ER, Cresswell P (2007) The interferon-inducible protein viperin inhibits influenza virus release by perturbing lipid rafts. Cell Host Microbe 2:96–105. doi:10.1016/j.chom.2007.06.009 S1931-3128(07)00135-7 [PII]

Watanabe Y, Hashimoto Y, Shiratsuchi A, Takizawa T, Nakanishi Y (2005) Augmentation of fatality of influenza in mice by inhibition of phagocytosis. Biochem Biophys Res Commun 337:881–886. doi:10.1016/j.bbrc.2005.09.133 S0006-291X(05)02132-7 (PII)

Welliver TP, Garofalo RP, Hosakote Y, Hintz KH, Avendano L, Sanchez K, Velozo L, Jafri H, Chavez-Bueno S, Ogra PL, McKinney L, Reed JL, Welliver RC Sr (2007) Severe human lower respiratory tract illness caused by respiratory syncytial virus and influenza virus is characterized by the absence of pulmonary cytotoxic lymphocyte responses. J Infect Dis 195:1126–1136. doi:10.1086/512615

White MR, Tecle T, Crouch EC, Hartshorn KL (2007) Impact of neutrophils on antiviral activity of human bronchoalveolar lavage fluid. Am J Physiol Lung Cell Mol Physiol 293:L1293–L1299. doi:10.1152/ajplung.00266.2007

Wilson IA, Cox NJ (1990) Structural basis of immune recognition of influenza virus hemagglutinin. Ann Rev Immunol 8:737–771. doi:10.1146/annurev.iy.08.040190.003513

Wisskirchen C, Ludersdorfer TH, Muller DA, Moritz E, Pavlovic J (2011) The cellular RNA helicase UAP56 is required for prevention of double-stranded RNA formation during influenza A virus infection. J Virol 85:8646–8655. doi:10.1128/JVI.02559-10

Wong JP, Christopher ME, Viswanathan S, Karpoff N, Dai X, Das D, Sun LQ, Wang M, Salazar AM (2009) Activation of toll-like receptor signaling pathway for protection against influenza virus infection. Vaccine 27:3481–3483. doi:10.1016/j.vaccine.2009.01.048 S0264-410X(09) 00126-1 [PII]

Woods CW, McClain MT, Chen M, Zaas AK, Nicholson BP, Varkey J, Veldman T, Kingsmore SF, Huang Y, Lambkin-Williams R, Gilbert AG, Hero AO 3rd, Ramsburg E, Glickman S, Lucas JE, Carin L, Ginsburg GS (2013) A host transcriptional signature for presymptomatic detection of infection in humans exposed to influenza H1N1 or H3N2. PLoS ONE 8:e52198. doi:10.1371/journal.pone.0052198

Wright PF, Neumann G, Kawaoka Y (2013) Orthomyxoviruses. In: Knipe DM, Howley PM (eds) Fields virology, 6th edn. Wolters Kluwer Health: Lippincott Willams and Wilkins, Philadelphia, PA pp 1691–1740

Yan N, Chen ZJ (2012) Intrinsic antiviral immunity. Nat Immunol 13:214–222. doi:10.1038/ni. 2229

Yu CI, Becker C, Wang Y, Marches F, Helft J, Leboeuf M, Anguiano E, Pourpe S, Goller K, Pascual V, Banchereau J, Merad M, Palucka K (2013) Human CD1c+ dendritic cells drive the differentiation of CD103+ CD8+ mucosal effector T cells via the cytokine TGF-beta. Immunity 38:818–830. doi:10.1016/j.immuni.2013.03.004 S1074-7613(13)00139-8 [PII]

Yu HB, Finlay BB (2008) The caspase-1 inflammasome: a pilot of innate immune responses. Cell Host Microbe 4:198–208. doi:10.1016/j.chom.2008.08.007

Yu WC, Chan RW, Wang J, Travanty EA, Nicholls JM, Peiris JS, Mason RJ, Chan MC (2011) Viral replication and innate host responses in primary human alveolar epithelial cells and alveolar macrophages infected with influenza H5N1 and H1N1 viruses. J Virol 85:6844–6855. doi:10.1128/JVI.02200-10

Zaslavsky E, Nudelman G, Marquez S, Hershberg U, Hartmann BM, Thakar J, Sealfon SC, Kleinstein SH (2013) Reconstruction of regulatory networks through temporal enrichment profiling and its application to H1N1 influenza viral infection. BMC Bioinformatics 14(Suppl 6):S1. doi:10.1186/1471-2105-14-S6-S1

Zeng H, Goldsmith C, Thawatsupha P, Chittaganpitch M, Waicharoen S, Zaki S, Tumpey TM, Katz JM (2007) Highly pathogenic avian influenza H5N1 viruses elicit an attenuated type i interferon response in polarized human bronchial epithelial cells. J Virol 81:12439–12449. doi:10.1128/JVI.01134-07

Zhou J, Law HK, Cheung CY, Ng IH, Peiris JS, Lau YL (2006) Differential expression of chemokines and their receptors in adult and neonatal macrophages infected with human or avian influenza viruses. J Infect Dis 194:61–70. doi:10.1086/504690 JID36098 [PII]

Ziegler-Heitbrock L, Ancuta P, Crowe S, Dalod M, Grau V, Hart DN, Leenen PJ, Liu YJ, MacPherson G, Randolph GJ, Scherberich J, Schmitz J, Shortman K, Sozzani S, Strobl H, Zembala M, Austyn JM, Lutz MB (2010) Nomenclature of monocytes and dendritic cells in blood. Blood 116:e74–e80. doi:10.1182/blood-2010-02-258558

Zimmermann P, Manz B, Haller O, Schwemmle M, Kochs G (2011) The viral nucleoprotein determines Mx sensitivity of influenza A viruses. J Virol 85:8133–8140. doi:10.1128/JVI. 00712-11

Wilson IA, Cox NJ (1990) Structural basis of immune recognition of influenza virus hemagglutinin. Annu Rev Immunol 8:737–771. doi:10.1146/annurev.iy.08.040190.003513
Wisskirchen C, Ludersdorfer TH, Muller DA, Moritz E, Pavlovic J (2011) The cellular RNA helicase UAP56 is required for prevention of double-stranded RNA formation during influenza A virus infection. J Virol 85:8646–8655. doi:10.1128/JVI.02559-10
Wong JP, Christopher ME, Viswanathan S, Karpoff N, Dai X, Das D, Sun LQ, Wang M, Salazar AM (2009) Activation of toll-like receptor signaling pathway for protection against influenza virus infection. Vaccine 27:3481–3483. doi:10.1016/j.vaccine.2009.01.048. S0264-410X(09)00125-1 [pii]
Woods CW, McClain MT, Chen M, Zaas AK, Nicholson BP, Varkey J, Veldman T, Kingsmore SF, Huang Y, Lambkin-Williams R, Gilbert AG, Hero AO 3rd, Ramsburg E, Glickman S, Lucas JE, Carin L, Ginsburg GS (2013) A host transcriptional signature for presymptomatic detection of infection in humans exposed to influenza H1N1 or H3N2. PLoS ONE 8:e52198. doi:10.1371/journal.pone.0052198
Wright PF, Neumann G, Kawaoka Y [illegible]

The NS1 Protein: A Multitasking Virulence Factor

Juan Aylon and Adolfo García-Sastre

Abstract The non-structural protein 1 of influenza virus (NS1) is a relatively small polypeptide with an outstanding number of ascribed functions. NS1 is the main viral antagonist of the innate immune response during influenza virus infection, chiefly by inhibiting the type I interferon system at multiple steps. As such, its role is critical to overcome the first barrier the host presents to halt the viral infection. However, the pro-viral activities of this well-studied protein go far beyond and include regulation of viral RNA and protein synthesis, and disruption of the host cell homeostasis by dramatically affecting general gene expression while tweaking the PI3K signaling network. Because of all of this, NS1 is a key virulence factor that impacts influenza pathogenesis, and adaptation to new hosts, making it an attractive target for control strategies. Here, we will overview the many roles that have been ascribed to the NS1 protein, and give insights into the sequence features and structural properties that make them possible, highlighting the need to understand how NS1 can actually perform all of these functions during viral infection.

Contents

J. Ayllon
Department of Microbiology, Global Health and Emerging Pathogens Institute, Icahn School of Medicine at Mount Sinai, New York, NY 10029, USA

A. García-Sastre (✉)
Department of Microbiology, Department of Medicine,
Division of Infectious Diseases; and Global Health and Emerging Pathogens Institute,
Icahn School of Medicine at Mount Sinai, New York, NY 10029, USA
e-mail: Adolfo.garcia-sastre@mssm.edu

Current Topics in Microbiology and Immunology (2015) 386: 73–107
DOI: 10.1007/82_2014_400

Published Online: 10 July 2014

1 The Road to Understanding NS1 Functions: The Non-Structural Protein that became Lindenmann's Reverse Interferon

When the influenza virus genome was originally mapped (Palese 1977; Shaw and Palese 2013), it became a challenge to assign a role for the non-structural proteins found in infected cells, but apparently not present in the virion. Among them was the non-structural protein 1 (NS1) (Lazarowitz et al. 1971), a highly expressed protein originated from the collinear mRNA transcribed from segment 8 in the influenza virus genome. The same segment also encoded another non-structural protein, NS2, generated by alternative splicing of segment 8 mRNAs and that was renamed NEP (nuclear export protein) after its functions became clearer and the protein was also found in virions (O'Neill et al. 1998). Some initial studies with temperature sensitive mutants (Koennecke et al. 1981; Shimizu et al. 1982) showed that segment 8 was required for the efficient replication of the virus, and hinted that NS1 might be playing a role in the regulation of viral gene expression, yet it was unclear how could be so given that NS1 was not necessary for in vitro replication of the viral segments, that only required the polymerase subunits and the nucleoprotein (Huang et al. 1990) (Fig. 1).

Among the first features that could be ascribed to NS1 was its ability to bind different species of RNA (vRNA, dsRNA, polyA tails and snRNA) (Hatada et al. 1992; Hatada and Fukuda 1992; Qiu and Krug 1994; Qiu et al. 1995) and, related to this, the NS1 was found to be a regulator of host gene expression by blocking splicing of pre-mRNA and export of polyadenylated mRNAs out of the nucleus (Alonso-Caplen and Krug 1991; Alonso-Caplen et al. 1992; Fortes et al. 1994;

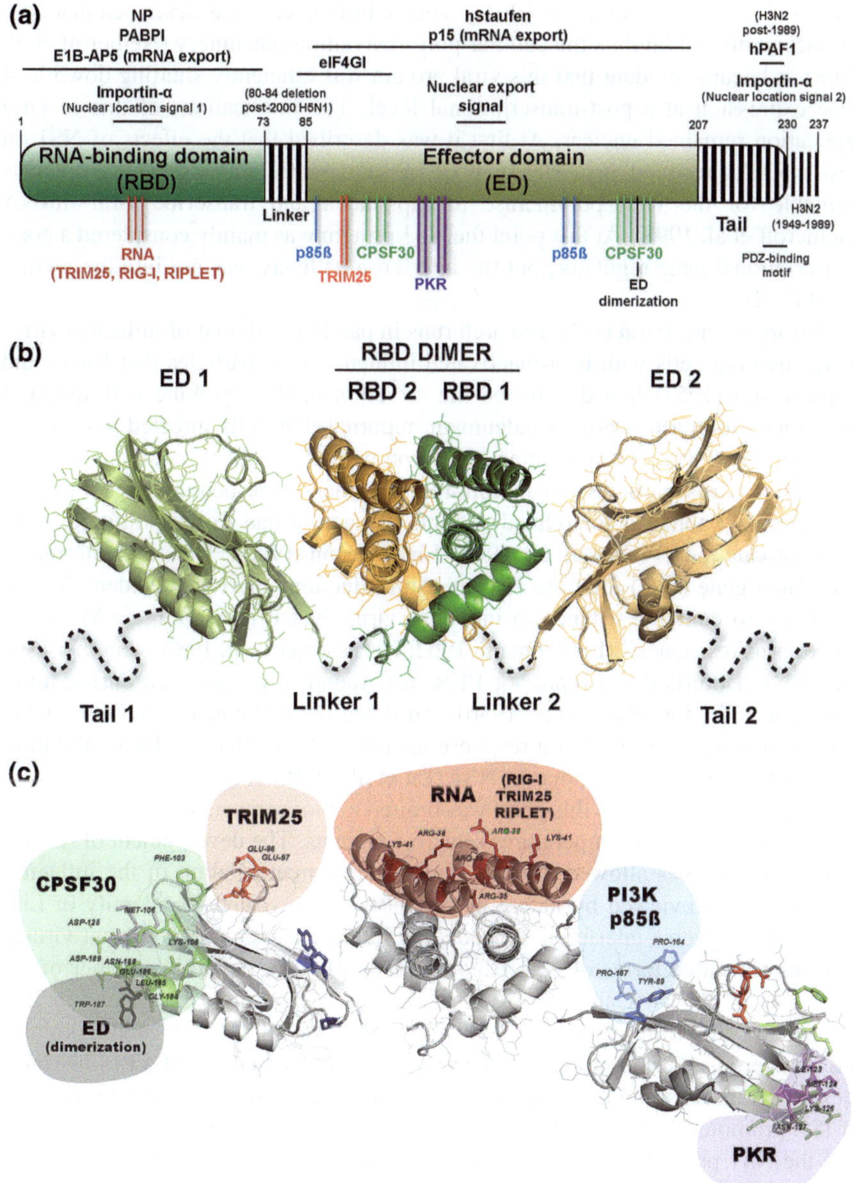

Fig. 1 **a–c** Features, interactors, and structure of the influenza A virus NS1 protein. **a** Schematic representation of the primary structure of an NS1 monomer, highlighting its most representative features and the regions known to be required for its multiple interactions. **b** The NS1 dimer, adapted from the X-ray structure described for the H5N1 A/Vietnam/1203/2004 NS1 (Bornholdt and Prasad 2008; PDB ID: 3F5T). The RNA-binding domains (RBD) are shown interacting, while the effector domains (ED) are in a monomeric state. Both the linker and the disordered tail regions of the protein, not present on the original structure, are hinted as a dashed line. **c** Residues and regions involved in the best characterized interactions of NS1. The color code is the same as in (**a**) for comparison purposes

Qian et al. 1994; Qiu and Krug 1994). When a little later it was described that NS1 interacts with and inhibits the cellular polyadenylation machinery (Nemeroff et al. 1998), it became evident that this viral protein was efficiently shutting down host gene expression at a post-transcriptional level. The implications of this in viral replication remained unclear. At first it was described that the effects of NS1 on host mRNAs resulted in a steady pool of sequestered mRNAs in the nucleus available for the viral polymerase to cap-snatch and transcribe viral mRNA (Nemeroff et al. 1998). At this point the NS1 protein was mainly considered a post-transcriptional gene regulator, but the interferon pathway was not into the picture yet (Fig. 2).

History of interferon (IFN) research runs in parallel with that of influenza virus. It was treating cells with heat-inactivated influenza viral particles that Isaacs and Lindenmann (1957) first discovered the secretion of this cytokine with antiviral properties. Soon afterwards, Lindenmann reported that cells infected with a live influenza virus were not producing interferon upon subsequent treatment with the inactivated virus particles, an inhibitory phenomenon he denominated "inverse interference": some factor related to viral replication had to be inhibiting interferon production (Weber et al. 2004; Lindenmann 1960). The first interferon-stimulated gene (ISG) found to prevent viral infections in vivo was identified for its ability to confer resistance to influenza virus, hence its naming as Mx, from "mixovirus resistance" (Lindenmann 1962; Horisberger et al. 1983). Another ISG, the antiviral translational repressor PKR, was found to be inhibited during influenza virus infection (Katze et al. 1986), and it was the first connection between the NS1 protein and the interferon response as it was shown that the PKR inhibitory effect was, at least in part, due to NS1 (Lu et al. 1995) (Fig. 3).

Research on NS1 up to this point was limited to biochemical assays, transfection studies, and the use of temperatures sensitive mutants. The development of reverse genetics techniques allowed directed and selective manipulation of the influenza virus genome (reviewed by Palese et al. 1996), and revealed the identity of Lindenmann's "inverse interferon" encoded by influenza virus. Recombinant viruses carrying truncated forms of NS1 (Egorov et al. 1998) or devoid altogether of the NS1 gene (delNS1) (García-Sastre et al. 1998) were severely attenuated in IFN competent cells while still growing efficiently in Vero cells, which cannot produce a/ß interferons. Furthermore, the delNS1 virus was lethal in STAT1−/− mice lacking a transcription factor required for IFN action, and induced higher activation of ISG promoter than its wild type counterpart. For the first time it was postulated that the NS1 protein was a virally encoded antagonist of the interferon response, and thus became the first of such inhibitors to be described for a negative-stranded RNA virus. While interferon-inhibitor accessory proteins had by then been described for other viruses (Weber et al. 2004), the limited genome size and small number of proteins encoded by influenza viruses had made it difficult to believe that one of them could be nonessential and mostly devoted to oppose the host innate immune response, as the delNS1 virus demonstrated. The exploration of the mechanisms by which NS1 exerts its inhibitory effect advanced in parallel with the increasing knowledge on the innate immune response pathways: the discovery

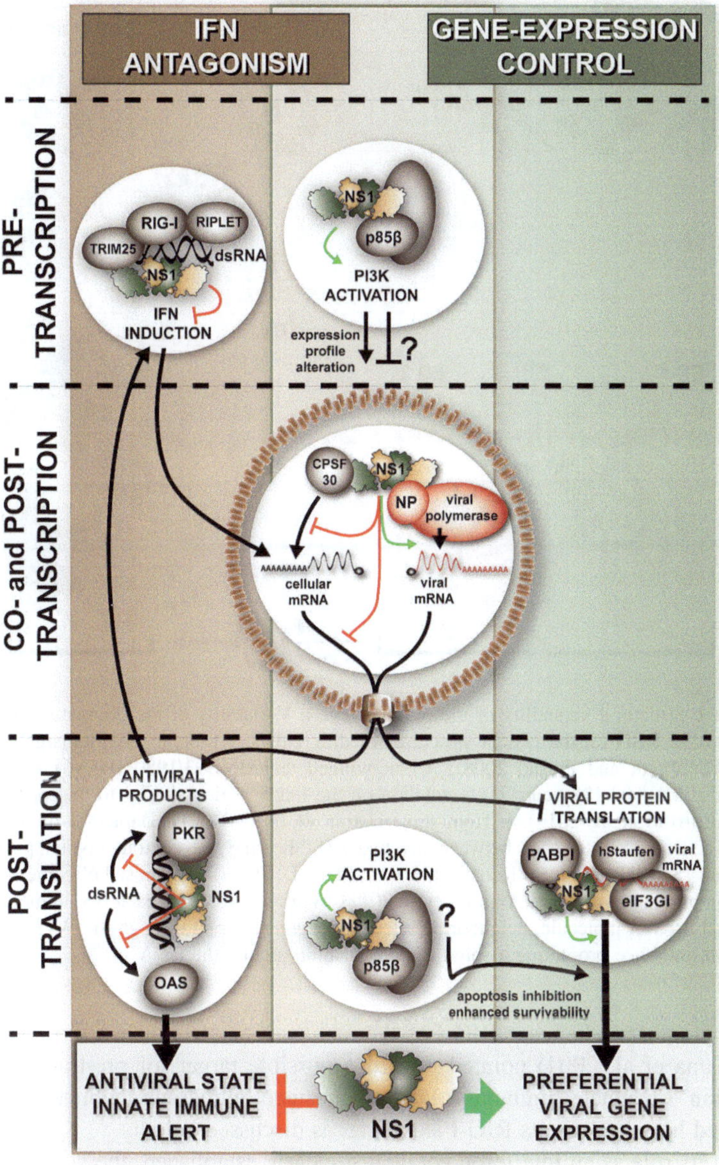

Fig. 2 Overview of the functions of the influenza A virus NS1 protein in the cytoplasm and nucleus of infected cells. NS1 is the main IFN antagonist of influenza virus, and also plays a critical role in the viral takeover of the cellular gene expression machinery. NS1 inhibits the IFN pathway at a pre-transcriptional level by blocking the activation of the RIG-I sensing and signaling platform, and at a post-translational level by repressing the activation of the anti-viral genes PKR and OAS. In the nucleus, NS1 inhibits the correct processing and export of mRNA, thus hindering all cellular gene expression including that of IFN-related genes. At the same time, NS1 enhances the production of viral mRNA, and in turn the specific translation of the latter by interacting with several translation-related factors. As a result of all these functions, NS1 renders the cell unable to properly respond to the viral infection or to alert neighboring cells of the danger. The reported activation of PI3K by NS1 may change the expression profile of the cell, inhibiting premature apoptosis or inducing other unknown changes on the cellular environment

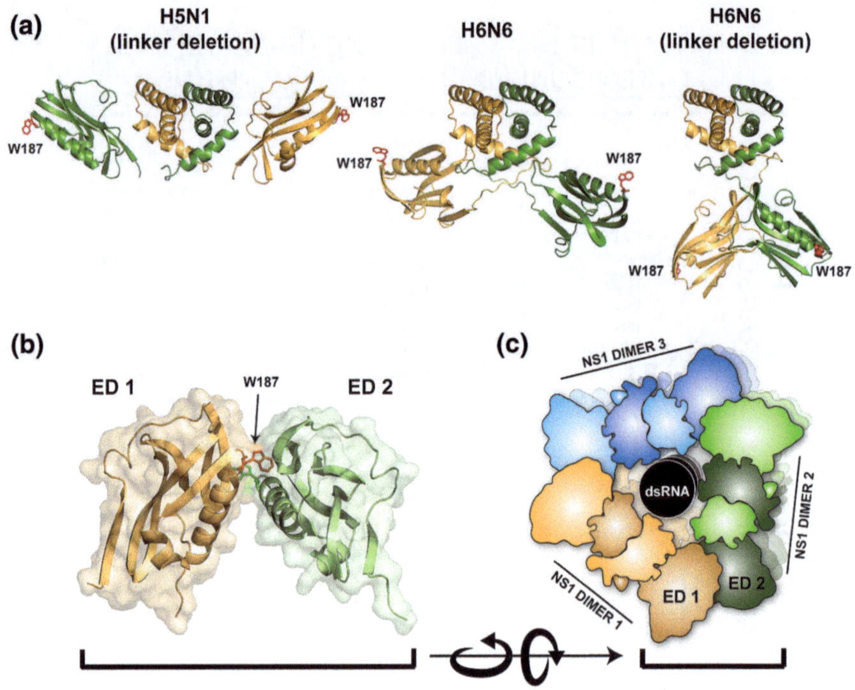

Fig. 3 **a–c** Structural versatility of the NS1 protein. **a** Variability of the orientation of the ED respect to the RBD on the crystal structures of different NS1 proteins: A/Vietnam/1203/2004 (H5N1)(Bornholdt and Prasad 2008), A/blue-winged teal/MN/993/1980 (H6N6) and A/blue-winged teal/MN/993/1980 carrying a deletion on the linker region similar to that of the H5N1 protein (Carrillo et al. 2014). **b** Homodimerization of the NS1 ED. Depiction of one of the variable helix-helix interfaces between the two ED, showing the central, pivotal position of tryptophan 187 (Adapted from Kerry et al. 2011; PDB ID: 3O9S). **c** Proposed oligomerization of NS1 upon binding to dsRNA (Aramini et al. 2011). While the RBD on each NS1 dimer binds to the central dsRNA molecule, neighboring effector domains interact through the W187-mediated helix-helix interface promoting a spiral oligomerization around the RNA

of the cytoplasmic helicase RIG-I as the main sensor of influenza virus infection (Yoneyama et al. 2004) pointed toward a possible target for pre-transcriptional repression of innate immunity, and ever since numerous publications have addressed how NS1 limits RIG-I signaling, as discussed below.

With its role as an interferon antagonist clearly established, the actual strategy used by NS1 remained unclear. Some experimental setups pointed toward a prevalence of the originally described general gene expression shut off (Nemeroff et al. 1998) as the main mechanism to prevent antiviral inducible gene expression, while others highlighted the pre-transcriptional inhibition of the RIG-I/IRF3 axis (Pichlmair et al. 2006; Mibayashi et al. 2007). This apparent dichotomy was resolved thanks to growing evidence of a strain-dependent behavior of the NS1 protein (Kochs et al. 2007). Indeed, the subtleties of NS1 performance were soon revealed as complex as the ever-growing array of functions it has been related to; including a very well structurally-characterized—but functionally obscure-activation of the PI3K signaling pathway (Hale et al. 2006), a critical regulator of cell fate. In the following paragraphs, we will summarize the broad scope of the NS1 functions, their regulation and the—still not completely understood—effects they have in influenza virus pathogenesis.

2 Sequence and Structure of NS1

The NS1 protein is encoded in the smallest of the genomic segments of influenza virus, denominated NS, and numbered as segment 8 in influenza A and B and segment 7 in influenza C viruses (Shaw and Palese 2013). Collinear transcription of the segment generates the NS1 mRNA, whereas its splicing leads to the generation of the NEP mRNA (Inglis et al. 1979; Lamb and Choppin 1979). As a result, NS1 and NEP share their first 10 aminoacids and bases 503–690 on the NS1 coding sequence overlap with bases 31–221 on NEP, though on a shifted reading frame (Lamb and Lai 1980). This partial sharing of genetic information makes difficult to mutate selectively certain residues of NS1 without affecting NEP. This remains both a caveat and a challenge when generating recombinant viruses with modified NS segments, though careful engineering can be used to circumvent the overlap by separating NS1 and NEP ORFs (Manicassamy et al. 2010; Varble et al. 2010; Marazzi et al. 2012). An alternative splicing product that would generate a third protein from the NS segment (NS3) has been described for certain isolates of influenza A virus. Though its function and relevance remain unclear, NS3 could be providing an adaptive advantage when jumping to a new host species (Selman et al. 2012).

NS1 mRNA translates into a ~26 kDa polypeptide whose length may vary slightly among different strains: for influenza A viruses (IAV) it ranges between 215–237 aminoacids (Hale et al. 2008c). Comparison of a large number of isolates from different strains revealed two subsets of NS1 proteins based on sequence homology that were named alleles A and B (Scholtissek and von Hoyningen-Huene 1980; Treanor et al. 1989; Ludwig et al. 1991). Among the same allele 90–100 % of the residues are conserved, while between alleles conservation can be as low as 60 %. All of NS1 proteins from human, swine, equine, and other mammal virus isolates belong to allele A. Allele A NS1s are also found in many avian strains, including those found to sporadically infect humans. Allele B comprises only avian-origin NS1, and reassortant human viruses with an allele B NS segment are attenuated in monkeys (Treanor et al. 1989), suggesting that allele A NS1, which underwent stronger evolutive pressures according to phylogenetic studies (Ludwig et al. 1991), provides specific advantages for infecting diverse host species.

The NS1 polypeptide comprises two functionally distinct globular domains: an N-terminal RNA binding domain (RBD) (amino acids 1–73), and a C-terminal effector domain (ED) (85-end), separated by a short linker region. Crystallographic data is available on both the individually expressed RBD and ED of several strains (Chien et al. 1997; Liu et al. 1997; Bornholdt and Prasad 2006; Hale et al. 2008a; Cheng et al. 2009; Kerry et al. 2011), as well as on the full length NS1 proteins of H5N1 and H6N6 avian viruses (Bornholdt and Prasad 2008; Carrillo et al. 2014). The RBD domain is formed by 3 α-helices and homodimerizes to constitute a six-helix antiparallel bundle, which sets up the tracks upon which dsRNA can sit (Liu et al. 1997; Cheng et al. 2009). Dimerization is absolutely required for RNA binding, and so is the conserved arginine in position 38, with some other charged residues being also important for stabilizing the interaction through hydrogen bonds and electrostatic contacts (R35, R37 and K41, among others) (Wang et al. 1999). Alanine substitutions of R38 and K41 have been extensively used as abrogators of the RNA-binding function of NS1 in different studies.

The C-terminal effector domain, formed by seven ß-strands and three α-helices, can also homodimerize independently (Bornholdt and Prasad 2006; Hale et al. 2008a). Interaction between the EDs takes place through the highly conserved tryptophan residues at position 187, which reciprocally embed into hydrophobic pockets resulting in a variable helix-helix interface. Biophysical data and in silico analysis suggest that the RBD association is highly stable and has the properties of an obligate dimer, whereas contacts between the monomers in the ED dimer are likely to be transient (Kerry et al. 2011; Aramini et al. 2011). The short linker region between the RBD and the ED is thought to be flexible allowing different conformations of the NS1 homodimer quaternary structure, in which the strong RBD dimer remains fixed and the effector domains change their relative position cycling between mono and dimeric statages. It is not clear whether dimerization of the ED takes place within the same NS1 RBD dimer, with neighbouring NS1 RBD dimers to generate oligomers, or both. In any case, the length of the linker and the exact amino acid composition of its sequence, as well as nearby residues, are probably important steric determinants of the tridimensional disposition that NS1 can adopt, and may influence in a strain specific manner the interactions of this viral protein with its cellular partners (Hale et al. 2010a; Kerry et al. 2011; Carrillo et al. 2014). While most of the NS1 proteins have an 11 amino acid long linker, highly pathogenic H5N1 strains isolated after 2000 carry a deletion of 5 amino acids in that region (residues 80–84), a genotype that is persistently found ever since and has replaced the full-length linker consensus, hinting toward a selective advantage for H5N1 influenza viruses that has not yet been identified (Dundon and Capua 2009).

The structure of the last residues of the C-terminal end of NS1 is not apparent in the NS1 crystals and they are thought to form a disordered and flexible "tail". Interestingly, this is one of the most variable regions among different NS1 proteins and the main reason for the diversity in their lengths, with successive truncations and elongations showing up through viral evolution (Suarez and Perdue 1998). As a noteworthy example, the NS1 of human-circulating viruses acquired seven additional residues in their C-terminus during the late 1940s due to a single point mutation, extending its length from 230 to 237 amino acids. For the following 40 years, the NS1 proteins of all human isolates were 237 residues long, including those of the 1957 and 1968 pandemic strains, with few and punctual exceptions (Hale et al. 2008c). Then, by the late 1980s a reversion of the original mutation brought the NS1 length back to 230 amino acid residues. Interestingly, shortening of the NS1 sequence happened in parallel and about the same time in H1N1 and H3N2 strains. There is no evidence of any clear evolutionary advantage associated with this convergence, and the only biological implication found with this change is that it could have allowed H3N2 strains to gain a novel function by unmasking a histone H3-like sequence, as discussed below (Marazzi et al. 2012).

3 The Great Antagonist: NS1 and the Innate Immune Response

Innate immunity is one of the first barriers a virus faces when infecting a host. Mammalian cells have evolved sophisticated antiviral mechanisms based on sensing intruding pathogen products and triggering of signaling cascades leading to the production of type I (IFNa and IFNß) and type III (IFNλ) interferons. Interferons are cytokines that act in an autocrine and paracrine manner to alert neighboring cells of the presence of the intruder, promoting changes in their expression profiles and leading ultimately to the establishment of an effective anti-viral state through the production of a myriad of interferon-stimulated genes (ISG) (García-Sastre 2011; Schneider et al. 2014). Furthermore, the interferon system not only limits the original spread of the pathogen, but is also linked to the activation of the slower, yet more specific, adaptive immune response (Schmolke and García-Sastre 2010; Iwasaki and Medzhitov 2010). Given such a formidable defense mechanism, it is not surprising that pathogens have developed a number of different strategies to overcome, limit, or hide from the interferon system and establish a successful infection.

The NS1 protein's main contribution to influenza virus pathogenesis is the inhibition of the host's innate immune response through repression of the type I/III interferon system. The virus encodes several other factors that have been described to limit to a certain degree this response, either directly by interacting with components of the interferon pathway (the case of the accessory PB1-F2 protein or the PB2 subunit of the viral polymerase) (Varga et al. 2011; Graef et al. 2010; Iwai et al. 2010), or indirectly by allowing the virus to outrun the interferon effects (the case of highly efficient polymerase complexes found in some virus strains) (Grimm et al. 2007). However, NS1 is the main viral interferon antagonist due to the large impact it has in this pathway, which can be inhibited by NS1 at multiple levels. Not all virus strains rely equally in all of the anti-interferon functions of NS1, nor are all these functions conserved among different strains, and yet the striking degree of redundancy in inhibiting the IFN system is a good proof of how relevant for the virus is to block the host's response. In the following paragraphs we will address the different stages of the anti-viral response at which NS1 exerts its antagonism.

3.1 Pre-Transcriptional Inhibition: NS1 and the RIG-I Signaling Axis

The interferon signaling cascade is triggered by the recognition of molecules bearing pathogen-associated molecular patterns (PAMPs): a series of alien or uncommon biological fingerprints that the cell can distinguish as "non-self," and thus, alert of the presence of an invading agent. This recognition is carried out by specialized molecular sensors known as pattern recognition receptors (PRRs) that can be classified into different families according to their subcellular location, the PAMPs they recognize and the origin of those PAMPs (Takeuchi and Akira 2009). The cytosolic RNA helicase RIG-I (retinoic acid-inducible gene I) is the PRR that accounts for detection of influenza virus in epithelial cells, the main targets for influenza virus infection in vivo. The PAMPs that RIG I detects upon infection are dsRNA structures with 5′-triphophates, which are specific for viral RNAs and not found in cytoplasmic cellular RNAs (Yoneyama et al. 2004; Pichlmair et al. 2006). Binding of RIG-I to its PAMP triggers an ATP-dependent conformational change on RIG-I, exposing two N-terminal caspase recruiting domains (CARD) (Myong et al. 2009). Upon this structural change different residues in RIG-I are ubiquitinated by the E3 ligases TRIM25 (Gack et al. 2007) and RIPLET (Oshiumi et al. 2009), and/or bound to free ubiquitin chains also produced by TRIM25 (Zeng et al. 2010), resulting in RIG-I oligomerization. The modified RIG-I CARDs can then bind to the CARD domains of the mitochondrial adaptor MAVS (mitochondrial antiviral signaling), which in turn leads to MAVS oligomerization and to the scaffolding of a multi-kinase signaling platform that ultimately leads to the phosphorylation and nuclear translocation of the transcription factors IRF3, AP-1(c-Jun/ATF-2) and NFκB. Once in the nucleus, these activated factors are the essential components of the enhanceosome that drives transcription of the IFN gene (McWhirter et al. 2005).

The NS1 protein of influenza A viruses has been reported to block the activation of IRF3 (Talon et al. 2000a), NFκB (Wang et al. 2000) and AP-1 (Ludwig et al. 2002), repressing pre-transcriptionally the expression of interferons. This inhibitory action takes place at the very origin of the RIG-I signaling pathway. NS1 forms a complex with RIG-I, detectable by co-immunoprecipitation (Pichlmair et al. 2006; Guo et al. 2007; Opitz et al. 2007; Mibayashi et al. 2007), but there is no clear evidence on whether this complex involves direct inhibitory contacts between the two protein or it is mediated through other interactions. Indeed, NS1 has been reported to also associate with two positive regulators of RIG-I: the ubiquitin ligases TRIM25 (Gack et al. 2009) and RIPLET (Rajsbaum et al. 2012). By binding the coiled coil domain of TRIM25 NS1 can block its oligomerization and subsequent E3 ligase activity on the CARD domains of RIG-I. Mutant NS1 proteins carrying E96A/E97A substitutions in a putative protein-protein interaction motif in the ED are unable to bind TRIM25 and cause viral attenuation and higher IFN induction (Gack et al. 2009). NS1 can also interact with RIPLET and prevent it from activating RIG-I, although E96/E97 residues are not involved in that inhibition (Rajsbaum et al. 2012). It is controversial whether RIPLET and TRIM25 can both ubiquitinate the same residues in the C-terminal CARD domains of RIG-I. Instead, RIPLET seems to be specifically driving a distinct modification of the N-terminus of the sensor, allowing its initial conformational change and the subsequent activation by TRIM25 (Oshiumi et al. 2013). According to this model, NS1 could be blocking independently two required regulatory steps on the activation of RIG-I. This apparent redundancy can be explained by the fact that interaction of NS1 with TRIM25, RIPLET or both is both viral strain- and host species-specific (Rajsbaum et al. 2012). As an example, human IAV NS1 proteins can bind both human RIPLET and TRIM25, whereas they are unable to bind murine TRIM25 and as such rely mostly on their inhibition through RIPLET to inhibit RIG-I in mice. The ability of different NS1 to interact with host-specific components of the RIG-I pathway may help in surpassing the interspecies barrier, and as such it could be a factor influencing this critical aspect of IAV epidemiology.

Additionally, the dsRNA binding ability of NS1 could also be playing a role in the pre-transcriptional inhibition of the interferon pathway by sequestering away the PAMPs that RIG-I recognizes. A fact weighting against this possibility is the very low affinity of the RBD of NS1 for dsRNA (Chien et al. 2004), that makes it unlikely to outcompete more efficient binders such as RIG-I. On the other hand, mutation of amino-acids R38 and K41, both pivotal for dsRNA binding (Wang et al. 1999), greatly impairs the ability to block interferon production (Pichlmair et al. 2006). Remarkably, R38/K41 substitutions also abrogate the aforementioned interactions of NS1 with RIG-I, TRIM25 and RIPLET (Pichlmair et al. 2006; Gack et al. 2009; Rajsbaum et al. 2012). Although it is not ruled out that those two amino acids could be specifically involved in direct protein-protein contact interfaces, it is tempting to propose that the RNA binding properties of NS1 help its localization into multicomponent and dynamic RNA-protein complexes in which the NS1 exerts its inhibition. Indeed, some pieces of data suggest that such complexes are formed during influenza virus infection (Onomoto et al. 2012). The actual role of RNA-binding on IFN antagonism of the RIG-I pathway by NS1 remains to be fully elucidated.

While the interaction of IAV NS1 with the components of the RIG-I signaling axis are conserved among virus isolates, the extent and efficiency of the inhibitory effect varies significantly among different viral strains. Several studies have addressed this issue (Hayman et al. 2006; Kochs et al. 2007; Kuo et al. 2010) and, despite discrepancies related to the different experimental approaches, all conclude that several strains of H1N1, H2N2, and H3N2 human-circulating viruses cannot block efficiently the pre-transcriptional steps of the IFN signaling cascade. The NS1 proteins of these viruses must then rely on a different strategy: crippling host gene expression, including that of IFN and IFN-stimulated genes, at a post-transcriptional level as discussed below.

3.2 Co- and Post-Transcriptional Inhibition: Limiting Host Gene Expression

The NS1 protein of a number of IAV strains can also efficiently suppress the expression of cellular genes by directly interfering with the pre-mRNA processing machinery of the host. In eukaryotic cells, the 3′ ends of primary transcripts are cleaved upon recognition of a conserved AAUAAA sequence some 10–30 bases upstream of the cleavage site. The Cleavage and Polyadenylation Specificity Factor (CPSF) is a polyprotein complex formed by four subunits that recognizes the AAUAAA sequence, binds to the nascent mRNA and catalyzes the endonucleolytic step and the subsequent addition of a poly(A) tail (Wahle and Keller 1996; Colgan and Manley 1997). The smallest of the components of CPSF is a 30 kDa protein (CPSF30) with five C3H zinc fingers (Barabino et al. 1997). The effector domain of NS1 binds to two of the CPSF30 zinc fingers (F2F3), and by doing so inhibits the binding of the whole CPSF complex to pre-mRNA and its consequent cleavage and polyadenylation (Nemeroff et al. 1998; Twu et al. 2006; Das et al. 2008). Additionally, the influenza virus replication machinery (the polymerase subunits PB1, PB2, and PA; as well as the nucleoprotein NP) contributes to stabilizing NS1-CPSF interactions in a strain-specific manner (Twu et al. 2007; Kuo and Krug 2009).

By blocking CPSF, NS1 inhibits cellular mRNA processing and the expression of cellular genes, including those of interferon and ISG that are involved in the anti-viral response. CPSF30 inhibition may also explain at least partially some other functional effects of NS1 expression: the suppression of nucleo-cytoplasmic transport of mRNA (Fortes et al. 1994; Qiu and Krug 1994), since this transport requires polyadenylation, and the inhibition of mRNA splicing (Alonso-Caplen and Krug 1991; Alonso-Caplen et al. 1992; Fortes et al. 1994; Qian et al. 1994), in which CPSF is also involved (Li et al. 2001). Viral transcripts are not affected by the repression of CPSF, however, because their polyadenylation is directly catalyzed by the viral polymerase (Shaw and Palese 2013). Moreover, it's been hypothesized that the sequestered pre-mRNA in the nucleus provides a steady pool of capped 5′ ends for cap snatching by the viral polymerase (Nemeroff et al. 1998).

Relevant residues involved in the NS1-CPSF30 interaction have been characterized by mutagenesis (Li et al. 2001; Noah et al. 2003; Kochs et al. 2007; Twu et al. 2007) and more recently by the X-ray crystal structure of the NS1 ED in complex with the F2F3 region of CPSF30, described for the A/Udorn/73 (H3N2) human seasonal strain (Ud) (Das et al. 2008). A patch of highly conserved hydrophobic residues at NS1 (184-188) embeds into a pocket on the F2F3 CPSF30 domain, with G184 standing in a central position. Substitution of G184 by an arginine effectively abrogates Ud NS1 binding to CPSF30 (Das et al. 2008). Interestingly, this NS1 residue is also required for virulence in mice independently of both the IFN system and CPSF30 interactions (Steidle et al. 2010). Another important NS1 residue that impact CPSF30 binding is W187, which is pivotal in driving the dimerization of the NS1 ED (Hale et al. 2008a; Kerry et al. 2011;

Aramini et al. 2011). In fact, W187 mediated NS1 ED dimerization is incompatible with NS1-CPSF30 binding based on crystal structures (Kerry et al. 2011). This fact, as discussed below, likely plays a role on the spatial-temporal regulation of the NS1 functions. Two additional amino acids are important for stabilizing the NS1-CPSF30 interaction although they are not strictly part of the binding interface: these are a phenylalanine in postion 103 (F103) and a methionine in position 106 (M106) (Kochs et al. 2007; Das et al. 2008).

As with the pre-transcriptional inhibition of the RIG-I signaling, the suppression of general gene expression is a variable feature among different influenza virus strains. The NS1 proteins of H1N1, H2N2, and H3N2 viruses seasonally circulating in humans during the last century share a strong binding capability to CPSF30. On the other hand, the widely used egg- and mouse-adapted PR8 strain lacks this property due to substitutions in the aforementioned amino acids residues at positions 103 and 106 (Kochs et al. 2007). Also, the highly pathogenic H5N1 avian viruses involved in the 1997 human outbreak in Hong Kong carried F103L and M106I substitutions in their NS1s, which then could not bind CPSF30 efficiently (Twu et al. 2007). Interestingly, H5N1 strains eventually acquired F103 and M106 NS1 amino acid residues and most avian (and all human) isolates reported from 1998 onward carry this signature of strong CPSF30 binding. Gain-of-function studies in which the H5N1 strain A/Hong Kong/483/1997 was mutated to carry F103 and M106 NS1 amino acid residues resulted in increased virulence and systemic spread in mice (Spesock et al. 2011). However, a similar approach rendered the opposite results with a different isolate (A/Hong Kong/456/1997) (Dankar et al. 2013).

Another relevant influenza virus whose NS1 is defective in binding to CPSF30 and repressing cellular gene expression is the 2009 pandemic (pH1N1) influenza virus. This strain carries three NS1 amino acid substitutions (K108R, D125E, D189G) that, like F103L and M106I, prevent optimal NS1 binding to CPSF30 (Hale et al. 2010b). In this case, restoring NS1 binding to CPSF30 slightly decreased replication and virulence in mice. As shown by these examples, dissecting the contribution of CPSF30 inhibition to pathogenesis is a difficult task, as it is most probably impacted by synergy versus competition with other NS1 functions depending on the strain,. Indeed, variations in CPSF30 binding seem to arise commonly upon influenza virus adaptation to different hosts (Hossain et al. 2008; Brown et al. 2001). In general, mouse-, egg- and swine-adapted viruses have NS1s that bind weakly to CPSF30, whereas those from human-circulating strains are strong binders (with the exception of the pH1N1 virus, whose NS1 is of swine origin) In the case of avian strains both NS1 phenotypes can be found (Twu et al. 2007; Hale et al. 2010b).

While the inhibition of CPSF30 is presumed to block unspecifically overall gene expression, some NS1 proteins may have evolved to repress expression of specific sets of genes. This is the case of influenza A H3N2 viruses isolated after 1989. As previously mentioned, the NS1 of these viruses reverted back to a length of 230 amino acids from a 237 amino acid length configuration (Hale et al. 2008c). As a result, their C-terminal residues became ARSKV, a very similar motif to the

ARTKQ motif found on histone H3. Consequently, the tail on these NS1 proteins acts as a histone tail mimic, repressing the expression of specific cellular genes through competition with H3 for binding to the PAF1 transcription-elongation complex (Marazzi et al. 2012). PAF1 regulated genes include those involved in the IFN response.

Additionally, the NS1 of the H1N1, A/WSN/33 (WSN) strain has been reported to interact with several components involved in mRNA export (NXF1, p15, Rae1, E1B-AP5) and block their function (Satterly et al. 2007). Although WSN NS1 is able to bind to CPSF30 (Twu et al. 2007), it lacks the D189 amino acid residue involved in optimal interaction (Hale et al. 2010b). Inhibition of cellular mRNA export proteins may give some specificity for inhibition of cellular gene expression to NS1, as different cellular mRNA use different export factors to translocate to the cytoplasm (Satterly et al. 2007).

3.3 Post-Translational Inhibition of Antiviral Genes: PKR and OAS

The anti-interferon antagonism of NS1 goes beyond the pre- and post-transcriptional repression of the interferon genes: NS1 also blocks directly the antiviral effects of some of the interferon-stimulated gene (ISG) products. The best studied of these are the Ser/Thr kinase PKR and the RNAse L-pathway activator OAS (2′-5′-oligo (A) synthetase).

PKR is an RNA-binding protein kinase constitutively expressed in an inactive conformation in mammalian cells that becomes upregulated upon interferon treatment (Hovanessian 1989). Overall, PKR is a sensor activated by dsRNA and other stimuli. Upon activation, it phosphorylates a number of substrates and activates different signal transduction pathways to counteract potential threats. In its best characterized role as an antiviral agent, PKR phosphorylates the alpha subunit of the eIF2 translation initiation factor, effectively repressing all protein synthesis in the cell (García et al. 2006). Proof of the relevance of this inhibition for the host *vs* pathogen arms race is that many different viruses have evolved specific proteins that inhibit PKR (reviewed by García et al. 2006).

Influenza A virus was found to inhibit PKR activity in early studies (Katze et al. 1986, 1988). In fact, influenza virus has been postulated to antagonize PKR during infection via two different mechanisms: (i) by regulating the function of p58IPK, a factor that in turns regulates PKR activity (Melville et al. 1999; Goodman et al. 2007) and (ii) by the action of the NS1 protein. The lack of PKR allows NS1-defective recombinant viruses (delNS1) to replicate efficiently in mice (Bergmann et al. 2000). Several studies suggested that the inhibitory effect caused by NS1 was due to sequestration of dsRNA away from PKR (Hatada et al. 1992; Lu et al. 1995). However, as commented earlier regarding RIG-I inhibition, the affinity of NS1 for dsRNA is much lower than that of PKR, so out-competition in vivo seems unlikely (Li et al. 2006). Furthermore, a recombinant influenza virus carrying RNA binding-defective R38A NS1 effectively represses PKR (Min and Krug 2006), and NS1 also blocks the dsRNA-independent activation of PKR by PACT (PKR-associated activator) (Li et al. 2006). In fact, NS1 binds PKR through an interaction that involves NS1 amino acids 123–127 and the N-terminal region of PKR (Min et al. 2007). Based upon these findings, it has been postulated that NS1 prevents the activating conformational change in PKR subsequent to PKR binding to dsRNA (Li et al. 2006).

Beyond its role in translational repression, PKR has also been involved in the activation of several signaling pathways, including the transcription factor NFκB that is pivotal for IFN gene expression (Williams 2001; Munir and Berg 2013). Indeed, PKR was believed to be of a major cytoplasmic PRR involved in the transcriptional activation of IFN, until the discovery of the RIG-I—like sensors (Pichlmair and Reis e Sousa 2007). However, the relevance of PKR as a sensor involved in antiviral gene expression should not be lightly ruled out.

The 2′-5′-oligo (A) synthetase (OAS) is an IFN-stimulated gene product that catalyzes the formation of 2′-5′-polyA chains from ATP. The main function of these oligomers is to activate the otherwise latent RNAse L, a potent repressor of viral infection due to its degradation of single-stranded RNA. By-products of this degradation might also be recognized by RIG-I like receptors and positively feedback the IFN response (Silverman 2007). Silencing and knock-down of RNAse-L greatly enhances the replication of a recombinant A/Udorn/72 virus encoding the NS1 RNA-binding unpaired mutant R38A (Min and Krug 2006). No direct interaction has been described between NS1 and OAS and/or RNAse L: the proposed mechanism of action for this inhibition is sequestration of dsRNA away from OAS. In this case, contrary to what happens with PKR or RIG-I, the dsRNA binding affinity of OAS is low enough for NS1 to outcompete it in vivo (Min and Krug 2006).

4 Additional Pro-Viral Functions of NS1

4.1 Activation of PI3K and Regulation of the Apoptotic Response

Phosphoinositide-3-kinases (PI3K) are ubiquitously expressed and highly conserved cytoplasmic heterodimeric enzymes (Engelman et al. 2006). Upon activation by a number of different stimuli, they catalyze the formation of PIP3 (phosphatidylinositol (3,4,5) trisphosphate), a membrane-embedded lipidic second messenger. PIP3 acts as docking platform for PH domain-containing proteins involved in signaling,—the best characterized being the Ser/Thr kinase Akt. Cellular responses that involve PI3K signaling include survival, proliferation, trafficking, and regulation of the immune function (Engelman et al. 2006). Because of its relevance as a checkpoint for cellular homeostasis, the PI3K network is very tightly regulated, and abnormalities in its behavior lie behind numerous hereditary and oncogenic pathologies (Kok et al. 2009).

Influenza A virus is known to activate PI3K signaling twice during infection, as detected by the phosphorylation state of its downstream effector Akt (Ehrhardt and Ludwig 2009; Ayllon et al. 2012a): a first, early, and transient PI3K activation peak takes place during viral attachment and entry, probably related to the required uptake by endocytosis (Ehrhardt et al. 2006), whereas a second, sustained activation appears 2–3 h post-infection and is due to NS1, which can directly bind to the PI3K complex (Hale et al. 2006; Shin et al. 2007b; Zhirnov and Klenk 2007). The structural and mechanistic basis for this activation has been well studied: the heterodimeric PI3K is kept at its basal state due to inhibitory contacts exerted by the regulatory subunit (termed p85) over the catalytic one (termed p110). This inhibition is mediated by two SH2 domains on p85. NS1 binds to p85 and displaces the N-terminal SH2 domain from its position on the heterodimer, thus releasing the inhibition over p110 (Hale et al. 2008b, 2010a). Several relevant sequential features and amino acids in NS1 involved in p85 binding have been mapped (Hale et al. 2006, 2010a; Shin et al. 2007a), including a highly conserved tyrosine in position 89 that settles in the center of the NS1-p85 interphase (Hale et al. 2006, 2010a). Conservative substitution of tyrosine 89 for phenylalanine (Y89F) abrogates p85 binding and PI3K/Akt activation.

Despite the knowledge on the activation mechanism of PI3K by NS1, its biological relevance remains obscure. By using the Y89F substitution in the PR8 backbone, it has been shown that PI3K activation improves viral replication in tissue culture and virulence in the mouse model (Ayllon et al. 2012b; Hrincius et al. 2012); although in a strain-dependent manner as it does not impact fitness of another H1N1 strain, A/WSN/33 (Ayllon et al. 2012b). Given the well-characterized role of PI3K signaling as anti-apoptotic, it was first suggested that by activating it NS1 would stimulate cell survival beneficially for the virus (Zhirnov et al. 2002; Ehrhardt et al. 2007; Zhirnov and Klenk 2007; Shin et al. 2007a). Although initial studies had pointed out that NS1 could actually be promoting apoptosis instead (Schultz-Cherry et al. 2001), it is possible that increased apoptosis is an indirect consequence of the many cellular-disturbing functions of the protein such as CPSF30 inhibition. Indeed, the use of a delNS1 virus showed clearly the anti-apoptotic role of NS1 (Zhirnov and Klenk 2007), although remains controversial whether this feature is a result of lack of PI3K/Akt activation: Y89F and other p85 binding-defective mutants are still anti-apoptotic, at least in the Ud backbone (Jackson et al. 2010). Activation of PI3K by NS1 has been shown to regulate cationic currents in the airway epithelium, the primary target of influenza virus infection, and thereby this influences liquid accumulation and pathogenicity (Gallacher et al. 2009).

A most noteworthy aspect of NS1 activation of PI3K it is its isotype specificity. Class IA PI3K comprises three different catalytic p110 isotypes (p110a, p110ß, and p110δ) and two main p85 ones: p85α and p85ß. Because PI3K is an obligate heterodimer, the different possible combinations of catalytic and regulatory subunits, each with distinct relative ratios of expression in different cell types and tissues, provides a complex diversity amplifier for the PI3K pathway whose research has become increasingly appealing given its relevance in human malignancies (Vanhaesebroeck et al. 2010). The NS1 protein binds very specifically to p85ß (Hale et al. 2006; Shin et al. 2007a): a remarkable feature unique among the numerous PI3K activators. It is unknown why influenza virus would only target p85ß complexes, as well as if there are also preferred p110 isotypes, but this may be the key for understanding of the biological relevance of PI3K activation by NS1.

4.2 Regulation of Viral RNA and Protein Synthesis

Early studies on temperature-sensitive mutant viruses had suggested that the NS3 was involved in the regulation of vRNA synthesis (Wolstenholme et al. 1980). Influenza virus gene expression has traditionally been divided into early and late stages, with the NS and NP vRNAs being selectively expressed during the former and all the eight genomic segments showing higher expression levels at the latter (Shapiro et al. 1987; Skehel 1973). Alanine substitutions of NS1 amino acids 123/124 of the Ud strain result in a temporal deregulation of vRNA synthesis, with late genes being generated earlier and in greater numbers (Min et al. 2007). Although residues 123/124 are required for binding to and inhibiting PKR, the observed phenotype was unrelated to any activation of PKR, as it could also be noted on PKR−/− mice. Further evidence that NS1 plays a role in regulating viral RNA synthesis came from recombinant PR8 viruses carrying deletions of their whole NS1 ED, which specifically impair the mRNA levels of HA (Maamary et al. 2012). The mechanism by which NS1 can influence vRNA temporal regulation is unknown, but it has been postulated to be related to the well-characterized interaction of NS1 with the viral ribonucleoprotein complex (Marion et al. 1997b; Kuo and Krug 2009) through its direct binding to NP (Robb et al. 2011). Complementary, very recent data suggests that NS1 inhibition of DDX21 may be the key for this process. DDX21 is a cellular helicase able to block the viral polymerase complex formation and an interacting partner of both NS1/CPSF30 and PB1 (Chen et al. 2014).

Influenza virus efficiently takes over the cellular protein production systems, so in infected cells there is a preferential translation of viral products over the host's own (Garfinkel and Katze 1993). The NS1 protein contributes to this phenomenon by selectively shutting off cellular gene expression at co- and post-transcriptional levels, as described earlier, but additionally has also shown to directly enhance the translation of viral mRNAs, a feature mapped to its N-terminal 113 amino acids (Marion et al. 1997a). NS1 can bind to the conserved 5′ UTR regions of the mRNA (Park and Katze 1995), as well as to different proteins involved in eukaryotic translation: the elongation initiation factor 4GI (eIF4GI) (Aragón et al. 2000), its interactor PABPI (Burgui et al. 2003) and hStaufen, a dsRNA binding protein involved in the transport of mRNA to active translation sites (Falcon et al. 1999). The proposed model for NS1 enhancing viral translation involves the selective recruitment of these factors to the 5′ viral UTRs in cytoplasmic polysomes that were actually one of the first subcellular locations in which NS1 was found (Krug and Etkind 1973).

4.3 Interactions with Other Host Cell Factors: the C-terminal PDZ Binding Motif

High-throughput screening strategies combined with bioinformatics analysis have been used to identify cellular pathways and components affected during influenza virus infection (Shapira et al. 2009; Pichlmair et al. 2012; de Chassey et al. 2013). In addition to confirming previously characterized interactions of NS1, these studies have also identified novel potential interactors of NS1, which will require further research. Another approach to discover additional functions and partners for NS1 has been the use of bioinformatics and sequence analysis to find common motifs in the protein's sequence (Obenauer et al. 2006). This identified a putative PDZ binding motif (PBM) in the C-terminus of many of 230 amino acid long NS1 proteins. PDZ domains are important protein recognition signals, relevant in the assembly of multi-component signaling complexes (Javier and Rice 2011). The most common C-terminus sequences in NS1 proteins of human (RSKV/RSEV) and avian (ESEV/EPEV) strains are putative PBMs, although only the latter has been found to interact with PDZ domain-containing proteins such as Scribble and Dlg1, which may be affecting cellular junctions and the apoptotic response (Liu et al. 2010; Javier and Rice 2011, Golebiewski et al. 2011). The relevance of this avian-specific motif is unclear: while it has been shown to increase replication of laboratory-adapted WSN strain (Jackson et al. 2008) and avian-H7N1 viruses (Soubies et al. 2010), when introduced into the highly pathogenic A/VN/1203/04 (H5N1) did not affect virulence, at least in a murine model (Zielecki et al. 2010).

5 Achieving Multifunctionality: Regulation of NS1

5.1 Intracellular Distribution

A quick overview of the plethora of activities associated to NS1 highlights that some of them must take place in the nucleus (CPSF30 binding), while others should happen in the cytoplasm (RIG-I signaling and PKR inhibition, PI3K activation). Therefore, the subcellular location of the protein and its regulation must play a role in determining which functions are executed at which time.

NS1 was originally described as a nuclear protein (Lazarowitz et al. 1971) and indeed can be predominantly found in the nucleus of infected cells, especially at early times post-infection. Up to two different nuclear location signals (NLS) can be found depending on the viral strain (Greenspan et al. 1988; Melen et al. 2007). Every NS1 protein of influenza A and influenza B viruses has a monopartite NLS signal in its N-terminus (amino acids 35–41), which overlaps with critical residues for dsRNA binding such as R38 and K41. Nuclear translocation due to this NLS is mediated by the karyopherin importin α (Melén et al. 2007). Additionally, those 237 residues-long NS1 proteins from H3N2 IAV, which gained an elongated tail between 1950 and 1989, have a second, bipartite NLS around positions 219-232 (Melén et al. 2007). Interestingly, this second NLS also encompasses a nucleolar location signal (NoLS), which remained functional after the loss of the seven amino acid extension on H3N2 (Melén et al. 2007). The nucleo-cytoplasmic location of NS1 can also be regulated by a nuclear export signal (NES) present on the ED and identified in the Ud strain (Li et al. 1998).

5.2 *Post-Translational Modifications*

Post-translational modification is a common mechanism to regulate multi-functional proteins. As such, several studies have been performed in order to address which of these modifications can affect NS1, and to what effect. Up to this date, NS1 has been found to be modified by phosphorylation and by coupling to the ubiquitin-like proteins ISG15 and SUMO.

Early studies showed that the NS1 protein of the A/WSN (H1N1) strain was phosphorylated soon after infection, probably in the nucleus (Privalsky and Penhoet 1978, 1981). Structural analysis suggested different serine and threonine residues available for modification (Bornholdt and Prasad 2006), and later those residues were experimentally identified in the H3N2 Ud strain as T215 (Hale et al. 2009), S42 and S48 (Hsiang et al. 2012). There is no clear role for these phosphorylation events, however, and even their presence seems to be strain-specific, as they could not be detected in the 2009 H1N1 pandemic virus (Hsiang et al. 2012). Threonine 215 is a distinctive feature of human-adapted strains, with avian-adapted viruses displaying a proline in the same position, and can be phosphorylated in vitro by CDK and ERK kinases (Hale et al. 2009). Recombinant Ud viruses carrying a T215A mutation are attenuated (Hale et al. 2009), however, this is probably due to other factors beyond phosphorylation, as other non-phosphorylable substitutions do not affect viral performance, including the avian-like T215P (Hsiang et al. 2012). Serine 48 is not totally conserved (e.g. the 2009 pandemic H1N1 and many H3N2 viruses do not carry it) and its substitution has no impact on viral replication (Hsiang et al. 2012). Only phosphorylation of serine 42, mediated by cellular PKCα, has been shown to play a relevant role for the virus, as its substitution on the Ud NS1 affects dsRNA binding and consequently replication (Hsiang et al. 2012).

Different studies have described covalent binding of NS1 to ISG15, a 15 kDa, interferon-stimulated ubiquitin homologue with an array of anti-viral properties (Zhao et al. 2013), and identified Herc5 as the E3 ligase involved in the process (Tang et al. 2010; Zhao et al. 2011). Though several lysine residues can be ISGylated after transfection of the NS1 protein (Tang et al. 2010), K41 seems to be the main target during an actual infection in the Ud and WSN strains (Zhao et al. 2011). As stated earlier, amino acid K41 is involved in both dsRNA binding and nuclear import, the latter through interaction with importin α. ISG15 modification of K41 impairs interaction of NS1 with the karyopherin without affecting its dsRNA-binding properties. Substitution of the K41 amino acid renders the same protective effect on viral growth kinetics against interferon treatment as siRNA knock-down of ISG15 (Zhao et al. 2011; Hsiang et al. 2012). Proposed mechanisms for ISG15-based suppression of the NS1 function, based on in vitro data, are prevention of PKR binding, abrogation of RBD dimerization and overall subpar antagonism of the IFN system (Tang et al. 2010). As with most other NS1-associated features, ISGylation has a strong strain-specific component: modification of K41 could not be detected in the PR8 NS1 (Tang et al. 2010); also, this anti-viral effect may have been counteracted by certain strains of H3N2 viruses with naturally occurring K41R substitutions (Zhao et al. 2013). Additionally, as described below, influenza B virus NS1 has evolved a unique pro-viral mechanism to inhibit ISGylation by directly binding to ISG15.

Another ubiquitin-like protein that can be conjugated to NS1 is SUMO (small ubiquitin-like modifier (Pal et al. 2010; Xu et al. 2011; Santos et al. 2013). SUMO proteins can regulate function, stability, location, and interactivity of numerous proteins, both cellular and from different pathogens, including viruses (Everett et al. 2013). The NS1 protein can be modified by the three main isotypes of SUMO (SUMO 1 and SUMO 2/3) (Santos et al. 2013). Again, SUMOylation of NS1 is strain-dependent, and none could be detected in the 2009 pH1N1 strain (Xu et al. 2011). On the PR8 strain, SUMOylation was found to be affecting lysines at positions 70 and 219. The role of SUMoylation on NS1 performance has not been fully elucidated yet: in some strains could be affecting the stability of the protein (Xu et al. 2011). While this is not the case of the PR8 NS1, proper levels of SUMOylation are still required for optimal IFN antagonism by this strain's protein (Santos et al. 2013).

5.3 Structural Versatility

The quaternary structure of NS1 may provide an additional route for the achievement of multifunctionality, on top of (and probably together with) sub-cellular location and post-translational modification. The modular constitution of NS1, with two independently dimerizable RBD and ED globular domains separated by a linker, allows for a variety of different structures. The RBD-RBD dimer, due to its strong nature, seems to be permanent, but the EDs may cycle between dimeric and monomeric states, and change their relative position respect to the RBD dimer (Kerry et al. 2011; Aramini et al. 2011). Recent structural studies have showed how residues close to the linker region and its overall length may dramatically affect the ED-to-RBD positioning (Carrillo et al. 2014), an interesting observation given the five amino acid deletion in the linker of many highly pathogenic H5N1 strains, whose relevance and contribution to virulence remains unclear. As commented earlier, the ED may dimerize through a weak helix-helix interface with the conserved tryptophan in position W187 being pivotal for the interaction. It is unclear whether the ED-ED interactions happen within the same NS1 dimer, between different dimers to promote the reported multimerization of NS1 (Nemeroff et al. 1995; Wang et al. 2002; Bornholdt and Prasad 2008), or both. In any case, the status of the ED probably has a great impact on the range of interactors available for binding the NS1 protein: the surface involved in dimerization is also involved in binding to CPS30 (Hale et al. 2008a, b), so both interactions are mutually exclusive unless in the context of a multimer. Similarly, allosteric considerations predict that a dimeric ED could not interact with a PI3K complex sitting in its canonical membrane location (Hale et al. 2010b). Additionally, the dimerization of the effector domain also has a key functional role: it contributes to strengthen dsRNA binding (Kerry et al. 2011; Aramini et al. 2011). An elegant model has been proposed to explain this by the cooperative binding of multiple NS1 monomers to the same dsRNA strand, spirally wrapping it through W187-mediated ED interactions (Aramini et al. 2011). Disruption of the ED-ED dimer by substitution of W187 results in attenuation of a recombinant PR8 virus in vivo, as well as an altered pattern of temporal and spatial distribution of the protein during infection (Ayllon et al. 2012c). The latter hints to different NS1 conformers playing distinct roles at specific times after infection: whether this is due to the interplay of expression levels, availability and affinity to different interactors, or there are more complex regulatory mechanisms underlying this phenomenon remains unknown.

6 The NS1 Protein of Influenza B and C viruses

Most of the work on characterizing the NS1 protein functions has been done on influenza A virus, and their counterpart on influenza B viruses is not as well understood. Sequence wise, A/NS1 and B/NS1 share less than 20 % amino acid identity. However, they seem to display a similar but not identical set of functional properties. B/NS1 can complement the growth of influenza A delNS1 virus (Donelan et al. 2004). B/NS1 is also an IFN antagonist that can bind dsRNA (Talon et al. 2000b; Donelan et al. 2004; Wang and Krug 1996) and can inhibit PKR (Dauber et al. 2004, 2006), although it lacks the post-transcriptional inhibitory properties of A/NS1 (Wang and Krug 1996) and does not activate PI3K (Ehrhardt et al. 2007). The most distinctive feature of B/NS1 is its ability to counteract the IFN-inducible ISG15 conjugation. As mentioned earlier, ISG15 is a small ubiquitine-like modifier with known anti-viral properties against a variety of viruses, and it has been described that A/NS1 can be conjugated to and modified by ISG15 (Tang et al. 2010; Zhao et al. 2011). The first report that ISG15 could function as an ubiquitin-like anti-viral modifier came from the finding that B/NS1, but not A/NS1, could bind ISG15 and sequester it away from its E1-activating enzyme, identified as Ube1L (Yuan and Krug 2001), a mechanism that later was found to be shared by vaccinia virus through its E3L protein (Guerra et al. 2008). Interestingly, this feature is host-dependent: ISG15 and Ube1L knock-out mice are still more susceptible to influenza B than wild type animals (Lai et al. 2009), and that is because B/NS1 can only bind to human and nonhuman primate ISG15, but not to murine or canine ISG15 (Sridharan et al. 2010; Versteeg et al. 2010). ISG15 comprises two ubiquitin-like domains spaced by a 5-amino acid linker region. This short inter-domain "hinge" is the key for the species specificity of the B/NS1-ISG15 interaction: only humans and other primates have the residues required for the binding (a DxCDE motif). This was first shown by mutagenesis studies (Sridharan et al. 2010) and confirmed by X-ray crystal analysis (Guan et al. 2011), and might be in part responsible for the restriction of influenza B to a human reservoir, as opposed to the wider spread in multiple host species of influenza A.

Very little is known about the NS1 protein of influenza C viruses. It has been described that C/NS1 can upregulate the splicing of viral RNAs (Muraki et al. 2010) and that it can also antagonize IFN production by inhibiting RIG-I signaling, probably by a dsRNA-independent mechanism (Pachler and Vlasak 2011).

7 Influenza Virus Control and NS1

7.1 Recombinant NS1-Modified Viruses as Vaccines

Given its aforementioned role as a virulence factor and IFN antagonist, lack of or truncation in the NS1 gene causes influenza virus to be attenuated in vivo and elicit a strong innate response, which in turn activates the antigen-presenting cells that trigger and direct the adaptive brunch of immunity (Schmolke and García-Sastre 2010; Iwasaki and Medzhitov 2010; Mueller et al. 2010). This combination of attenuation, limited replication ability, and intrinsic adjuvant properties is the main rationale that originally led to the consideration of recombinant NS1-modified viruses as potential live attenuated vaccines, designed against both influenza A and influenza B (Richt and García-Sastre 2009). A number of studies using live attenuated influenza virus strains with deletions on the C-terminus of NS1 have shown protective effect on mice (Talon et al. 2000b; Hai et al. 2008; Pica et al. 2012), pigs (Solorzano et al. 2005; Richt et al. 2006; Vincent et al. 2007), horses (Quinlivan et al. 2005), birds (Wang et al. 2008; Steel et al. 2009), ferrets (Zhou et al. 2010), and macaques (Baskin et al. 2009). Phase I trials in healthy volunteers aged 18–50 have also shown safety and immunogenicity of a virus lacking NS1 (Wacheck et al. 2010). Although attenuation of the recombinant viruses carrying modified NS1 is a potential caveat for the industrial production of vaccines, the growth of these viruses in IFN-incompetent cell- and egg- based systems may be a way to circumvent this issue (Talon et al. 2000b; Richt and García-Sastre 2009).

7.2 Antiviral Compounds Targeting NS1

NS1 has also been considered a promising target for small antiviral molecules that could hinder one or more of its associated functions. Structural knowledge and an extensive availability of sequences from different NS1 strains have allowed in silico identification of potential binding sites for inhibitory compounds (Darapaneni et al. 2009; Krug and Aramini 2009), and a number of approaches have been used in order to screen for them (Engel 2013; Beyleveld et al. 2013). In vitro the dsRNA-binding capability of NS1, being the most conserved feature among different NS1, has been the target of two different studies that have used fluorescently- (Cho et al. 2012) or radiactively-labeled RNA species (Maroto et al. 2008) to monitor the inhibition of binding upon screening with compound collections, with promising results. Additionally, high-throughput cell-based reporter screenings have been performed focusing on NS1 inhibition of the IFNβ promoter induction (Ortigoza et al. 2012) or its repression of general gene expression (Mata et al. 2011). Although serendipitously both studies identified two promising antiviral compounds, neither of them are direct inhibitors of NS1 and their antiviral function is mediated through interference with the viral polymerase function (Ortigoza et al. 2012) or through repression of the proviral mTORC1 pathway (Mata et al. 2011). An alternative strategy used a yeast-based phenotype complementation assay to identify several small molecules that could revert NS1-mediated growth arrest in yeast (Basu et al. 2009). A leading compound from this study was shown to mediate its antiviral activity by allowing RNA-induced IFN to be produced during infection despite the presence of NS1, and to require RNase L to be functional (Basu et al. 2009; Walkiewicz et al. 2011). This compound was further optimized chemically to increase its potency (Walkiewicz et al. 2011; Jablonski et al. 2012). However, whether its activity is directly mediated by NS1 inhibition during viral infection or not remains to be elucidated.

Despite all the aforementioned efforts, finding an effective and clinically viable inhibitor for NS1 remains a formidable challenge, given the degree of redundancy on the NS1 functions, the high level of inter-strain variability on their outcome and the relative easiness with which influenza virus generates escape mutants.

8 Concluding Remarks

The NS1 protein is an accessory factor of influenza virus. It is not required for the production of infectious influenza virus particles and the whole NS1 gene can be removed without turning the virus unviable, unlike any other viral gene with the exception of those that encode small peptides like PB1-F2. And yet, influenza viruses dedicate around 5% of their coding resources on NS1 and its overall function is well conserved not only among different strains, but even among the three influenza virus genera/types. The reason behind this conservation resides on the very specialized role of the NS1 as the main viral disruptor of the host cell antiviral response.

NS1 blocks the innate immune response by targeting the IFN system at different steps, thus rendering the infected cell unable to counteract the virus or to alert of its presence to other cells susceptible to infection or involved in immunity. Complementarily, NS1 helps taking over the cellular machinery shutting down the cells' own production while promoting viral-only gene expression, and increases the infected cell survivability, so cellular resources are available longer.

One of the main challenges for influenza researchers is to understand how such a small protein can do so many different things. NS1 has no known enzymatic activities, so all its functions seem to be based on interactions and interference with different complexes. Many of the interactions of NS1 have been structurally characterized, but a single NS1 monomer cannot interact with all of its partners simultaneously for simple allosteric reasons. Oligomerization and a relative plasticity on the positioning of the domains of NS1 could provide with structurally different pools of NS1, and allow this protein to be involved on different interactions. The subcellular location of NS1 is also relevant as many of its partners are strictly nuclear or cytoplasmic. It is unknown how the different conformational and/or spatial states of NS1 are regulated during infection. A balance between NS1 expression levels and the availability of interactors may drive the protein to a certain status and function. Moreover, post-translational regulatory mechanisms (phosphorylation or conjugation to ubiquitin-like proteins), might also regulate NS1 function.

The outstanding volume of knowledge built around NS1 during the last couple of decades has brought light into this remarkable viral polypeptide, unveiling the complexities of the interactions between virus and host. Further understanding of these interactions will help designing new antiviral strategies and surveilling potential threats emerging from animal reservoirs. Ultimately, the study of the virus-cell interface through factors like NS1 may enlighten us about many critical cellular processes whose relevance in health and disease does not need to be solely restricted to viral infection.

Acknowledgments Work in AG-S laboratory is partially funded by NIH grants U19AI106754, U19AI083025, P01AI090935, P01AI097092, U19AI089987, R01AI088770, R01AI079110, R01AI089539, U01AI095611, R01DA033773; NIH contracts HHSN272201000054C, HHSN-272200900032C, HHSN272201300023C; and by CRIP (Center for Research on Influenza Pathogenesis), and NIAID funded Center of Excellence in Influenza Research and Surveillance (CEIRS, contract # HHSN272201400008C).

References

Alonso-Caplen FV, Krug RM (1991) Regulation of the extent of splicing of influenza virus NS1 mRNA: role of the rates of splicing and of the nucleocytoplasmic transport of NS1 mRNA. Mol Cell Biol 11:1092–1098

Alonso-Caplen FV, Nemeroff ME, Qiu Y, Krug RM (1992) Nucleocytoplasmic transport: the influenza virus NS1 protein regulates the transport of spliced NS2 mRNA and its precursor NS1 mRNA. Genes Dev 6:255–267

Aragón T, de la Luna S, Novoa I, Carrasco L, Ortin J, Nieto A (2000) Eukaryotic translation initiation factor 4GI is a cellular target for NS1 protein, a translational activator of influenza virus. Mol Cell Biol 20:6259–6268

Aramini JM, Ma LC, Zhou L, Schauder CM, Hamilton K, Amer BR, Mack TR, Lee HW, Ciccosanti CT, Zhao L, Xiao R, Krug RM, Montelione GT (2011) Dimer interface of the effector domain of non-structural protein 1 from influenza A virus: an interface with multiple functions. J Biol Chem 286:26050–26060

Ayllon J, García-Sastre A, Hale BG (2012a) Influenza A viruses and PI3K: are there time, place and manner restrictions? Virulence 3:411–414

Ayllon J, Hale BG, García-Sastre A (2012b) Strain-specific contribution of NS1-activated phosphoinositide 3-kinase signaling to influenza A virus replication and virulence. J Virol 86:5366–5370

Ayllon J, Russell RJ, García-Sastre A, Hale BG (2012c) Contribution of NS1 effector domain dimerization to influenza A virus replication and virulence. J Virol 86:13095–13098

Barabino SM, Hubner W, Jenny A, Minvielle-Sebastia L, Keller W (1997) The 30-kD subunit of mammalian cleavage and polyadenylation specificity factor and its yeast homolog are RNA-binding zinc finger proteins. Genes Dev 11:1703–1716

Baskin CR, Bielefeldt-Ohmann H, Tumpey TM, Sabourin PJ, Long JP, García-Sastre A, Tolnay AE, Albrecht R, Pyles JA, Olson PH, Aicher LD, Rosenzweig ER, Murali-Krishna K, Clark EA, Kotur MS, Fornek JL, Proll S, Palermo RE, Sabourin CL, Katze MG (2009) Early and sustained innate immune response defines pathology and death in nonhuman primates infected by highly pathogenic influenza virus. Proc Natl Acad Sci USA 106:3455–3460

Basu D, Walkiewicz MP, Frieman M, Baric RS, Auble DT, Engel DA (2009) Novel influenza virus NS1 antagonists block replication and restore innate immune function. J Virol 83:1881–1891

Bergmann M, García-Sastre A, Carnero E, Pehamberger H, Wolff K, Palese P, Muster T (2000) Influenza virus NS1 protein counteracts PKR-mediated inhibition of replication. J Virol 74:6203–6206

Beyleveld G, White KM, Ayllon J, Shaw ML (2013) New-generation screening assays for the detection of anti-influenza compounds targeting viral and host functions. Antiviral Res 100:120–132

Bornholdt ZA, Prasad BV (2006) X-ray structure of influenza virus NS1 effector domain. Nat Struct Mol Biol 13:559–560

Bornholdt ZA, Prasad BV (2008) X-ray structure of NS1 from a highly pathogenic H5N1 influenza virus. Nature 456:985–988

Brown EG, Liu H, Kit LC, Baird S, Nesrallah M (2001) Pattern of mutation in the genome of influenza A virus on adaptation to increased virulence in the mouse lung: identification of functional themes. Proc Natl Acad Sci USA 98:6883–6888

Burgui I, Aragon T, Ortin J, Nieto A (2003) PABP1 and eIF4GI associate with influenza virus NS1 protein in viral mRNA translation initiation complexes. J Gen Virol 84:3263–3274

Carrillo B, Choi JM, Bornholdt ZA, Sankaran B, Rice AP, Prasad BV (2014) The influenza A virus protein NS1 displays structural polymorphism. J Virol 88:4113–4122

Chen G, Liu CH, Zhou L, Krug RM (2014) Cellular DDX21 RNA Helicase inhibits influenza A virus replication but is counteracted by the viral NS1 protein. Cell Host Microbe 15:484–493

Cheng A, Wong SM, Yuan YA (2009) Structural basis for dsRNA recognition by NS1 protein of influenza A virus. Cell Res 19:187–195

Chien CY, Tejero R, Huang Y, Zimmerman DE, Rios CB, Krug RM, Montelione GT (1997) A novel RNA-binding motif in influenza A virus non-structural protein 1. Nat Struct Biol 4:891–895

Chien CY, Xu Y, Xiao R, Aramini JM, Sahasrabudhe PV, Krug RM, Montelione GT (2004) Biophysical characterization of the complex between double-stranded RNA and the N-terminal domain of the NS1 protein from influenza A virus: evidence for a novel RNA-binding mode. Biochemistry 43:1950–1962

Cho EJ, Xia S, Ma LC, Robertus J, Krug RM, Anslyn EV, Montelione GT, Ellington AD (2012) Identification of influenza virus inhibitors targeting NS1A utilizing fluorescence polarization-based high-throughput assay. J Biomol Screen 17:448–459

Colgan DF, Manley JL (1997) Mechanism and regulation of mRNA polyadenylation. Genes Dev 11:2755–2766

Dankar SK, Miranda E, Forbes NE, Pelchat M, Tavassoli A, Selman M, Ping J, Jia J, Brown EG (2013) Influenza A/Hong Kong/156/1997(H5N1) virus NS1 gene mutations F103L and M106I both increase IFN antagonism, virulence and cytoplasmic localization but differ in binding to RIG-I and CPSF30. Virol J 10:243

Darapaneni V, Prabhaker VK, Kukol A (2009) Large-scale analysis of influenza A virus sequences reveals potential drug target sites of non-structural proteins. J Gen Virol 90:2124–2133

Das K, Ma LC, Xiao R, Radvansky B, Aramini J, Zhao L, Marklund J, Kuo RL, Twu KY, Arnold E, Krug RM, Montelione GT (2008) Structural basis for suppression of a host antiviral response by influenza A virus. Proc Natl Acad Sci USA 105:13093–13098

Dauber B, Heins G, Wolff T (2004) The influenza B virus nonstructural NS1 protein is essential for efficient viral growth and antagonizes beta interferon induction. J Virol 78:1865–1872

Dauber B, Schneider J, Wolff T (2006) Double-stranded RNA binding of influenza B virus nonstructural NS1 protein inhibits protein kinase R but is not essential to antagonize production of alpha/beta interferon. J Virol 80:11667–11677

de Chassey B, Aublin-Gex A, Ruggieri A, Meyniel-Schicklin L, Pradezynski F, Davoust N, Chantier T, Tafforeau L, Mangeot PE, Ciancia C, Perrin-Cocon L, Bartenschlager R, Andre P, Lotteau V (2013) The interactomes of influenza virus NS1 and NS2 proteins identify new host factors and provide insights for ADAR1 playing a supportive role in virus replication. PLoS Pathog 9:e1003440

Donelan NR, Dauber B, Wang X, Basler CF, Wolff T, García-Sastre A (2004) The N- and C-terminal domains of the NS1 protein of influenza B virus can independently inhibit IRF-3 and beta interferon promoter activation. J Virol 78:11574–11582

Dundon WG, Capua I (2009) A closer look at the NS1 of influenza virus. Viruses 1:1057–1072

Egorov A, Brandt S, Sereinig S, Romanova J, Ferko B, Katinger D, Grassauer A, Alexandrova G, Katinger H, Muster T (1998) Transfectant influenza A viruses with long deletions in the NS1 protein grow efficiently in vero cells. J Virol 72:6437–6441

Ehrhardt C, Ludwig S (2009) A new player in a deadly game: influenza viruses and the PI3K/Akt signalling pathway. Cell Microbiol 11:863–871

Ehrhardt C, Marjuki H, Wolff T, Nurnberg B, Planz O, Pleschka S, Ludwig S (2006) Bivalent role of the phosphatidylinositol-3-kinase (PI3K) during influenza virus infection and host cell defence. Cell Microbiol 8:1336–1348

Ehrhardt C, Wolff T, Ludwig S (2007) Activation of phosphatidylinositol 3-kinase signaling by the nonstructural NS1 protein is not conserved among type A and B influenza viruses. J Virol 81:12097–12100

Engel DA (2013) The influenza virus NS1 protein as a therapeutic target. Antiviral Res 99:409–416

Engelman JA, Luo J, Cantley LC (2006) The evolution of phosphatidylinositol 3-kinases as regulators of growth and metabolism. Nat Rev Genet 7:606–619

Everett RD, Boutell C, Hale BG (2013) Interplay between viruses and host sumoylation pathways. Nat Rev Microbiol 11:400–411

Falcon AM, Fortes P, Marion RM, Beloso A, Ortin J (1999) Interaction of influenza virus NS1 protein and the human homologue of Staufen in vivo and in vitro. Nucleic Acids Res 27:2241–2247

Fortes P, Beloso A, Ortin J (1994) Influenza virus NS1 protein inhibits pre-mRNA splicing and blocks mRNA nucleocytoplasmic transport. EMBO J 13:704–712

Gack MU, Albrecht RA, Urano T, Inn KS, Huang IC, Carnero E, Farzan M, Inoue S, Jung JU, García-Sastre A (2009) Influenza A virus NS1 targets the ubiquitin ligase TRIM25 to evade recognition by the host viral RNA sensor RIG-I. Cell Host Microbe 5:439–449

Gack MU, Shin YC, Joo CH, Urano T, Liang C, Sun L, Takeuchi O, Akira S, Chen Z, Inoue S, Jung JU (2007) TRIM25 RING-finger E3 ubiquitin ligase is essential for RIG-I-mediated antiviral activity. Nature 446:916–920

Gallacher M, Brown SG, Hale BG, Fearns R, Olver RE, Randall RE, Wilson SM (2009) Cation currents in human airway epithelial cells induced by infection with influenza A virus. J Physiol 587:3159–3173

García MA, Gil J, Ventoso I, Guerra S, Domingo E, Rivas C, Esteban M (2006) Impact of protein kinase PKR in cell biology: from antiviral to antiproliferative action. Microbiol Mol Biol Rev 70:1032–1060

García-Sastre A (2011) Induction and evasion of type I interferon responses by influenza viruses. Virus Res 162:12–18

García-Sastre A, Egorov A, Matassov D, Brandt S, Levy DE, Durbin JE, Palese P, Muster T (1998) Influenza A virus lacking the NS1 gene replicates in interferon-deficient systems. Virology 252:324–330

Garfinkel MS, Katze MG (1993) Translational control by influenza virus. Selective translation is mediated by sequences within the viral mRNA 5′-untranslated region. J Biol Chem 268:22223–22226

Golebiewski L, Liu H, Javier RT, Rice AP (2011) The avian influenza virus NS1 ESEV PDZ binding motif associates with Dlg1 and Scribble to disrupt cellular tight junctions. J Virol 85:10639–10648

Goodman AG, Smith JA, Balachandran S, Perwitasari O, Proll SC, Thomas MJ, Korth MJ, Barber GN, Schiff LA, Katze MG (2007) The cellular protein P58IPK regulates influenza virus mRNA translation and replication through a PKR-mediated mechanism. J Virol 81:2221–2230

Graef KM, Vreede FT, Lau YF, McCall AW, Carr SM, Subbarao K, Fodor E (2010) The PB2 subunit of the influenza virus RNA polymerase affects virulence by interacting with the mitochondrial antiviral signaling protein and inhibiting expression of beta interferon. J Virol 84:8433–8445

Greenspan D, Palese P, Krystal M (1988) Two nuclear location signals in the influenza virus NS1 nonstructural protein. J Virol 62:3020–3026

Grimm D, Staeheli P, Hufbauer M, Koerner I, Martinez-Sobrido L, Solorzano A, García-Sastre A, Haller O, Kochs G (2007) Replication fitness determines high virulence of influenza A virus in mice carrying functional Mx1 resistance gene. Proc Natl Acad Sci USA 104:6806–6811

Guan R, Ma LC, Leonard PG, Amer BR, Sridharan H, Zhao C, Krug RM, Montelione GT (2011) Structural basis for the sequence-specific recognition of human ISG15 by the NS1 protein of influenza B virus. Proc Natl Acad Sci USA 108:13468–13473

Guerra S, Caceres A, Knobeloch KP, Horak I, Esteban M (2008) Vaccinia virus E3 protein prevents the antiviral action of ISG15. PLoS Pathog 4:e1000096

Guo Z, Chen LM, Zeng H, Gomez JA, Plowden J, Fujita T, Katz JM, Donis RO, Sambhara S (2007) NS1 protein of influenza A virus inhibits the function of intracytoplasmic pathogen sensor, RIG-I. Am J Respir Cell Mol Biol 36:263–269

Hai R, Martinez-Sobrido L, Fraser KA, Ayllon J, García-Sastre A, Palese P (2008) Influenza B virus NS1-truncated mutants: live-attenuated vaccine approach. J Virol 82:10580–10590

Hale BG, Barclay WS, Randall RE, Russell RJ (2008a) Structure of an avian influenza A virus NS1 protein effector domain. Virology 378:1–5

Hale BG, Batty IH, Downes CP, Randall RE (2008b) Binding of influenza A virus NS1 protein to the inter-SH2 domain of p85 suggests a novel mechanism for phosphoinositide 3-kinase activation. J Biol Chem 283:1372–1380

Hale BG, Randall RE, Ortin J, Jackson D (2008c) The multifunctional NS1 protein of influenza A viruses. J Gen Virol 89:2359–2376

Hale BG, Jackson D, Chen YH, Lamb RA, Randall RE (2006) Influenza A virus NS1 protein binds p85beta and activates phosphatidylinositol-3-kinase signaling. Proc Natl Acad Sci USA 103:14194–14199

Hale BG, Kerry PS, Jackson D, Precious BL, Gray A, Killip MJ, Randall RE, Russell RJ (2010a) Structural insights into phosphoinositide 3-kinase activation by the influenza A virus NS1 protein. Proc Natl Acad Sci USA 107:1954–1959

Hale BG, Steel J, Medina RA, Manicassamy B, Ye J, Hickman D, Hai R, Schmolke M, Lowen AC, Perez DR, García-Sastre A (2010b) Inefficient control of host gene expression by the 2009 pandemic H1N1 influenza A virus NS1 protein. J Virol 84:6909–6922

Hale BG, Knebel A, Botting CH, Galloway CS, Precious BL, Jackson D, Elliott RM, Randall RE (2009) CDK/ERK-mediated phosphorylation of the human influenza A virus NS1 protein at threonine-215. Virology 383:6–11

Hatada E, Fukuda R (1992) Binding of influenza A virus NS1 protein to dsRNA in vitro. J Gen Virol 73(Pt 12):3325–3329

Hatada E, Takizawa T, Fukuda R (1992) Specific binding of influenza A virus NS1 protein to the virus minus-sense RNA in vitro. J Gen Virol 73(Pt 1):17–25

Hayman A, Comely S, Lackenby A, Murphy S, McCauley J, Goodbourn S, Barclay W (2006) Variation in the ability of human influenza A viruses to induce and inhibit the IFN-beta pathway. Virology 347:52–64

Horisberger MA, Staeheli P, Haller O (1983) Interferon induces a unique protein in mouse cells bearing a gene for resistance to influenza virus. Proc Natl Acad Sci USA 80:1910–1914

Hossain MJ, Hickman D, Perez DR (2008) Evidence of expanded host range and mammalian-associated genetic changes in a duck H9N2 influenza virus following adaptation in quail and chickens. PLoS One 3:e3170

Hovanessian AG (1989) The double stranded RNA-activated protein kinase induced by interferon: dsRNA-PK. J Interferon Res 9:641–647

Hrincius ER, Hennecke AK, Gensler L, Nordhoff C, Anhlan D, Vogel P, McCullers JA, Ludwig S, Ehrhardt C (2012) A single point mutation (Y89F) within the non-structural protein 1 of influenza A viruses limits epithelial cell tropism and virulence in mice. Am J Pathol 180:2361–2374

Hsiang TY, Zhou L, Krug RM (2012) Roles of the phosphorylation of specific serines and threonines in the NS1 protein of human influenza A viruses. J Virol 86:10370–10376

Huang TS, Palese P, Krystal M (1990) Determination of influenza virus proteins required for genome replication. J Virol 64:5669–5673

Inglis SC, Barrett T, Brown CM, Almond JW (1979) The smallest genome RNA segment of influenza virus contains two genes that may overlap. Proc Natl Acad Sci USA 76:3790–3794

Isaacs A, Lindenmann J (1957) Virus interference. I. The interferon. Proc R Soc Lond B Biol Sci 147:258–267

Iwai A, Shiozaki T, Kawai T, Akira S, Kawaoka Y, Takada A, Kida H, Miyazaki T (2010) Influenza A virus polymerase inhibits type I interferon induction by binding to interferon beta promoter stimulator 1. J Biol Chem 285:32064–32074

Iwasaki A, Medzhitov R (2010) Regulation of adaptive immunity by the innate immune system. Science 327:291–295

Jablonski JJ, Basu D, Engel DA, Geysen HM (2012) Design, synthesis, and evaluation of novel small molecule inhibitors of the influenza virus protein NS1. Bioorg Med Chem 20:487–497

Jackson D, Hossain MJ, Hickman D, Perez DR, Lamb RA (2008) A new influenza virus virulence determinant: the NS1 protein four C-terminal residues modulate pathogenicity. Proc Natl Acad Sci USA 105:4381–4386

Jackson D, Killip MJ, Galloway CS, Russell RJ, Randall RE (2010) Loss of function of the influenza A virus NS1 protein promotes apoptosis but this is not due to a failure to activate phosphatidylinositol 3-kinase (PI3K). Virology 396:94–105

Javier RT, Rice AP (2011) Emerging theme: cellular PDZ proteins as common targets of pathogenic viruses. J Virol 85:11544–11556

Katze MG, Detjen BM, Safer B, Krug RM (1986) Translational control by influenza virus: suppression of the kinase that phosphorylates the alpha subunit of initiation factor eIF-2 and selective translation of influenza viral mRNAs. Mol Cell Biol 6:1741–1750

Katze MG, Tomita J, Black T, Krug RM, Safer B, Hovanessian A (1988) Influenza virus regulates protein synthesis during infection by repressing autophosphorylation and activity of the cellular 68,000-Mr protein kinase. J Virol 62:3710–3717

Kerry PS, Ayllon J, Taylor MA, Hass C, Lewis A, García-Sastre A, Randall RE, Hale BG, Russell RJ (2011) A transient homotypic interaction model for the influenza A virus NS1 protein effector domain. PLoS One 6:e17946

Kochs G, García-Sastre A, Martinez-Sobrido L (2007) Multiple anti-interferon actions of the influenza A virus NS1 protein. J Virol 81:7011–7021

Koennecke I, Boschek CB, Scholtissek C (1981) Isolation and properties of a temperature-sensitive mutant (ts 412) of an influenza A virus recombinant with a ts lesion in the gene coding for the nonstructural protein. Virology 110:16–25

Kok K, Geering B, Vanhaesebroeck B (2009) Regulation of phosphoinositide 3-kinase expression in health and disease. Trends Biochem Sci 34:115–127

Krug RM, Aramini JM (2009) Emerging antiviral targets for influenza A virus. Trends Pharmacol Sci 30:269–277

Krug RM, Etkind PR (1973) Cytoplasmic and nuclear virus-specific proteins in influenza virus-infected MDCK cells. Virology 56:334–348

Kuo RL, Krug RM (2009) Influenza a virus polymerase is an integral component of the CPSF30-NS1A protein complex in infected cells. J Virol 83:1611–1616

Kuo RL, Zhao C, Malur M, Krug RM (2010) Influenza A virus strains that circulate in humans differ in the ability of their NS1 proteins to block the activation of IRF3 and interferon-beta transcription. Virology 408:146–158

Lai C, Struckhoff JJ, Schneider J, Martinez-Sobrido L, Wolff T, García-Sastre A, Zhang DE, Lenschow DJ (2009) Mice lacking the ISG15 E1 enzyme UbE1L demonstrate increased susceptibility to both mouse-adapted and non-mouse-adapted influenza B virus infection. J Virol 83:1147–1151

Lamb RA, Choppin PW (1979) Segment 8 of the influenza virus genome is unique in coding for two polypeptides. Proc Natl Acad Sci USA 76:4908–4912

Lamb RA, Lai CJ (1980) Sequence of interrupted and uninterrupted mRNAs and cloned DNA coding for the two overlapping nonstructural proteins of influenza virus. Cell 21:475–485

Lazarowitz SG, Compans RW, Choppin PW (1971) Influenza virus structural and nonstructural proteins in infected cells and their plasma membranes. Virology 46:830–843

Li S, Min JY, Krug RM, Sen GC (2006) Binding of the influenza A virus NS1 protein to PKR mediates the inhibition of its activation by either PACT or double-stranded RNA. Virology 349:13–21

Li Y, Chen ZY, Wang W, Baker CC, Krug RM (2001) The 3′-end-processing factor CPSF is required for the splicing of single-intron pre-mRNAs in vivo. RNA 7:920–931

Li Y, Yamakita Y, Krug RM (1998) Regulation of a nuclear export signal by an adjacent inhibitory sequence: the effector domain of the influenza virus NS1 protein. Proc Natl Acad Sci USA 95:4864–4869

Lindenmann J (1960) Interferon and inverse interference. Z Haut Geschlechtskr 146:287–309

Lindenmann J (1962) Resistance of mice to mouse-adapted influenza A virus. Virology 16:203–204

Liu J, Lynch PA, Chien CY, Montelione GT, Krug RM, Berman HM (1997) Crystal structure of the unique RNA-binding domain of the influenza virus NS1 protein. Nat Struct Biol 4:896–899

Liu H, Golebiewski L, Dow EC, Krug RM, Javier RT, Rice AP (2010) The ESEV PDZ-binding motif of the avian influenza A virus NS1 protein protects infected cells from apoptosis by directly targeting Scribble. J Virol 84:11164–11174

Lu Y, Wambach M, Katze MG, Krug RM (1995) Binding of the influenza virus NS1 protein to double-stranded RNA inhibits the activation of the protein kinase that phosphorylates the elF-2 translation initiation factor. Virology 214:222–228

Ludwig S, Schultz U, Mandler J, Fitch WM, Scholtissek C (1991) Phylogenetic relationship of the nonstructural (NS) genes of influenza A viruses. Virology 183:566–577

Ludwig S, Wang X, Ehrhardt C, Zheng H, Donelan N, Planz O, Pleschka S, García-Sastre A, Heins G, Wolff T (2002) The influenza A virus NS1 protein inhibits activation of Jun N-terminal kinase and AP-1 transcription factors. J Virol 76:11166–11171

Maamary J, Pica N, Belicha-Villanueva A, Chou YY, Krammer F, Gao Q, García-Sastre A, Palese P (2012) Attenuated influenza virus construct with enhanced hemagglutinin protein expression. J Virol 86:5782–5790

Manicassamy B, Manicassamy S, Belicha-Villanueva A, Pisanelli G, Pulendran B, García-Sastre A (2010) Analysis of in vivo dynamics of influenza virus infection in mice using a GFP reporter virus. Proc Natl Acad Sci USA 107:11531–11536

Marazzi I, Ho JS, Kim J, Manicassamy B, Dewell S, Albrecht RA, Seibert CW, Schaefer U, Jeffrey KL, Prinjha RK, Lee K, García-Sastre A, Roeder RG, Tarakhovsky A (2012) Suppression of the antiviral response by an influenza histone mimic. Nature 483:428–433

Marion RM, Aragon T, Beloso A, Nieto A, Ortin J (1997a) The N-terminal half of the influenza virus NS1 protein is sufficient for nuclear retention of mRNA and enhancement of viral mRNA translation. Nucleic Acids Res 25:4271–4277

Marion RM, Zurcher T, de la Luna S, Ortin J (1997b) Influenza virus NS1 protein interacts with viral transcription-replication complexes in vivo. J Gen Virol 78(Pt 10):2447–2451

Maroto M, Fernandez Y, Ortin J, Pelaez F, Cabello MA (2008) Development of an HTS assay for the search of anti-influenza agents targeting the interaction of viral RNA with the NS1 protein. J Biomol Screen 13:581–590

Mata MA, Satterly N, Versteeg GA, Frantz D, Wei S, Williams N, Schmolke M, Pena-Llopis S, Brugarolas J, Forst CV, White MA, García-Sastre A, Roth MG, Fontoura BM (2011) Chemical inhibition of RNA viruses reveals REDD1 as a host defense factor. Nat Chem Biol 7:712–719

McWhirter SM, Tenoever BR, Maniatis T (2005) Connecting mitochondria and innate immunity. Cell 122:645–647

Melen K, Kinnunen L, Fagerlund R, Ikonen N, Twu KY, Krug RM, Julkunen I (2007) Nuclear and nucleolar targeting of influenza A virus NS1 protein: striking differences between different virus subtypes. J Virol 81:5995–6006

Melville MW, Tan SL, Wambach M, Song J, Morimoto RI, Katze MG (1999) The cellular inhibitor of the PKR protein kinase, P58(IPK), is an influenza virus-activated co-chaperone that modulates heat shock protein 70 activity. J Biol Chem 274:3797–3803

Mibayashi M, Martinez-Sobrido L, Loo YM, Cardenas WB, Gale M Jr, García-Sastre A (2007) Inhibition of retinoic acid-inducible gene I-mediated induction of beta interferon by the NS1 protein of influenza A virus. J Virol 81:514–524

Min JY, Krug RM (2006) The primary function of RNA binding by the influenza A virus NS1 protein in infected cells: Inhibiting the 2′-5′ oligo (A) synthetase/RNase L pathway. Proc Natl Acad Sci USA 103:7100–7105

Min JY, Li S, Sen GC, Krug RM (2007) A site on the influenza A virus NS1 protein mediates both inhibition of PKR activation and temporal regulation of viral RNA synthesis. Virology 363:236–243

Mueller SN, Langley WA, Carnero E, García-Sastre A, Ahmed R (2010) Immunization with live attenuated influenza viruses that express altered NS1 proteins results in potent and protective memory CD8+ T-cell responses. J Virol 84:1847–1855

Munir M, Berg M (2013) The multiple faces of proteinkinase R in antiviral defense. Virulence 4:85–89

Muraki Y, Furukawa T, Kohno Y, Matsuzaki Y, Takashita E, Sugawara K, Hongo S (2010) Influenza C virus NS1 protein upregulates the splicing of viral mRNAs. J Virol 84:1957–1966

Myong S, Cui S, Cornish PV, Kirchhofer A, Gack MU, Jung JU, Hopfner KP, Ha T (2009) Cytosolic viral sensor RIG-I is a 5′-triphosphate-dependent translocase on double-stranded RNA. Science 323:1070–1074

Nemeroff ME, Barabino SM, Li Y, Keller W, Krug RM (1998) Influenza virus NS1 protein interacts with the cellular 30 kDa subunit of CPSF and inhibits 3′end formation of cellular pre-mRNAs. Mol Cell 1:991–1000

Nemeroff ME, Qian XY, Krug RM (1995) The influenza virus NS1 protein forms multimers in vitro and in vivo. Virology 212:422–428

Noah DL, Twu KY, Krug RM (2003) Cellular antiviral responses against influenza A virus are countered at the posttranscriptional level by the viral NS1A protein via its binding to a cellular protein required for the 3′ end processing of cellular pre-mRNAS. Virology 307:386–395

Obenauer JC, Denson J, Mehta PK, Su X, Mukatira S, Finkelstein DB, Xu X, Wang J, Ma J, Fan Y, Rakestraw KM, Webster RG, Hoffmann E, Krauss S, Zheng J, Zhang Z, Naeve CW (2006) Large-scale sequence analysis of avian influenza isolates. Science 311:1576–1580

O'Neill RE, Talon J, Palese P (1998) The influenza virus NEP (NS2 protein) mediates the nuclear export of viral ribonucleoproteins. EMBO J 17:288–296

Onomoto K, Jogi M, Yoo JS, Narita R, Morimoto S, Takemura A, Sambhara S, Kawaguchi A, Osari S, Nagata K, Matsumiya T, Namiki H, Yoneyama M, Fujita T (2012) Critical role of an antiviral stress granule containing RIG-I and PKR in viral detection and innate immunity. PLoS One 7:e43031

Opitz B, Rejaibi A, Dauber B, Eckhard J, Vinzing M, Schmeck B, Hippenstiel S, Suttorp N, Wolff T (2007) IFNbeta induction by influenza A virus is mediated by RIG-I which is regulated by the viral NS1 protein. Cell Microbiol 9:930–938

Ortigoza MB, Dibben O, Maamary J, Martinez-Gil L, Leyva-Grado VH, Abreu P Jr, Ayllon J, Palese P, Shaw ML (2012) A novel small molecule inhibitor of influenza A viruses that targets polymerase function and indirectly induces interferon. PLoS Pathog 8:e1002668

Oshiumi H, Matsumoto M, Hatakeyama S, Seya T (2009) Riplet/RNF135, a RING finger protein, ubiquitinates RIG-I to promote interferon-beta induction during the early phase of viral infection. J Biol Chem 284:807–817

Oshiumi H, Miyashita M, Matsumoto M, Seya T (2013) A distinct role of Riplet-mediated K63-Linked polyubiquitination of the RIG-I repressor domain in human antiviral innate immune responses. PLoS Pathog 9:e1003533

Pachler K, Vlasak R (2011) Influenza C virus NS1 protein counteracts RIG-I-mediated IFN signalling. Virol J 8:48

Pal S, Rosas JM, Rosas-Acosta G (2010) Identification of the non-structural influenza A viral protein NS1A as a bona fide target of the small ubiquitin-like Modifier by the use of dicistronic expression constructs. J Virol Methods 163:498–504

Palese P (1977) The genes of influenza virus. Cell 10:1–10

Palese P, Zheng H, Engelhardt OG, Pleschka S, García-Sastre A (1996) Negative-strand RNA viruses: genetic engineering and applications. Proc Natl Acad Sci USA 93:11354–11358

Park YW, Katze MG (1995) Translational control by influenza virus. Identification of cis-acting sequences and trans-acting factors which may regulate selective viral mRNA translation. J Biol Chem 270:28433–28439

Pica N, Langlois RA, Krammer F, Margine I, Palese P (2012) NS1-truncated live attenuated virus vaccine provides robust protection to aged mice from viral challenge. J Virol 86:10293–10301

Pichlmair A, Reis e Sousa C (2007) Innate recognition of viruses. Immunity 27:370–383

Pichlmair A, Schulz O, Tan CP, Naslund TI, Liljestrom P, Weber F, Reis e Sousa C (2006) RIG-I-mediated antiviral responses to single-stranded RNA bearing 5′-phosphates. Science 314:997–1001

Pichlmair A, Kandasamy K, Alvisi G, Mulhern O, Sacco R, Habjan M, Binder M, Stefanovic A, Eberle CA, Goncalves A, Burckstummer T, Muller AC, Fauster A, Holze C, Lindsten K, Goodbourn S, Kochs G, Weber F, Bartenschlager R, Bowie AG, Bennett KL, Colinge J, Superti-Furga G (2012) Viral immune modulators perturb the human molecular network by common and unique strategies. Nature 487:486–490

Privalsky ML, Penhoet EE (1978) Influenza virus proteins: identity, synthesis, and modification analyzed by two-dimensional gel electrophoresis. Proc Natl Acad Sci USA 75:3625–3629

Privalsky ML, Penhoet EE (1981) The structure and synthesis of influenza virus phosphoproteins. J Biol Chem 256:5368–5376

Qian XY, Alonso-Caplen F, Krug RM (1994) Two functional domains of the influenza virus NS1 protein are required for regulation of nuclear export of mRNA. J Virol 68:2433–2441

Qiu Y, Krug RM (1994) The influenza virus NS1 protein is a poly(A)-binding protein that inhibits nuclear export of mRNAs containing poly(A). J Virol 68:2425–2432

Qiu Y, Nemeroff M, Krug RM (1995) The influenza virus NS1 protein binds to a specific region in human U6 snRNA and inhibits U6-U2 and U6-U4 snRNA interactions during splicing. RNA 1:304–316

Quinlivan M, Zamarin D, García-Sastre A, Cullinane A, Chambers T, Palese P (2005) Attenuation of equine influenza viruses through truncations of the NS1 protein. J Virol 79:8431–8439

Rajsbaum R, Albrecht RA, Wang MK, Maharaj NP, Versteeg GA, Nistal-Villan E, García-Sastre A, Gack MU (2012) Species-specific inhibition of RIG-I ubiquitination and IFN induction by the influenza A virus NS1 protein. PLoS Pathog 8:e1003059

Richt JA, García-Sastre A (2009) Attenuated influenza virus vaccines with modified NS1 proteins. Curr Top Microbiol Immunol 333:177–195

Richt JA, Lekcharoensuk P, Lager KM, Vincent AL, Loiacono CM, Janke BH, Wu WH, Yoon KJ, Webby RJ, Solorzano A, García-Sastre A (2006) Vaccination of pigs against swine influenza viruses by using an NS1-truncated modified live-virus vaccine. J Virol 80:11009–11018

Robb NC, Chase G, Bier K, Vreede FT, Shaw PC, Naffakh N, Schwemmle M, Fodor E (2011) The influenza A virus NS1 protein interacts with the nucleoprotein of viral ribonucleoprotein complexes. J Virol 85:5228–5231

Santos A, Pal S, Chacon J, Meraz K, Gonzalez J, Prieto K, Rosas-Acosta G (2013) SUMOylation affects the interferon blocking activity of the influenza A nonstructural protein NS1 without affecting its stability or cellular localization. J Virol 87:5602–5620

Satterly N, Tsai PL, van Deursen J, Nussenzveig DR, Wang Y, Faria PA, Levay A, Levy DE, Fontoura BM (2007) Influenza virus targets the mRNA export machinery and the nuclear pore complex. Proc Natl Acad Sci USA 104:1853–1858

Schmolke M, García-Sastre A (2010) Evasion of innate and adaptive immune responses by influenza A virus. Cell Microbiol 12:873–880

Schneider WM, Chevillotte MD, Rice CM (2014) Interferon-stimulated genes: a complex web of host defenses. Annu Rev Immunol 32:513–545

Scholtissek C, von Hoyningen-Huene V (1980) Genetic relatedness of the gene which codes for the nonstructural (NS) protein of different influenza A strains. Virology 102:13–20

Schultz-Cherry S, Dybdahl-Sissoko N, Neumann G, Kawaoka Y, Hinshaw VS (2001) Influenza virus ns1 protein induces apoptosis in cultured cells. J Virol 75:7875–7881

Selman M, Dankar SK, Forbes NE, Jia J-J, Brown EG (2012) Adaptive mutation in influenza A virus non-structural gene is linked to host switching and induces a novel protein by alternative splicing. Emerg Microbes Infect 1:e42

Shapira SD, Gat-Viks I, Shum BO, Dricot A, de Grace MM, Wu L, Gupta PB, Hao T, Silver SJ, Root DE, Hill DE, Regev A, Hacohen N (2009) A physical and regulatory map of host-influenza interactions reveals pathways in H1N1 infection. Cell 139:1255–1267

Shapiro GI, Gurney T Jr, Krug RM (1987) Influenza virus gene expression: control mechanisms at early and late times of infection and nuclear-cytoplasmic transport of virus-specific RNAs. J Virol 61:764–773

Shaw ML, Palese P (2013) Orthomyxoviridae. In: Knipe D.M. HPH (ed) Fields Virology Sixth Edition, vol 1. Wolters Kluwer Health/Lippincott Williams & Wilkins, Philadelphia, pp 1151–1185

Shimizu K, Mullinix MG, Chanock RM, Murphy BR (1982) Temperature-sensitive mutants of influenza A/Udorn/72 (H3N2) virus. I. Isolation of temperature-sensitive mutants some of which exhibit host-dependent temperature sensitivity. Virology 117:38–44

Shin YK, Li Y, Liu Q, Anderson DH, Babiuk LA, Zhou Y (2007a) SH3 binding motif 1 in influenza A virus NS1 protein is essential for PI3K/Akt signaling pathway activation. J Virol 81:12730–12739

Shin YK, Liu Q, Tikoo SK, Babiuk LA, Zhou Y (2007b) Influenza A virus NS1 protein activates the phosphatidylinositol 3-kinase (PI3K)/Akt pathway by direct interaction with the p85 subunit of PI3K. J Gen Virol 88:13–18

Silverman RH (2007) Viral encounters with 2′, 5′-oligoadenylate synthetase and RNase L during the interferon antiviral response. J Virol 81:12720–12729

Skehel JJ (1973) Early polypeptide synthesis in influenza virus-infected cells. Virology 56:394–399

Solorzano A, Webby RJ, Lager KM, Janke BH, García-Sastre A, Richt JA (2005) Mutations in the NS1 protein of swine influenza virus impair anti-interferon activity and confer attenuation in pigs. J Virol 79:7535–7543

Soubies SM, Volmer C, Croville G, Loupias J, Peralta B, Costes P, Lacroux C, Guerin JL, Volmer R (2010) Species-specific contribution of the four C-terminal amino acids of influenza A virus NS1 protein to virulence. J Virol 84:6733–6747

Spesock A, Malur M, Hossain MJ, Chen LM, Njaa BL, Davis CT, Lipatov AS, York IA, Krug RM, Donis RO (2011) The virulence of 1997 H5N1 influenza viruses in the mouse model is increased by correcting a defect in their NS1 proteins. J Virol 85:7048–7058

Sridharan H, Zhao C, Krug RM (2010) Species specificity of the NS1 protein of influenza B virus: NS1 binds only human and non-human primate ubiquitin-like ISG15 proteins. J Biol Chem 285:7852–7856

Steel J, Lowen AC, Pena L, Angel M, Solorzano A, Albrecht R, Perez DR, García-Sastre A, Palese P (2009) Live attenuated influenza viruses containing NS1 truncations as vaccine candidates against H5N1 highly pathogenic avian influenza. J Virol 83:1742–1753

Steidle S, Martinez-Sobrido L, Mordstein M, Lienenklaus S, García-Sastre A, Staheli P, Kochs G (2010) Glycine 184 in nonstructural protein NS1 determines the virulence of influenza A virus strain PR8 without affecting the host interferon response. J Virol 84:12761–12770

Suarez DL, Perdue ML (1998) Multiple alignment comparison of the non-structural genes of influenza A viruses. Virus Res 54:59–69

Takeuchi O, Akira S (2009) Innate immunity to virus infection. Immunol Rev 227:75–86

Talon J, Horvath CM, Polley R, Basler CF, Muster T, Palese P, García-Sastre A (2000a) Activation of interferon regulatory factor 3 is inhibited by the influenza A virus NS1 protein. J Virol 74:7989–7996

Talon J, Salvatore M, O'Neill RE, Nakaya Y, Zheng H, Muster T, García-Sastre A, Palese P (2000b) Influenza A and B viruses expressing altered NS1 proteins: a vaccine approach. Proc Natl Acad Sci USA 97:4309–4314

Tang Y, Zhong G, Zhu L, Liu X, Shan Y, Feng H, Bu Z, Chen H, Wang C (2010) Herc5 attenuates influenza A virus by catalyzing ISGylation of viral NS1 protein. J Immunol 184:5777–5790

Treanor JJ, Snyder MH, London WT, Murphy BR (1989) The B allele of the NS gene of avian influenza viruses, but not the A allele, attenuates a human influenza A virus for squirrel monkeys. Virology 171:1–9

Twu KY, Kuo RL, Marklund J, Krug RM (2007) The H5N1 influenza virus NS genes selected after 1998 enhance virus replication in mammalian cells. J Virol 81:8112–8121

Twu KY, Noah DL, Rao P, Kuo RL, Krug RM (2006) The CPSF30 binding site on the NS1A protein of influenza A virus is a potential antiviral target. J Virol 80:3957–3965

Vanhaesebroeck B, Guillermet-Guibert J, Graupera M, Bilanges B (2010) The emerging mechanisms of isoform-specific PI3K signalling. Nat Rev Mol Cell Biol 11:329–341

Varble A, Chua MA, Perez JT, Manicassamy B, Garcia-Sastre A, tenOever BR (2010) Engineered RNA viral synthesis of microRNAs. Proc Natl Acad Sci USA 107:11519–11524

Varga ZT, Ramos I, Hai R, Schmolke M, García-Sastre A, Fernandez-Sesma A, Palese P (2011) The influenza virus protein PB1-F2 inhibits the induction of type I interferon at the level of the MAVS adaptor protein. PLoS Pathog 7:e1002067

Versteeg GA, Hale BG, van Boheemen S, Wolff T, Lenschow DJ, García-Sastre A (2010) Species-specific antagonism of host ISGylation by the influenza B virus NS1 protein. J Virol 84:5423–5430

Vincent AL, Ma W, Lager KM, Janke BH, Webby RJ, García-Sastre A, Richt JA (2007) Efficacy of intranasal administration of a truncated NS1 modified live influenza virus vaccine in swine. Vaccine 25:7999–8009

Wacheck V, Egorov A, Groiss F, Pfeiffer A, Fuereder T, Hoeflmayer D, Kundi M, Popow-Kraupp T, Redlberger-Fritz M, Mueller CA, Cinatl J, Michaelis M, Geiler J, Bergmann M, Romanova J, Roethl E, Morokutti A, Wolschek M, Ferko B, Seipelt J, Dick-Gudenus R, Muster T (2010) A novel type of influenza vaccine: safety and immunogenicity of replication-deficient influenza virus created by deletion of the interferon antagonist NS1. J Infect Dis 201:354–362

Wahle E, Keller W (1996) The biochemistry of polyadenylation. Trends Biochem Sci 21:247–250

Walkiewicz MP, Basu D, Jablonski JJ, Geysen HM, Engel DA (2011) Novel inhibitor of influenza non-structural protein 1 blocks multi-cycle replication in an RNase L-dependent manner. J Gen Virol 92:60–70

Wang L, Suarez DL, Pantin-Jackwood M, Mibayashi M, García-Sastre A, Saif YM, Lee CW (2008) Characterization of influenza virus variants with different sizes of the non-structural (NS) genes and their potential as a live influenza vaccine in poultry. Vaccine 26:3580–3586

Wang W, Krug RM (1996) The RNA-binding and effector domains of the viral NS1 protein are conserved to different extents among influenza A and B viruses. Virology 223:41–50

Wang W, Riedel K, Lynch P, Chien CY, Montelione GT, Krug RM (1999) RNA binding by the novel helical domain of the influenza virus NS1 protein requires its dimer structure and a small number of specific basic amino acids. RNA 5:195–205

Wang X, Basler CF, Williams BR, Silverman RH, Palese P, García-Sastre A (2002) Functional replacement of the carboxy-terminal two-thirds of the influenza A virus NS1 protein with short heterologous dimerization domains. J Virol 76:12951–12962

Wang X, Li M, Zheng H, Muster T, Palese P, Beg AA, García-Sastre A (2000) Influenza A virus NS1 protein prevents activation of NF-kappaB and induction of alpha/beta interferon. J Virol 74:11566–11573

Weber F, Kochs G, Haller O (2004) Inverse interference: how viruses fight the interferon system. Viral Immunol 17:498–515

Williams BR (2001) Signal integration via PKR. Sci STKE 89:re2

Wolstenholme AJ, Barrett T, Nichol ST, Mahy BW (1980) Influenza virus-specific RNA and protein syntheses in cells infected with temperature-sensitive mutants defective in the genome segment encoding nonstructural proteins. J Virol 35:1–7

Xu K, Klenk C, Liu B, Keiner B, Cheng J, Zheng BJ, Li L, Han Q, Wang C, Li T, Chen Z, Shu Y, Liu J, Klenk HD, Sun B (2011) Modification of nonstructural protein 1 of influenza A virus by SUMO1. J Virol 85:1086–1098

Yoneyama M, Kikuchi M, Natsukawa T, Shinobu N, Imaizumi T, Miyagishi M, Taira K, Akira S, Fujita T (2004) The RNA helicase RIG-I has an essential function in double-stranded RNA-induced innate antiviral responses. Nat Immunol 5:730–737

Yuan W, Krug RM (2001) Influenza B virus NS1 protein inhibits conjugation of the interferon (IFN)-induced ubiquitin-like ISG15 protein. EMBO J 20:362–371

Zeng W, Sun L, Jiang X, Chen X, Hou F, Adhikari A, Xu M, Chen ZJ (2010) Reconstitution of the RIG-I pathway reveals a signaling role of unanchored polyubiquitin chains in innate immunity. Cell 141:315–330

Zielecki F, Semmler I, Kalthoff D, Voss D, Mauel S, Gruber AD, Beer M, Wolff T (2010) Virulence determinants of avian H5N1 influenza A virus in mammalian and avian hosts: role of the C-terminal ESEV motif in the viral NS1 protein. J Virol 84:10708–10718

Zhao C, Collins MN, Hsiang TY, Krug RM (2013) Interferon-induced ISG15 pathway: an ongoing virus-host battle. Trends Microbiol 21:181–186

Zhao C, Hsiang TY, Kuo RL, Krug RM (2011) ISG15 conjugation system targets the viral NS1 protein in influenza A virus-infected cells. Proc Natl Acad Sci USA 107:2253–2258

Zhirnov OP, Klenk HD (2007) Control of apoptosis in influenza virus-infected cells by up-regulation of Akt and p53 signaling. Apoptosis 12:1419–1432

Zhirnov OP, Konakova TE, Wolff T, Klenk HD (2002) NS1 protein of influenza A virus down-regulates apoptosis. J Virol 76:1617–1625

Zhou B, Li Y, Belser JA, Pearce MB, Schmolke M, Subba AX, Shi Z, Zaki SR, Blau DM, García-Sastre A, Tumpey TM, Wentworth DE (2010) NS-based live attenuated H1N1 pandemic vaccines protect mice and ferrets. Vaccine 28:8015–8025

Role of NK Cells in Influenza Infection

Stacey Schultz-Cherry

Abstract Within days after infection, natural killer (NK) cells are recruited to the lungs and play an essential role in the immune response against influenza infection. Through interactions with the virus itself, as well as viral-infected cells, NK cells secrete a variety of cytokines and can contain viral replication by killing infected cells early after influenza infection. However, the virus has means of evading NK cell responses, including escaping NK cell recognition through mutation of the viral hemagglutinin (HA) protein, regulating HA levels, and by directly infecting and destroying NK cells. Although much of our understanding of NK cell role in influenza infection has come from animal models, there is increasing information from human infection. Studies conducted during the 2009 H1N1 pandemic provided much needed information on the importance of NK cells during human infection and suggest that NK lymphopenia may correlate with increased disease severity. However, more information on how different influenza virus subtypes influence NK cell levels and activities, the role of the different NK cell receptors in infection, and the impact of NK cells on human infection, particularly in high risk populations is needed.

Abbreviations

Dpi	Days post-infection
HA	Hemagglutinin
HPAI	Highly pathogenic avian influenza
IFN	Interferon
KIR	Killer immunoglobulin-like receptor
LPAI	Low pathogenic avian influenza
NA	Neuraminidase
NCR	Natural cytotoxicity receptor

S. Schultz-Cherry (✉)
Department of Infectious Diseases, St. Jude Children's Research Hospital, Danny Thomas Place, Memphis, TN, USA
e-mail: stacey.schultz-cherry@stjude.org

Current Topics in Microbiology and Immunology (2015) 386: 109–120 109
DOI: 10.1007/82_2014_403

Published Online: 4 July 2014

NK	Natural Killer
PBMC	Peripheral blood mononuclear cell
PR8	A/Puerto Rico/8/34 virus
Th2	T helper type-2

Contents

1 Introduction

Natural killer (NK) cells are large granular lymphocytes that are traditionally viewed as the first line of defense against viral infections. Although widely distributed throughout the body, NK cells make up 10 % of the resident lymphocytes in the lung where their survival may be promoted by cytokines and type 1 interferons (IFN) produced by bronchial epithelial cells (Culley 2009; Ge et al. 2004). Within days of infection, or hours after initiation of inflammatory responses, NK cells are recruited to the lung from the blood and become activated to secrete a variety of cytokines, including IFN-γ, through interactions with dendritic cells and macrophages. NK cell signature genes are readily detectable at the early, innate immune response phase and continue into the intermediate phase with a peak at 5 days post-infection (Pommerenke et al. 2012). NK cells not only contain viral replication by killing infected cells early after influenza infection (Stein-Streilein et al. 1983) prior to the development of adaptive immunity, but also play a critical role in the development of the adaptive immune response (Altfeld et al. 2011; Vivier et al. 2008). Our understanding of NK cells is increasing rapidly and their functions go beyond simply being innate "killers." They are potent and early sources of cytokines including T helper type-2 (Th2)-associated cytokines and

IL-10 (Culley 2009). Intriguingly, the existence of NK cell memory, i.e. long-term alteration of NK cell responses according to previous experience, has been recently described (Cooper et al. 2009; Sun et al. 2009).

2 NK Cell Receptors

There is no unifying receptor that identifies all NK cells across different species. Although all are CD3 negative, murine NK cells can be identified by NK1.1 or CD49b, depending on the mouse strain, and further subdivided into four subsets with distinct maturation levels according to their surface expression of CD27 and CD11b (Hayakawa et al. 2010), while human NK cells are typically defined as $CD3^{-}CD56^{+}$, with further subdivision into $CD56^{bright}$ (lack CD16 and killer immunoglobulin-like receptor (KIR)) and $CD56^{dim}$ (express CD16 and KIR) (Jost and Altfeld 2013).

NK cells, unlike B and T cells, also do not appear to express unique receptors for specific antigens. However, they do possess a cache of distinct stimulatory and inhibitory receptors belonging to three major families of molecules involved in the regulation of human and murine NK cell functions. These include the Ig-like transmembrane natural cytotoxicity receptors (NCRs), the C-type lectin-like Ly49 (mice) and KIR receptors (humans), and the NKG2 receptors (Table 1). Engagement of these specific receptors by corresponding ligands results in signal transduction cascades regulating NK functions, including cytolysis by (1) exocytosis of cytoplasmic granules containing perforin and granzyme, (2) Fas ligand-mediated induction of apoptosis, and (3) antibody-dependent cellular cytotoxicity as well as cytokine/chemokine production (Cooper et al. 2001; Jost and Altfeld 2013).

3 NK Cells During Influenza Infection

In both humans and mice, NK cells initially represent a substantial portion of the resident lymphocyte population in healthy lungs, and within days, further cells are recruited to the respiratory tract (van Helden et al. 2012; Wang et al. 2012). Defects in NK cell activity or depletion results in delayed viral clearance and increased morbidity and mortality (Dong et al. 2000; Liu et al. 2004; Nogusa et al. 2008; O'Brien et al. 2011; Stein-Streilein and Guffee 1986; Stein-Streilein et al. 1988). They have also been shown to be involved in osteopontin and *Toxoplasma gondii*-mediated protection against severe influenza infection (O'Brien et al. 2011; Sato et al. 2012). More recently, Kumar et al. demonstrated that conventional NK cells produce IL-22 in response to influenza virus, which is important for tissue regeneration (Kumar et al. 2013).

However, there have been examples of NK cells exacerbating morbidity and pathology during influenza virus infection in mice. Studies from Zhou et al.

Table 1 NK receptors

Receptor family	Species	Receptor	Function
NCR	Mouse	NCR1	Activating
		NKp46(?)	
	Human	NKp46	
		NKp30	
		NKp44	
C-type lectin	Mouse	Ly49A	Inhibitory
		Ly49C	Inhibitory
		Ly49D	Activating
		Ly49H	Activating
		Ly49I	Inhibitory
		Ly49P	Inhibitory
KIR	Human	KIR2DL1	Inhibitory
		KIR2DL2/3	Inhibitory
		KIR2DL/4	Activating
		KIR2DL5	Inhibitory
		KIR2DS1	Activating
		KIR2DS2	Activating
		KIR2DS3	Activating
		KIR2DS4	Activating
		KIR2DS5	Activating
		KIR3DL1	Inhibitory
		KIR3DS2	Activating
		KIR3DL2	Inhibitory
C-type lectin/NKG2	Human, mouse	CD94/NKG2A	Inhibitory
		CD94/NKG2C	Activating
		CD94/NKG2E	Activating
		NKG2D	Activating
	Mouse	NKR-P1	Activating/inhibitory
	Human	NKR-P1A	Inhibitory

suggest that the viral dose may influence NK cell activity. They found that depletion of NK cells from mice infected with a high dose of A/Puerto Rico/8/34 (PR8) virus led to increased survival in contrast to depletion from mice infected with 10-fold less virus who had decreased survival as compared to non-depleted mice (Zhou et al. 2013). Further, adoptive transfer of NK cells from the high dose-infected mice led to increased morbidity and mortality. Although no mechanism was defined, they speculated that enhanced pathology could be a contributing factor. In support of the Zhou studies, Abdul-Careem et al. demonstrated that NK1.1$^+$ cell-depleted mice infected with a high dose of the PR8 virus showed increased resistance to influenza virus-induced pathology (Abdul-Careem et al. 2012). These studies raise the interesting possibility that NK cells may play dual roles during influenza infection, conferring protection or inducing pathology, depending on the viral dose. Further studies are needed to better understand these findings, especially with influenza subtypes associated with differing levels of pathogenicity for mammals.

3.1 NK Cells in Mouse Models of Influenza Infection

Murine models and in vitro experiments have demonstrated that the murine NKp46/NCR1 receptor (Walzer et al. 2007), equivalent to NKp46 in humans, can interact with the hemagglutinin (HA) protein through the sialic acid moieties on the receptor itself, leading to enhanced cytotoxicity against infected cells (Arnon et al. 2004; Gazit et al. 2006; Glasner et al. 2012). It appears that the 3 branched *O*-glycan sequences on the NKp46 glycosylation site are important for recognizing H1 strains (Mendelson et al. 2010). However, given the variability amongst the HA subtypes, the interaction with the NKp46 receptor can vary. For example, NKp46 recognition of H5 viruses was insufficient to mediate direct killing of infected cells in vitro (Achdout et al. 2010). Regardless, H1 and H5 viral infection of NCR1 KO mice resulted in increased viral titers as compared to wild-type control mice, highlighting the importance of NCR1/NKp46 in protection against influenza infection (Achdout et al. 2010), although the interaction of HA with NKp46 is likely more complicated than previously appreciated. Little is known about the influence of other murine NK cell receptors on influenza infection.

3.2 NK Cells in Human Influenza Infection

Although the importance of NK cells in the control of influenza infection is well-documented in mice, less is known about human infection. In vitro studies showed that human NK cells require the interaction between an inhibitory KIR and its ligand to become engaged. Specifically, KIR2DL3+ NK cells obtained from HLA-C1-positive individuals exhibited strong anti-influenza activity. Information from in vivo studies is more limited, although the 2009 H1N1 pandemic afforded a unique opportunity to monitor human NK cell levels.

Jost et al. demonstrated that the absolute numbers of peripheral blood NK cells, particularly CD56^{bright} cells, decreased during acute seasonal or pandemic H1N1 infection as compared to healthy unvaccinated individuals (Jost et al. 2011). CD56^{bright} NK cells have an increased capacity to produce cytokines and proliferate than other NK cell subsets (Bjorkstrom et al. 2010) suggesting that influenza infection may impact the production of cytokines required to promote effective anti-influenza immune responses rather than of other NK cytolytic functions. In a small cohort study in Viet Nam, NK lymphopenia was significantly more common in previously healthy adults that developed severe versus mild pandemic H1N1 influenza virus illness from days 4–11 post-onset and accompanied by decreased CD4 counts (Fox et al. 2012). In support of these studies, additional work showed that the percentage of NK cells among peripheral blood mononuclear cells (PBMCs) was low in three pandemic H1N1 patients with underlying conditions compared to four mild patients, while a subsequent study found a decreased percentage of NK cells in children with moderate and severe infection (Heltzer et al. 2009). Given the many different NK cell subsets, it is possible that particular subsets are more/less associated with disease severity. Indeed, recent work demonstrated that patients with severe pandemic H1N1 infection had significant increases in the percentage of $NKp46^+$ $NKp44^+$ NK cells and proportions of NK cells expressing KIR2DL1 and KIR3DL1, with reductions in the percentages of $NKp46^+$ $NKp44^-$ cells compared to healthy controls (Juarez-Reyes et al. 2013). Combined, these studies suggest that human influenza infection leads to reduced NK cell levels and this may impact disease severity, although further longitudinal cohort studies are needed to verify these findings and define the complex alterations of NK cells that might contribute to influenza pathogenesis.

3.2.1 NK Cells in High Risk Populations

Arguably, the best evidence for the importance of NK cells in human influenza virus infections comes from studies in high risk populations. Neonates, especially small-for-gestational-age (SGA) neonates, have lower NK cells than adults. In response to influenza virus stimulation, neonatal NK cells, especially SGA baby cells, expressed lower antiviral cytokines than adult NK cells. These studies suggest that depressed antiviral activity and lower frequency of NK cells in neonates may play a role in the increased susceptibility to infections seen in this group (Li et al. 2013). Genetic studies of a First Nations community that was severely affected during the first wave of the 2009 H1N1 pandemic revealed that KIR3DL1/S1 allotypes, 3DL1/S1 and 2DL1 ligand-negative pairs, and 2DL2/L3 ligand-positive pairs were enriched among ICU patients, relative to Caucasian populations and ICU non-Aboriginal patients, suggesting possible association with NK cell dysfunction in patients with overactive immune responses to H1N1/09, leading to severe disease (La et al. 2011). Again, further studies are needed in targeted populations to expand upon these preliminary findings.

4 Evasion of NK Cell Activity by Influenza Virus

Although it is evident that NK cells contribute to the immune control of influenza infection, the virus is able to replicate and spread within the infected host, suggesting that it can evade NK cell-mediated immune responses. An early means of escape is through rapid viral replication overwhelming the limited numbers of resident lung NK cells. NK cell infiltration does not typically occur until 5 days post-infection (dpi) (Guo and Topham 2010; Toapanta and Ross 2009; Weiss et al. 2010) while viral replication peaks within 3 dpi (Doherty et al. 2006) allowing sufficient time for the virus to spread in the host. The virus has also evolved numerous mechanisms to specifically evade or escape NK recognition (Guo et al. 2011).

4.1 Mutation of Viral HA

Interaction of NKp46 with the HA protein allows NK cells to recognize and kill influenza virus-infected targets. Yet, HA mutates frequently and rapidly allowing for a possible means to escape recognition by NK cells. For example, cells infected with human H3N2 influenza viruses isolated between 1999 and 2003 are lysed less effectively by NK cells than cells infected with viruses isolated between 1969 and 1996, due to the acquisition of two new glycosylation sites in the HA of the recent viruses. Deletion of either of these potential glycosylation sites from the HA led to increased NK lysis indicating that HA glycosylation may impact NK cell recognition of influenza virus-infected cells (Owen et al. 2007). Further, O-linked glycosylation sites on the NKp46 are also involved in the interaction of H1N1 HA (Glasner et al. 2012; Mendelson et al. 2010) highlighting the complexity of the NK cell receptor-HA interaction and the need to monitor these interactions with diverse and rapidly evolving influenza strains, for example, the highly pathogenic avian (HPAI) H5N1 or the H7N9 viruses.

4.2 Role for Viral Neuraminidase (NA)

As discussed, NKp44 and NKp46 recognize the HA expressed on viral infected cells or when the virus adheres to cells in a sialic-acid dependent mechanism leading to NK cell-mediated killing. Removing NRKp46 sialic acid residues, specifically Thr 225, reduces HA binding (Arnon et al. 2004). Thus, it is not surprising that removal of NK cell sialic acids by the viral NA is another means of escaping NK cell antiviral responses. Elegant studies by Bar-On et al. demonstrated that the viral NA can remove NKp46/NCR1 sialic acids leading to decreased binding to HA and infected cells (Bar-On et al. 2013). Intriguingly, oseltamivir carboxylate treatment of infected cells or mice increased NKp46 binding to recombinant HA and infected cells, and protected PR8 virus-infected mice. Subsequent studies demonstrated that NA had a similar impact on NKp44 (Bar-On et al. 2014). These studies provide another mechanism by which influenza virus can evade NK cell antiviral activity and provide intriguing insight into potential immune modulatory activities of Tamiflu.

4.3 Modulating HA Levels

Sufficient quantities of HA protein must be expressed on the infected target cell surface or on the surface of the free virions for effective interactions with NK cells. In vitro studies demonstrated that the amount of HA affects the binding of the NKp46 and NKp44 receptors to HA (Arnon et al. 2004; Ho et al. 2008). This could be important during replication in vivo where HA levels may be low early and late in infection, leading to decreased NK cytotoxicity. However, high concentrations of viral particles or HA can impair NK cell function (Ali et al. 1984; Mao et al. 2010). In vitro pre-incubating NK cells with 1–10 μg/ml HA concentrations inhibited cell killing potentially by interfering with NKp46-mediated signaling. One can envision where this biphasic effect could significantly impact NK cell activities, where the levels of HA may be too low early in infection allowing for "escaped notice" by NK cells or overwhelming and potentially toxic to NK cells in the case of subtypes that replicate to very high titers quickly, for example, the HPAI H5N1 viruses.

4.4 Seek and Destroy

One of the most effective means to escape an antiviral immune response is to infect and kill immune cells. Indeed, influenza viruses can inhibit NK cells functions by infecting and destroying human (Mao et al. 2009) and murine (Guo et al. 2011) NK cells. In vitro studies with two distinct H1N1 viruses, PR8 with mouse cells and A/Hong Kong/54/98 with human cells, demonstrated that the virus bound to NK cells via sialic acid receptors then underwent clathrin- and caveolin-dependent endocytosis. Although virus replication was abortive, the cells underwent apoptosis resulting in reduced NK cytotoxicity. In vivo, anti-M2 straining in the lung co-localized with NKp46 and lysosome-associated membrane protein 1, a marker for NK cell lytic granules (Alter et al. 2004) and infection of mice with a GFP reporter virus confirmed that a significant proportion of NK cells were GFP positive suggesting that influenza virus may be able to enter cells in vivo (Manicassamy et al. 2010). These studies provide compelling evidence that influenza virus can disarm NK cells through direct infection.

5 Role of NK Cells in Non-mouse, Non-human Influenza Infection

Influenza A viruses have a wide species-tropism where they pose continual public health risks by "jumping" from animal or bird species into humans. Yet, little is known about the role of NK cells in influenza infection in its natural hosts: birds and swine. Intriguingly, similar to the work in mice and humans, it appears that activation and levels of lung NK cells in infected birds may correlate with pathogenicity (Jansen et al. 2013). Chickens infected with low pathogenic avian influenza viruses (LPAI), which exhibit mild clinical signs of infection, had a rapid increase in $CD56^{+}$ NK cells within 1 day post-infection that was complemented with increased CD107 expression. In contrast, infection with a HPAI virus did not lead to increased activation of lung NK cells, although there were similar levels of the virus, and birds died within 36–48 h post-infection. These results suggest that NK cells may be important in disease severity in influenza infected birds, although more work is needed in both avian and swine models.

6 Conclusions and Ways Forward

In contrast to the vast literature on adaptive immune responses against influenza virus infection, we are only beginning to understand the role of innate cellular immunity. Among the first cells recruited to the lung after infection, NK cells are essential for the immune response against influenza infection. Upon recognition of the infected cells or virions by interplay between the NK cell receptors and viral HA, NK cells are poised to destroy infected cells and kick-start the adaptive immune response. However, the virus can counterattack NK cytotoxicity through a variety of mechanisms, highlighting the complexity of the NK cell-virus relationship. However, more information on how different influenza virus subtypes influence NK cell levels and activities, the role for the different NK cell receptors in infection, and the impact of NK cells on human infection, particularly in high-risk populations is needed. Beyond the virus-mediated suppression of NK cell function, we need to understand how factors like age, genetic expression, nutrition, and even immune status/underlying infections impact NK cell functions. In support of this, recent studies in mice highlighted that caloric restriction alters NK cell cytotoxicity during influenza infection potentially by reducing the pool of mature NK cell subsets (Clinthorne et al. 2013; Gardner 2005; Ritz et al. 2008). Further, aged mice have reduced mature NK cells in their periphery, defective IFN-γ production, and impaired degranulation in response to influenza infection. Thus, defects in NK cell function could impair the ability of aged mice to induce an effective antiviral response to influenza (Beli 2011). Finally, we need to define the impact of influenza therapeutics including vaccines, vaccine adjuvants, and antivirals on NK cell activities. Great progress has been made in our understanding of NK cell biology during influenza infection but there is still much to be studied, including the impact of NK cells on influenza infection in swine and birds.

References

Abdul-Careem MF, Mian MF, Yue G, Gillgrass A, Chenoweth MJ, Barra NG, Chew MV, Chan T, Al-Garawi AA, Jordana M, Ashkar AA (2012) Critical role of natural killer cells in lung immunopathology during influenza infection in mice. J Infect Dis 206:167–177. doi:10.1093/infdis/jis340

Achdout H, Meningher T, Hirsh S, Glasner A, Bar-On Y, Gur C, Porgador A, Mendelson M, Mandelboim M, Mandelboim O (2010) Killing of avian and Swine influenza virus by natural killer cells. J Virol 84:3993–4001. doi:10.1128/JVI.02289-09

Ali SA, Rees RC, Oxford J (1984) Modulation of human natural killer cytotoxicity by influenza virus and its subunit protein. Immunology 52:687–695

Alter G, Malenfant JM, Altfeld M (2004) CD107a as a functional marker for the identification of natural killer cell activity. J Immunol Methods 294:15–22. doi:10.1016/j.jim.2004.08.008

Altfeld M, Fadda L, Frleta D, Bhardwaj N (2011) DCs and NK cells: critical effectors in the immune response to HIV-1. Nat Rev Immunol 11:176–186. doi:10.1038/nri2935

Arnon TI, Achdout H, Lieberman N, Gazit R, Gonen-Gross T, Katz G, Bar-Ilan A, Bloushtain N, Lev M, Joseph A, Kedar E, Porgador A, Mandelboim O (2004) The mechanisms controlling the recognition of tumor- and virus-infected cells by NKp46. Blood 103:664–672. doi:10.1182/blood-2003-05-1716

Bar-On Y, Glasner A, Meningher T, Achdout H, Gur C, Lankry D, Vitenshtein A, Meyers AFA, Mandelboim M, Mandelboim O (2013) Neuraminidase-mediated, NKp46-dependent immune-evasion mechanism of influenza viruses. Cell Rep 3:1044–1050. doi:10.1016/j.celrep.2013.03.034

Bar-On Y, Seidel E, Tsukerman P, Mandelboim M, Mandelboim O (2014) Influenza virus uses its neuraminidase protein to evade the recognition of two activating NK cell receptors. J Infect Dis. doi:10.1093/infdis/jiu094

Beli E, Clinthorne JF, Duriancik DM, Hwang I, Kim S, Gardner EM (2011) Natural killer cell function is altered during the primary response of aged mice to influenza infection. Mech Ageing Dev 132:503–510

Bjorkstrom NK, Ljunggren HG, Sandberg JK (2010) CD56 negative NK cells: origin, function, and role in chronic viral disease. Trends Immunol 31:401–406. doi:10.1016/j.it.2010.08.003

Clinthorne JF, Beli E, Duriancik DM, Gardner EM (2013) NK cell maturation and function in C57BL/6 mice are altered by caloric restriction. J Immunol 190:712–722. doi:10.4049/jimmunol.1201837

Cooper MA, Elliott JM, Keyel PA, Yang L, Carrero JA, Yokoyama WM (2009) Cytokine-induced memory-like natural killer cells. Proc Natl Acad Sci USA 106:1915–1919. doi:10.1073/pnas.0813192106

Cooper MA, Fehniger TA, Turner SC, Chen KS, Ghaheri BA, Ghayur T, Carson WE, Caligiuri MA (2001) Human natural killer cells: a unique innate immunoregulatory role for the CD56(bright) subset. Blood 97:3146–3151

Culley FJ (2009) Natural killer cells in infection and inflammation of the lung. Immunology 128:151–163. doi:10.1111/j.1365-2567.2009.03167.x

Doherty PC, Turner SJ, Webby RG, Thomas PG (2006) Influenza and the challenge for immunology. Nat Immunol 7:449–455. doi:10.1038/ni1343

Dong L, Mori I, Hossain MJ, Kimura Y (2000) The senescence-accelerated mouse shows aging-related defects in cellular but not humoral immunity against influenza virus infection. J Infect Dis 182:391–396. doi:10.1086/315727

Fox A, Le NM, Horby P, van Doorn HR, Nguyen VT, Nguyen HH, Nguyen TC, Vu DP, Nguyen MH, Diep NT, Bich VT, Huong HT, Taylor WR, Farrar J, Wertheim H, Nguyen VK (2012) Severe pandemic H1N1 2009 infection is associated with transient NK and T deficiency and aberrant CD8 responses. PLoS One 7:e31535. doi:10.1371/journal.pone.0031535

Gardner EM (2005) Caloric restriction decreases survival of aged mice in response to primary influenza infection. J Gerontol A Biol Sci Med Sci 60:688–694

Gazit R, Gruda R, Elboim M, Arnon TI, Katz G, Achdout H, Hanna J, Qimron U, Landau G, Greenbaum E, Zakay-Rones Z, Porgador A, Mandelboim O (2006) Lethal influenza infection in the absence of the natural killer cell receptor gene Ncr1. Nat Immunol 7:517–523. doi:10.1038/ni1322

Ge N, Nishioka Y, Nakamura Y, Okano Y, Yoneda K, Ogawa H, Sugita A, Yanagawa H, Sone S (2004) Synthesis and secretion of interleukin-15 by freshly isolated human bronchial epithelial cells. Int Arch Allergy Immunol 135:235–242. doi:10.1159/000081309

Glasner A, Zurunic A, Meningher T, Lenac Rovis T, Tsukerman P, Bar-On Y, Yamin R, Meyers AF, Mandeboim M, Jonjic S, Mandelboim O (2012) Elucidating the mechanisms of influenza virus recognition by Ncr1. PloS One 7:e36837. doi:10.1371/journal.pone.0036837

Guo H, Kumar P, Malarkannan S (2011) Evasion of natural killer cells by influenza virus. J Leukoc Biol 89:189–194. doi:10.1189/jlb.0610319

Guo H, Topham DJ (2010) Interleukin-22 (IL-22) production by pulmonary natural Killer cells and the potential role of IL-22 during primary influenza virus infection. J Virol 84:7750–7759. doi:10.1128/JVI.00187-10

Hayakawa Y, Andrews DM, Smyth MJ (2010) Subset analysis of human and mouse mature NK cells. Methods Mol Biol 612:27–38. doi:10.1007/978-1-60761-362-6_3

Heltzer ML, Coffin SE, Maurer K, Bagashev A, Zhang Z, Orange JS, Sullivan KE (2009) Immune dysregulation in severe influenza. J Leukoc Biol 85:1036–1043. doi:10.1189/jlb.1108710

Ho JW, Hershkovitz O, Peiris M, Zilka A, Bar-Ilan A, Nal B, Chu K, Kudelko M, Kam YW, Achdout H, Mandelboim M, Altmeyer R, Mandelboim O, Bruzzone R, Porgador A (2008) H5-type influenza virus hemagglutinin is functionally recognized by the natural killer-activating receptor NKp44. J Virol 82:2028–2032. doi:10.1128/JVI.02065-07

Jansen CA, de Geus ED, van Haarlem DA, van de Haar PM, Londt BZ, Graham SP, Gobel TW, van Eden W, Brookes SM, Vervelde L (2013) Differential lung NK cell responses in avian influenza virus infected chickens correlate with pathogenicity. Sci Rep 3:2478. doi:10.1038/srep02478

Jost S, Altfeld M (2013) Control of human viral infections by natural killer cells. Annu Rev Immunol 31:163–194. doi:10.1146/annurev-immunol-032712-100001

Jost S, Quillay H, Reardon J, Peterson E, Simmons RP, Parry BA, Bryant NN, Binder WD, Altfeld M (2011) Changes in cytokine levels and NK cell activation associated with influenza. PLoS One 6:e25060. doi:10.1371/journal.pone.0025060

Juarez-Reyes A, Noyola DE, Monsivais-Urenda A, Alvarez-Quiroga C, Gonzalez-Amaro R (2013) Influenza virus infection but not H1N1 influenza virus immunization is associated with changes in peripheral blood NK cell subset levels. Clin Vaccine Immunol 20:1291–1297. doi:10.1128/CVI.00194-13

Kumar P, Thakar MS, Ouyang W, Malarkannan S (2013) IL-22 from conventional NK cells is epithelial regenerative and inflammation protective during influenza infection. Mucosal Immunol 6:69–82. doi:10.1038/mi.2012.49

La D, Czarnecki C, El-Gabalawy H, Kumar A, Meyers AF, Bastien N, Simonsen JN, Plummer FA, Luo M (2011) Enrichment of variations in KIR3DL1/S1 and KIR2DL2/L3 among H1N1/09 ICU patients: an exploratory study. PLoS One 6:e29200. doi:10.1371/journal.pone.0029200

Li J, Li H, Mao H, Yu M, Yang F, Feng T, Fan Y, Lu Q, Shen C, Yin Z, Mao M, Tu W (2013) Impaired NK cell antiviral cytokine response against influenza virus in small-for-gestational-age neonates. Cell Mol Immunol 10:437–443. doi:10.1038/cmi.2013.31

Liu B, Mori I, Hossain MJ, Dong L, Takeda K, Kimura Y (2004) Interleukin-18 improves the early defence system against influenza virus infection by augmenting natural killer cell-mediated cytotoxicity. J Gen Virol 85:423–428

Manicassamy B, Manicassamy S, Belicha-Villanueva A, Pisanelli G, Pulendran B, Garcia-Sastre A (2010) Analysis of in vivo dynamics of influenza virus infection in mice using a GFP reporter virus. Proc Natl Acad Sci USA 107:11531–11536. doi:10.1073/pnas.0914994107

Mao H, Tu W, Liu Y, Qin G, Zheng J, Chan PL, Lam KT, Peiris JS, Lau YL (2010) Inhibition of human natural killer cell activity by influenza virions and hemagglutinin. J Virol 84:4148–4157. doi:10.1128/JVI.02340-09

Mao H, Tu W, Qin G, Law HK, Sia SF, Chan PL, Liu Y, Lam KT, Zheng J, Peiris M, Lau YL (2009) Influenza virus directly infects human natural killer cells and induces cell apoptosis. J Virol 83:9215–9222. doi:10.1128/JVI.00805-09

Mendelson M, Tekoah Y, Zilka A, Gershoni-Yahalom O, Gazit R, Achdout H, Bovin NV, Meningher T, Mandelboim M, Mandelboim O, David A, Porgador A (2010) NKp46 O-glycan sequences that are involved in the interaction with hemagglutinin type 1 of influenza virus. J Virol 84:3789–3797. doi:10.1128/JVI.01815-09

Nogusa S, Ritz BW, Kassim SH, Jennings SR, Gardner EM (2008) Characterization of age-related changes in natural killer cells during primary influenza infection in mice. Mech Ageing Dev 129:223–230. doi:10.1016/j.mad.2008.01.003

O'Brien KB, Schultz-Cherry S, Knoll LJ (2011) Parasite-mediated upregulation of NK cell-derived gamma interferon protects against severe highly pathogenic H5N1 influenza virus infection. J Virol 85:8680–8688. doi:10.1128/JVI.05142-11

Owen RE, Yamada E, Thompson CI, Phillipson LJ, Thompson C, Taylor E, Zambon M, Osborn HM, Barclay WS, Borrow P (2007) Alterations in receptor binding properties of recent human influenza H3N2 viruses are associated with reduced natural killer cell lysis of infected cells. J Virol 81:11170–11178. doi:10.1128/JVI.01217-07

Pommerenke C, Wilk E, Srivastava B, Schulze A, Novoselova N, Geffers R, Schughart K (2012) Global transcriptome analysis in influenza-infected mouse lungs reveals the kinetics of innate and adaptive host immune responses. PLoS One 7:e41169. doi:10.1371/journal.pone.0041169

Ritz BW, Aktan I, Nogusa S, Gardner EM (2008) Energy restriction impairs natural killer cell function and increases the severity of influenza infection in young adult male C57BL/6 mice. J Nutr 138:2269–2275. doi:10.3945/jn.108.093633

Sato K, Iwai A, Nakayama Y, Morimoto J, Takada A, Maruyama M, Kida H, Uede T, Miyazaki T (2012) Osteopontin is critical to determine symptom severity of influenza through the regulation of NK cell population. Biochem Biophys Res Commun 417:274–279. doi:10.1016/j.bbrc.2011.11.100

Stein-Streilein J, Bennett M, Mann D, Kumar V (1983) Natural killer cells in mouse lung: surface phenotype, target preference, and response to local influenza virus infection. J Immunol 131:2699–2704

Stein-Streilein J, Guffee J (1986) In vivo treatment of mice and hamsters with antibodies to asialo GM1 increases morbidity and mortality to pulmonary influenza infection. J Immunol 136:1435–1441

Stein-Streilein J, Guffee J, Fan W (1988) Locally and systemically derived natural killer cells participate in defense against intranasally inoculated influenza virus. Reg Immunol 1:100–105

Sun JC, Beilke JN, Lanier LL (2009) Adaptive immune features of natural killer cells. Nature 457:557–561. doi:10.1038/nature07665

Toapanta FR, Ross TM (2009) Impaired immune responses in the lungs of aged mice following influenza infection. Respir Res 10:112. doi:10.1186/1465-9921-10-112

van Helden MJ, Zaiss DM, Sijts AJ (2012) CCR2 defines a distinct population of NK cells and mediates their migration during influenza virus infection in mice. PLoS One 7:e52027. doi:10.1371/journal.pone.0052027

Vivier E, Tomasello E, Baratin M, Walzer T, Ugolini S (2008) Functions of natural killer cells. Nat Immunol 9:503–510. doi:10.1038/ni1582

Walzer T, Blery M, Chaix J, Fuseri N, Chasson L, Robbins SH, Jaeger S, Andre P, Gauthier L, Daniel L, Chemin K, Morel Y, Dalod M, Imbert J, Pierres M, Moretta A, Romagne F, Vivier E (2007) Identification, activation, and selective in vivo ablation of mouse NK cells via NKp46. Proc Natl Acad Sci USA 104:3384–3389. doi:10.1073/pnas.0609692104

Wang J, Li F, Zheng M, Sun R, Wei H, Tian Z (2012) Lung natural killer cells in mice: phenotype and response to respiratory infection. Immunology 137:37–47. doi:10.1111/j.1365-2567.2012.03607.x

Weiss ID, Wald O, Wald H, Beider K, Abraham M, Galun E, Nagler A, Peled A (2010) IFN-gamma treatment at early stages of influenza virus infection protects mice from death in a NK cell-dependent manner. J Interferon Cytokine Res 30:439–449. doi:10.1089/jir.2009.0084

Zhou G, Juang SW, Kane KP (2013) NK cells exacerbate the pathology of influenza virus infection in mice. Eur J Immunol 43:929–938. doi:10.1002/eji.201242620

Host Detection and the Stealthy Phenotype in Influenza Virus Infection

Pradyot Dash and Paul G. Thomas

Abstract The innate host response to influenza virus infection plays a critical role in determining the subsequent course of infection and the clinical outcome of disease. The host has a diverse array of detection and effector mechanisms that are able to recognize and initiate effective antiviral responses. In opposition, the virus utilizes a number of distinct mechanisms to evade host detection and effector activity in order to remain "stealthy" throughout its replication cycle. In this review, we describe these host and viral mechanisms, including the major pattern recognition receptor families (the TLRs, NLRs, and RLRs) in the host and the specific viral proteins such as NS1 that are key players in this interaction. Additionally, we explore nonreductive mechanisms of viral immune evasion and propose areas important for future inquiry.

Contents

P. Dash · P.G. Thomas (✉)
Department of Immunology, St. Jude Children's Research Hospital,
Memphis, TN 38105, USA
e-mail: paul.thomas@stjude.org

Current Topics in Microbiology and Immunology (2015) 386: 121–147

DOI: 10.1007/82_2014_412

Published Online: 20 July 2014

1 Introduction

Influenza virus is a pleomorphic enveloped virus of approximately 100 nm in diameter, containing a single-stranded negative sense segmented genome. The genus *Influenzavirus* belongs to the family *Orthomyxoviridae* and consists of three serotypes: Influenza A, B, and C. Influenza A viruses show considerable sequence variation in their surface glycoproteins, hemagglutinin (HA) and neuraminidase (NA). Based on phylogenetic and serological analyses, Influenza A virus (IAV) is known to contain 17 HA and 10 NA subtypes (Shaw and Palese 2007). Only H1, H2, H3 and N1 and N2 subtypes have been known to cause sustained human-human infection and transmission. Occasionally, animal viruses such as H5N1, H9N2, and H7N9 infected humans as well and are capable of causing severe disease; additional, subclinical infections likely occur with other strains but are not detected due to the absence of symptoms (Wang et al. 2009; Uyeki et al. 2012; Imai et al. 2012; Herfst et al. 2012; Gao et al. 2013; Song et al. 2014). The influenza B virus (IBV) is structurally similar to IAV but only one subtype of HA has been found. IAV and IBV each contain eight segments in their genomes, whereas Influenza C virus (ICV) consists of only seven segments. Influenza C virus (ICV) has a surface glycoprotein known as the hemagglutinin-esterase-fusion (HEF) protein that mediates both binding and fusion and possesses an additional receptor destroying enzymatic activity (analogous to the NA of IAV and IBV) that destroys the HEF-9-O-acetylated sialic acid by enzymatic removal of the acetyl group. Thus, the ICV do not have a separate protein with neuraminidase activity (Luo 2012).

The eight segments of influenza A virus encodes 13 proteins (Palese and Shaw 2007). Of these 8 segments, segment 1, 4, 5, 6 are monocistronic and encode for PB2, HA, NP, and NA proteins, respectively. The other segments (2, 3, 7, and 8) in addition to their primary transcripts and proteins, also generate additional proteins by alternative splicing or frame shifts. Segment 2 that encodes the polymerase subunit PB1 also expresses two other proteins in some strains by ribosomal frame shift due to leaky ribosomal scanning: PB1-F2 and PB1-N40 (Chen et al. 2001; Wise et al. 2009). PB1-F2 is 87 amino acids in length and has been described as a virulence factor causing cell death. However, the contribution of PB1-F2 to virulence is still not clear since the protein is normally found to be expressed in avian strains and eliminated by truncation when adapted to mammalian hosts (Zell et al. 2007). Notably, the swine strains of IAV lack expression of PB1-F2 (Chen et al. 2001; Zell et al. 2007; McAuley et al. 2010). In addition, the effect of PB1-F2 on cell death was found to be cell (Chen et al. 2001; Yamada et al. 2004) and strain specific (McAuley et al. 2010). For some strains, an additional virulence factor, PB1-N40, was recently identified (Wise et al. 2009), although the function of this protein is not well-known. In vitro, though not essential, it has been reported to support virus replication (Wise et al. 2009). The third segment of IAV primarily expresses the viral protein PA, and recently has been reported to express an alternate product termed PA-X (Jagger et al. 2012). Additionally, the mRNA from segments 7 and 8 of IAV that encode for M1 and NS1, respectively, also give rise to alternatively spliced mRNA that express M2 and NS2, also known as NEP (Palese and Shaw 2007).

2 Influenza Virus Infection of Host Cell

The primary target cells for influenza virus infection are the respiratory epithelial cells of the upper respiratory (e.g., nasal airways and trachea) and the lower respiratory (small airways and lungs) tracts (Sanders et al. 2011). The prevailing view is that infection by the virus is achieved by HA-binding to these cells via sialic acid moieties on the cell surface, which triggers internalization of the virus via endocytosis. Early studies on influenza virus entry using electron microscopy and radioisotope-labeled viruses suggested that phagocytosis (perhaps indistinguishable from receptor-mediated endocytosis at that time) is a major route for virus entry (Patterson et al. 1979; Matlin et al. 1981). The endocytic pathway involves both clathrin-mediated and nonclathrin-, noncaveolin-mediated endocytosis (Sieczkarski and Whittaker 2002; Rust et al. 2004). An alternative pathway, macropinocytosis, has been described for entry of large filamentous and spherical influenza virions (de Vries et al. 2011; Rossman et al. 2012). Though it is speculated that internalization of viruses through pinocytic vesicles will converge with the endocytic pathway at some point, the exact route and kinetics of merging is not known (de Vries et al. 2011). Apart from endocytosis and pinocytosis, reports have described influenza virus infection of cells by attachment to the plasma membrane followed by direct release of the viral contents into the cytoplasm (Hoyle and Finter 1957; Morgan and Rose 1968; White et al. 1981). This pathway is similar to a mechanism used by many other viruses, e.g., SFV (White et al. 1980), HIV (27, 28), CMV (Compton et al. 1992), RSV (Srinivasakumar et al. 1991), and HSV (Sarmiento et al. 1979). It was shown that, in mildly acidic pH conditions, influenza virus can fuse to the plasma membrane of MDCK cells (Matlin et al. 1981). Another study observed direct fusion by electron microscopy in infected chorioallantoic membrane (an ex vivo, polarized, epithelial structure), suggesting that viral entry pathways may be dependent on the type and differentiation of the target cells (Morgan and Rose 1968). Indeed, work with well-differentiated human airway epithelial cell cultures found that broad-spectrum neuraminidase treatment did not affect influenza virus entry, though it did alter the entry of hPIV3, another sialic acid receptor-using virus (Kogure et al. 2006; Thompson et al. 2006). Further, cells lacking sialylated N-glycans can be infected with influenza virus (Stray et al. 2000; Thompson et al. 2006; Nicholls et al. 2007; Oshansky et al. 2011; de Vries et al. 2012) suggesting an alternative, nonsialic acid receptor-dependent route exists.

However, in most cell types and experimental systems that have been studied, the influenza virus HA initiates host cell infection by binding to sialic acid receptors. The HA subtypes of the well-adapted human IAV have been described to bind to α (2, 6)-sialic acid linkages preferentially. In contrast, the avian-adapted HA subtypes preferentially bind to α (2, 3)-sialic acid linkages. In polarized cells, influenza virus infection through the endocytic route results in internalization of the virus into early endosomes in an actin-dependent manner (Sun and Whittaker 2007) followed by trafficking through the endocytic network in a multistep process (Lakadamyali et al. 2003, 2006; Sieczkarski and Whittaker 2003). Release of viral nucleic acids from the endosome following binding and endocytosis of the virus is a key step in initiating productive infection and requires trafficking of virus containing endosomes. During this trafficking to the late endosomal stage, the interior pH of the endosome drops, which is sensed by the tetrameric viral M2 protein causing the M2 ion channel to assume an open configuration (Pinto et al. 1992). The H^+ ions enter into the virion through this opening causing destabilization of the M1 protein from the ribonucleic protein (RNP) complex of the virus. Lowering of pH further induces conformational changes of the HA2 subunit resulting in exposure of the hydrophobic fusion peptide motif of the HA. When the fusion peptide comes in close apposition of the endosomal membrane, the peptide is inserted into the membrane (White and Wilson 1987; Xu and Wilson 2011; Fontana et al. 2012). Several HA molecules come together to form a cluster known as the "fusogenic unit" and the individual HA unit undergoes further conformational changes resulting in fusion of the viral envelope and capsid with the endosomal membrane and formation of the pore (Hamilton et al. 2012). The pH of activation of HA varies among IAV strains, thus playing an important role in determining the fitness of the virus in the infection process.

Following the pH-dependent fusion and formation of the pore between the virion and endosomal membranes, the viral RNPs are released into the cytoplasm (frequently described as uncoating). The RNPs are then transported to the nucleus where transcription of the viral genome occurs using the viral RNA-dependent RNA polymerase (RdRp), generating 5′ cap structures with short nucleotides derived from host cell mRNA. This is achieved by the binding of the PB2 subunit of the viral RdRp to the 5′ cap of host mRNAs and subsequent cleaving by the PA subunit approximately 10–15 nt downstream of the cap structure. The elongation of the mRNA from the viral genome is carried out by the PB1 subunit using the 5′cap + nucleotides as primers, which also adds a polyadenylated [poly(A)] tail by means of a stuttering mechanism on a sequence of uridine residues near the 5′ end of the negative-strand genome. The viral mRNAs are transported back to the cytoplasm for translation. In the nucleus, the genome of the virus is also replicated through an intermediate RNA template (cRNA) step by the RdRp. This intermediate lacks the poly (A) tail or any 5′ modification. In the nucleus, newly synthesized genomes are encapsidated with NP, RdRP subunits, PB2, PB1, and PA to form RNPs and are transported to the cytoplasm by binding with M1 and NEP. Other viral components such as HA, NA, and M2 are transported to the plasma membrane via the Golgi network and assemble with RNPs to form mature virus particles that are released from the cell via budding (Palese and Shaw 2007)

3 Host Cell Response to Influenza Virus

Upon infection of respiratory epithelial cells with influenza virus, the host rapidly initiates an innate immune response. The first responder to the virus infection is the infected cell itself, which plays a major role in coordinating the ensuing innate immune response. Viral induction of the innate immune response can be divided into early (initiation and amplification) and late responses (local systemic response) that cause the recruitment of innate cells to the site of infection. Sensors on the cell surface, endosomes, and cytosol have been found to detect ligands such as incoming virus particles or their unique molecular signatures. These sensors activate downstream signaling and induce two types of responses: an antiviral response and a proinflammatory response. Subsequently, concurrent viral replication generates more of these ligands (within the first few hours) which amplify these responses in infected (in the first replication cycle of the virus) and neighboring cells (following release of progeny virus). Production of a variety of cytokines and chemokines in the initiation phase of the early response locally attracts other cellular mediators of the innate response including neutrophils, macrophages, monocytes, and NK cells. In this review, we discuss the early innate immune response to IAV and the viral strategies and characteristics that evade this host cell response.

As mentioned above, the host cell possesses an array of innate immune sensors to detect components of invading pathogens that are nonself. Alternatively, there are also sensors that recognize host cell-derived components under certain pathologic conditions such as the cellular stress response often associated with infection, metabolic disorders, and cancer. These sensors are collectively termed as pattern recognition receptors (PRRs). The PRRs recognize unique molecular signatures known as pathogen-associated molecular patterns (PAMPs), which are nonself. The self-derived molecular patterns arising following pathogen infection and/or cellular stress responses, such as reactive oxygen species (ROS), ATP, changes in ion flux, and denatured cytosolic and nuclear contents, including DNA from necrotic cells, are broadly termed danger-associated molecular patterns (DAMPs). Thus, PRRs, by sensing DAMPs, can also play a role in tissue homeostasis (Marshak-Rothstein 2006). To date, known PRRs have been classified into five major groups: Toll-like receptors (TLRs), retinoic acid-inducible gene-I (RIG-I) like receptors (RLRs), nucleotide oligomerization and binding domain (NOD) like receptors (NLRs), C-type lectin receptors (CLRs) and the Pyrin-HIN (PYHIN) domain containing family that includes AIM2. It has been shown that at least three (TLRs, RLRs and NLRs) out of the above five PRR families play a role in innate immunity to influenza virus infection (Lupfer and Kanneganti 2013). We will discuss them in detail below.

There is considerable variation in the expression pattern of the PRRs in tissues and at the cellular level. In general, the TLRs are both intracellular (compartmentalized and cytosolic) and on the cell surface, whereas the RLRs and NLRs are exclusively cytosolic. Consequently, these PRRs demonstrate differential recognition for various PAMPs and DAMPs.

3.1 Toll-Like Receptors

Among the PRRs, the Toll receptor in Drosophila was first shown to be important for protection against fungal infection (Lemaitre et al. 1996). Subsequently, the mammalian homologue of the Toll receptors, the TLRs, were described for humans and mice (Kawai and Akira 2011). Thus far, there have been 10 and 12 TLRs described for humans and mice, respectively. Based on sequence comparisons of several vertebrate genomes, the TLRs are classified into six major families based on PAMP recognition (Roach et al. 2005). They are: TLR1 (TLR 1, TLR2, TLR6 and TLR10 (only in human)), TLR3 (TLR3), TLR4 (TLR4), TLR5 (TLR5), TLR7 (TLR7, TLR8 (human-only) and TLR9) and TLR11 (mouse only, including TLR11, TLR12 and TLR13). Each family recognizes a general class of PAMPs (Roach et al. 2005). The TLRs reported to play a role in antiviral immunity include TLR3, TLR7, TLR8, and TLR9. TLR expression varies across different cell types. There have been differing reports on the location of TLR3 on epithelial cells, perhaps resulting from the differentiation status of the cells in cultures across different experiments. Using primary cell cultures, it was shown that TLR3 expression is limited to the cell surface in human bronchial epithelial cell lines (BEAS-2B) (Hewson et al. 2005) and fibroblasts (Matsumoto et al. 2002). Expression was upregulated upon rhinovirus infection and active virus replication (Hewson et al. 2005). In contrast, Guilott et al., showed intracellular expression of TLR3 in uninfected BEAS-2B cells and the human lung carcinoma cell line A549 (Guillot et al. 2005). Expression of TLRs 1 to 6 has been reported in polarized mouse uterine epithelial cells (Soboll et al. 2006). Similarly, cervical epithelial cells of female mice express mRNA for TLR3, TLR9, and TLR7, but had only a weak signal for TLR8 (Andersen et al. 2006). Macrophages, fibroblasts, and some epithelial cell lines express TLR3 both on the cell surface and in the early endosome (Cario and Podolsky 2000). Recently, using an immunofluorescence technique on an in vitro polarized model of human alveolar epithelial cells (AEC) and frozen human tracheal tissues, which are important cells for influenza virus infection, Ioannidis et al. reported that TLR1 and TLR3 are expressed on both apical and basolateral surfaces of the hAEC (Ioannidis et al. 2013). In contrast, TLR2 and TLR6 were predominantly expressed basolaterally. TLR4, TLR5, TLR7, TLR9, and TLR10 were expressed weakly on the apical side or the luminal surface of the epithelial cells. It was also reported that TLR3, TLR7, and TLR9, which have been reported to be expressed only on the endosomal compartment of the DC (Muzio et al. 2000; Matsumoto et al. 2003; Funami et al. 2004), were found to be present in both intracellular and apical surfaces mostly restricted to the cilial border of human tracheal epithelium (Ioannidis et al. 2013). No TLR8 expression was found in respiratory epithelial cells in vivo and in vitro (Ioannidis et al. 2013).

The TLRs are classified as type I trans-membrane proteins with extracellular leucine-rich repeats that recognize cognate ligands, a trans-membrane domain, and a cytoplasmic domain consisting of a conserved signaling Toll/interleukin-1 receptor (TIR) domain. It has been reported that endosomal acidification is required for the activation of TLRs such as TLR3 (Ioannidis et al. 2013) and TLR9 (Macfarlane and Manzel 1998). Stimulation of TLRs with PAMPs can lead to downstream signaling in two main pathways: the MyD88 signaling pathway (proinflammatory) and the TRIF signaling pathway (antiviral). All TLRs except TLR3 activate NFκB and the IRF3/7 response in a MyD88-dependent manner for signaling. TLR3 exclusively uses the TRIF-dependent pathway, whereas TLR4 uses both the TRIF and MyD88 pathways (Takeuchi and Akira 2007).

The prominent cytokines of the antiviral response are the type I and type III interferons (IFN). In humans, the type I IFNs comprises IFN-α, IFN-β, IFN-ω, IFN-ε, and IFN-κ (Samuel 2001). There are 13 different subtypes of IFN-α and only one IFN-β characterized in human (Díaz and Testa 1996). The type III IFNs consist of IFN-λ1, λ2, and λ3 (also known as IL29, IL28A and IL28B, respectively) (Kotenko et al. 2003; Sheppard et al. 2003) and have been described to play important roles in epithelial antiviral responses (Durbin et al. 2013).

Since IAV infects through the endocytic route, one might expect that TLR3, TLR7, and TLR8 should be major sensors for IFN induction by viral infection. Early studies showed that TLR7 plays a major role in sensing influenza viral RNA (Diebold et al. 2004; Lund et al. 2004). pDC derived from mice deficient in TLR7 showed marked decreases in IFNα production in tissue culture supernatants after infection (Diebold et al. 2004; Lund et al. 2004). Since uncoating of the viral RNA from the endocytosed virion into the cytoplasm occurs in a carefully orchestrated maturation process, the precise mechanisms by which the IAV RNA exposure to TLR7 occurs in the endosome is currently not known. It was suggested that proteosomal degradation of some virions in the endosomes may lead to exposure of the viral RNA to TLR7 (Diebold et al. 2004). It also can be speculated that following viral replication de novo generated viral RNA is released from dead or dying cells or by phagocytosis of dead cells allowing the viral RNA to enter the endocytic route, resulting in TLR7 mediated recognition and signaling. Alternatively, differential entry such as pinocytosis or isolated endocytic vesicles containing virions that failed to achieve the optimal pH of activation (see discussion below) may lead to lysosomal degradation, thus exposing the viral RNA to TLR7.

The role for TLR3 in recognition of IAV was shown to be more proinflammatory than antiviral. It was found that after TLR3 stimulation the BEAS-B2 cells produced more of the proinflammatory cytokines IL6 and IL8 and less IFN-β (Le Goffic et al. 2007). Interestingly, TLR3-/- mice were shown to have a survival advantage after infection with IAV, despite higher viral loads and lower viral clearance (Le Goffic et al. 2006) indicating that perhaps these proinflammatory cytokines are not essential for effective viral clearance. A similar phenomenon was seen in TLR4 knockout mice, which had better survival than the TLR4 sufficient animals after IAV infection (Imai et al. 2008; Nhu et al. 2010). Though a specific ligand derived from IAV is not known for TLR4, it was shown that endogenous oxidized phospholipids (Imai et al. 2008) and proteins such as S100A9 (Tsai et al. 2014) produced in response to the acute lung injury in IAV infection can act as DAMPs and stimulate the TLR4-TRIF-NF-κB signaling pathway. The authors of these two reports went on to demonstrate that enhanced acute lung injury was alleviated by the elimination of IL6 in H5N1 and IAV PR8 infected mice, though contributions by cytokines other than IL6 cannot be ruled out.

A role for TLR10 has recently been described in influenza infection (Lee et al. 2014). The authors reported that H1N1 and H5N1 infection of primary human macrophages and a human monocyte cell line induced type I and III IFNs and proinflammatory cytokines IL8 and IL6 in a TLR10-dependent manner. H5N1 virus infection induced robust TLR10 expression, indicating that the severe inflammation seen in influenza infection can be amplified by positive feedback through TLR10. TLR10 induction required active replication of the virus; however, the viral component(s) that induced the TLR10-dependent inflammatory response have not been identified. Although TLR10-knockdown reduced the expression of IFNs and cytokines, it did not have any effect on viral replication (Lee et al. 2014), suggesting that TLR10 signaling may play a role in shaping local innate effectors such as monocytes and macrophages and influencing the adaptive immune response, rather than modulating the antiviral response within the epithelial cell. While these reports highlight a negative role in clinical outcomes for TLR3 and TLR4 in mice and TLR10 in in vitro cultures, associated with heightened inflammation, it is possible that at least one PRR is necessary for effective control of the virus through initiation of an appropriate inflammatory response leading to functional wound healing. These situations might represent a special case of virulent viruses, as is the case for both pathogenic H5N1 and to a lesser extent PR8, where stimulation of these TLRs results in an inappropriate inflammatory response and pathogenesis.

Finally, the nonclassical PRR PAR2 (proteinase-activated receptor) is expressed on epithelial cells of the respiratory and gastrointestinal tract and works synergistically with TLR4 to suppress TLR3—mediated IRF3 activation and induction of ISGs. Mice deficient in PAR2 or TLR4 were protected from influenza–associated disease, potentially as a result of derepression of the TLR3-IRF3 signaling pathway (Nhu et al. 2010).

3.2 *RIG-I-Like Receptors (RLRs)*

The RIG-I-like receptors or the RLRs consist of three members identified in humans and mice: the Retinoic acid-inducible gene-I (RIG-I, also known as DDX58), melanoma differentiation-associated gene 5 (MDA5), and laboratory of genetics and physiology 2 (LGP2, also known as DHX58). RIG-I and MDA5 consist of two N-terminal caspase recruitment domains (CARD), a central DExD/H box helicase with RNA binding and ATPase functions, and a C-terminal domain consisting of a regulatory domain (absent in MDA-5). In contrast, the LGP-2 does not have the CARD domain but contains a DExD/H box helicase and a regulatory domain similar to that of RIG-I, which is absent in MDA-5. The regulatory domain keeps the molecule in a closed conformation, inhibiting downstream signaling prior to activation. Upon ligand interaction, RIG-I and LGP are thought to undergo a conformational change leading to activation of antiviral signaling (Saito et al. 2007). The RLRs have been reported to be expressed in most tissue types and are maintained typically at low levels (Loo and Gale 2011). However, following infection or interferon exposure, the expression of the RLRs was shown to be greatly increased (Kang et al. 2004; Yoneyama et al. 2004; Tatsuta et al. 2012). Increased expression following ectopic overexpression (Yoneyama et al. 2005) or infection in the absence of IFN signaling (Yount et al. 2007) suggests that this low intrinsic basal expression pattern in part regulates unnecessary and potentially detrimental RLR activation in the homeostatic condition.

RIG-I and MDA-5 are key sensors of infection mediated by RNA viruses. They share structural and functional similarities but detect mostly nonoverlapping groups of viruses. Over the last few years, RIG-I has been shown to play a role in triggering innate immune responses to infection by negative-strand viruses such as paramyxoviruses, orthomyxoviruses, rhabdoviruses such as vesicular stomatitis virus, Ebola virus, and EBER RNA, carried by the Epstein-Barr virus (Kato et al. 2006; Cárdenas et al. 2006; Samanta et al. 2006; Yoneyama and Fujita 2007). In contrast, MDA-5 has been implicated in sensing positive strand RNA viruses such as picornaviruses (Kato et al. 2006; Gitlin et al. 2006). Certain flaviviruses induce innate immune responses via RIG-I and MDA5 (Sumpter et al. 2005; Chang et al. 2006; Fredericksen and Gale 2006; Kato et al. 2006; Loo et al. 2008). The ligands for both RIG-I and MDA-5 have been identified primarily through infection with a variety of viruses or transfection with viral or synthetic RNA such as Poly (I)(C) (Sumpter et al. 2005; Kato et al. 2006; Saito et al. 2007; Liu et al. 2007). Using RIG-I-deficient animals, Kato et al. showed that RIG-I plays an important role in initiating antiviral responses in fibroblasts and conventional DC but not plasmacytoid DC (Kato et al. 2005). Conversely, TLRs drive the initiation of antiviral responses in pDC with no contribution from RIG-I (Kato et al. 2005). Initially it was suggested that RIG-I and MDA5 were involved in sensing dsRNA generated from viral infection (Kang et al. 2002; Yoneyama et al. 2004; Andrejeva et al. 2004; Yoneyama et al. 2005; Rothenfusser et al. 2005). It was further shown that while RIG-I may be involved in recognition of short dsRNAs of less than 1 kb, MDA-5 is responsible for sensing long dsRNA (>1 kb) (Kato et al. 2008). Subsequently, it was reported that the 5′ triphosphate-linked ssRNA characteristic of viral RNA products can be recognized by RIG-I (Hornung et al. 2006; Pichlmair et al. 2006). Later, it was found that RIG-I responds to short dsRNAs with a triphosphorylated 5′ terminus and poly-U/A-rich sequences, while MDA5 activation is more dependent on complex dsRNA structures (Hornung et al. 2006; Kato et al. 2008; Saito and Gale 2008; Schlee et al. 2009; Schmidt et al. 2009; Pichlmair et al. 2009; Binder et al. 2011). A role for RIG-I in the detection of RNA products from DNA virus infections has also been described. Cellular RNA polymerase III can convert double-stranded DNA poly(dA-dT) to a short dsRNA species with a 5′-triphosphate that triggers the RIG-I pathway in human and mouse cells (Chiu et al. 2009).

In contrast, LGP2 which lacks signaling CARDs, binds to both dsRNA (Pippig et al. 2009) and single-stranded RNA with 5′-triphosphates via its C-terminal regulatory domain with greater affinity than RIG-I and MDA5 (Takahasi et al. 2009). There have been contrasting reports on the role of LGP2 in viral RNA sensing and signaling by RLR. While it was suggested that LGP2 inhibits RIG-I signaling and activity both in vitro (Yoneyama et al. 2005) and in vivo (Rothenfusser et al. 2005), augmentation of MDA5 signaling by LGP2 was also shown (Venkataraman et al. 2007; Satoh et al. 2010). LGP2 functions in cDC but not in pDC (Satoh et al. 2010) and is dispensable for the recognition of synthesized dsRNA and 5′ triphosphate RNA (Saito et al. 2007).

While many of the above studies involved chemically synthesized or virus-derived RNA, the exact molecular signature of the RNA (analogous to the specific epitope in adaptive immunity) is poorly studied. Saito et al mapped these unique signatures to two regions of the HCV genome: nucleotides 2406–3256 and 8872–9616, by measuring IFN-β promoter activity (Saito et al. 2008). Similarly, in IAV, single stranded viral RNA with a 5′ triphosphate derived from in vitro RNP reconstitution assays were shown to be the ligand for RIG-I, with the strength of IFNβ induction similar for all IAV gene segments (Rehwinkel et al. 2010). Surprisingly, in the absence of mRNA transcription, IFNβ induction was enhanced, suggesting the vRNA and cRNA (which do not have 5′ triphosphate), but not the mRNA, are potent inducers of IFN via RIG-I pathway (Rehwinkel et al. 2010) indicating molecular signatures in the termini may be playing a role. Indeed, recently a short region (27 nt) of 5′ UTR and a longer region of 3′ UTR of the IAV NS gene segment was shown to induce RIG-I dependent IFN-β induction (Davis et al. 2012). Further, a U/A rich region within the 3′ UTR was shown to be a potent inducer in a 5′ triphosphate-independent manner (Davis et al. 2012).

Interestingly, it was shown that infection of mice with a virus (PR8) stock containing high defective interfering (DI) particle content had increased protection compared to the group infected with low DI content (Tapia et al. 2013). The DI influenza particles are incomplete virus particles with shorter genome segments but identical termini (Tapia et al. 2013). In the case of influenza, the DI genome is mostly enriched for PB2, PB1, PA (Saira et al. 2013), and M gene (Noble and Dimmock 1995). Tapia and colleagues showed Sendai virus DI particles generated in cells during the course of a normal infection induced stronger antiviral responses than the cells with full length virus genomes (Tapia et al. 2013). Though a direct measurement of the antiviral cytokines produced between the high and low DI particle-containing IAV infections was not shown in those studies, it is tempting to assume that the 3′ and 5′ termini of the IAV DI may be a better stimulant of RIG-I and thus cause greater IFN production. More recently, direct recognition of IAV RNPs by RIG-I has been reported (Weber et al. 2013) suggesting that our knowledge of the nature of the ligands that activate these sensors is incomplete.

3.3 Nod-Like Receptors (NLRs)

The NLR family consists of a large number (20) of intracellular sensors with a conserved nucleotide oligomerization domain (NOD) (Lupfer and Kanneganti 2013). At the N-terminus, the NLRs contain a protein interacting caspase activation and recruitment (CARD) or pyrin domain (PYD) that drive recruitment and binding to the protein caspase-1 directly, or through an intermediate interaction with the adaptor protein, apoptosis-associated speck-like protein containing a CARD (ASC) . At the C-terminus, NLRs contain a variable leucine-rich repeat (LRR) involved in PAMP sensing (Strowig et al. 2012). The NLRs have been shown to be expressed in a variety of cells and are also induced after influenza infection (Ichinohe et al. 2009; Allen et al. 2009).

Of the known NLRs, stimulation of NLRP1, NLRP3, and NLRC4 with PAMPs and DAMPs causes activation of the caspase-1 containing inflammasome (Thomas et al. 2009; Malireddi et al. 2010; Masters et al. 2012). The activated caspase-1 cleaves inactive pro-IL1β and pro-IL18 to their active form (Black et al. 1989) which then signals through target cell receptors to induce an array of proinflammatory cytokines, including, KC, MIP1α, IL6, TNFα, and IFN-γ (Dinarello et al. 1998; Allen et al. 2009; Thomas et al. 2009). Alternatively, caspase-1 activation can lead to a cell death known as pyroptosis (Bergsbaken et al. 2009). Other NLRs such as NLRP12 (Zaki et al. 2011) and NLRP6 (Anand et al. 2012), have been implicated in down-modulating canonical NF-κB signaling, thus acting as anti-inflammatory stimuli.

The ligands that induce NLR signaling are thus far not well-defined. Initially, it was suggested that dsRNA but not ssRNA could induce activation of the NLRP3 inflammasome in a TLR3-independent manner (Kanneganti et al. 2006; Rajan et al. 2010). Infection of NLRP3-deficient macrophages with the IAV PR8 strain did not activate caspase-1, while wild type macrophages had robust activation (Kanneganti et al. 2006). However, it is known that influenza virus does not generate dsRNA during replication (Weber et al. 2006). Indeed, intraperitoneal injection of NLRP3-deficient mice with influenza viral RNA derived from stock virus resulted in reduced IL1β and Il18 production compared to wild type animals (Allen et al. 2009; Thomas et al. 2009). Additionally, our own studies and related work observed decreased survival to influenza virus infection in NLRP3-deficient mice (Allen et al. 2009; Thomas et al. 2009). Another report using similar mice found defective adaptive immune responses to IAV, but failed to see any difference in mortality (Ichinohe et al. 2009). This work used a different infection dose than the other studies, which may account for the difference in mortality. The absence of NLRP3 also caused reduced cellular infiltration to the lungs and an improper wound healing response, but did not compromise type IFN induction (Thomas et al. 2009).

While direct recognition of the RNA ligands by NLRs is still under investigation, other viral components have been reported to induce antiviral responses. The IAV M2 protein ion channel activates the inflammasome in an NLRP3-dependent manner (Ichinohe et al. 2010). Other chemical stimuli such as uric acid crystals (Martinon et al. 2006), silica, and asbestos, (Dostert et al. 2008; Hornung et al. 2008), changes in intracellular ion flux (Franchi et al. 2007; Pétrilli et al. 2007), abnormal reactive oxygen species (ROS) (Dostert et al. 2008; Allen et al. 2009), and abnormal protein aggregates such as amyloid-β (Halle et al. 2008) have been suggested to activate NLRs as second messengers. Endosomal destabilization has also been implicated in the activation of NLRP3 inflammasome (Hornung and Latz 2010; Tschopp 2011). The absence of a known ligand and the diverse nature of the ligands that have found to stimulate NLRs have led to a two signal model for inflammasome activation (Meylan et al. 2006; Ogura et al. 2006). In this model, initial upstream signals such as TLR, RLR, or the cellular stress response (ATP/ROS/endosomal destabilization) induces transcription and translation of proIL1β, proIL18, and NLRP3 as a part of the proinflammatory program, which is followed by a second signal triggering NLRP3 to activate caspase-1 and produce active IL1β and IL18.

Apart from these indirect roles in inflammasome activation, recent reports have suggested a direct interaction of the PRRs in the assembly of the inflammasome that does not require NLRs. Poeck et al. showed that after infection with the negative-strand virus VSV, RIG-I, rather than initiating its canonical sensing of ssRNA and signaling through MAVS, instead interacts with CARD9–Bcl-10-ASC causing inflammasome assembly and caspase-1 activation in an NLRP3-independent manner (Poeck et al. 2010). Similar observations were also found by Pothichet et al., who reported an overlapping TLR3/RIG-I/NLRP3 pathway in inflammasome activation by IAV in normal human bronchial epithelial cells (Pothlichet et al. 2013). The authors suggest that RIG-I occupies the most upstream position in this pathway. When it senses viral ssRNA, it induces the MAVS-IFN pathway. In addition, as shown by Poeck et al., they also found RIG-I interactions with ASC and caspase-1. They went on to suggest that IFN-driven upregulation of TLR3 and NLRP3 sets off a positive feedback loop of inflammasome activation (Pothlichet et al. 2013). This provided a direct example of a two signal model of NLR activation as suggested before.

NLRC1 (NOD1) and NLRC2 (NOD2) have been known to signal through the adapter protein RIPK2 (also known as RICK or RIP2) and induce NFκB and MAPK signaling. A role for NOD2 as a viral PRR has been shown. Transfection of viral genomes derived from RSV, IAV and PIV into A549 cells showed IRF3 activation in a NOD2-dependent manner (Sabbah et al. 2009). Another indirect role for NOD2 in inhibition of viral replication has been described (Dugan et al. 2009). NOD2 increases the enzymatic activity of OAS2 which in turn enhances the activity of RNAse L to degrade viral RNA (Malathi et al. 2007; Dugan et al. 2009). Finally, Lupfer et al. showed that IAV infection results in RIPK2-induced mitophagy in infected cells. This process is not NFkB or MAPK dependent (Lupfer et al. 2013).

4 Evasion Strategy by Influenza Virus

Due to their clinical importance, significant work has been conducted to understand how influenza viruses can evade effective antiviral responses. The NS1 protein has received most of the attention, along with contributions from some other viral determinants. However, other "nonreductive" features of the viral life cycle also appear to contribute to a stealthy phenotype but cannot be easily ascribed to an isolate feature of the viral genome. We discuss both types of strategies below.

4.1 Viral Determinant of Innate Immune Evasion

The eighth segment of influenza virus encodes the NS gene, consisting of two separate products: NS1 and NEP (NS2). NS1 plays a major role in regulating the host cell response (García-Sastre 2011). It has been implicated in the inhibition of dsRNA sensors such as TLR3 by sequestering dsRNA intermediates (Talon et al. 2000). Though a known dsRNA ligand from IAV infection has not been detected (Weber et al. 2006), it is possible that NS1 may be targeting downstream pathways and RNA sensors, including RIG-I (Guo et al. 2007; Rehwinkel et al. 2010) to inhibit antiviral responses. NS1 has been shown to interact directly with RIG-I (Mibayashi et al. 2007) and indirectly via binding to ligand RNA (Pichlmair et al. 2006; Rehwinkel et al. 2010). However, NS1 inhibition of the ubiquitin ligase tripartite motif containing protein 25 (TRIM25) has been observed, preventing the ubiquitination of RIG-I which limits its signal transduction activity (Gack et al. 2009). This suggests there are multiple, possibly overlapping, pathways for NS1 to inhibit RIG-I activation. Further downstream, NS1 has also been found to inhibit activation and nuclear translocation of the transcription factors IRF3 (Talon et al. 2000), NF-κB (Wang et al. 2000) and ATF-2/c-Jun (Ludwig et al. 2002). In vivo infections of mice and pigs with IAV NS1 mutants have demonstrated reduced pathogenesis (Garcia-Sastre et al. 1998; Talon et al. 2000; Donelan et al. 2003; Falcon et al. 2005; Solórzano et al. 2005).

Limiting host cell protein synthesis as a viral evasion strategy has been described for multiple viruses (157), reducing the antiviral response and channeling the host cell protein synthesis machinery for replication of the virus. IAV has been observed to utilize this strategy via the viral protein PA-X, which is translated from the PA gene segment in an alternative reading frame (Desmet et al. 2013). Similarly, NS1 has been implicated in the alteration of host cell mRNA by binding to cleavage and polyadenylation specificity factor (CPSF30) (Nemeroff et al. 1998; Noah et al. 2003). Other polymerase proteins have been implicated in suppression of host cell protein synthesis. The well-described "cap snatching mechanism" involving PB2 and PA for viral mRNA transcription (Plotch et al. 1981; Dias et al. 2009) has been suggested to reduce the levels of capped host mRNAs, attenuating host cell gene expression including the antiviral response (Nakhaei et al. 2009).

The phosphatidylinositol-3-kinases (PI3K) are a family of enzymes involved in cellular functions such as cell growth, proliferation, differentiation, motility, survival, and intracellular trafficking (Datta et al. 1999). IAV NS1 has been shown to induce PI3K activation by direct binding of the p85 subunit (Hale et al. 2006). Later in the infection, NS1 induced activation of PI3K and its downstream effector AKT/Protein kinase B prevents premature apoptosis and favors viral replication.

Recombinant IAV with a deletion of NS1 induces a stronger caspase-1 activity and higher IL1-β and IL18 levels in primary human macrophages (Stasakova et al. 2005). This result indicates a role for NS1 in antagonizing the NLR pathway. Although the precise mechanism of such antagonism is not known, it is possible that NS1, by virtue of its ability to perturb PKR and RIG-I pathways, can eliminate the priming signal for subsequent NLRP3 inflammasome activation.

Apart from NS1 and PA-X, the other protein that has been well studied for a role in innate immune evasion is PB1-F2. PB1-F2 is a small protein of 87aa encoded by an alternate reading frame within the PB1 gene and originally described to be proapoptotic (Chen et al. 2001). Later, it was shown that PB1-F2 mediates cell death via interaction with the mitochondrial proteins ANT3 and VDAC1 (Zamarin et al. 2005). Murine infection with IAV deficient in PB1-F2 showed reduced pathogenesis in mice (Zamarin et al. 2006). It was further shown that the N66S amino acid residue may contribute to the increased virulence associated with H5N1 and the 1918 pandemic H1N1 (Conenello and Palese 2007; McAuley et al. 2007). However, the recent pandemic 2009 H1N1 strain lacked a functional PB1-F2, yet showed increased virulence over prior seasonal strains. Engineering PB1-F2 into the 2009 strain had a minimal effect on virulence in animal models (Hai et al. 2010; Pena et al. 2012) indicating that virulence can represent a strain-specific combination of multiple determinants of host and viral factors. Additionally, PB1-F2 has been described to decrease mitochondrial membrane potential by binding to MAVS and inhibiting induction of IFN (Varga et al. 2012).

4.2 Nonreductive Determinants of Viral Fitness

Apart from specific viral proteins and domains that play a role in the evasion of the innate immune response, other features of the virus such as its spherical or elongated shape, its replication fitness, which represents a compound result of many specific features, its secondary RNA structure may also play a role in the ability of the virus to be stealthy and establish infection without detection by host cell recognition machinery.

Role of HA in Entry

The HA in different virus subtypes and strains can vary with regard to the optimum pH of activation (Mittal et al. 2003). For example, the HA molecule of H2 subtype undergoes a slow pH-dependent conformational change compared to the H3-HA molecule (Puri et al. 1990; Leikina et al. 2002). Similarly, the stability of the pH dependent conformational change has also been reported to be influenced by the density of the surface HA molecules (Markovic et al. 2001; Leikina et al. 2002). Experimental work with H5N1 viruses and mutants in the A/chicken/Vietnam/C58/04 (H5N1) background found that the optimal pH of activation is a key contributor to the observed increased pathogenesis. Using mutants that differ only, or primarily, in their optimum pH of activation, Zarket et al. showed that a higher pH of activation is highly pathogenic in avian species whereas a lower pH of activation favors pathogenesis in mice (Zaraket et al. 2013b). In another study, the same group showed that a mutant IAV (VN/1203-K58I) whose pH of activation is 5.5 compared to the wild type strain's pH of 6.0 grew to similar titers as the wild type virus in MDCK and NHBE cells, but not in A549 cells (which have a lower endosomal pH than either of those cell types), resulting in reduced growth (Zaraket et al. 2013a). Interestingly, they found that an increase in acid stability resulted in increased virus growth in the upper respiratory tract. However, the mutation was not sufficient to confer transmission in ferrets, indicating that additional cell type specific features of endosomal pH activation may be playing a role in this in vivo model. Thus, it is clear that the HA sequence determine the stability of the HA with regard to pH, and by extension the genetic and environmental stability of the virus and its replication potential (Reed et al. 2010).

Role of HA in Exit

The HA also plays a role in the exit of the virus from the cell by budding. HA proteins in infected cells are synthesized as polypeptides (HA0) which lack membrane fusion activity (Skehel and Wiley 2000). To acquire this functionality, the HA0 must be cleaved by host cell proteases at the linker sequence between the HA1 and HA2 subunits, which are then reorganized to the mature HA molecule that is expressed on the surface of the virion (Garten and Klenk 1999). Thus, the expression pattern of host cell proteases has been suggested to play a critical role in the tissue restriction of IAV replication. Although the array of proteases that can mediate cleavage of HA0 is only beginning to be detailed, the established role of specific proteases in tissue tropism and pathogenesis provides an illustrative example. It has been reported that the HA in low pathogenic avian influenza viruses (LPAIV) can only be cleaved by certain trypsin like proteases expressed exclusively in the respiratory tract (of terrestrial birds) or the gastrointestinal tract (of water fowl and other terrestrial birds), resulting in the restriction of viral replication in those tissue compartments (Bertram et al. 2010). In contrast, the highly pathogenic avian influenza virus (HPAIV) contains a polybasic cleave site in its HA that is readily cleaved by a ubiquitously expressing protease, furin, in the trans-golgi network, resulting in systemic infection and severe disease (Bosch et al. 1981; Webster and Rott 1987; Perdue et al. 1997). However, it appears that the cleavability of the HA is not the only determinant of pathogenesis as HPAIV and known pandemic strains lacking furin multibasic cleavage sites have caused severe disease in human populations (Bertram et al. 2010).

RNA Accessibility

One may hypothesize that influenza virus infections utilizing distinct methods of entry (endocytosis, macropinocytosis, or penetration of RNP by plasma membrane fusion) may result in very different host responses, considering the localization of innate immune receptor distribution. Especially in the physiological setting with a low multiplicity of infection, such differential entry into the target cells will result in a variation in the kinetics of accessibility of the viral RNA to the host cytoplasmic sensors. It has been reported that IAV entering by endocytosis localizes to early endosome within 10 min and to the late endosome by 40 min after infection in HeLa cells (Sieczkarski and Whittaker 2003). However, the entry kinetics appear to vary by cell type. Viral fusion with the endosome has been detected as early as 10 min in MDCK and CHO cells (Yoshimura et al. 1982; Yoshimura and Ohnishi 1984; Lakadamyali et al. 2003). It is interesting to note that influenza infection of HeLa cells is found to be inefficient (Lohmeyer et al. 1979; Gujuluva et al. 1994). In contrast, we might speculate that virus internalized by macropinocytosis may take an even longer time (compared to endocytosis in HeLa cells) to reach the optimum low pH for virus uncoating. Another consideration is that the endocytic vesicle, regardless of the method of internalization, may fail to achieve fusion with the virus particle as a result of stochastic processes, resulting in diversion of the virion into the lysosomal pathway and autophagic destruction. It has been suggested that autophagy can present viral nucleic acid to TLRs in endolysomes (Kawai and Akira 2009). Thus, viruses with increased HA acid stability may enter endolysomes and the autophagy pathway, resulting in induction of IFN via TLR7/RIG I pathway. On the other hand, viruses that fuse at the plasma membrane and release RNPs may be more likely to encounter the RIG-I pathway (Weber et al. 2013) and initiate the antiviral response more quickly. Of note, differentiated human bronchial epithelial cells derived from asthmatic patients mounted an enhanced activation of the inflammasome and innate immune signaling after IAV infection (Bauer et al. 2012). It is reported that the pH of the bronchial tree mucous in asthmatic patients is around 5.3 (Ryley and Brogan 1968) as opposed to the normal range of 6.9–9.0 in the trachea (Karnad et al. 1990). Although apical pH data from these cultures was not reported, it has been suggested that cultures from cystic fibrosis patients also exhibit a more acidic pH than those from healthy individuals (Coakley et al. 2003). In summary, under acidic pH conditions, IAV can fuse directly to the plasma membrane (Matlin et al. 1981) and release RNPs to the cytosol directly (Morgan and Rose 1968). Thus, we can hypothesize that those viral genomes may be recognized faster than viruses entering through the endocytic route, resulting in faster initiation of the innate immune response. However, very little research has been done on the role of such differential entry affecting the proinflammatory and antiviral responses, and further investigation is warranted.

Genomic Features

Another aspect of RNA accessibility in determining the stealthy phenotype of influenza virus is the viral genome itself. Detection by both RIG-I and MDA-5 of flaviviruses suggests that these viruses may have genomic features that trigger both sensors (Loo et al. 2008). Similarly, within a given virus, distinct strains may have more "innate immunogenic" features by virtue of different sequences. Limited studies attempting to define the exact features of the RNA ligand stimulating immune responses from HCV (Saito et al. 2008) and IAV (Davis et al. 2012) indicated that certain regions of the genome may be more immunogenic than others. While studies from Davis et al., suggested that the 3′ and 5′ UTR of the IAV containing U/A tracts are potent innate immune inducers, little is known about the rest of the viral genome. It can be assumed that certain subtypes and strains may have more of these immunogenic features (potentially defined by secondary structures and sequence composition) than others.

Another factor that may contribute to viral stealthiness is the presence of defective interfering (DI) particle, which, until recently, has been shown to be a phenomenon of in vitro viral propagation (Von Magnus 1954; Nayak 1980). Recently, the presence of DI particles in human samples infected with pandemic H1N1 has been described (Saira et al. 2013). Another group has also described the presence of "semi infectious" particles in vitro as well as in vivo propagated virus inoculums (Brooke et al. 2013). Using immunofluorescence staining for four different viral proteins, the authors proposed that 90 % of infectious inocula failed to establish productive infection by lacking expression of one or more viral proteins (Brooke et al. 2013). This was independent of cell type in the presence of an intact IFN system, though presence of partial RNA similar to DI particles in this "semi-infectious" population could not be ruled out (Brooke et al. 2013). We can imagine that the presence or absence of DI particles or "semi-infectious" particles in inocula may play an important role in determining in the outcome of infection and the efficiency of transmission.

5 Conclusion and Future Direction

In sum, multiple compound features of viral entry, trafficking and replication can combine to allow the virus to evade host recognition to greater or lesser extents. Given the exponential growth of the virus with each round of replication, even a slight advantage in early replication kinetics can result in a significant alteration in viral titers and clinical and pathological outcomes (Askovich et al. 2013). Dissecting these "whole virus" features presents a new challenge for influenza research, which made great strides in the last decade using reverse genetics technology. Systems biology and other high-throughput approaches will be necessary to provide insights into these areas of influenza virus biology.

Acknowledgment The authors were supported by NIH/NIAID Contracts HHSN266200700005C (St. Jude Center of Excellence for Influenza Research and Surveillance) and HHSN272200800058C (Systems Influenza).

References

Allen IC, Scull MA, Moore CB et al (2009) The NLRP3 inflammasome mediates in vivo innate immunity to influenza A virus through recognition of viral RNA. Immunity 30:556–565. doi:10.1016/j.immuni.2009.02.005

Anand PK, Malireddi RKS, Lukens JR et al (2012) NLRP6 negatively regulates innate immunity and host defence against bacterial pathogens. Nature 488:389–393. doi:10.1038/nature11250

Andersen JM, Al-Khairy D, Ingalls RR (2006) Innate immunity at the mucosal surface: role of toll-like receptor 3 and toll-like receptor 9 in cervical epithelial cell responses to microbial pathogens. Biol Reprod 74:824–831. doi:10.1095/biolreprod.105.048629

Andrejeva J, Childs KS, Young DF et al (2004) The V proteins of paramyxoviruses bind the IFN-inducible RNA helicase, mda-5, and inhibit its activation of the IFN-β promoter. Proc Natl Acad Sci U S A 101:17264–17269. doi:10.1073/pnas.0407639101

Askovich PS, Sanders CJ, Rosenberger CM et al (2013) Differential host response, rather than early viral replication efficiency, correlates with pathogenicity caused by influenza viruses. PloS One 8:e74863. doi:10.1371/journal.pone.0074863

Bauer RN, Brighton LE, Mueller L et al (2012) Influenza enhances caspase-1 in bronchial epithelial cells from asthmatic volunteers and is associated with pathogenesis. J Allergy Clin Immunol 130:958–967 e14. doi:10.1016/j.jaci.2012.07.013

Bergsbaken T, Fink SL, Cookson BT (2009) Pyroptosis: host cell death and inflammation. Nat Rev Microbiol 7:99–109. doi:10.1038/nrmicro2070

Bertram S, Glowacka I, Steffen I et al (2010) Novel insights into proteolytic cleavage of influenza virus hemagglutinin. Rev Med Virol 20:298–310. doi:10.1002/rmv.657

Binder M, Eberle F, Seitz S et al (2011) Molecular mechanism of signal perception and integration by the innate immune sensor retinoic acid-inducible gene-I (RIG-I). J Biol Chem 286:27278–27287. doi:10.1074/jbc.M111.256974

Black RA, Kronheim SR, Sleath PR (1989) Activation of interleukin-1 beta by a co-induced protease. FEBS Lett 247:386–390

Bosch FX, Garten W, Klenk HD, Rott R (1981) Proteolytic cleavage of influenza virus hemagglutinins: primary structure of the connecting peptide between HA1 and HA2 determines proteolytic cleavability and pathogenicity of Avian influenza viruses. Virology 113:725–735

Brooke CB, Ince WL, Wrammert J et al (2013) Most influenza a virions fail to express at least one essential viral protein. J Virol 87:3155–3162. doi:10.1128/JVI.02284-12

Cárdenas WB, Loo Y-M, Gale M Jr et al (2006) Ebola virus VP35 protein binds double-stranded RNA and inhibits alpha/beta interferon production induced by RIG-I signaling. J Virol 80:5168–5178. doi:10.1128/JVI.02199-05

Cario E, Podolsky DK (2000) Differential alteration in intestinal epithelial cell expression of toll-like receptor 3 (TLR3) and TLR4 in inflammatory bowel disease. Infect Immun 68:7010–7017

Chang T-H, Liao C-L, Lin Y-L (2006) Flavivirus induces interferon-beta gene expression through a pathway involving RIG-I-dependent IRF-3 and PI3K-dependent NF-kappaB activation. Microbes Infect Inst Pasteur 8:157–171. doi:10.1016/j.micinf.2005.06.014

Chen W, Calvo PA, Malide D et al. (2001) A novel influenza A virus mitochondrial protein that induces cell death. Nat Med 7:1306–1312. http://dx.doi.org/10.1038/nm1201-1306

Chiu Y-H, Macmillan JB, Chen ZJ (2009) RNA polymerase III detects cytosolic DNA and induces type I interferons through the RIG-I pathway. Cell 138:576–591. doi:10.1016/j.cell.2009.06.015

Coakley RD, Grubb BR, Paradiso AM et al (2003) Abnormal surface liquid pH regulation by cultured cystic fibrosis bronchial epithelium. Proc Natl Acad Sci U S A 100:16083–16088. doi:10.1073/pnas.2634339100

Compton T, Nepomuceno RR, Nowlin DM (1992) Human cytomegalovirus penetrates host cells by pH-independent fusion at the cell surface. Virology 191:387–395

Conenello GM, Palese P (2007) Influenza A virus PB1-F2: a small protein with a big punch. Cell Host Microbe 2:207–209. http://dx.doi.org/10.1016/j.chom.2007.09.010

Datta SR, Brunet A, Greenberg ME (1999) Cellular survival: a play in three Akts. Genes Dev 13:2905–2927

Davis WG, Bowzard JB, Sharma SD et al (2012) The 3' untranslated regions of influenza genomic sequences are 5'PPP-independent ligands for RIG-I. PloS One 7:e32661. doi:10.1371/journal.pone.0032661

Desmet EA, Bussey KA, Stone R, Takimoto T (2013) Identification of the N-terminal domain of the influenza virus PA responsible for the suppression of host protein synthesis. J Virol 87:3108–3118. doi:10.1128/JVI.02826-12

Dias A, Bouvier D, Crépin T et al (2009) The cap-snatching endonuclease of influenza virus polymerase resides in the PA subunit. Nature 458:914–918. doi:10.1038/nature07745

Díaz MO, Testa D (1996) Type I interferon genes and proteins. Biotherapy Dordr Neth 8:157–162

Diebold SS, Kaisho T, Hemmi H et al (2004) Innate antiviral responses by means of TLR7-mediated recognition of single-stranded RNA. Science 303:1529–1531. doi:10.1126/science.1093616

Dinarello CA, Novick D, Puren AJ et al (1998) Overview of interleukin-18: more than an interferon-gamma inducing factor. J Leukoc Biol 63:658–664

Donelan NR, Basler CF, Garcia-Sastre A (2003) A recombinant influenza A virus expressing an RNA-binding-defective NS1 protein induces high levels of beta interferon and is attenuated in mice. J Virol 77:13257–13266

Dostert C, Pétrilli V, Van Bruggen R et al (2008) Innate immune activation through Nalp3 inflammasome sensing of asbestos and silica. Science 320:674–677. doi:10.1126/science.1156995

Dugan JW, Albor A, David L et al (2009) Nucleotide oligomerization domain-2 interacts with 2'-5'-oligoadenylate synthetase type 2 and enhances RNase-L function in THP-1 cells. Mol Immunol 47:560–566. doi:10.1016/j.molimm.2009.09.025

Durbin RK, Kotenko SV, Durbin JE (2013) Interferon induction and function at the mucosal surface. Immunol Rev 255:25–39. doi:10.1111/imr.12101

Falcon AM, Fernandez-Sesma A, Nakaya Y, et al. (2005) Attenuation and immunogenicity in mice of temperature-sensitive influenza viruses expressing truncated NS1 proteins. J Gen Virol 86:2817–2821. http://dx.doi.org/10.1099/vir.0.80991-0

Fontana J, Cardone G, Heymann JB et al (2012) Structural changes in Influenza virus at low pH characterized by cryo-electron tomography. J Virol 86:2919–2929. doi:10.1128/JVI.06698-11

Franchi L, Kanneganti T-D, Dubyak GR, Núñez G (2007) Differential requirement of P2X7 receptor and intracellular K+ for caspase-1 activation induced by intracellular and extracellular bacteria. J Biol Chem 282:18810–18818. doi:10.1074/jbc.M610762200

Fredericksen BL, Gale M Jr (2006) West Nile virus evades activation of interferon regulatory factor 3 through RIG-I-dependent and -independent pathways without antagonizing host defense signaling. J Virol 80:2913–2923. doi:10.1128/JVI.80.6.2913-2923.2006

Funami K, Matsumoto M, Oshiumi H et al (2004) The cytoplasmic "linker region" in Toll-like receptor 3 controls receptor localization and signaling. Int Immunol 16:1143–1154. doi:10.1093/intimm/dxh115

Gack MU, Albrecht RA, Urano T et al (2009) Influenza A virus NS1 targets the ubiquitin ligase TRIM25 to evade recognition by the host viral RNA sensor RIG-I. Cell Host Microbe 5:439–449. doi:10.1016/j.chom.2009.04.006

Gao H-N, Lu H-Z, Cao B et al (2013) Clinical findings in 111 cases of influenza A (H7N9) virus infection. N Engl J Med 368:2277–2285. doi:10.1056/NEJMoa1305584

García-Sastre A (2011) Induction and evasion of type I interferon responses by influenza viruses. Virus Res 162:12–18. doi:10.1016/j.virusres.2011.10.017

Garcia-Sastre A, Egorov A, Matassov D et al (1998) Influenza A virus lacking the NS1 gene replicates in interferon-deficient systems. Virology 252:324–330

Garten W, Klenk HD (1999) Understanding influenza virus pathogenicity. Trends Microbiol 7:99–100

Gitlin L, Barchet W, Gilfillan S et al (2006) Essential role of mda-5 in type I IFN responses to polyriboinosinic: polyribocytidylic acid and encephalo myocarditis picornavirus. Proc Natl Acad Sci U S A 103:8459–8464. doi:10.1073/pnas.0603082103

Le Goffic R, Balloy V, Lagranderie M et al (2006) Detrimental contribution of the Toll-like receptor (TLR)3 to influenza A virus-induced acute pneumonia. PLoS Pathog 2:e53. doi:10.1371/journal.ppat.0020053

Le Goffic R, Pothlichet J, Vitour D et al (2007) Cutting Edge: Influenza A virus activates TLR3-dependent inflammatory and RIG-I-dependent antiviral responses in human lung epithelial cells. J Immunol Baltim Md 1950 178:3368–3372

Guillot L, Le Goffic R, Bloch S et al (2005) Involvement of toll-like receptor 3 in the immune response of lung epithelial cells to double-stranded RNA and influenza A virus. J Biol Chem 280:5571–5580. doi:10.1074/jbc.M410592200

Gujuluva CN, Kundu A, Murti KG, Nayak DP (1994) Abortive replication of influenza virus A/WSN/33 in HeLa229 cells: defective viral entry and budding processes. Virology 204:491–505. doi:10.1006/viro.1994.1563

Guo Z, Chen L, Zeng H et al (2007) NS1 protein of influenza A virus inhibits the function of intracytoplasmic pathogen sensor, RIG-I. Am J Respir Cell Mol Biol 36:263–269. doi:10.1165/rcmb.2006-0283RC

Hai R, Schmolke M, Varga ZT et al (2010) PB1-F2 Expression by the 2009 Pandemic H1N1 Influenza Virus Has Minimal Impact on Virulence in Animal Models. J Virol 84:4442–4450. doi:10.1128/JVI.02717-09

Hale BG, Jackson D, Chen Y-H et al (2006) Influenza A virus NS1 protein binds p85beta and activates phosphatidylinositol-3-kinase signaling. Proc Natl Acad Sci U S A 103:14194–14199. doi:10.1073/pnas.0606109103

Halle A, Hornung V, Petzold GC et al (2008) The NALP3 inflammasome is involved in the innate immune response to amyloid-beta. Nat Immunol 9:857–865. doi:10.1038/ni.1636

Hamilton BS, Whittaker GR, Daniel S (2012) Influenza virus-mediated membrane fusion: determinants of hemagglutinin fusogenic activity and experimental approaches for assessing virus fusion. Viruses 4:1144–1168. doi:10.3390/v4071144

Herfst S, Schrauwen EJA, Linster M et al (2012) Airborne transmission of influenza A/H5N1 virus between ferrets. Science 336:1534–1541. doi:10.1126/science.1213362

Hewson CA, Jardine A, Edwards MR et al (2005) Toll-like receptor 3 is induced by and mediates antiviral activity against rhinovirus infection of human bronchial epithelial cells. J Virol 79:12273–12279. doi:10.1128/JVI.79.19.12273-12279.2005

Hornung V, Bauernfeind F, Halle A et al (2008) Silica crystals and aluminum salts activate the NALP3 inflammasome through phagosomal destabilization. Nat Immunol 9:847–856. doi:10.1038/ni.1631

Hornung V, Ellegast J, Kim S et al (2006) 5′-Triphosphate RNA is the ligand for RIG-I. Science 314:994–997. doi:10.1126/science.1132505

Hornung V, Latz E (2010) Critical functions of priming and lysosomal damage for NLRP3 activation. Eur J Immunol 40:620–623. doi:10.1002/eji.200940185

Hoyle L, Finter NB (1957) The use of influenza virus labelled with radio-sulphur in studies of the early stages of the interaction of virus with the host cell. J Hyg (Lond) 55:290–297

Ichinohe T, Lee HK, Ogura Y et al (2009) Inflammasome recognition of influenza virus is essential for adaptive immune responses. J Exp Med 206:79

Ichinohe T, Pang IK, Iwasaki A (2010) Influenza virus activates inflammasomes via its intracellular M2 ion channel. Nat Immunol 11:404–410. doi:10.1038/ni.1861

Imai M, Watanabe T, Hatta M et al (2012) Experimental adaptation of an influenza H5 HA confers respiratory droplet transmission to a reassortant H5 HA/H1N1 virus in ferrets. Nature 486:420–428. doi:10.1038/nature10831

Imai Y, Kuba K, Neely GG et al (2008) Identification of oxidative stress and Toll-like receptor 4 signaling as a key pathway of acute lung injury. Cell 133:235–249. doi:10.1016/j.cell.2008.02.043

Ioannidis I, Ye F, McNally B et al (2013) Toll-like receptor expression and induction of type I and type III interferons in primary airway epithelial cells. J Virol 87:3261–3270. doi:10.1128/JVI.01956-12

Jagger BW, Wise HM, Kash JC et al (2012) An overlapping protein-coding region in influenza A virus segment 3 modulates the host response. Science 337:199–204. doi:10.1126/science.1222213

Kang D, Gopalkrishnan RV, Wu Q et al (2002) mda-5: An interferon-inducible putative RNA helicase with double-stranded RNA-dependent ATPase activity and melanoma growth-suppressive properties. Proc Natl Acad Sci U S A 99:637–642. doi:10.1073/pnas.022637199

Kang D-C, Gopalkrishnan RV, Lin L et al (2004) Expression analysis and genomic characterization of human melanoma differentiation associated gene-5, mda-5: a novel type I interferon-responsive apoptosis-inducing gene. Oncogene 23:1789–1800. doi:10.1038/sj.onc.1207300

Kanneganti T-D, Body-Malapel M, Amer A et al (2006) Critical role for Cryopyrin/Nalp3 in activation of caspase-1 in response to viral infection and double-stranded RNA. J Biol Chem 281:36560–36568. doi:10.1074/jbc.M607594200

Karnad DR, Mhaisekar DG, Moralwar KV (1990) Respiratory mucus pH in tracheostomized intensive care unit patients: Effects of colonization and pneumonia. Crit Care Med 18:699–701

Kato H, Sato S, Yoneyama M et al (2005) Cell type-specific involvement of RIG-I in antiviral response. Immunity 23:19–28. doi:10.1016/j.immuni.2005.04.010

Kato H, Takeuchi O, Mikamo-Satoh E et al (2008) Length-dependent recognition of double-stranded ribonucleic acids by retinoic acid-inducible gene-I and melanoma differentiation-associated gene 5. J Exp Med 205:1601–1610. doi:10.1084/jem.20080091

Kato H, Takeuchi O, Sato S et al (2006) Differential roles of MDA5 and RIG-I helicases in the recognition of RNA viruses. Nature 441:101–105. doi:10.1038/nature04734

Kawai T, Akira S (2011) Toll-like receptors and their crosstalk with other innate receptors in infection and immunity. Immunity 34:637–650. doi:10.1016/j.immuni.2011.05.006

Kawai T, Akira S (2009) The roles of TLRs, RLRs and NLRs in pathogen recognition. Int Immunol 21:317–337. doi:10.1093/intimm/dxp017

Kogure T, Suzuki T, Takahashi T et al (2006) Human trachea primary epithelial cells express both sialyl(alpha2-3)Gal receptor for human parainfluenza virus type 1 and avian influenza viruses, and sialyl(alpha2-6)Gal receptor for human influenza viruses. Glycoconj J 23:101–106. doi:10.1007/s10719-006-5442-z

Kotenko SV, Gallagher G, Baurin VV et al (2003) IFN-lambdas mediate antiviral protection through a distinct class II cytokine receptor complex. Nat Immunol 4:69–77. doi:10.1038/ni875

Lakadamyali M, Rust MJ, Babcock HP, Zhuang X (2003) Visualizing infection of individual influenza viruses. Proc Natl Acad Sci U A 100:9280–9285. http://dx.doi.org/10.1073/pnas.0832269100

Lakadamyali M, Rust MJ, Zhuang X (2006) Ligands for clathrin-mediated endocytosis are differentially sorted into distinct populations of early endosomes. Cell 124:997–1009. doi:10.1016/j.cell.2005.12.038

Lee SMY, Kok K-H, Jaume M et al (2014) Toll-like receptor 10 is involved in induction of innate immune responses to influenza virus infection. Proc Natl Acad Sci U S A 111:3793–3798. doi:10.1073/pnas.1324266111

Leikina E, Ramos C, Markovic I et al (2002) Reversible stages of the low-pH-triggered conformational change in influenza virus hemagglutinin. EMBO J 21:5701–5710

Lemaitre B, Nicolas E, Michaut L et al (1996) The dorsoventral regulatory gene cassette spatzle/Toll/cactus controls the potent antifungal response in Drosophila adults. Cell 86:973–983

Liu P, Jamaluddin M, Li K et al (2007) Retinoic acid-inducible gene i mediates early antiviral response and toll-like receptor 3 expression in respiratory syncytial virus-infected airway epithelial cells. J Virol 81:1401–1411. doi:10.1128/JVI.01740-06

Lohmeyer J, Talens LT, Klenk H-D (1979) Biosynthesis of the influenza virus envelope in abortive infection. J Gen Virol 42:73–88. doi:10.1099/0022-1317-42-1-73

Loo Y-M, Fornek J, Crochet N et al (2008) Distinct RIG-I and MDA5 signaling by RNA viruses in innate immunity. J Virol 82:335–345. doi:10.1128/JVI.01080-07

Loo Y-M, Gale M Jr (2011) Immune signaling by RIG-I-like receptors. Immunity 34:680–692. doi:10.1016/j.immuni.2011.05.003

Ludwig S, Wang X, Ehrhardt C et al (2002) The influenza A virus NS1 protein inhibits activation of Jun N-terminal kinase and AP-1 transcription factors. J Virol 76:11166–11171

Lund JM, Alexopoulou L, Sato A et al (2004) Recognition of single-stranded RNA viruses by Toll-like receptor 7. Proc Natl Acad Sci U S A 101:5598–5603. doi:10.1073/pnas.0400937101

Luo M (2012) Influenza virus entry. In: Rossmann MG, Rao VB (eds) Viral Molecular Machines. Springer, Boston, pp 201–221

Lupfer C, Kanneganti T-D (2013) The expanding role of NLRs in antiviral immunity. Immunol Rev 255:13–24. doi:10.1111/imr.12089

Lupfer C, Thomas PG, Anand PK et al (2013) Receptor interacting protein kinase 2-mediated mitophagy regulates inflammasome activation during virus infection. Nat Immunol 14:480–488. doi:10.1038/ni.2563

Macfarlane DE, Manzel L (1998) Antagonism of immunostimulatory CpG-oligodeoxynucleotides by quinacrine, chloroquine, and structurally related compounds. J Immunol Baltim Md 1950 160:1122–1131

von Magnus P (1954) Incomplete forms of influenza virus. Adv Virus Res 2:59–79

Malathi K, Dong B, Gale M Jr, Silverman RH (2007) Small self-RNA generated by RNase L amplifies antiviral innate immunity. Nature 448:816–819. doi:10.1038/nature06042

Malireddi RKS, Ippagunta S, Lamkanfi M, Kanneganti T-D (2010) Cutting edge: proteolytic inactivation of poly(ADP-ribose) polymerase 1 by the Nlrp3 and Nlrc4 inflammasomes. J Immunol Baltim Md 185:3127–3130. doi:10.4049/jimmunol.1001512

Markovic I, Leikina E, Zhukovsky M et al (2001) Synchronized activation and refolding of influenza hemagglutinin in multimeric fusion machines. J Cell Biol 155:833–844. doi:10.1083/jcb.200103005

Marshak-Rothstein A (2006) Toll-like receptors in systemic autoimmune disease. Nat Rev Immunol 6:823–835. doi:10.1038/nri1957

Martinon F, Pétrilli V, Mayor A et al (2006) Gout-associated uric acid crystals activate the NALP3 inflammasome. Nature 440:237–241. doi:10.1038/nature04516

Masters SL, Gerlic M, Metcalf D et al (2012) NLRP1 inflammasome activation induces pyroptosis of hematopoietic progenitor cells. Immunity 37:1009–1023. doi:10.1016/j.immuni.2012.08.027

Matlin KS, Reggio H, Helenius A, Simons K (1981) Infectious entry pathway of influenza virus in a canine kidney cell line. J Cell Biol 91:601–613

Matsumoto M, Funami K, Tanabe M et al (2003) Subcellular localization of Toll-like receptor 3 in human dendritic cells. J Immunol Baltim Md 1950 171:3154–3162

Matsumoto M, Kikkawa S, Kohase M et al (2002) Establishment of a monoclonal antibody against human Toll-like receptor 3 that blocks double-stranded RNA-mediated signaling. Biochem Biophys Res Commun 293:1364–1369. doi:10.1016/S0006-291X(02)00380-7

McAuley JL, Hornung F, Boyd KL, et al. (2007) Expression of the 1918 influenza A virus PB1-F2 enhances the pathogenesis of viral and secondary bacterial pneumonia. Cell Host Microbe 2:240–249. http://dx.doi.org/10.1016/j.chom.2007.09.001

McAuley JL, Zhang K, McCullers JA (2010) The effects of influenza A virus PB1-F2 protein on polymerase activity are strain specific and do not impact pathogenesis. J Virol 84:558–564. doi:10.1128/JVI.01785-09

Meylan E, Tschopp J, Karin M (2006) Intracellular pattern recognition receptors in the host response. Nature 442:39–44

Mibayashi M, Martinez-Sobrido L, Loo Y-M, et al. (2007) Inhibition of retinoic acid-inducible gene I-mediated induction of beta interferon by the NS1 protein of influenza A virus. J Virol 81:514–524. http://dx.doi.org/10.1128/JVI.01265-06

Mittal A, Leikina E, Chernomordik LV, Bentz J (2003) Kinetically differentiating influenza hemagglutinin fusion and hemifusion machines. Biophys J 85:1713–1724. doi:10.1016/S0006-3495(03)74601-3

Morgan C, Rose HM (1968) Structure and development of viruses as observed in the electron microscope. 8 Entry of influenza virus. J Virol 2:925–936

Muzio M, Bosisio D, Polentarutti N et al (2000) Differential expression and regulation of toll-like receptors (TLR) in human leukocytes: selective expression of TLR3 in dendritic cells. J Immunol Baltim Md 1950 164:5998–6004

Nakhaei P, Genin P, Civas A, Hiscott J (2009) RIG-I-like receptors: sensing and responding to RNA virus infection. Semin Immunol 21:215–222. doi:10.1016/j.smim.2009.05.001

Nayak DP (1980) Defective interfering influenza viruses. Annu Rev Microbiol 34:619–644. doi:10.1146/annurev.mi.34.100180.003155

Nemeroff ME, Barabino SM, Li Y et al (1998) Influenza virus NS1 protein interacts with the cellular 30 kDa subunit of CPSF and inhibits 3′ end formation of cellular pre-mRNAs. Mol Cell 1:991–1000

Nhu QM, Shirey K, Teijaro JR et al (2010) Novel signaling interactions between proteinase-activated receptor 2 and Toll-like receptors in vitro and in vivo. Mucosal Immunol 3:29–39. doi:10.1038/mi.2009.120

Nicholls JM, Chan MCW, Chan WY et al (2007) Tropism of avian influenza A (H5N1) in the upper and lower respiratory tract. Nat Med 13:147–149. doi:10.1038/nm1529

Noah DL, Twu KY, Krug RM (2003) Cellular antiviral responses against influenza A virus are countered at the posttranscriptional level by the viral NS1A protein via its binding to a cellular protein required for the 3' end processing of cellular pre-mRNAS. Virology 307:386–395

Noble S, Dimmock NJ (1995) Characterization of putative defective interfering (DI) A/WSN RNAs isolated from the lungs of mice protected from an otherwise lethal respiratory infection with influenza virus A/WSN (H1N1): a subset of the inoculum DI RNAs. Virology 210:9–19. doi:10.1006/viro.1995.1312

Ogura Y, Sutterwala FS, Flavell RA (2006) The inflammasome: first line of the immune response to cell stress. Cell 126:659–662. doi:10.1016/j.cell.2006.08.002

Oshansky CM, Pickens JA, Bradley KC et al (2011) Avian influenza viruses infect primary human bronchial epithelial cells unconstrained by sialic acid α2,3 residues. PloS One 6:e21183. doi:10.1371/journal.pone.0021183

Palese P, Shaw ML (2007) Orthomyxoviridae: the viruses and their replication, 5th ed. Lippincott Williams and Wilkins, Philadelphia

Patterson S, Oxford JS, Dourmashkin RR (1979) Studies on the mechanism of influenza virus entry into cells. J Gen Virol 43:223–229

Pena L, Vincent AL, Loving CL et al (2012) Restored PB1-F2 in the 2009 pandemic H1N1 influenza virus has minimal effects in swine. J Virol 86:5523–5532. doi:10.1128/JVI.00134-12

Perdue ML, García M, Senne D, Fraire M (1997) Virulence-associated sequence duplication at the hemagglutinin cleavage site of avian influenza viruses. Virus Res 49:173–186

Pétrilli V, Papin S, Dostert C et al (2007) Activation of the NALP3 inflammasome is triggered by low intracellular potassium concentration. Cell Death Differ 14:1583–1589. doi:10.1038/sj.cdd.4402195

Pichlmair A, Schulz O, Tan CP et al (2006) RIG-I-mediated antiviral responses to single-stranded RNA bearing 5′-phosphates. Science 314:997–1001. doi:10.1126/science.1132998

Pichlmair A, Schulz O, Tan C-P et al (2009) Activation of MDA5 requires higher-order RNA structures generated during virus infection. J Virol 83:10761–10769. doi:10.1128/JVI.00770-09

Pinto LH, Holsinger LJ, Lamb RA (1992) Influenza virus M2 protein has ion channel activity. Cell 69:517–528

Pippig DA, Hellmuth JC, Cui S et al (2009) The regulatory domain of the RIG-I family ATPase LGP2 senses double-stranded RNA. Nucleic Acids Res 37:2014–2025. doi:10.1093/nar/gkp059

Plotch SJ, Bouloy M, Ulmanen I, Krug RM (1981) A unique cap(m7G pppXm)-dependent influenza virion endonuclease cleaves capped RNAs to generate the primers that initiate viral RNA transcription. Cell 23:847–858

Poeck H, Bscheider M, Gross O et al (2010) Recognition of RNA virus by RIG-I results in activation of CARD9 and inflammasome signaling for interleukin 1 beta production. Nat Immunol 11:63–69. doi:10.1038/ni.1824

Pothlichet J, Meunier I, Davis BK et al (2013) Type I IFN triggers RIG-I/TLR3/NLRP3-dependent inflammasome activation in influenza A virus infected cells. PLoS Pathog 9:e1003256. doi:10.1371/journal.ppat.1003256

Puri A, Booy FP, Doms RW et al (1990) Conformational changes and fusion activity of influenza virus hemagglutinin of the H2 and H3 subtypes: effects of acid pretreatment. J Virol 64:3824–3832

Rajan JV, Warren SE, Miao EA, Aderem A (2010) Activation of the NLRP3 inflammasome by intracellular poly I:C. FEBS Lett 584:4627–4632. doi:10.1016/j.febslet.2010.10.036

Reed ML, Bridges OA, Seiler P et al (2010) The pH of activation of the hemagglutinin protein regulates H5N1 influenza virus pathogenicity and transmissibility in ducks. J Virol 84:1527–1535. doi:10.1128/JVI.02069-09

Rehwinkel J, Tan CP, Goubau D et al (2010) RIG-I detects viral genomic RNA during negative-strand RNA virus infection. Cell 140:397–408. doi:10.1016/j.cell.2010.01.020

Roach JC, Glusman G, Rowen L et al (2005) The evolution of vertebrate Toll-like receptors. Proc Natl Acad Sci U S A 102:9577–9582. doi:10.1073/pnas.0502272102

Rossman JS, Leser GP, Lamb RA (2012) Filamentous influenza virus enters cells via macropinocytosis. J Virol 86:10950–10960. doi:10.1128/JVI.05992-11

Rothenfusser S, Goutagny N, DiPerna G et al (2005) The RNA helicase Lgp2 inhibits TLR-independent sensing of viral replication by retinoic acid-inducible gene-I. J Immunol Baltim Md 1950 175:5260–5268

Rust MJ, Lakadamyali M, Zhang F, Zhuang X (2004) Assembly of endocytic machinery around individual influenza viruses during viral entry. Nat Struct Mol Biol 11:567–573. http://dx.doi.org/10.1038/nsmb769

Ryley HC, Brogan TD (1968) Variation in the composition of sputum in chronic chest diseases. Br J Exp Pathol 49:625–633

Sabbah A, Chang TH, Harnack R et al (2009) Activation of innate immune antiviral responses by Nod2. Nat Immunol 10:1073–1080. doi:10.1038/ni.1782

Saira K, Lin X, DePasse JV et al (2013) Sequence analysis of in vivo defective interfering-like RNA of influenza A H1N1 pandemic virus. J Virol 87:8064–8074. doi:10.1128/JVI.00240-13

Saito T, Gale M Jr (2008) Differential recognition of double-stranded RNA by RIG-I-like receptors in antiviral immunity. J Exp Med 205:1523–1527. doi:10.1084/jem.20081210

Saito T, Hirai R, Loo Y-M et al (2007) Regulation of innate antiviral defenses through a shared repressor domain in RIG-I and LGP2. Proc Natl Acad Sci U S A 104:582–587. doi:10.1073/pnas.0606699104

Saito T, Owen DM, Jiang F et al (2008) Innate immunity induced by composition-dependent RIG-I recognition of hepatitis C virus RNA. Nature 454:523–527. doi:10.1038/nature07106

Samanta M, Iwakiri D, Kanda T et al (2006) EB virus-encoded RNAs are recognized by RIG-I and activate signaling to induce type I IFN. EMBO J 25:4207–4214. doi:10.1038/sj.emboj.7601314

Samuel CE (2001) Antiviral actions of interferons. Clin Microbiol Rev 14:778–809. http://dx.doi.org/10.1128/CMR.14.4.778-809.2001

Sanders CJ, Doherty PC, Thomas PG (2011) Respiratory epithelial cells in innate immunity to influenza virus infection. Cell Tissue Res 343:13–21. doi:10.1007/s00441-010-1043-z

Sarmiento M, Haffey M, Spear PG (1979) Membrane proteins specified by herpes simplex viruses. III. Role of glycoprotein VP7(B2) in virion infectivity. J Virol 29:1149–1158

Satoh T, Kato H, Kumagai Y et al (2010) LGP2 is a positive regulator of RIG-I- and MDA5-mediated antiviral responses. Proc Natl Acad Sci U S A 107:1512–1517. doi:10.1073/pnas.0912986107

Schlee M, Roth A, Hornung V et al (2009) Recognition of 5′ triphosphate by RIG-I helicase requires short blunt double-stranded RNA as contained in panhandle of negative-strand virus. Immunity 31:25–34. doi:10.1016/j.immuni.2009.05.008

Schmidt A, Schwerd T, Hamm W et al (2009) 5′-triphosphate RNA requires base-paired structures to activate antiviral signaling via RIG-I. Proc Natl Acad Sci U S A 106:12067–12072. doi:10.1073/pnas.0900971106

Shaw M, Palese P (2007) Orthomyxoviridae: The Viruses and Their Replication, 6th ed. Lippincott Williams and Wilkins, Philadelphia

Sheppard P, Kindsvogel W, Xu W et al (2003) IL-28, IL-29 and their class II cytokine receptor IL-28R. Nat Immunol 4:63–68. doi:10.1038/ni873

Sieczkarski SB, Whittaker GR (2003) Differential requirements of Rab5 and Rab7 for endocytosis of influenza and other enveloped viruses. Traffic Cph Den 4:333–343

Sieczkarski SB, Whittaker GR (2002) Influenza virus can enter and infect cells in the absence of clathrin-mediated endocytosis. J Virol 76:10455–10464. doi:10.1128/JVI.76.20.10455-10464.2002

Skehel JJ, Wiley DC (2000) Receptor binding and membrane fusion in virus entry: the influenza hemagglutinin. Annu Rev Biochem 69:531–569. doi:10.1146/annurev.biochem.69.1.531

Soboll G, Shen L, Wira CR (2006) Expression of Toll-like receptors (TLR) and responsiveness to TLR agonists by polarized mouse uterine epithelial cells in culture. Biol Reprod 75:131–139. doi:10.1095/biolreprod.106.050690

Solórzano A, Webby RJ, Lager KM et al (2005) Mutations in the NS1 protein of swine influenza virus impair anti-interferon activity and confer attenuation in pigs. J Virol 79:7535–7543. doi:10.1128/JVI.79.12.7535-7543.2005

Song R, Pang X, Yang P et al (2014) Surveillance of the first case of human avian influenza A (H7N9) virus in Beijing, China. Infection 42:127–133. doi:10.1007/s15010-013-0533-9

Srinivasakumar N, Ogra PL, Flanagan TD (1991) Characteristics of fusion of respiratory syncytial virus with HEp-2 cells as measured by R18 fluorescence dequenching assay. J Virol 65:4063–4069

Stasakova J, Ferko B, Kittel C et al (2005) Influenza A mutant viruses with altered NS1 protein function provoke caspase-1 activation in primary human macrophages, resulting in fast apoptosis and release of high levels of interleukins 1beta and 18. J Gen Virol 86:185–195. doi:10.1099/vir.0.80422-0

Stray SJ, Cummings RD, Air GM (2000) Influenza virus infection of desialylated cells. Glycobiology 10:649–658

Strowig T, Henao-Mejia J, Elinav E, Flavell R (2012) Inflammasomes in health and disease. Nature 481:278–286. doi:10.1038/nature10759

Sumpter R Jr, Loo Y-M, Foy E et al (2005) Regulating intracellular antiviral defense and permissiveness to hepatitis C virus RNA replication through a cellular RNA helicase, RIG-I. J Virol 79:2689–2699. doi:10.1128/JVI.79.5.2689-2699.2005

Sun X, Whittaker GR (2007) Role of the actin cytoskeleton during influenza virus internalization into polarized epithelial cells. Cell Microbiol 9:1672–1682. doi:10.1111/j.1462-5822.2007.00900.x

Takahasi K, Kumeta H, Tsuduki N et al (2009) Solution structures of cytosolic RNA sensor MDA5 and LGP2 C-terminal domains: identification of the RNA recognition loop in RIG-I-like receptors. J Biol Chem 284:17465–17474. doi:10.1074/jbc.M109.007179

Takeuchi O, Akira S (2007) Signaling pathways activated by microorganisms. Curr Opin Cell Biol 19:185–191. doi:10.1016/j.ceb.2007.02.006

Talon J, Horvath CM, Polley R et al (2000) Activation of interferon regulatory factor 3 is inhibited by the influenza A virus NS1 protein. J Virol 74:7989–7996

Tapia K, Kim W-K, Sun Y et al (2013) Defective viral genomes arising in vivo provide critical danger signals for the triggering of lung antiviral immunity. PLoS Pathog 9:e1003703. doi:10.1371/journal.ppat.1003703

Tatsuta T, Imaizumi T, Shimoyama T et al (2012) Expression of melanoma differentiation associated gene 5 is increased in human gastric mucosa infected with Helicobacter pylori. J Clin Pathol 65:839–843. doi:10.1136/jclinpath-2011-200590

Thomas PG, Dash P, Aldridge JR Jr et al (2009) The intracellular sensor NLRP3 mediates key innate and healing responses to influenza A virus via the regulation of caspase-1. Immunity 30:566–575. doi:10.1016/j.immuni.2009.02.006

Thompson CI, Barclay WS, Zambon MC, Pickles RJ (2006) Infection of human airway epithelium by human and avian strains of influenza a virus. J Virol 80:8060–8068. doi:10.1128/JVI.00384-06

Tsai S-Y, Segovia JA, Chang T-H et al (2014) DAMP molecule S100A9 acts as a molecular pattern to enhance inflammation during influenza A virus infection: role of DDX21-TRIF-TLR4-MyD88 pathway. PLoS Pathog 10:e1003848. doi:10.1371/journal.ppat.1003848

Tschopp J (2011) Mitochondria: Sovereign of inflammation? Eur J Immunol 41:1196–1202. doi:10.1002/eji.201141436

Uyeki TM, Nguyen DC, Rowe T et al (2012) Seroprevalence of antibodies to avian influenza A (H5) and A (H9) viruses among market poultry workers, Hanoi, Vietnam, 2001. PloS One 7:e43948. doi:10.1371/journal.pone.0043948

Varga ZT, Grant A, Manicassamy B, Palese P (2012) Influenza virus protein PB1-F2 inhibits the induction of type I interferon by binding to MAVS and decreasing mitochondrial membrane potential. J Virol 86:8359–8366. doi:10.1128/JVI.01122-12

Venkataraman T, Valdes M, Elsby R et al (2007) Loss of DExD/H box RNA helicase LGP2 manifests disparate antiviral responses. J Immunol Baltim Md 1950 178:6444–6455

De Vries E, Tscherne DM, Wienholts MJ et al (2011) Dissection of the influenza A virus endocytic routes reveals macropinocytosis as an alternative entry pathway. PLoS Pathog 7:e1001329. doi:10.1371/journal.ppat.1001329

De Vries E, de Vries RP, Wienholts MJ et al (2012) Influenza A virus entry into cells lacking sialylated N-glycans. Proc Natl Acad Sci U S A 109:7457–7462. doi:10.1073/pnas.1200987109

Wang M, Fu C-X, Zheng B-J (2009) Antibodies against H5 and H9 avian influenza among poultry workers in China. N Engl J Med 360:2583–2584. doi:10.1056/NEJMc0900358

Wang X, Li M, Zheng H et al (2000) Influenza A virus NS1 protein prevents activation of NF-kappaB and induction of alpha/beta interferon. J Virol 74:11566–11573

Weber F, Wagner V, Rasmussen SB et al (2006) Double-stranded RNA is produced by positive-strand RNA viruses and DNA viruses but not in detectable amounts by negative-strand RNA viruses. J Virol 80:5059–5064. doi:10.1128/JVI.80.10.5059-5064.2006

Weber M, Gawanbacht A, Habjan M et al (2013) Incoming RNA virus nucleocapsids containing a 5′-triphosphorylated genome activate RIG-I and antiviral signaling. Cell Host Microbe 13:336–346. doi:10.1016/j.chom.2013.01.012

Webster RG, Rott R (1987) Influenza virus A pathogenicity: the pivotal role of hemagglutinin. Cell 50:665–666

White J, Kartenbeck J, Helenius A (1980) Fusion of Semliki forest virus with the plasma membrane can be induced by low pH. J Cell Biol 87:264–272

White J, Matlin K, Helenius A (1981) Cell fusion by Semliki Forest, influenza, and vesicular stomatitis viruses. J Cell Biol 89:674–679

White JM, Wilson IA (1987) Anti-peptide antibodies detect steps in a protein conformational change: low-pH activation of the influenza virus hemagglutinin. J Cell Biol 105:2887–2896

Wise HM, Foeglein A, Sun J et al (2009) A complicated message: Identification of a novel PB1-related protein translated from influenza A virus segment 2 mRNA. J Virol 83:8021–8031. doi:10.1128/JVI.00826-09

Xu R, Wilson IA (2011) Structural characterization of an early fusion intermediate of influenza virus hemagglutinin. J Virol 85:5172–5182. doi:10.1128/JVI.02430-10

Yamada H, Chounan R, Higashi Y et al (2004) Mitochondrial targeting sequence of the influenza A virus PB1-F2 protein and its function in mitochondria. FEBS Lett 578:331–336. doi:10.1016/j.febslet.2004.11.017

Yoneyama M, Fujita T (2007) Function of RIG-I-like receptors in antiviral innate immunity. J Biol Chem 282:15315–15318. doi:10.1074/jbc.R700007200

Yoneyama M, Kikuchi M, Matsumoto K et al (2005) Shared and unique functions of the DExD/H-box helicases RIG-I, MDA5, and LGP2 in antiviral innate immunity. J Immunol Baltim Md 1950 175:2851–2858

Yoneyama M, Kikuchi M, Natsukawa T et al (2004) The RNA helicase RIG-I has an essential function in double-stranded RNA-induced innate antiviral responses. Nat Immunol 5:730–737. doi:10.1038/ni1087

Yoshimura A, Kuroda K, Kawasaki K et al (1982) Infectious cell entry mechanism of influenza virus. J Virol 43:284

Yoshimura A, Ohnishi S (1984) Uncoating of influenza virus in endosomes. J Virol 51:497–504

Yount JS, Moran TM, López CB (2007) Cytokine-independent upregulation of MDA5 in viral infection. J Virol 81:7316–7319. doi:10.1128/JVI.00545-07

Zaki MH, Vogel P, Malireddi RKS et al (2011) The NOD-like receptor NLRP12 attenuates colon inflammation and tumorigenesis. Cancer Cell 20:649–660. doi:10.1016/j.ccr.2011.10.022

Zamarin D, Garcia-Sastre A, Xiao X, et al. (2005) Influenza virus PB1-F2 protein induces cell death through mitochondrial ANT3 and VDAC1. PLoS Pathog 1:e4. http://dx.doi.org/10.1371/journal.ppat.0010004

Zamarin D, Ortigoza MB, Palese P (2006) Influenza A virus PB1-F2 protein contributes to viral pathogenesis in mice. J Virol 80:7976–7983. http://dx.doi.org/10.1128/JVI.00415-06

Zaraket H, Bridges OA, Duan S et al (2013a) Increased acid stability of the hemagglutinin protein enhances H5N1 influenza virus growth in the upper respiratory tract but is insufficient for transmission in ferrets. J Virol 87:9911–9922. doi:10.1128/JVI.01175-13

Zaraket H, Bridges OA, Russell CJ (2013b) The pH of activation of the hemagglutinin protein regulates H5N1 influenza virus replication and pathogenesis in mice. J Virol 87:4826–4834. doi:10.1128/JVI.03110-12

Zell R, Krumbholz A, Eitner A et al (2007) Prevalence of PB1-F2 of influenza A viruses. J Gen Virol 88:536–546. doi:10.1099/vir.0.82378-0

Part II
Vaccines and Adaptive Immunity

Inactivated and Adjuvanted Influenza Vaccines

Giuseppe Del Giudice and Rino Rappuoli

Abstract Inactivated influenza vaccines are produced every year to fight against the seasonal epidemics of influenza. Despite the nonoptimal coverage, even in subjects at risk like the elderly, pregnant women, etc., these vaccines significantly reduce the burden of mortality and morbidity linked to the influenza infection. Importantly, these vaccines have also contributed to reduce the impact of the last pandemics. Nevertheless, the performance of these vaccines can be improved mainly in those age groups, like children and the elderly, in which their efficacy is suboptimal. The use of adjuvants has proven effective to this scope. Oil-in-water adjuvants like MF59 and AS03 have been licensed and widely used, and shown efficacious in preventing influenza infection in the last pandemic. MF59-adjuvanted inactivated vaccine was more efficacious than non-adjuvanted vaccine in preventing influenza infection in young children and in reducing hospitalization due to the influenza infection in the elderly. Other adjuvants are now at different stages of development and some are being tested in clinical trials. The perspective remains to improve the way inactivated vaccines are prepared and to accelerate their availability, mainly in the case of influenza pandemics, and to enhance their efficacy/effectiveness for a more successful impact at the public health level.

Contents

G. Del Giudice · R. Rappuoli (✉)
Research and Development, Novartis Vaccines, Via Fiorentina 1, 53100 Siena, Italy
e-mail: rino.rappuoli@novartis.com

G. Del Giudice
e-mail: giuseppe.del_giudice@novartis.com

Current Topics in Microbiology and Immunology (2015) 386: 151–180
DOI: 10.1007/82_2014_406

Published Online: 20 July 2014

1 Introduction

Despite the availability of vaccines licensed for all age groups and despite their proven benefits, influenza remains a major problem for public health because of both seasonal epidemics and pandemics, which can occur periodically. Every year in the United States alone, more than 200,000 hospitalizations and up to 49,000 deaths are attributed to influenza infection (Thompson et al. 2003, 2004, 2010). Most of the hospitalizations occur in children younger than 2 years, while the highest mortality rates are observed in subjects older than 65. Subjects at any age with various conditions such as pregnancy, chronic and metabolic diseases, HIV infection, and immunosuppressive treatments, are at increased risk of influenza hospitalization and death (Mertz et al. 2013). Several reasons can contribute to this.

First, the perception of the danger of the influenza infection varies enormously in the general population. The relatively milder-than-expected nature of the last pandemic (swine-origin A/H1N1 2009) has not significantly and broadly enhanced the awareness of this danger. For example, influenza vaccination is still mainly perceived as a need for the elderly, underscoring the huge need for vaccinating young children who represent the major reservoir of the infection in the community (Esposito et al. 2012), and of pregnant women (Karlsson et al. 2012). Indeed, the WHO SAGE in 2012 issued the new recommendations for influenza vaccination, putting pregnant women, health care professionals, and 6–59-month-old children at the top (WHO 2012). This is on the basis of the yearly adaptation of the composition of the vaccines as recommended by the WHO (WHO 2013).

Second, despite these recommendations that were already issued by some national authorities, such as the US authorities (Committee on Infectious Diseases 2013), the coverage still remains suboptimal, even in the elderly groups for whom the cost of vaccination is covered by health insurances in many countries (Centers for Disease Control 2013).

Third, despite this care in adapting the influenza vaccines to the circulating strains, mismatching is not uncommon. Influenza A viruses have a high propensity to recombine, giving rise to a panoply of drifted strains, i.e., strains carrying mutations in the amino acid sequence of the major surface proteins, which represent the major constituents of the inactivated vaccines, namely, the hemagglutinin (HA) and the neuraminidase (NA). Although these mutations affect only a few amino acids as compared to stronger mutations that lead to new (shifted) virus strains that cause pandemics, they are poorly recognized by functionally active, hemagglutination-inhibiting (HI) antibodies directed against the original strains, with a consequent reduction of the efficacy/effectiveness of the influenza vaccine during the years of mismatch between the vaccine and circulating virus strains (Carrat and Flahault 2007).

Lastly, currently available seasonal influenza vaccines exhibit a lower immunogenicity and efficacy in those age groups with a greater need to be vaccinated against influenza, i.e., young children and the elderly (Goodwin et al. 2006; Osterholm et al. 2012; Jefferson et al. 2012).

For all these reasons, a very active work is in progress in order to improve the efficacy/effectiveness of inactivated influenza vaccines, for example, by producing strains better matched with the wild type viruses, by administering the vaccine subcutaneously, by increasing the dose of the antigens in the vaccine, by changing the composition of the vaccine from a trivalent to a quadrivalent vaccine, and by formulating the vaccine with appropriate adjuvants.

2 The Inactivated Influenza Vaccines

The vast majority of the inactivated influenza vaccines registered for use in humans are obtained by growing the influenza viruses in embryonated eggs, a methodology developed by Macfarlane Burnet in 1937. The first vaccine was licensed in the US in 1945: it was bivalent, containing the A/PR8 (H1N1) and the B strains adapted to grow in eggs. This A/H1N1 strain was changed in 1958 with the A/H2N2 virus strain, which during the pandemic had completely replaced the A/H1N1, and then in 1968, with the appearance of the A/H3N2 pandemic virus which wiped out the A/H2N2. The vaccine became trivalent only in 1978 with the reappearance of the A/H1N1 from Russia, a strain which did not replace the A/H3N2, but instead continued to circulate, and even to represent the strain more frequently, was isolated seasonally. The first generation vaccines were based on whole virions that had been chemically inactivated using formalin or β-propio lactone. Very few vaccines are still based on inactivated whole virions (Barrett et al. 2011; van der Velden et al. 2014). In all the others, inactivated viruses undergo treatment to further disrupt the viral particle (split vaccines), or are submitted to further steps of purification to remove most of the adventitious and of non-superficial antigens (subunit vaccines) (Fiore et al. 2009; Oxford et al. 2011; Hannoun 2013).

New inactivated influenza vaccines have been developed by growing the influenza viruses in continuous cell lines, for example, the MDCK cell line (Dormitzer et al. 2012). This procedure has several advantages. Not all influenza strains recommended for seasonal vaccines grow equally well in eggs, while the vast majority of them can be cultured in cell lines. In addition, highly pathogenic avian viruses are lethal for embryonated eggs, rendering difficult, if not impossible, their use to prepare pandemic vaccines, and rendering necessary the use of strains obtained with reverse genetics (Engelhardt 2013). On the contrary, highly pathogenic avian influenza virus strains grow efficiently in cell lines. Finally, and importantly, when influenza isolates are passaged in eggs, they undergo amino acid changes, which may affect their immunogenicity and finally their efficacy when used as . Indeed, cell-derived vaccines have been shown to confer a higher level of protection in ferrets than egg-derived vaccines (Katz and Webster 1989). Some of these vaccines derived from MDCK cells (European Medicines Agency 2008; Food and Drug Administration 2012), from Vero cells (European Medicines Agency 2009), or from insect cells (Food and Drug Administration 2013), have now been licensed in Europe and/or the USA, or in the rest of the world.

Most of the vaccines available today contain three virus strains: two A (H1N1 and H3N2) and one B, belonging to the Victoria or to the Yamagata lineages. The frequent observation of co-circulation of the two B lineages and the frequent mismatch between the vaccine component and the circulating strains have prompted vaccine manufacturers to produce quadrivalent inactivated influenza vaccines (QIV) containing two A and two B strains (Belshe 2010) that have now been licensed in some countries.

The amount of antigen of an influenza-inactivated vaccine is calculated on the content of HA. Each dose must contain not less than 15 μg of each of the three (or four) HAs. This does not mean that other components are not present. The second component is NA; various amounts of internal proteins, like M1 and NP, can also be detected (Co et al. 2009). In any case, the amount of NA and of other viral components is nor required by regulatory agencies for registering the vaccines. This implies that not all inactivated vaccines are equal. Whole-virion, split and subunit vaccines appear very different when analyzed with electron microscopy (Renfrey and Watts 1994; Oxford et al. 2011) and, as said, their non-HA composition can vary from one vaccine to another, and even from one batch to another in the same vaccine. For these reasons, most of the analysis of the immune response to influenza vaccines is focused on HA, which is the only antigen onto which all influenza vaccines are standardized and, importantly, the major target of the protective antibody response (see below).

3 The Immune Response to Inactivated Influenza Vaccines

Seasonal inactivated influenza vaccines are given before or at the beginning of the influenza season as a single dose (15 μg of each component) in adolescents, adults and elder subjects, and as two half-doses (7.5 μg of each component) 3–4 weeks apart in young children never vaccinated before. This regimen of vaccination is dictated by the fact that the vast majority of subjects have been immunologically primed to influenza via continuous clinically overt or subclinical contacts with the virus and/or via yearly vaccinations. The situation is different in children younger than 2–3 years of age which require two doses of the vaccine to achieve a substantial priming. Indeed, in several studies carried out in pediatric populations it has been shown that the percentage of children positive for anti-influenza viral antibodies increases with age, this percentage being very low during the first year of life and progressively increasing later on (Zaman et al. 2007). This is in line with the observation that more than one dose is needed for effective priming against avian influenza virus strains, even when the vaccine is administered together with strong adjuvants, because individuals of all ages are immunologically naïve to them (see below).

Several lines of evidence based on human challenge studies and also on vaccines containing only recombinant HA, but not other antigens, support the notion that the antibody response against HA, as detected by HI and by MN, represents the major protective effector arm against influenza, since these antibodies are known to prevent the infection (Montomoli et al. 2011). Indeed, levels of antibodies >1:40 as detected by HI are considered to correlate with protection in adults and in the elderly, and are currently accepted by regulatory agencies for registering vaccines (Hobson et al. 1972; Coudeville et al. 2010). Results derived from efficacy studies strongly suggest, however, that this threshold of 1:40 should be significantly higher when applied to young children, who are mostly immunologically naïve to influenza (Black et al. 2011).

Human challenge studies and studies in schoolchildren receiving a vaccine that matched the NA but not the HA of circulating strains indicate that NA-inhibiting antibodies may also contribute to protection (Beutner et al. 1979; Clements et al. 1986). During the pandemic of 1968, when H3N2 influenza replaced H2N2 strains, the antigenic similarity of NA in the seasonal and new pandemic strains did not prevent a pandemic; individuals with higher pre-existing titers of NA-inhibiting antibodies had a lower frequency of H3N2 infection and less severe disease (Monto and Kendal 1973). Thus, anti-NA immunity appears to play a sizeable role in protection as compared to anti-HA immunity, leading to some consideration of including anti-NA antibody assays in vaccine evaluations (Marcelin et al. 2012). However, the poor physical stability of NA limits its utility in inactivated influenza vaccines (Kendal et al 1980).

Cellular immunity after vaccination with inactivated influenza vaccines is much less frequently investigated. Unlike the situation encountered after infection with the virus when CD4+ or CD8+ T cells against internal non-structural proteins appear to play an important role in protection (Wilkinson et al. 2012; Sridhar et al. 2013), a direct role of cell-mediated immunity in the protective response against the infection is less expected after vaccination with vaccines containing soluble antigens. For example, the frequency of granzyme B-positive T cells after vaccination with a split vaccine has been suggested to correlate with protection against ILI in the elderly better than the antibody response (McElhaney et al. 2006). These data have to be taken with some caution since in vitro restimulation of cells was done with the whole virus, which could have restimulated cell population primed by previous encounters with the virus more than by the vaccine. Nevertheless, achieving high and sustained titers of high affinity antibodies through immunization requires coordinated innate and adaptive responses, including CD4+ T-cell-mediated help for B-cell activation and affinity maturation through somatic hypermutation. Recent data have shown that T follicular helper (Tfh) CD4+ cells can be detected in the bloodstream after vaccination with inactivated influenza vaccines, although some controversy still exists on their exact phenotype concerning the expression of CXCR5, in addition to ICOS-1 and IL-21. These cells exert a strong helper function on the production of influenza-specific antibodies by B cells (Bentebibel et al. 2013; Spensieri et al. 2013). Interestingly, their frequency correlated with the titers of neutralizing antibodies detected in the serum of vaccinated subjects (Spensieri et al. 2013).

4 Towards Better Inactivated Influenza Vaccines

Existing data clearly show that influenza vaccination programs have saved millions of lives, especially in the elderly where these programs are more widely applied (Poland and Morse 2010). However, when looking at the efficacy of existing vaccines in preventing influenza infection, the figures can vary significantly based on the age and on the endpoints considered in the various studies. As said above, the efficacy of these vaccines is higher in immunologically fully competent adults (e.g. 70–90 %), and much lower in young children, in the elderly, and in adults with underlying conditions like immunosuppression, chronic metabolic diseases, etc (e.g. around 50 % or even lower, especially at the extreme of ages when, based on some recent meta analyses, the efficacy of existing inactivated, non-adjuvanted vaccines can be very low, mainly in very young children) (Osterholm et al. 2012; Jefferson et al. 2012). As anticipated, these figures can be dramatically affected during the influenza seasons when the circulating virus strains do not match with the strains contained in the vaccines (Carrat and Flahault 2007). For these reasons, several attempts are being made to develop new influenza vaccine or to improve the existing vaccines through different technological approaches.

One approach followed by all influenza vaccine manufacturers has been the development of quadrivalent vaccines (QIV), containing 2 A and 2 B strains. Both inactivated and live attenuated QIVs have been tested in all age groups and have been licensed in some countries (Domachowske et al. 2013; Greenberg et al. 2013; Kieninger et al. 2013; Langley et al. 2013; McKeage 2013; Pépin et al. 2013). In all these studies, the presence of the second B strain did not interfere with the immunogenicity of the other 3 components. While these vaccines are expected to enhance the coverage, thanks to the inclusion of the second B strain, it is still unclear whether their efficacy against infection would be improved as compared to their trivalent counterparts, unless several more virus strains equally circulate in the population. For example, in a multinational, phase 3, observer-blinded study, the absolute efficacy of a split QIV was evaluated in about 5,000 3–8 year-old children, half of whom received the QIV, and the other half a control (hepatitis A vaccine).

The QIV showed an efficacy of 59.3 % against RT-PCR-confirmed influenza of any severity and due to any influenza virus strain (Jain et al. 2013). Unfortunately, the relative efficacy of the QIV versus the conventional TIV was not investigated, although it is likely that it would not to be different since in this large study, only strains belonging to the B/Victoria lineage circulated. This conclusion is also supported by previous efficacy studies with the TIV from the same manufacturers that had shown an efficacy of 66.9 % in healthy adults against culture-confirmed influenza A and/or B (Beran et al. 2009). The results of this efficacy study underline the fact that in front of various studies claiming about the need for developing QIV (Belshe 2010; Dolin 2013), the potential net impact of QIV on influenza-associated outcomes is expected to vary seasonally, depending on annual incidence of cases caused by the two B lineages, vaccine coverage, etc (Reed et al. 2012). It is likely that QIV may exert a stronger impact on public health when they will be developed together with strong adjuvants like the oil-in-water adjuvants (see below). Data published so far have shown that QIV adjuvanted with MF59 strongly enhanced the immunogenicity of the subunit vaccine in healthy 3 to <36 month-old children as compared to the unadjuvanted counterpart (Della Cioppa et al. 2011). Analogous enhancement of the antibody response was reported in adults receiving the split QIV adjuvanted with AS03B, containing a half dose of α-tocopherol as compared to the conventional AS03A adjuvant (Beran et al. 2013) (see below for details on these adjuvants).

Intradermal delivery of vaccines offers the advantage of favoring the migration of antigens to lymph nodes with consequent stimulation of resident dendritic cells (DC), and at the same time inducing the activation of resident Langerhans cells (LC) as well as the activation and migration of dermal DCs, which synergistically result in the activation of antigen-specific T cells in the lymph nodes. By delivering the antigen at an anatomical site rich in professional antigen-presenting cells, the intradermal vaccination also has the potential of allowing to reduce the amount of vaccine antigen to achieve protection. The interest for the intradermal route for vaccination against influenza dates back to the 1940s and 1950s (Halperin et al. 1979). More recently, a substantial number of clinical studies have been carried out to evaluate the intradermal route for administration of influenza vaccine to individuals of all ages, including the elderly. Two studies in adults and in the elderly showed that 20 or 40 % of a regular human dose of a subunit or a split influenza vaccine induced immune responses comparable to, or higher than, those induced by the conventional full-dose vaccine (Belshe et al. 2004; Kenney et al. 2004). In all these studies, however, the comparison with equally low doses of the vaccine given intramuscularly was missing. When a study with such controls was conducted, the better immune response of the intradermally administered influenza vaccine disappeared, since all low doses (3, 6, or 9 μg) given either intradermally or intramuscularly were almost as immunogenic as the standard dose of 15 μg given intramuscularly (Belshe et al. 2007). Nevertheless, a split influenza vaccine given intradermally in 0.1 ml volume containing 9 μg of HA of each virus strain, has been licensed for use in adults of 18–64 years. All studies carried out with this vaccine have consistently shown a non-inferiority of the antibody response (measured by HI) as compared to the intramuscular vaccine containing 15 μg of each HA, and good tolerability, except for a significantly more frequent local reaction such as erythema, induration, swelling, pruritus, and ecchymosis (Gorse et al. 2013; Leroux-Roels et al. 2008; Moro et al. 2013).

Another approach to improve the protection conferred by influenza vaccines in older adults has been to increase the amount of antigen contained in each vaccine dose. More than 40 years ago using a whole-virion H2N2 vaccine, it was shown that increasing the antigen dosage by 15 times in healthy adults increased the HI antibody titers from 7- to 35-fold (Mostow et al. 1970). Similar enhancement of the immunogenicity was observed later by various groups using both monovalent and trivalent split influenza vaccines, with an effect more evident in the elderly than in nonelderly (Sullivan et al. 2010; Chen et al. 2011; Tsang et al. 2013). This has led to the registration in 2009 of a high dose influenza vaccine (60 mg of each HA) for adults aged more than 65 years.

5 Adjuvanted Influenza Vaccines

Adjuvants represent the best known way to enhance the immune response to vaccines. Most vaccines licensed worldwide contain adjuvants. Seasonal influenza vaccines are among the few which do not contain adjuvants. This is because individuals — mainly adults, are already immunologically experienced with influenza antigens, thanks to previous annual vaccinations and/or previous contacts (clinically overt or not) with the influenza virus. In such a context, the vaccination acts through the expansion of an already existing pool of memory cells without any need for further "help" from an adjuvant.

Aluminum salts are the most utilized vaccine adjuvants worldwide. However, the use of these adjuvants with both seasonal and pandemic (avian) influenza vaccines has mostly failed. Adsorption of the influenza virus HA onto aluminum phosphate increased the immunogenicity of the vaccine in mice (Davenport 1968), but it failed to enhance an antibody response over a nonadjuvanted vaccine in healthy military recruits (Davenport et al. 1968). Despite this failure, during the 1960s and the 1970s, many inactivated influenza vaccines (whole-virion, split or subunit) commercially available both in Europe and in the USA were still prepared together with aluminum salts. They were not removed until the 1980s, based on the overwhelming evidence that the adjuvant did not increase the immunogenicity of the vaccine while it increased its reactogenicity.

The potential use of aluminum salts was reconsidered for the development of vaccines against the avian influenza virus A/H5N1. Some controversial results have been reported. Indeed, if some enhancement was observed, it was lower than that provided by the oil-in-water adjuvants in dose sparing and in increasing the responsiveness to the vaccine at all ages, including elderly individuals (Leroux-Roels and Leroux-Roels 2009).

The enhancement of the immunogenicity of influenza vaccines by mineral oil adjuvants was already shown in the 1950s. These adjuvants allowed significant dose sparing, enhancement of the antigen-specific antibody response, and persistence of these antibodies for at least 2–9 years (Hennessy and Davenport 1961; Salk et al. 1952; Salk 1953; Davis et al. 1961; Davenport et al. 1962). However, mineral oils were non-metabolizable and non-excretable, causing serious adverse events such as sterile abscesses in almost 3 % of the vaccinees, and raised concerns about possible long-term effects. An almost 20-year follow up of these subjects did not show any increased mortality attributable to the mineral oil adjuvant, not even in those subjects who had had sterile abscesses (Beebe et al. 1972).

Nevertheless, the unacceptably high frequency of local side effects prevented for several years the development of novel, potent oil-based adjuvants. We had to wait until the mid-1990s to see the development of the first oil-in-water adjuvant, referred to as MF59, which was finally licensed for use together with an inactivated subunit influenza vaccine in >65-year-old subjects. The successful approach to the development of a strong and safe adjuvant such as MF59 was to reduce the amount of the oil in the emulsion from 50 to 4–5 % and to replace the non-metabolizable oil with a fully metabolizable, such as squalene, which is a physiological component of the human body, being the precursor of cholesterol and of corticosteroid hormones (O'Hagan et al. 2013). The development of MF59-adjuvanted influenza vaccine prompted other groups to develop other emulsion adjuvants based on squalene plus other ingredients, for example the AS03, containing α-tocopherol as the major component and licensed with the pandemic A/H1N1 vaccine and with the avian A/H5N1 vaccine (Garçon et al. 2012), and the AF03, licensed with the pandemic A/H1N1 vaccine (Klucker et al. 2012) (Table 1).

5.1 *MF59-Adjuvanted Seasonal, Pandemic and Avian Vaccines*

After extensive studies in animals showing its safety and strong adjuvanticity (O'Hagan et al. 2013), MF59 was first licensed in 1997 in Italy and later in more than 20 countries worldwide, in association with the seasonal inactivated subunit influenza virus vaccine for individuals aged 65 years or more. This was based on the results of an extensive clinical development plan which included more than 20,000 subjects (mostly elderly individuals) and which showed that the MF59 adjuvanted vaccine was more immunogenic than conventional non-adjuvanted influenza vaccines, and well tolerated, inducing a low incidence of local mild reactions which did not increase following subsequent vaccinations. Noteworthy, the enhancement of the antibody response to the vaccine remained unaltered upon further immunizations, suggesting that the enhanced antibody response in previous years did not affect the immunogenicity of the adjuvanted vaccine in the following

Table 1 Squalene-containing oil-in-water emulsions licensed or in phase of development with inactivated influenza vaccines

Adjuvant (source)	Emulsion prepared squalene (% v/v)	Injected dose squalene % v/v (mg)	Additional components	Tween (% mg)	Span	Buffer	Size (nm)	Year Licensed (vaccine)	Reference
MF59 (Novartis)	4.3	2.15(9.75)	Nil	0.5(1.17)	0.5 % (mg)	Citrate pH 6.5	160	(seasonal, H1N1 pandemic, H5N1 avian)	O'Hagan et al. 2013
AS03A (GSK)	4.5	2.25(10.68)	2.50 % α-tocopherol (mg)	2.0(4.85)	Nil	PBS pH 6.8	160	(H1N1 pandemic, H5N1 avian)	Garçon et al. 2012
AS03B (GSK)	4.5	2.25(10.68)	1.25 % α-tocopherol (mg)	2.0(4.85)	Nil	PBS pH 6.8	160	Clinical stage (Phase II–III seasonal)	Rümke et al. 2013; Beran et al. 2013; McElhaney et al. 2013
AF03 (Sanofi-Pasteur)	32.5	5.0(25)	Polyoxyethylene cetostearyl ether (1 %); mannitol	None	Sorbitan monooleate (0.75 %)	PBS pH 7.2	90	(H1N1 pandemic influenza)	Klucker et al. 2012
Stable emulsion (IDRI)	10	2(9.3)	Lecithin (0.4 %); pluronic F68 (0.4 %); α-tocopherol (0.03 %); glycerol (2 %)	Nil	Nil	Ammonium phosphate buffer 25 mM pH 5.5	100–130	Clinical stage (Phase I H5N1 avian)	Treanor et al. 2013

years (Podda 2001). The adjuvant effect of MF59 was particularly strong in subsets of elderly populations who had a higher risk of developing influenza and influenza-triggered complications. This includes elderly subjects with low pre-immunization antibody titers (1:40) (Baldo et al. 2006) and subjects with chronic underlying diseases, such as cardiovascular, respiratory, and metabolic diseases (Banzhoff et al. 2003). More recently, MF59-adjuvanted seasonal vaccine induced higher seroprotection rates in adults >65-year-old as compared to non-adjuvanted vaccines and intradermal vaccines (Scheifele et al. 2013).

In addition to immunosenescence, antigenic mismatch between the vaccine virus strains and the circulating virus strains can affect the influenza vaccine efficacy and effectiveness (Carrat and Flahault 2007). Mismatch is caused by the accumulation of point mutations at antigenic sites on the HA and NA proteins (antigenic drift) occurring between the time that the World Health Organization (WHO) makes its recommendation for vaccine composition and subsequent exposure to the circulating strain. This leads to the appearance new antigenic determinants. Although occurring in both type A and type B viruses, the antigenic drift occurs more frequently in the influenza A (H3N2) viral subtype (Carrat and Flahault 2007). In older subjects with a high (≥80 %) post-vaccination seroprotection rate against the homologous vaccine strain, the rate of sero-protection against the drifted circulating strains can drop to 4–75 %, based on the circulating and on the vaccine strains, and on the age groups (Giuseppe Del Giudice et al. 2006; Ansaldi et al. 2008). In addition, antigenic mismatch can have a strong impact on vaccine effectiveness, as demonstrated by a study for the period 1995–2005, when the vaccine effectiveness among older adults (≥65 years of age) dropped during the seasons with a drifted strain (1997–1998 and 2002–2003) to values below 30 % (Legrand et al. 2006). Several clinical studies have shown that the seasonal MF59-adjuvanted influenza vaccine induces statistically significant stronger antibody responses against heterovariant influenza A virus strains and against the two B lineages as compared to non-adjuvanted vaccines. These results have been consistently reported in adults and in the elderly (Giuseppe Del Giudice et al. 2006; Ansaldi et al. 2008, 2010; Camilloni et al. 2009; Baldo et al. 2010), as well as in 6–36- and in 6–72-month-old children (Vesikari et al. 2009a, 2011).

The enhancement of the immunogenicity induced by MF59 (as compared to conventional adjuvants such as aluminum salts [Bernstein et al. 2008]) has also been shown with the vaccine against the avian H5N1 influenza virus in children, adults and in >65-year-old individuals, and also in all these age groups against the pandemic H1N1 virus (Giuseppe Del Giudice et al. 2013; O'Hagan et al. 2013). A key finding of several clinical studies has been that the use of MF59 also induced a wide breadth of cross-reactivity against all the H5N1 drifted virus strains tested in adults, the elderly and children (Alberini et al. 2009; Banzhoff et al. 2009; Vesikari et al. 2012a, b). The enhanced breadth of cross-clade antibody neutralization provided by MF59 was further underlined in a prime-boost study in which priming and boosting vaccines contained heterovariant virus strains. Indeed, the MF59 adjuvant induced a priming with a vaccine based on a virus (e.g. H5N3, non-pathogenic, of duck origin) that was very different from the virus strain (e.g. the pathogenic H5N1 clade 1, isolated in Vietnam in 2004) used for the boosting 6–8 years later. One booster dose allowed very rapid increase in the neutralizing antibody titers not only against the homologous clade 1 virus strain, but also against all the drifted virus strains belonging to clade 1 and to various clade 2 subclades (Stephenson et al. 2008; Galli et al. 2009a).

The availability of H5N1 vaccines adjuvanted (or not) with MF59 allowed investigating how the adjuvant contributed to the priming of antigen-specific CD4+ T-cell responses in healthy subjects. After a single immunization with the MF59-adjuvanted H5N1 vaccine (clade 1), there was a significant increase of the frequency of HA-specific central memory CD4+ T cells committed to produce IL-2 (with or without TNF-α), but not IFN-γ. The frequency of these cells did not increase after the second dose of the vaccine 3 weeks later, and persisted at frequencies higher than baseline for 6 months, when it increased after a booster dose and was maintained at high levels later on (Galli et al. 2009b). It is interesting to note that these CD4+ T cells induced by the MF59-adjuvanted vaccines were mostly directed against epitopes which were conserved among the HAs of the various H5N1 clades. Nevertheless, these cells also recognized sequences that contained epitopes which varied in the HA of clade 2.1 and of H5N3 virus strains. It is remarkable that a threefold increase in the frequency of H5-specific memory CD4+ T cells after a single dose of MF59-adjuvanted vaccine was predictive of a rise of neutralizing antibody titers above 1:80 after the booster dose 6 months after the first dose, and also of their persistence over time after the booster dose (Galli et al. 2009b).

As already mentioned above, the MF59-adjuvanted trivalent seasonal vaccine is highly immunogenic in children, much more so than conventional non-adjuvanted vaccines with antibodies persisting at protective levels for longer periods (Vesikari et al. 2009a, b). More recently, these data were extended to show that higher antibody response translated into a significantly higher efficacy in preventing polymerase chain reaction (PCR)-detected influenza infection, as compared to placebo and as compared to conventional non-adjuvanted split influenza vaccines approved for use in the pediatric population, with a satisfactory safety profile (Vesikari et al. 2011). This study also allowed defining a correlate of protection in this young age group. The correlate turns out to be higher (1:110 for 50 % efficacy, or 1:629 for 90 % efficacy) than that conventionally accepted for adults and the elderly (1:40) (Black et al. 2011). This could be expected based on the consideration that children are mostly immunologically naïve to influenza, and the only protective mechanisms against infection are those triggered by vaccination with the inactivated vaccine, i.e. the functionally active antibodies. In contrast, adults and the elderly have had the opportunity during their life to mount effector mechanisms triggered by infections (subclinical or clinically overt) involving internal viral antigens that are not the main components of inactivated vaccines and that are able to induce cell-mediated mechanisms of protection, different from the mechanisms mediated by antibodies mostly directed against HA. This has recently been shown in a challenge study in human volunteers (Wilkinson et al. 2012), and after infection with pandemic H1N1 (Sridhar et al. 2013). In these two studies, in healthy adults, the frequency of CD4+ or CD8+ T cells, respectively, directed against internal viral proteins inversely correlated with the clinical outcome of the influenza infection, although cell-mediated immunity was unable by itself to prevent the infection.

The enhanced immunogenicity of the seasonal inactivated influenza vaccines translated into evident clinical benefits also in the elderly. Vaccination using MF59-adjuvanted vaccines was shown to significantly reduce the probability of being hospitalized for pneumonia in the elderly over 64 years of age (Puig-Barberà et al. 2004). In subsequent case-control studies, it was shown that during peak virus circulation, immunization with MF59-adjuvanted vaccines was associated with an 87 % relative risk reduction in hospitalization for acute coronary syndrome, 93 % for cerebrovascular accidents and 69 % for pneumonia (Puig-Barberà et al. 2007). Superior clinical protection against influenza-like illness has also been reported (Iob et al. 2005). Most recently, a large, prospective, randomized, observational study (~ 170,000 subjects) carried out over three consecutive influenza seasons has shown that the use of the MF59-adjuvanted vaccine allows a reduction of 23 % of hospitalization for influenza and pneumonia in subjects over 65 years of age (Mannino et al. 2012). The stronger effectiveness of MF59-adjuvanted inactivated vaccine as compared to non-adjuvanted vaccine in preventing laboratory confirmed influenza in the elderly was reported in a recent study in the elderly in Canada (Van Buynder et al. 2013).

The mechanism(s) of the basis of the increased breadth of antibody response mediated by the MF59 adjuvant are still under investigation. The data obtained so far clearly show that MF59 not only influences the quantity of anti-influenza antigen antibodies, but it also, and more importantly, dramatically affects the quality of these antibodies, shaping the B-cell epitopes recognized by specific, neutralizing antibodies, which are now directed against functional epitopes located in the HA1 region of HA and near the catalytic site of NA. This was demonstrated in studies in which serum samples from subjects vaccinated with non-adjuvanted, with aluminum hydroxide adjuvanted, or with MF59-adjuvanted H5N1 vaccines were analyzed by whole-genome-fragment phage display libraries (GFPDL), followed by surface plasmon resonance technologies (Khurana et al. 2010). While sera from subjects vaccinated with non-adjuvanted or alum-adjuvanted vaccines mostly recognized fragments of the HA2 region, the presence of MF59 in the vaccine induced epitope spreading from HA2 to HA1 and allowed the appearance of antibodies to NA. Moreover, a nearly 20-fold increase in the frequency of HA1/HA2-specific phage clones was observed in sera after Aflunov administration, when compared to responses after the unadjuvanted or alum-adjuvanted H5N1 vaccines. Additionally, MF59-adjuvanted vaccines induced a 2- to 3-fold increase in the frequency of antibodies reactive with properly folded HA1 (28–319), a fragment that absorbed most neutralizing activity in immune sera (Khurana et al. 2010), and that was known to be recognized by cross-reacting neutralizing monoclonal antibodies, and by sera from immune subjects who had recovered from a natural infection with the H5N1 virus (Khurana et al. 2009). The adjuvant-dependent increased binding to conformational HA1 epitopes paralleled the broadening of cross-clade neutralization and predicted improved in vivo protection. Finally, antibodies against potentially protective epitopes in the C-terminal region of NA, close to the sialic acid-binding enzymatic site, were also induced primarily following vaccination with MF59-adjuvanted H5N1 vaccine, but not with non-adjuvanted nor with alum-adjuvanted vaccines (Khurana et al. 2010). More recent studies have shown that the spreading of the epitopes recognized by MF59-adjuvanted vaccines, with an increased number of regions recognized in the HA1 globular head as compared to the HA2 fragment, is a general phenomenon and also applies to 2009 A/H1N1 pandemic immunization of toddlers, adolescents and adults. In addition, MF59 significantly enhances the avidity of the induced antibodies, especially in toddlers and adolescents, as compared to non-adjuvanted vaccines (Khurana et al. 2011a, b).

In the past few years, several groups have shown that it is possible to isolate monoclonal antibodies (mAbs) from infected or vaccinated subjects boadly reactive against a large panel of influenza virus strains, and recognizing epitopes residing in the stem region of the HA (Corti and Lanzavecchia 2013). These observations and the intrinsic property of the stem region of being highly conserved among the known HAs has prompted several groups to consider the development of "universal" influenza vaccines using the stem region as the key immunogen (Pica and Palese 2013). Recently, however, data have been reported showing that antibody response exquisitely directed against the HA2 region can enhance the severity of the influenza infection in pigs following challenge with an heterovariant virus via an enhancement of the fusion of the virus to target cells (Khurana et al. 2013). If these data are confirmed, one should be cautious about the potential risks of "universal" influenza vaccines (Crowe 2013). A corollary of this is that MF59-adjuvanted vaccine would offer a significant risk of disease enhancement because of its propensity to direct the antibody response toward the globular head of the HA and much less to the HA2 moiety of the HA.

The exact mechanism through which MF59 exerts its adjuvanticity is only partially understood. From in vivo studies using genome wide microarray analysis in mice, we now know that MF59 is more potent than CpG and aluminum salts in inducing a wide range of genes linked with the immune response. In addition, MF59 induces the upregulation of IL1β and of other genes involved in IL1β processing, such as caspase 1, and of genes coding for Ccr2 and its ligands (Ccl2, Ccl7 and Ccl8). Furthermore, MF59 promotes a rapid influx of CD11b$^+$ cells into the muscle compared to other adjuvants. MHC class II$^+$ cells were also recruited in the muscle at 4 days, suggesting that CD11b$^+$ cells differentiate into functional inflammatory DCs, expressing high levels of MHC class II (Mosca et al. 2008). In summary, MF59, although not capable of activating directly DCs in vitro, can trigger a local immunostimulatory environment characterized by the expression of several cytokines, which may indirectly activate DCs through a TLR-independent mechanism. In addition to recruitment and activation of cells at the site of injects, MF59 also favors the uptake of the antigen by antigen-presenting cells and its transport to the draining luymph nodes (Calabro et al. 2011). Interestingly, enough recent data have clearly shown that no one of the components of MF59, not even the most abundant component, squalene, mediate the adjuvant effect of this adjuvant. This activity requires the presence of the emulsion, which needs the orchestrated presence of all constituents (Calabro et al. 2013). Very recent data have shown that MF59, but not other adjuvants like incomplete Freund's adjuvant, aluminum hydroxide or calcium phosphate, induced the release of extracellular ATP from the muscle, and this release represented the "danger signal" specifically triggered by this adjuvant and able to enhance the antibody response to the co-administered antigens (Vono et al. 2013).

Since 1997, both meta-analysis of controlled clinical trials in adults, adolescents, and children (Pellegrini et al. 2009; Black et al. 2010), and postmarketing pharmacovigilance surveillance (Schultze et al. 2008) have demonstrated that the addition of MF59 does not change the incidence of autoimmune syndromes, chronic diseases, death or neurological conditions, and so on. The safety profile of MF59-adjuvanted influenza vaccine was recently confirmed in the large effectiveness study carried out in Lombardy, Italy (Villa et al. 2013). Moreover, the excellent safety profile has now been confirmed after the widespread use of MF59-adjuvanted vaccines against the 2009 A/H1N1 pandemic influenza (Banzhoff et al. 2011; Tsai et al. 2013), including pregnant women (Heikkinen et al. 2012; Rubinstein et al. 2013) and subjects of various ages with various underlying pathological conditions (O'Hagan et al. 2013).

5.2 AS03-Adjuvanted Influenza Vaccines

In addition to squalene, the AS03 adjuvant contains α-tocopherol which acts as an immunostimulat (Garçon et al. 2012) (Table 1). Despite the fact that all these oil-in-water adjuvants contain squalene, the behavior in vivo varies due to the presence of the other components. For example, unlike MF59, which only activates the mouse transcriptome at the site of injection in the muscle (Caproni et al. 2012), AS03 is able to strongly induce upregulation of genes encoding inflammatory cytokines and chemokines at distant sites, such as in the draining lymph nodes, and this effect is specifically mediated by α-tocopherol (Morel et al. 2011).

AS03 has been licensed together with pandemic A/H1N1 and with avian A/H5N1 split inactivated monovalent vaccines. With both vaccines, AS03 allowed a significant antigen dose sparing, showed a strong activation of antigen-specific CD4+ T cells (Moris et al. 2011), and an acceptable safety profile, including in pregnant women (Ludvigsson et al. 2013). In the very few clinical studies where A/H1N1 monovalent vaccines adjuvanted with the AS03 or with the MF59 adjuvants , the AS03-adjuvanted vaccines induced higher titers of antibodies but also higher reactogenicity, while the MF59-adjuvanted vaccines induced a lower but acceptable antibody response, and exhibited a significantly better safety profile (Meier et al. 2011; Rahier et al. 2011).

Clinical studies were carried out recently using seasonal trivalent influenza vaccine together with various preparations of AS03 containing lower amounts of α-tocopherol with or without monophosphoryl lipid A (MPL), in an attempt to improve the adjuvanticity of the AS03 adjuvant and to reduce, at the same time, its reactogenicity. The AS03 preparation with the best balance between improved immunogenicity and acceptable reactogenicity turned out to be the AS03B containing half (5.93 mg) of the amount of α-tocopherol as compared to the amount used for the pandemic A/H1N1 vaccine (AS03A) (Rümke et al. 2013). The AS03B adjuvant was used to enhance the immunogenicity of a QIV in healthy adults (Beran et al. 2013), and to carry out a randomized phase 3 efficacy trial with a seasonal trivalent split vaccine in the elderly aged at least 65 years, which involved 43,802 subjects in 15 countries who received either the adjuvanted vaccine or the same non-adjuvanted vaccine during two consecutive influenza seasons (2008–2009 and 2009–2010) (McElhaney et al. 2013). The influenza attack rate (590 cases confirmed as influenza A, B or both) was lightly lower in the groups given the adjuvanted vaccine than in the group given non-adjuvanted vaccine, not meeting the statistically significance for superiority criterion, however. A similar non-significant result ($p = 0.1205$) was obtained when PCRs were carried out in swabs taken as a result of fever. A relative efficacy of 22 % for the adjuvanted vaccine was observed only against A/H3N2 influenza in the post-hoc analysis and of 17 % against influenza A in the exploratory analysis (McElhaney et al. 2013).

The AS03-adjuvanted monovalent vaccine against the pandemic A/H1N1 influenza virus has been extensively used in many European countries and in Canada. In March 2010, the first cases of narcolepsy with cataplexy were reported by Sweden and Finland as being associated with the use of this vaccine. An increased risk of narcolepsy with cataplexy after vaccination with the AS03-adjuvanted pandemic A/H1N1 vaccine, mainly in subjects aged between 5 and 19 years of age, has been reported from Finland, Sweden, England, Ireland, France, and Norway (Nohynek et al. 2012; Partinen et al. 2012; National Narcolepsy Study Steering Committee Ireland 2012; Heier et al 2012 Szakács et al. 2013; Miller et al. 2013; Dauvilliers et al. 2013). The mechanisms behind this increased risk of narcolepsy remain unclear. For example, the incidence of narcolepsy in China has a pattern of seasonality, with peaks during the influenza season, more evident during the 2009 A/H1N1 pandemic (Han et al. 2011). It should be noted that adjuvanted pandemic vaccines were not used and this peak of incidence of narcolepsy cannot be ascribed to it. Data from Finland do not support the hypothesis that the increased risk of narcolepsy could be due to the concomitant use of the vaccine during the peak of the influenza pandemic (Melén et al. 2013). It has been recently hypothesized that in genetically susceptible subjects (HLA-DQA1*01:02/DQB1*06:02 [DQ0602]) narcolepsy could have been caused by a phenomenon of molecular mimicry, via the induction of CD4+ T cells reacting with two epitopes of the neuropeptide hypocretin ($HCRT_{56–68}$ and $HCRT_{87–99}$) that shared some homology with the amino acid sequence 275–287 of the HA of the pandemic A/H1N1 virus strain (De la Herrán-Arita et al. 2013). The lack of association between narcolepsy and the use of influenza vaccines containing other oil-in-water adjuvants such as MF59 rules out the ingredients common to all the adjuvants (e.g. squalene) as a trigger of this severe complication

(Tsai et al. 2013). Additional in-depth studies are required to unveil the cause-effect relationship observed in several countries between the use of the AS03-adjuvanted pandemic vaccine and the insurgence of narcolepsy.

5.3 AF03-Adjuvanted Influenza Vaccines

As compared to MF59 and AS03, AF03-adjuvanted influenza vaccines (Klucker et al. 2012, Table 1) have been used much less. As in the case of MF59 and AS03, AF03 also allowed significant dose sparing of the A/H5N1 avian influenza vaccine to allow a significantly enhanced antibody response (Levie et al. 2008). In a trial carried out in 6 month- to 7-year-old subjects, AF03-adjuvanted pandemic A/H1N1 vaccine induced very strong antibody responses reaching the conventional level of seroprotection (HI titer ≥1:40) after a single dose in children older than 3 years of age. However, two doses were required in children aged 6–35 months (Vesikari et al. 2012b).

6 Other Adjuvants

If only inactivated influenza vaccines adjuvanted with oil-in-water emulsions have been licensed so far, the 2009 pandemic, the thread of avian influenza infections, mainly with A/H5N1 viruses but more recently with A/H7N9 viruses, and the widely recognized low performance of inactivated vaccines at the extremes of age, have prompted various groups to test their adjuvants with influenza vaccines.

The adjuvants under testing are at different stages of development, from pre-clinical to phase I trials in humans belong to various families. They include, for example, TLR agonists, such as TLR-3 (poly-I:C), TLR-4 (MPL and its derivatives), TLR-5 (flagellin), and TLR-9 (CpG) agonists, Iscoms and Iscomatrix, virus-like-particles (VLP), various sorts of liposomes, etc. (Table 2).

The synthetic MPL-like molecule glucopyranosyl-lipid A (GLA), formulated in a stable oil-in-water emulsion (SE), is a TLR-4 agonist which has been widely tested in several preclinical models and recently used to enhance the immunogenicity of a recombinant A/H5N1 HA protein in almost 400 healthy adults. Two administrations of 3.8–45 μg of a recombinant, baculovirus-derived HA were well tolerated and induced levels of HI antibodies above 1:40 in 72–82% of subjects (Treanor et al. 2013). In other studies, GLA-SE was shown to activate myeloid dendritic cells to produce high levels of TNF-a, IL-6 and IL-12 with an enhancement of the Th1-type response and suppression of Il-10 production (Behzad et al. 2012).

The TLR-5 agonist flagellin from *Salmonella typhimurium* was fused with tandem copies of the extracellular domain of the M2 protein (M2e) or with the globular head of the HA. In both cases, the presence of flagellin significantly enhanced the antibody response to these antigens (Taylor et al. 2012; Turley et al. 2011).

Table 2 Some adjuvants currently tested for enhancing the immune response to inactivated influenza vaccines and at different stages of development

Adjuvant	Source	Stage of development	Reference
Virosomes	Crucell/Johnson & Johnson Solvay/Abbott	Licensed	Moser et al. 2011; Wilschut 2009
CAF01: Cationic liposomes	Statens Serum Institut	Preclinical	Christensen et al. 2011
CCS/C: Cationic liposomes	NasVax	Phase I	Ben-Yehuda et al. 2003
TLR-9 agonist: CpG not conjugated to antigens	Coley/Pfizer	Phase I	Cooper et al. 2004
TLR-9 agonist: CpG conjugated to antigens	Dynavax	Phase I	Livingston et al. 2006
TLR-9 agonist: IC31	Intercell/Valneva	Phase I	Riedl et al. 2008
TLR-5 agonist: *S. typhimurium* flagellin	Vaxinnate	Phase I	Turley et al. 2011; Taylor et al. 2012
TLR-4 agonist: glucopyranosyl-lipid A (GLA) with stable oil-in-water emulsion (SE)	IDRI	Phase I	Treanor et al. 2013
TLR-3 agonist: poly(I:C)	Hemispherx Biopharma	Phase I	Hafner et al. 2013
Iscoms: Matrix-M	Isconova	Phase I	Rimmelzwaan et al. 2000; Pedersen et al. 2012
Alpha-galactosylceramide	Various sources	Preclinical	Galli et al. 2007

Variable levels of immune enhancement have been reported in clinical trials with TLR-9 agonists (Cooper et al. 2004), various forms of Iscoms (Rimmelzwaan et al. 2000; Pedersen et al. 2012), various forms of liposomes (Ben-Yehuda et al. 2003; Wilschut 2009; Moser et al. 2011; Christensen et al. 2011), etc (Table 2). Interesting results have been reported with recombinant virus-like particles (VLP) produced in insect cells or in plant cells and including in their composition HA, NA and M1. These constructs have been amply tested in animals where they showed good efficacy against lethal challenge with infectious viruses. In humans, these VLPs were well tolerated and induced good antibody responses against pandemic A/H1N1 and avian A/H5N1 viruses at levels that are considered protective (Khurana et al. 2011b; López-Macías et al. 2011). VLPs can also offer the opportunity to blend together HAs from various influenza virus strains to widen the breadth of protective antibody response against multiple influenza viruses (Pushko et al. 2011). VLPs containing antigens from the avian A/H7N9 influenza virus have recently shown very good immunogenicity in clinical trials in healthy adults (Fries et al. 2013).

In general, as compared to the oil-in-water adjuvants MF59 and AS03 licensed for several years, the experience with these adjuvants is still limited. Larger databases are required in order to establish their unequivocal safety and their immunogenicity, and possibly the efficacy/effectiveness in various age groups before they can become a reality in the influenza vaccine landscape.

7 Conclusions and Perspectives

It is undeniable that inactivated influenza vaccines have an illustrious history (Oxford et al. 2011) and have contributed during the past several decades to reduce the mortality and the morbidity due to the seasonal epidemics of influenza, mainly in older adults, and to attenuate the deleterious impact of the last influenza pandemics. Nevertheless, their efficacy and effectiveness is far to be optimal. The use of adjuvants, like the oil-in-water emulsions, have significantly improved their efficacy in young children (Vesikari et al. 2011) and their effectiveness in the elderly (Mannino et al. 2012; Van Buynder et al. 2013). These adjuvants have allowed significant dose sparing, enhancement of the immunogenicity, strong priming, and long lasting immunological memory with pandemic and avian influenza vaccines. The advent of novel generation adjuvants can even improve the beneficial effects of inactivated influenza vaccines. However, several areas still need a significant improvement in the field of influenza vaccine development in order to achieve the ultimate goal of wide coverage and public health impact in all age groups.

1. The majority of inactivated influenza vaccines are still produced in embryonated eggs using reassorted virus strains that do not necessarily produce the desired yield of viruses to allow efficient and timely vaccine production. This is experienced every year for seasonal vaccines (even twice a year if the virus strains recommended by WHO for the Southern Hemisphere are different from those recommended for the Northern Hemisphere), but the situation can be dramatic in case of a pandemic. The registration of influenza vaccines produced by cell culture (European Medicines Agency 2008, 2009; Food and Drug Administration 2012) or using recombinant HA (Food and Drug Administration 2013) can change the landscape and allow the preparation of vaccines more closely reproducing the circulating strains.
2. Furthermore, the potency of the inactivated vaccines is still based on the content of HA which is measured using the single radial immunodiffusion, a methodology developed during the 1970s (Schild et al. 1975), that requires strain-specific antisera, the preparation of which in sheep is time consuming and can further delay the vaccine production. In addition, the measurement of the content of other viral antigens, such as NA, M1, NP, etc, is not required, and it is known that the content of these proteins can not only vary significantly

from one vaccine to another (Co et al. 2009), but also in various batches of the same vaccine. If it is well established that the protection against influenza infection is primarily mediated by antibodies directed against the HA, the relative contribution of the immune response against the other viral components still remains unknown.

3. The antibody response induced by inactivated influenza vaccines is measured with methodologies like HI that, despite the requirement for the registration of vaccines, are far to give reproducible results in different laboratories. Other methods, like MN, are not standardized yet (Montomoli et al. 2011). This implies that results with different vaccines from different trials and with assays carried out in different laboratories cannot be readily compared. As a corollary, the HI antibody titer of 1:40, commonly considered as a correlate of protection against influenza (Hobson et al. 1972), should be reconsidered (i) because of the intrinsic variability of the assay used; (ii) because it determines the level of 50 % efficacy of the vaccine, which is not ideal in a public health perspective; (iii) because it applies to immunologically primed subjects like young and old adults, but not children, for whom much higher threshold of seroprotection have been proposed (Black et al. 2011).
4. Inactivated influenza vaccines, as the majority of vaccines based on soluble proteins, exquisitely induce antigen-specific antibody responses and CD4+ T cell responses with various reported functional phenotypes (depending on the assays used to measure them), and with a proven ability to help B cells to produce antigen-specific antibodies (Spensieri et al. 2013). The ability of these vaccines to induce cell-mediated immunity directly involved in the effector mechanisms of protection is still a matter of debate. Adjuvants like oil-in-water MF59 are unable to induce antigen-specific CD8+ T cells (Galli et al. 2009b). Other methods are required in order to prime and expand influenza-specific T cells able to participate in the protection against the infection or against the disease. Furthermore, antigens other than the surface antigens like HA and NA are likely required in order to achieve this goal. This is the reason why attempts are being made to use internal proteins like NP and M1, delivered in an appropriate manner, to induce CD8+ T cells to be functionally active against the virus (Powell et al. 2013).
5. Vaccines against the influenza pandemic must be produced quickly to become available prior to the pandemic. During the last H1N1 pandemic, the production of the vaccine started only in June because of the lack of reassortants and specific reagents; the vaccine was available at the peak of the pandemic, and mass vaccination had been implemented when transmission already declined (Centers for Disease Control 2010). A prompter response to a pandemic has become feasible due to in vitro synthesis of genomes (Gibson et al. 2010). As a prerequisite, sequences of the viruses isolated must be provided to the vaccine manufacturer as soon as they are available. A combination of enzymatic, cell-free assembly techniques with enzymatic error correction allows for the rapid and accurate synthesis of genes that are then used to transfect cell lines qualified for vaccine manufacturing, from which viruses can be rescued for vaccine preparation. This process takes as few as 5 days with the recovery of synthetic

viruses antigenically identical to the wild-type viruses. This synthetic process has been successfully used to generate influenza strains including H1N1, seasonal and swine-origin H3N2, H5N1 and H7N9 (Dormitzer et al. 2013). The process of vaccine development can be further accelerated if, instead of subunit vaccines, vaccines are created based on self-amplifying viral mRNA, recently shown to be highly immunogenic in animals (Hekele et al. 2013).

References

Alberini I, Del Tordello E, Fasolo A, Temperton N, Galli G, Gentile C, Montomoli E, Hilbert AK, Banzhoff A, Giuseppe Del Giudice G, Donnelly J, Rappuoli R, Capecchi B (2009) Pseudoparticle neutralization is a reliable assay to measure immunity and cross-reactivity to H5N1 influenza viruses. Vaccine 27:5998–6003

Ansaldi F, Bacilieri S, Durando P, Sticchi L, Valle L, Montomoli E, Icardi G, Gasparini R, Crovari P (2008) Cross-protection by MF59-adjuvanted influenza vaccine: neutralizing and hemagglutination-inhibiting antibody activity against A(H3N2) drifted influenza viruses. Vaccine 26:1525–1529

Ansaldi F, Zancolli F, Durando P, Montomoli E, Sticchi L, Giuseppe Del Giudice G, Icardi G (2010) Antibody response against heterogeneous circulating influenza virus strains elicited by MF59-and non-adjuvanted vaccines during seasons with good or partical matching between vaccine strain and clinical isolates. Vaccine 28:4123–4129

Baldo V, Baldovin T, Floreani A, Minuzzo M, Trivello R (2006) Response to influenza vaccine in people with non-protective HI antibody titers. Eur J Epidemiol 21:843–845

Baldo V, Baldovin T, Pellegrini M, Angiolelli G, Majori S, Floreani A, Busana MC, Bertoncello C, Trivello R (2010) Immunogenicity of three different influenza vaccines against homologous and heterologous strains in nursing home elderly residents. Clin Dev Immunol 2010:517198. doi: 10.1155/2010/517198. Epub 2010 Mar 29

Banzhoff A, Nacci P, Podda A (2003) A new MF59-adjuvanted influenza vaccine enhances the immune response in the elderly with chronic diseases: Results from an immunogenicity meta-analysis. Gerontology 49:177–184

Banzhoff A, Gasparini R, Laghi-Pasini F, Staniscia T, Durando P, Montomoli E, Capecchi PL, Di Giovanni P, Sticchi L, Gentile C, Hilbert A, Brauer V, Tilman S, Podda A (2009) MF59-adjuvanted H5N1 vaccine induces immunologic memory and heterotypic antibody responses in non-elderly and elderly adults. PLoS ONE 4(2):e4384

Banzhoff A, Haertel S, Praus M (2011) Passive surveillance of adverse events of an MF59-adjuvanted H1N1v vaccine during the pandemic mass vaccinations. Hum Vaccin 7:539–548

Barrett PN, Berezuk G, Fritsch S, Aichinger G, Hart MK, El-Amin W, Kistner O, Ehrlich HJ (2011) Efficacy, safety, and immunogenicity of a Vero-cell-culture-derived trivalent influenza vaccine: a multicentre, double-blind, randomised, placebo-controlled trial. Lancet 377:751–759

Beebe GW, Simon AH, Vivona S (1972) Long-term mortality follow-up of Army recruits who received adjuvant influenza virus vaccine in 1951-1953. Am J Epidemiol 95:337–346

Behzad H, Huckriede AL, Haynes L, Gentleman B, Coyle K, Wilschut JC, Kollmann TR, Reed SG, McElhaney JE (2012) GLA-SE, a synthetic toll-like receptor 4 agonist, enhances T-cell responses to influenza vaccine in older adults. J Infect Dis 205:466–473

Belshe RB (2010) The need for quadrivalent vaccine against seasonal influenza. Vaccine 28(Suppl 4):D45–D53

Belshe RB, Newman FK, Cannon J, Duane C, Treanor J, Van Hoecke C, Howe BJ, Dubin G (2004) Serum antibody responses after intradermal vaccination against influenza. N Engl J Med 351:2286–2294

Belshe RB, Newman FK, Wilkins K, Graham IL, Babusis E, Ewell M, Frey SE (2007) Comparative immunogenicity of trivalent influenza vaccine administered by intradermal or intramuscular route in healthy adults. Vaccine 25:6755–6763

Bentebibel SE, Lopez S, Obermoser G, Schmitt N, Mueller C, Harrod C, Flano E, Mejias A, Albrecht RA, Blankenship D, Xu H, Pascual V, Banchereau J, Garcia-Sastre A, Palucka AK, Ramilo O, Ueno H (2013) Induction of ICOS + CXCR3 + CXCR5 + TH cells correlates with antibody responses to influenza vaccination. Sci Transl Med 5:176ra32

Ben-Yehuda A, Joseph A, Zeira E, Even-Chen S, Louria-Hayon I, Babai I, Zakay-Rones Z, Greenbaum E, Barenholz Y, Kedar E (2003) Immunogenicity and safety of a novel liposomal influenza subunit vaccine (INFLUSOME-VAC) in young adults. J Med Virol 69:560–567

Beran J, Vesikari T, Wertzova V, Karvonen A, Honegr K, Lindblad N, Van Belle P, Peeters M, Innis BL, Devaster JM (2009) Efficacy of inactivated split-virus influenza vaccine against culture-confirmed influenza in healthy adults: a prospective randomized, placebo-controlled trial. J Infect Dis 200:1861–1869

Beran J, Peeters M, Dewé W, Raupachova J, Hobzova L, Devaster JM (2013) Immunogenicity and safety of quadrivalent versus trivalent inactivated vaccine: a randomized, controlled trial in adults. BMC Infect Dis 13:224

Bernstein DI, Edwards KM, Dekker CL, Belshe R, Talbot HK, Graham IL, Noah DL, He F, Hill H (2008) Effects of adjuvants on the safety and immunogenicity of an avian influenza H5N1 vaccine in adults. J Infect Dis 197:667–675

Beutner KR, Chow T, Rubi E, Strussenberg J, Clement J, Ogra PL (1979) Evaluation of a neuraminidase-specific influenza A virus vaccine in children: antibody responses and effects on two successive outbreaks of natural infection. J Infect Dis 140:844–850

Black S, Della Cioppa G, Malfroot A, Nacci P, Nicolay U, Pellegrini M, Sokal E, Vertruyen A (2010) Safety of MF59-adjuvanted versus non-adjuvanted influenza vaccines in children and adolescents: an integrated analysis. Vaccine 28:7331–7336

Black S, Nicolay U, Vesikari T, Knuf M, Giuseppe Del Giudice G, Della Cioppa G, Tsai T, Clemens R, Rappuoli R (2011) Hemagglutination inhibition antibody titers as a correlate of protection for inactivated influenza vaccines in children. Pediatr Infect Dis J 30:1081–1085

Calabro S, Tortoli M, Baudner BC, Pacitto A, Cortese M, O'Hagan DT, De Gregorio E, Seubert A, Wack A (2011) Vaccine adjuvants alum and MF59 induce rapid recruitment of neutrophils and monocytes that participate in antigen transport to draining lymph nodes. Vaccine 29:1812–1823

Calabro S, Tritto E, Pezzotti A, Taccone M, Muzzi A, Bertholet S, De Gregorio E, O'Hagan DT, Baudner B, Seubert A (2013) The adjuvant effect of MF59 is due to the oil-in-water emulsion formulation, none of the individual components induce a comparable adjuvant effect. Vaccine 31:3363–3369

Camilloni B, Neri M, Lepri E, Iorio AM (2009) Cross-reactive antibodies in middle-aged and elderly volunteers after MF59-adjuvanted subunit trivalent influenza vaccine against B viruses of the B/Victoria or B/Yamagata lineages. Vaccine 27:4099–4103

Caproni E, Tritto E, Cortese M, Muzzi A, Mosca F, Monaci E, Baudner B, Seubert A, De Gregorio E (2012) MF59 and Pam3CSK4 boost adaptive responses to influenza subunit vaccine through an IFN type I-independent mechanism of action. J Immunol 188:3088–3098

Carrat F, Flahault A (2007) Influenza vaccine: the challenge of antigenic drift. Vaccine 25:6852–6862

Centers for Disease Control (2010). Updated CDC estimates of 2009 H1N1 influenza cass, hospitalizations and deaths in the United States, April 2009–April 2010

Centers for Disease control (2013) Flu vaccination coverage. http://www.cdc.gov/flu/fluvaxview/coverage-1213estimates.htm. Accessed 23 Dec 2013

Chen WH, Cross AS, Edelman R, Sztein M, Blackwelder WC, Pasetti MF (2011) Antibody and Th1-type cell-mediated immune responses in elderly and young adults immunized with standard or a high dose influenza vaccine. Vaccine 29:2865–2873

Christensen D, Korsholm KS, Andersen P, Agger EM (2011) Cationic liposomes as vaccine adjuvants. Expert Rev Vaccines 10:513–521

Clements ML, Betts RF, Tierney EL, Murphy BR (1986) Serum and nasal wash antibodies associated with resistance to experimental challenge with influenza A wild-type virus. J Clin Microbiol 24:157–160

Co MDT, Orphin L, Cruz J, Pazoles P, Green KM, Potts J, Leporati AM, Babon JAB, Evans JE, Ennis FA, Terajima M (2009) In vitro evidence that commercial influenza vaccines are not similar in their ability to activate human T cell responses. Vaccine 27:319–327

Committee on Infectious Diseases (2013) Recommendations for prevention and control of influenza in children, 2013-2014. Pediatrics 132:e1089–e1104

Cooper CL, Davis HL, Morris ML, Efler SM, Krieg AM, Li Y, Laframboise C, Al Adhami MJ, Khaliq Y, Seguin I, Cameron DW (2004) Safety and immunogenicity of CPG 7909 injection as an adjuvant to Fluarix influenza vaccine. Vaccine 22:3136–3143

Corti D, Lanzavecchia A (2013) Broadly neutralizing antiviral antibodies. Annu Rev Immunol 31:705–742

Coudeville L, Bailleux F, Riche B, Megas F, Andre P, Ecochard R (2010) Relationship between haemagglutinin-inhibiting antibody titres and clinical protection against influenza: development and application of a Bayesian random effects model. BMC Med Res Methodol 10:18

Crowe JE Jr (2013) Universal flu vaccines: primum non nocere. Sci Transl Med 5:200fs34

Dauvilliers Y, Arnulf I, Lecendreux M, Monaca Charley C, Franco P, Drouot X, d'Ortho MP, Launois S, Lignot S, Bourgin P, Nogues B, Rey M, Bayard S, Scholz S, Lavault S, Tubert-Bitter P, Saussier C, Pariente A, Narcoflu-VF study group (2013) Increased risk of narcolepsy in children and adults after pandemic H1N1 vaccination in France. Brain 136:2486–2496

Davenport FM (1968) Antigenic enhancement of ether-extracted influenza virus vaccines by $AlPO_4$. Proc Soc Exp Biol Med 127:587–590

Davenport FM, Hennessy AV, Bell JA (1962) Immunologic advantages of emulsified influenza virus vaccines. Mil Med 127:95–100

Davenport DM, Hennessy AV, Askin FB (1968) Lack of adjuvant effect of $AlPO_4$ on purified influenza virus hemagglutining in man. J Immunol 100:1139–1140

Davis DJ, Philip RN, Bell JA, Voegel JE, Jensen DV (1961) Epidemiological studies on influenza in familiar and general population groups 1951-1956. III. Laboratory observations. Am J Hyg 73:138–147

De la Herrán-Arita AK, Kornum BR, Mahlios J, Jiang W, Lin L, Hou T, Macaubas C, Einen M, Plazzi G, Crowe C, Newell EW, Davis MM, Mellins ED, Mignot E (2013) CD4+ T Cell autoimmunity to hypocretin/orexin and cross-reactivity to a 2009 H1N1 influenza A epitope in narcolepsy. Sci Transl Med 5:216ra176

Giuseppe Del Giudice G, Hilbert AK, Bugarini R, Minutello A, Popova O, Toneatto D, Schoendorf I, Borkowski A, Rappuoli R, Podda A (2006) An MF59-adjuvanted inactivated influenza vaccine containing A/Panama/1999 (H3N2) induced broader serological protection against heterovariant influenza virus strain A/Fujian/2002 than a subunit and a split influenza vaccine. Vaccine 24:3063–3065

Giuseppe Del Giudice G, Fragapane E, Della Cioppa G, Rappuoli R (2013) Aflunov®: a vaccine tailored for pre-pandemic and pandemic approaches against influenza. Expert Opin Biol Ther 13:121–135

Della Cioppa G, Vesikari T, Sokal E, Lindert K, Nicolay U (2011) Trivalent and quadrivalent MF59®-adjuvanted influenza vaccine in young children: a dose-and schedule-finding study. Vaccine 29:8696–8704

Dolin R (2013) The quadrivalent approach to influenza vaccination. J Infect Dis 208:539–540

Domachowske JB, Pankow-Culot H, Bautista M, Geng Y, Claeys C, Peeters M, Innis BL, Jain V (2013) A randomized trial of candidate inactivated quadrivalent influenza vaccine versus trivalent influenza vaccines in children aged 3-17 years. J Infect Dis 207:1878–1887

Dormitzer PR, Tsai TF, Giuseppe Del Giudice G (2012) New technologies for influenza vaccines. Hum Vaccin Immunother 8:45–58

Dormitzer PR, Suphaphiphat P, Gibson DG, Wentworth DE, Stockwell TB, Algire MA, Alperovich N, Barro M, Brown DM, Craig S, Dattilo BM, Denisova EA, De Souza I, Eickmann M, Dugan VG, Ferrari A, Gomila RC, Han L, Judge C, Mane S, Matrosovich M,

Merryman C, Palladino G, Palmer GA, Spencer T, Strecker T, Trusheim H, Uhlendorff J, Wen Y, Yee AC, Zaveri J, Zhou B, Becker S, Donabedian A, Mason PW, Glass JI, Rappuoli R, Venter JC (2013) Synthetic generation of influenza vaccine viruses for rapid response to pandemics. Sci Transl Med 5:185ra68

Engelhardt OG (2013) Many ways to make an influenza virus–review of influenza virus reverse genetics methods. Influenza Other Respir Viruses 7:249–256

Esposito S, Tagliabue C, Tagliaferri L, Semino M, Longo MR, Principi N (2012) Preventing influenza in younger children. Clin Microbiol Infect 18(Suppl 5):42–49

European Medicines Agency (2008) Optaflu. http://www.ema.europa.eu/ema/index.jsp?curl=pages/medicines/human/medicines/000758/human_med_000952.jsp&mid=WC0b01ac058001d124. Accessed 23 Dec 2013

European Medicines Agency (2009) Celvaplan. http://www.ema.europa.eu/ema/index.jsp?curl=pages/medicines/human/medicines/000982/human_med_000690.jsp&mid=WC0b01ac058001d124. Accessed 23 Dec 2013

Fiore AE, Bridges CB, Cox NJ (2009) Seasonal influenza vaccines. Curr Top Microbiol Immunol 333:43–82

Food and Drug Administration (2012) Flucelvax. http://www.fda.gov/BiologicsBloodVaccines/Vaccines/ApprovedProducts/ucm328629.htm. Accessed 23 Dec 2013

Food and Drug Administration (2013) Flublok. http://www.fda.gov/BiologicsBloodVaccines/Vaccines/ApprovedProducts/ucm335836.htm. Accessed 23 Dec 2013

Fries LF, Smith GE, Glenn GM (2013) A recombinant virus-like particle influenza A (H7N9) vaccine. N Engl J Med 369:2564–2566

Galli G, Pittoni P, Tonti E, Malzone C, Uematsu Y, Tortoli M, Maione D, Volpini G, Finco O, Nuti S, Tavarini S, Dellabona P, Rappuoli R, Casorati G, Abrignani S (2007) Invariant NKT cells sustain specific B cell responses and memory. Proc Natl Acad Sci USA 104:3984–3989

Galli G, Hancock K, Hoschler K, DeVos J, Praus M, Bardelli M, Malzone C, Castellino F, Gentile C, McNally T, Giuseppe Del Giudice G, Banzhoff A, Brauer V, Montomoli E, Zambon M, Katz J, Nicholson K, Stephenson I (2009a) Fast rise of broadly cross-reactive antibodies after boosting long-lived human memory B cells primed by an MF59 adjuvanted prepandemic vaccine. Proc Natl Acad Sci USA 106:7962–7967

Galli G, Medini D, Borgogni E, Zedda L, Bardelli M, Malzone C, Nuti S, Tavarini S, Sammicheli C, Hilbert AK, Brauer V, Banzhoff A, Rappuoli R, Giuseppe Del Giudice G, Castellino F (2009b) Adjuvanted H5N1 vaccine induces early CD4+ T cell response that predicts long-term persistence of protective antibody levels. Proc Natl Acad Sci USA 106:3877–3882

Garçon N, Vaughn DW, Didierlaurent AM (2012) Development and evaluation of AS03, an adjuvant system containing α-tocopherol and squalene in an oil-in-water emulsion. Expert Rev Vaccines 11:349–366

Gibson DG, Smith HO, Hutchison CA III, Venter JC, Merryman C (2010) Chemical synthesis of the mouse mitochondrial genome. Nat Methods 7:901–903

Goodwin K, Viboud C, Simonsen L (2006) Antibody response to influenza vaccination in the elderly: a quantitative review. Vaccine 24:1159–1169

Gorse GJ, Falsey AR, Johnson CM, Morrison D, Fried DL, Ervin JE, Greenberg DP, Ozol-Godfrey A, Landolfi V, Tsang PH (2013) Safety and immunogenicity of revaccination with reduced dose intradermal and standard dose intramuscular influenza vaccines in adults 18-64 years of age. Vaccine 31:6034–6040

Greenberg DP, Robertson CA, Noss MJ, Blatter MM, Biedenbender R, Decker MD (2013) Safety and immunogenicity of a quadrivalent inactivated influenza vaccine compared to licensed trivalent inactivated influenza vaccines in adults. Vaccine 31:770–776

Hafner AM, Corthésy B, Merkle HP (2013) Particulate formulations for the delivery of poly(I:C) as vaccine adjuvant. Adv Drug Deliv Rev 65:1386–1399

Halperin W, Weiss WI, Altman R, Diamond MA, Black KJ, Iaci AW, Black HC, Goldfield M (1979) A comparison of the intradermal and subcutaneous routes of influenza vaccination with A/New Jersey/76 (Swine flu) and A/Victoria/75: Report of a study and review of the literature. Am J Public Health 69:1247–1250

Han F, Lin L, Warby SC, Faraco J, Li J, Dong SX, An P, Zhao L, Wang LH, Li QY, Yan H, Gao ZC, Yuan Y, Strohl KP, Mignot E (2011) Narcolepsy onset is seasonal and increased following the 2009 H1N1 pandemic in China. Ann Neurol 70:410–417

Hannoun C (2013) The evolving history of influenza viruses and influenza vaccines. Expert Rev Vaccines 12:1085–1094

Heier MS, Gautvik KM, Wannag E, Bronder KH, Midtlyng E, Kamaleri Y, Storsaeter J (2012) Incidence of narcolepsy in Norwegian children and adolescents after vaccination against H1N1 influenza A. Sleep Med 14:867–871

Heikkinen T, Young J, van Beek E, Franke H, Verstraeten T, Weil JG, Della Cioppa G (2012) Safety of MF59-adjuvanted A/H1N1 influenza vaccine in pregnancy: a comparative cohort study. Am J Obstet Gynecol 207(3):177.e1-8

Hekele A, Bertholet S, Archer J, Gibson DG, Palladino G, Brito LA, Otten GR, Brazzoli M, Buccato S, Bonci A, Casini D, Maione D, Qi ZQ, Gill JE, Caiazza NC, Urano J, Hubby B, Gao GF, Shu Y, De Gregorio E, Mandl CW, Mason PW, Settembre EC, Ulmer JB, Venter JC, Dormitzer PR, Rappuoli R, Geall AJ (2013) Rapidly produced SAM® vaccine against H7N9 influenza is immunogenic in mice. Emerg Microb Infect 2:e52

Hennessy AV, Davenport FM (1961) Relative merits of aqueous and adjuvant influenza vaccines when used in a two-dose schedule. Public Health Rep 76:411–419

Hobson D, Curry RL, Beare AS, Ward-Gardner A (1972) The role of serum haemagglutination-inhibiting antibody in protection against challenge infection with influenza A2 and B virus. J Hyg (Lond) 70:767–777

Iob A, Brianti G, Zamparo E, Gallo T (2005) Evidence of increased clinical protection of an MF59-adjuvant influenza vaccine compared to a non-adjuvant vaccine among elderly residents of long-term care facilities in Italy. Epidemiol Infect 133:687–693

Jain V, Rivera L, Zaman K, Espos RA Jr, Sirivichayakul C, Quiambao BP, Rivera-Medina DM, Kerdpanich P, Ceyhan M, Dinleyici EC, Cravioto A, Yunus M, Chanthavanich P, Linkittikul K, Kurugol Z, Alhan E, Caplanusi A, Durviaux S, Boutet P, Ofori-Anyinam O, Chandrasekaran V, Dbaibo G, Innis BL (2013) Vaccine for prevention of mild and moderate-to-severe influenza in children N Engl J Med Epub. doi:10.1056/NEJMoa1215817

Jefferson T, Rivetti A, Di Pietrantonj C, Demicheli V, Ferroni E (2012) Vaccines for preventing influenza in healthy children. Cochrane Database Syst Rev 8:CD004879

Karlsson EA, Marcelin G, Webby RJ, Schultz-Cherry S (2012) Review on the impact of pregnancy and obesity on influenza virus infection. Influenza Other Respir Viruses 6:449–460

Katz JM, Webster RG (1989) Efficacy of inactivated influenza A virus (H3N2) vacvcines grown in mammalian cells or embryonated eggs. J Infect Dis 160:191–198

Kendal AP, Bozeman FM, Ennis FA (1980) Further studies of the neuraminidase content of inactivated influenza vaccines and the neuraminidase antibody responses after vaccination of immunologically primed and unprimed populations. Infect Immun 29:966–971

Kenney RT, Frech SA, Muenz LR, Villar CP, Glenn GM (2004) Dose sparing with intradermal injection of influenza vaccine. N Engl J Med 351:2295–2301

Khurana S, Suguitan A Jr, Rivera Y, Simmons CP, Lanzavecchia A, Sallusto F, Manischewitz J, King LR, Subbarao K, Golding H (2009) Antigenic fingerprinting of H5N1 avian influenza using convalescent sera and monoclonal antibodies reveals potential vaccine and diagnostic tools. PLoS Med 6:e1000049. doi: 10.1371/journal.pmed.1000049

Khurana S, Chearwae W, Castellino F, Manischewitz J, King LR, Honorkiewicz A, Rock MT, Edwards KM, Giuseppe Del Giudice G, Rappuoli R, Golding H (2010) MF59-adjuvanted vaccines expand antibody repertoires targeting protective sites of pandemic H5N1 influenza virus. Sci Transl Med 2:15ra5

Khurana S, Verma N, Yewdell JW, Hilbert AK, Castellino F, Lattanzi M, Giuseppe Del Giudice G, Rappuoli R, Golding H (2011) MF59 adjuvant enhances diversity and affinity of antibody-mediated immune response to pandemic influenza viruses. Sci Transl Med 3:85ra48

Khurana S, Wu J, Verma N, Verma S, Raghunandan R, Manischewitz J, King LR, Kpamegan E, Pincus S, Smith G, Glenn G, Golding H (2011b) H5N1 virus-like particle vaccine elicits cross-reactive neutralizing antibodies that preferentially bind to the oligomeric form of influenza virus hemagglutinin in humans. J Virol 85:10945–10954

Khurana S, Loving CL, Manischewitz J, King LR, Gauger PC, Henningson J, Vincent AL, Golding H (2013) Vaccine-induced anti-HA2 antibodies promote virus fusion and enhance influenza virus respiratory disease. Sci Transl Med 5:200ra114

Kieninger D, Sheldon E, Lin WY, Yu CJ, Bayas JM, Gabor JJ, Esen M, Fernandez Roure JL, Narejos Perez S, Alvarez Sanchez C, Feng Y, Claeys C, Peeters M, Innis BL, Jain V (2013) Immunogenicity, reactogenicity and safety of an an inactivated quadrivalent influenza vaccine candidate versus inactivated trivalent influenza vaccine: a phase III, randomized trial in adults aged ≥18 years. BMC Infect Dis 13(1):343

Klucker MF, Dalençon F, Probeck P, Haensler J (2012) AF03, an alternative squalene emulsion-based vaccine adjuvant prepared by phase inversion temperature method. J Pharm Sci 101:4490–4500

Langley JM, Carmona Martinez A, Chatterjee A, Halperin SA, McNeil S, Reisinger KS, Aggarwal N, Haung LM, Peng CT, Garcia-Sicilia J, Salamanca de la Cueva I, Cabañas F, Treviño-Garza C, Rodriguez-Weber MA, de la OM, Chandrasekaran V, Dewé W, Liu A, Innis BL, Jain V (2013) Immunogenicity and safety of an inactivated quadrivalent influenza vaccine candidate: a phase III randomized controlled trial in children. J Infect Dis 208:544–553

Legrand J, Vergu E, Flahault A (2006) Real-time monitoring of the influenza vaccine field effectiveness. Vaccine 24:6605–6611

Leroux-Roels I, Leroux-Roels G (2009) Current status and progress of prepandemic and pandemic influenza vaccine development. Expert Rev Vaccines 8:401–423

Leroux-Roels I, Vets E, Freese R, Seiberling M, Weber F, Salamand C, Leroux-Roels G (2008) Seasonal influenza vaccine delivered by intradermal microinjection: a randomized controlled safety and immunogenicity trial in adults. Vaccine 26:6614–6619

Levie K, Leroux-Roels I, Hoppenbrouwers K, Kervyn AD, Vandermeulen C, Forgus S, Leroux-Roels G, Pichon S, Kusters I (2008) An adjuvanted, low-dose, pandemic influenza A (H5N1) vaccine candidate is safe, immunogenic, and induces cross-reactive immune responses in healthy adults. J Infect Dis 198:642–649

Livingston BD, Higgins D, Van Nest G (2006) Evolving strategies for the prevention of influenza infection: potential for multistrain targeting. BioDrugs 6:335–340

López-Macías C, Ferat-Osorio E, Tenorio-Calvo A, Isibasi A, Talavera J, Arteaga-Ruiz O, Arriaga-Pizano L, Hickman SP, Allende M, Lenhard K, Pincus S, Connolly K, Raghunandan R, Smith G, Glenn G (2011) Safety and immunogenicity of a virus-like particle pandemic influenza A (H1N1) 2009 vaccine in a blinded, randomized, placebo-controlled trial of adults in Mexico. Vaccine 29:7826–7834

Ludvigsson JF, Zugna D, Cnattingius S, Richiardi L, Ekbom A, Örtqvist Å, Persson I, Stephansson O (2013) Influenza H1N1 vaccination and adverse pregnancy outcome. Eur J Epidemiol 28:579–588

Mannino S, Villa M, Apolone G, Weiss NS, Groth N, Aquino I, Boldori L, Caramaschi F, Gattinoni A, Malchiodi G, Rothman KJ (2012) Effectiveness of adjuvanted influenza vaccination in elderly subjects in northern Italy. Am J Epidemiol 176:527–533

Marcelin G, Sandbulte MR, Webby RJ (2012) Contribution of antibody production against neuraminidase to the protection afforded by influenza vaccines. Rev Med Virol 22:267–279

McElhaney JE, Xie D, Hager WD, Barry MB, Wang Y, Kleppinger A, Ewen C, Kane KP, Bleackley RC (2006) T cell responses are better correlates of vaccine protection in the elderly. J Immunol 176:6333–6339

McElhaney JE, Beran J, Devaster JM, Esen M, Launay O, Leroux-Roels G, Ruiz-Palacios GM, van Essen GA, Caplanusi A, Claeys C, Durand C, Duval X, El Idrissi M, Falsey AR, Feldman G, Frey SE, Galtier F, Hwang SJ, Innis BL, Kovac M, Kremsner P, McNeil S, Nowakowski A, Richardus JH, Trofa A, Oostvogels L, Influence65 study group (2013) AS03-adjuvanted versus non-adjuvanted inactivated trivalent influenza vaccine against seasonal influenza in elderly people: a phase 3 randomised trial. Lancet Infect Dis 13:485–496

McKeage K (2013) Inactivated quadrivalent split-virus seasonal influenza vaccine (Fluarix® quadrivalent): a review of its use in the prevention of disease caused by influenza A and B. Drugs 73:1587–1594

Meier S, Bel M, L'huillier A, Crisinel PA, Combescure C, Kaiser L, Grillet S, Pósfay-Barbe K, Siegrist CA; H1N1 Epidemiology Study Group of Geneva (2011) Antibody responses to natural influenza A/H1N1/09 disease or following immunization with adjuvanted vaccines, in immunocompetent and immunocompromised children. Vaccine 29:3548–3557

Melén K, Partinen M, Tynell J, Sillanpää M, Himanen SL, Saarenpää-Heikkilä O, Hublin C, Olsen P, Ilonen J, Nohynek H, Syrjänen R, Kilpi T, Vuorela A, Kirjavainen T, Vaarala O, Julkunen I (2013) No serological evidence of influenza A H1N1pdm09 virus infection as a contributing factor in childhood narcolepsy after Pandemrix vaccination campaign in Finland. PLoS ONE 8:e68402

Mertz D, Kim TH, Johnstone J, Lam PP, Science M, Kuster SP, Fadel SA, Tran D, Fernandez E, Bhatnagar N, Loeb M (2013) Populations at risk for severe or complicated influenza illness: systematic review and meta-analysis. BMJ 347:f5061. doi:10.1136/bmj.f5061

Miller E, Andrews N, Stellitano L, Stowe J, Winstone AM, Shneerson J, Verity C (2013) Risk of narcolepsy in children and young people receiving AS03 adjuvanted pandemic A/H1N1 2009 influenza vaccine: retrospective analysis. BMJ 346:f794

Monto AS, Kendal AP (1973) Effect of neuraminidase antibody on Hong Kong influenza. Lancet 1:623–625

Montomoli E, Capecchi B, Hoschler K (2011) Correlates of protection against influenza. In: Rappuoli R, Giuseppe Del Giudice G (eds) Influenza vaccines for the future, 2nd edn. Springer, Basel, pp 199–222

Morel S, Didierlaurent A, Bourguignon P, Delhaye S, Baras B, Jacob V, Planty C, Elouahabi A, Harvengt P, Carlsen H, Kielland A, Chomez P, Garçon N, Van Mechelen M (2011) Adjuvant system AS03 containing α-tocopherol modulates innate immune response and leads to improved adaptive immunity. Vaccine 29:2461–2473

Moris P, van der Most R, Leroux-Roels I, Clement F, Dramé M, Hanon E, Leroux-Roels G, Van Mechelen M (2011) H5N1 influenza vaccine formulated with AS03a induces strong cross-reactive and polyfunctional CD4 T-cell responses. J Clin Immunol 31:443–454

Moro PL, Harrington T, Shimabukuro T, Cano M, Museru OI, Menschik D, Broder K (2013) Adverse events after Fluzone® intradermal vaccine reported to the Vaccine Adverse Event Reporting System (VAERS), 2011-2013. Vaccine 31:4984–4987

Mosca F, Tritto E, Muzzi A, Monaci E, Bagnoli F, Iavarone C, O'Hagan D, Rappuoli R, De Gregorio E (2008) Molecular and cellular signatures of human vaccine adjuvants. Proc Natl Acad Sci USA 105:10501–10506

Moser C, Amacker M, Zurbriggen R (2011) Influenza virosomes as a vaccine adjuvant and carrier system. Expert Rev Vaccines 10:437–446

Mostow SR, Schoenbaum SC, Dowdle WR, Coleman MT, Kaye HS, Hierholzer JC (1970) Studies on inactivated influenza vaccines. II. Effect of increasing dosage on antibody response and adverse reactions in man. Am J Epidemiol 92:248–256

National Narcolepsy Study Steeting Committee Ireland (2012) Investigation of an increase in the incidence of narcolepsy in children and adolescents in 2009 and 2010. http://healthupdate.gov.ie/wp-content/uploads/2012/04/Final_Report_of_National_Narcolepsy_Study_Steering_Committee-latest1.pdf. Accessed 27 Dec 2013

Nohynek H, Jokinen J, Partinen M, Vaarala O, Kirjavainen T, Sundman J, Himanen SL, Hublin C, Julkunen I, Olsén P, Saarenpää-Heikkilä O, Kilpi T (2012) AS03 adjuvanted AH1N1 vaccine associated with an abrupt increase in the incidence of childhood narcolepsy in Finland. PLoS ONE 7:e33536

O'Hagan DT, Ott GS, Nest GV, Rappuoli R, Giuseppe Del Giudice G (2013) The history of MF59® adjuvant: a phoenix that arose from the ashes. Expert Rev Vaccines 12:13–30

Osterholm MT, Kelley NS, Sommer A, Belongia EA (2012) Efficacy and effectiveness of influenza vaccines: a systematic review and meta-analysis. Lancet Infect Dis 12:36–44

Oxford J, Gilbert A, Lambkin-Williams R (2011) Influenza vaccines have a short but illustrious history of dedicated science enabling the rapid global production of A/swine (H1N1) vaccine in the current pandemic. In: Rappuoli R, Giuseppe Del Giudice G (eds) Influenza vaccines for the future, 2nd edition, Springer, Basel, pp 115–147

Partinen M, Saarenpää-Heikkilä O, Ilveskoski I, Hublin C, Linna M, Olsén P, Nokelainen P, Alén R, Wallden T, Espo M, Rusanen H, Olme J, Sätilä H, Arikka H, Kaipainen P, Julkunen I, Kirjavainen T (2012) Increased incidence and clinical picture of childhood narcolepsy following the 2009 H1N1 pandemic vaccination campaign in Finland. PLoS ONE 7:e33723

Pedersen GK, Madhun AS, Breakwell L, Hoschler K, Sjursen H, Pathirana RD, Goudsmit J, Cox RJ (2012) T-helper 1 cells elicited by H5N1 vaccination predict seroprotectioN. J Infect Dis 206:158–166

Pellegrini M, Nicolay U, Lindert K, Groth N, Della Cioppa G (2009) MF59-adjuvanted versus non-adjuvanted influenza vaccines: integrated analysis from a large safety database. Vaccine 27:6959–6965

Pépin S, Donazzolo Y, Jambrecina A, Salamand C, Saville M (2013) Safety and immunogenicity of a quadrivalent inactivated influenza vaccine in adults. Vaccine 31:5572–5578

Pica N, Palese P (2013) Toward a universal influenza virus vaccine: prospects and challenges. Annu Rev Med 64:189–202

Podda A (2001) The adjuvanted influenza vaccines with novel adjuvants: Experience with the MF59-adjuvanted vaccine. Vaccine 19:2673–2680

Poland G, Morse D (2010) Improving the public health: the US recommendation for universal influenza immunization. Vaccine 28:2799–2800

Powell TJ, Peng Y, Berthoud TK, Blais ME, Lillie PJ, Hill AV, Rowland-Jones SL, McMichael AJ, Gilbert SC, Dong T (2013) Examination of influenza specific T cell responses after influenza virus challenge in individuals vaccinated with MVA-NP + M1 vaccine. PLoS ONE 8:e62778

Puig-Barberà J, Diez-Domingo J, Pérez Hoyos S, Belenguer Varea A, González Vidal D (2004) Effectiveness of the MF59-adjuvanted influenza vaccine in preventing emergency admissions for pneumonia in the elderly over 64 years of age. Vaccine 23:283–289

Puig-Barberà J, Díez-Domingo J, Varea AB, Chavarri GS, Rodrigo JA, Hoyos SP, Vidal DG (2007) Effectiveness of MF59-adjuvanted subunit influenza vaccine in preventing hospitalisations for cardiovascular disease, cerebrovascular disease and pneumonia in the elderly. Vaccine 25:7313–7321

Pushko P, Pearce MB, Ahmad A, Tretyakova I, Smith G, Belser JA, Tumpey TM (2011) Influenza virus-like particle can accommodate multiple subtypes of hemagglutinin and protect from multiple influenza types and subtypes. Vaccine 29:5911–5918

Rahier JF, Papay P, Salleron J, Sebastian S, Marzo M, Peyrin-Biroulet L, Garcia-Sanchez V, Fries W, van Asseldonk DP, Farkas K, de Boer NK, Sipponen T, Ellul P, Louis E, Peake ST, Kopylov U, Maul J, Makhoul B, Fiorino G, Yazdanpanah Y, Chaparro M, European Crohn's Colitis Organisation (ECCO) (2011) H1N1 vaccines in a large observational cohort of patients with inflammatory bowel disease treated with immunomodulators and biological therapy. Gut 60:456–462

Reed C, Metzer MI, Finelli L, Fiore A (2012) Public health impact of including two lineages of influenza B in a quadrivalent seasonal influenza vaccine. Vaccine 30:1993–1998

Renfrey S (1994) Watts A (1994) Morphological and biochemical characterization of influenza vaccines commercially available in the United Kingdom. Vaccine 12:747–752

Riedl K, Riedl R, von Gabain A, Nagy E, Lingnau K (2008) The novel adjuvant IC31 strongly improves influenza vaccine-specific cellular and humoral immune responses in young adult and aged mice. Vaccine 26:3461–3468

Rimmelzwaan GF, Nieuwkoop N, Brandenburg A, Sutter G, Beyer WE, Maher D, Bates J, Osterhaus AD (2000) A randomized, double blind study in young healthy adults comparing cell mediated and humoral immune responses induced by influenza ISCOM vaccines and conventional vaccines. Vaccine 19:1180–1187

Rubinstein F, Micone P, Bonotti A, Wainer V, Schwarcz A, Augustovski F, Pichon Riviere A, Karolinski A; EVA Study Research Group Estudio Embarazo y Vacuna Antigripal (2013) Influenza A/H1N1 MF59 adjuvanted vaccine in pregnant women and adverse perinatal outcomes: multicentre study. BMJ 346:f393

Rümke HC, Richardus JH, Rombo L, Pauksens K, Plassmann G, Durand C, Devaster JM, Dewé W, Oostvogels L (2013) Selection of an adjuvant for seasonal influenza vaccine in elderly people: modelling immunogenicity from a randomized trial. BMC Infect Dis 13:348

Salk JE (1953) Use of adjuvants in studies on influenza immunization. III. Degree of persistence of antibody in subjects two years after vaccination. JAMA 151:1169–1175

Salk JE, Bailey ML, Laurel AM (1952) The use of adjuvants in studies on influenza immunization. II. Increased antibody formation in human subjects inoculated with influenza virus vaccine in a water-in-oil emulsion. Am J Hyg 55:439–456

Scheifele DW, McNeil SA, Ward BJ, Dionne M, Cooper C, Coleman B, Loeb M, Rubinstein E, McElhaney J, Hatchette T, Li Y, Montomoli E, Schneeberg A, Bettinger JA, Halperin SA, Research Network CI (2013) Safety, immunogenicity, and tolerability of three influenza vaccines in older adults: Results of a randomized, controlled comparison. Hum Vaccin Immunother 9:2460–2473

Schild GC, Wood JM, Newman RW (1975) A single-radial-immunodiffusion technique for the assay of influenza haemagglutinin antigen. Proposals for an assay method for the haemagglutinin content of influenza vaccines. Bull World Health Organ 52:223–231

Schultze V, D'Agosto V, Wack A, Novicki D, Zorn J, Hennig R (2008) Safety of MF59 adjuvant. Vaccine 26:3209–3222

Spensieri F, Borgogni E, Zedda L, Bardelli M, Buricchi F, Volpini G, Fragapane E, Tavarini S, Finco O, Rappuoli R, Giuseppe Del Giudice G, Galli G, Castellino F (2013) Human circulating influenza-CD4+ ICOS1+IL-21 + T cells expand after vaccination, exert helper function, and predict antibody responses. Proc Natl Acad Sci USA 110:14330–14335

Sridhar S, Begom S, Bermingham A, Hoschler K, Adamson W, Carman W, Bean T, Barclay W, Deeks JJ, Lalvani A (2013) Cellular immune correlates of protection against symptomatic pandemic influenza. Nat Med 19:1305–1312

Stephenson I, Nicholson KG, Hoschler K, Zambon MC, Hancock K, DeVos J, Katz JM, Praus M, Banzhoff A (2008) Antigenically distinct MF59-adjuvanted vaccine to boost immunity to H5N1. N Engl J Med 359:1631–1633

Sullivan SJ, Jacobson R, Poland GA (2010) Advances in the vaccination of the elderly against influenza: role of a high-dose vaccine. Expert Rev Vaccines 9:1127–1133

Szakács A, Darin N, Hallböök T (2013) Increased childhood incidence of narcolepsy in western Sweden after H1N1 influenza vaccination. Neurology 80:1315–1321

Taylor DN, Treanor JJ, Sheldon EA, Johnson C, Umlauf S, Song L, Kavita U, Liu G, Tussey L, Ozer K, Hofstaetter T, Shaw A (2012) Development of VAX128, a recombinant hemagglutinin (HA) influenza-flagellin fusion vaccine with improved safety and immune response. Vaccine 30:5761–5769

Thompson WW, Shay DK, Weintraub E, Brammer L, Cox N, Anderson LJ, Fukuda K (2003) Mortality associated with influenza and RSV. JAMA 289:179–186

Thompson WW, Shay DK, Weintraub E, Brammer L, Bridges CB, Cox NJ, Fukuda K (2004) Influenza-associated hospitalizations in the United States. JAMA 292:1333–1340

Thompson MG, Shay DK, Zhou H, Bridges CB, Cheng PY, Burns E, Bresee JS, Cox NJ (2010) Estimates of deaths associated with seasonal influenza – United States 1976-2007. MMWR 59:1057–1062

Treanor JJ, Essink B, Hull S, Reed S, Izikson R, Patriarca P, Goldenthal KL, Kohberger R, Dunkle LM (2013) Evaluation of safety and immunogenicity of recombinant influenza hemagglutinin (H5/Indonesia/05/2005) formulated with and without a stable oil-inwater emulsion containing glucopyranosyl-lipid A (SE+GLA) adjuvant. Vaccine 31(48):5760–5765

Tsai T, Giuseppe Del Giudice G, Crucitti A, Weil J, Narasimhan V (2013) Is the adjuvant solely to blame? BMJ 346:f2375. doi:10.1136/bmj.f2375

Tsang P, Gorse GJ, Strout CB, Sperling M, Greenberg DP, Ozol-Godfrey A, Diazgranados C, Landolfi V (2013) Immunogenicity and safety of Fluzone® intradermal and high-dose influenza vaccines in older adults ≥ 65 years of age: A randomized, controlled, phase II trial. Vaccine Epub. doi:10.1016/j.vaccine.2013.09.074

Turley CB, Rupp RE, Johnson C, Taylor DN, Wolfson J, Tussey L, Kavita U, Stanberry L, Shaw A (2011) Safety and immunogenicity of a recombinant M2e-flagellin influenza vaccine (STF2.4xM2e) in healthy adults. Vaccine 29:5145–5152

Van Buynder PG, Konrad S, Van Buynder JL, Brodkin E, Krajden M, Ramler G, Bigham M (2013) The comparative effectiveness of adjuvanted and unadjuvanted trivalent inactivated influenza vaccine (TIV) in the elderly. Vaccine 31:6122–6128

van der Velden MV, Fritz R, Pöllabauer EM, Portsmouth D, Howard MK, Kreil TR, Dvorak T, Fritsch S, Vesikari T, Diez-Domingo J, Richmond P, Lee BW, Kistner O, Ehrlich HJ, Barrett PN, Aichinger G (2014) Safety and Immunogenicity of a Vero Cell Culture-Derived Whole-Virus Influenza A(H5N1) Vaccine in a Pediatric Population. J Infect Dis 209:12–23

Vesikari T, Pellegrini M, Karvonen A, Groth N, Borkowski A, O'Hagan DT, Podda A (2009a) Enhanced immunogenicity of seasonal influenza vaccines in young children using MF59 adjuvant. Pediatr Infect Dis J 28:563–571

Vesikari T, Groth N, Karvonen A, Borkowski A, Pellegrini M (2009b) MF59-adjuvanted influenza vaccine (Fluad®) in children: safety and immunogenicity following a second year seasonal vaccination. Vaccine 27:6291–6295

Vesikari T, Knuf M, Wutzler P, Karvonen A, Kieninger-Baum D, Schmitt HJ, Baehner F, Borkowski A, Tsai TF, Clemens R (2011) Oil-in-water emulsion adjuvant with influenza vaccine in young children. N Engl J Med 365:1406–1416

Vesikari T, Forstén A, Borkowski A, Gaitatzis N, Banzhoff A, Clemens R (2012a) Homologous and heterologous antibody responses to a one-year booster dose of an MF59® adjuvanted A/H5N1 pre-pandemic influenza vaccine in pediatric subjects. Hum Vaccin Immunother 8:921–928

Vesikari T, Pepin S, Kusters I, Hoffenbach A, Denis M (2012b) Assessment of squalene adjuvanted and non-adjuvanted vaccines against pandemic H1N1 influenza in children 6 months to 17 years of age. Hum Vaccin Immunother 8:1283–1292

Villa M, Black S, Groth N, Rothman KJ, Apolone G, Weiss NS, Aquino I, Boldori L, Caramaschi F, Gattinoni A, Malchiodi G, Crucitti A, Della Cioppa G, Scarpini E, Mavilio D, Mannino S (2013) Safety of MF59-adjuvanted influenza vaccination in the elderly: results of a comparative study of MF59-adjuvanted vaccine versus nonadjuvanted influenza vaccine in northern Italy. Am J Epidemiol 178:1139–1145

Vono M, Taccone M, Caccin P, Gallotta M, Donvito G, Falzoni S, Palmieri E, Pallaoro M, Rappuoli R, Di Virgilio F, De Gregorio E, Montecucco C, Seubert A (2013) The adjuvant MF59 induces ATP release from muscle that potentiates response to vaccination. Proc Natl Acad Sci USA 110:21095–21100

Wilkinson TM, Li CK, Chui CS, Huang AK, Perkins M, Liebner JC, Lambkin-Williams R, Gilbert A, Oxford J, Nicholas B, Staples KJ, Dong T, Douek DC, McMichael AJ, Xu XN (2012) Preexisting influenza-specific CD4+ T cells correlate with disease protection against influenza challenge in humans. Nat Med 18:274–280

Wilschut J (2009) Influenza vaccines: the virosome concept. Immunol Lett 122:118–121

World Health Organization (2012) Meeting of the Strategic Advisory Group of Experts on immunization, April 2012 – conclusions and recommendations. Weekly Epidemiol Rec 87:201–216

World Health Organization (2013) http://www.who.int/influenza/vaccines/virus/recommendations/201309_recommendation.pdf. Accessed 23 Dec 2013

Zaman A, Holmes TH, Stamatis S, Tu WW, He XS, Bouvier N, Kemble G, Greenberg HB, Lewis DB, Arvin AM, Dekker CL (2007) Humoral and cellular immune responses in children given annual immunization with trivalent inactivated influenza vaccine. Pediatr Infect Dis J 26:107–115

Live Attenuated Influenza Vaccine

Hong Jin and Kanta Subbarao

Abstract Cold-adapted Ann Arbor based live attenuated influenza vaccine (LAIV) has been available in the USA since 2003. The vaccine is efficacious against influenza infection. Features of LAIV include: easy administration suitable for mass immunization, cross-reactivity to drifted strains for broader coverage, and establishment of herd immunity for control of influenza spread. Annual seasonal LAIV now contains four strains against influenza A H1N1, H3N2, influenza B-Victoria, and B-Yamagata lineages that are co-circulating in humans. LAIV played a significant role in protecting the public from the 2009 H1N1 pandemic and has been evaluated for pandemic preparedness. Pandemic vaccines including influenza H2, H5, H6, H7, and H9 subtypes have been produced and evaluated in preclinical and small-scale phase I clinical studies. This review summarizes the current status and perspectives of seasonal and pandemic LAIV.

Abbreviations

LAIV	Live attenuated influenza vaccine
T/LAIV	Trivalent live attenuated influenza vaccine
Q/LAIV	Quadrivalent live attenuated influenza vaccine
pLAIV	Pandemic live attenuated influenza vaccine
TIV	Trivalent inactivated influenza vaccine
IIV	Inactivated influenza vaccine
MDV-A	Master donor virus for influenza A vaccines
MDV-B	Master donor virus for influenza B vaccines
ca	Cold adapted
ts	Temperature sensitive
att	Attenuated

H. Jin
MedImmune LLC, 297 North Bernardo Avenue, Mountain View, CA 94043, USA
e-mail: jinh@medimmune.com

K. Subbarao (✉)
Laboratory Infectious Diseases, NIAID, NIH, Bethesda, MD 20892, USA
e-mail: ksubbarao@niaid.nih.gov

Current Topics in Microbiology and Immunology (2015) 386: 181–204
DOI: 10.1007/82_2014_410

Published Online: 25 July 2014

wt	Wild-type
RG	Reverse genetics
PCKC	Primary chicken kidney cells
NT	Nasal turbinates
HAI	Hemagglutination inhibition
NW	Nasal wash

Contents

1 Introduction

Influenza viruses cause significant morbidity and mortality, leading to more than 100,000 hospitalizations and 3,000–49,000 deaths annually (Thompson et al. 2003). Influenza viruses undergo constant genetic drift resulting in emergent antigenic variants that can escape immunity to HA and NA antigens of previously circulating strains. Therefore, influenza vaccines must be updated annually to match the contemporary strains in order to provide optimal protection. Trivalent LAIV (T/LAIV, H1N1, H3N2, one B strain) in a frozen formulation was approved by the US FDA in 2003 for healthy persons 5–49 years of age and the next generation of a liquid formulation was approved for 2–49 year olds in 2007. LAIV is the first new influenza vaccine, as well as the first nasally administered vaccine of any kind for human use, in the USA since the introduction of injectable trivalent influenza vaccine (TIV) in the 1940s (Grabenstein et al. 2006). The formulation of the vaccine was recently changed from trivalent to quadrivalent to account for the epidemiology of B strains in circulation. Two antigenically distinct lineages of influenza B viruses have circulated globally since 1985 and vaccines against one lineage do not offer cross-protection against the other lineage (Rota et al. 1990). In order to provide broader coverage of influenza B viruses an additional B strain is now included in the vaccine. T/LAIV was therefore discontinued in 2013 with the approval and marketing of a quadrivalent LAIV (Q/LAIV, H1N1, H3N2, two B strains).

The development of LAIV is the culmination of over 40 years of collaborative research and development between University of Michigan and scientists from the National Institutes of Health (NIH) and the biopharmaceutical industry (Wyeth, Aviron, and MedImmune). Following the approval in the USA in 2003, T/LAIV was approved in Israel, South Korea, United Arab Emirates, Mexico, and Macau for individuals 2–49 years of age, in Canada for individuals 2–59 years of age and in the European Union for individuals 2–17 years of age. In June 2014, the Advisory Committee on Immunization Practices (ACIP) made a preferential recommendation of LAIV for healthy children ages 2 to 8 years old in the USA.

2 Development of Cold-Adapted Ann Arbor Donor Viruses

LAIV is developed based on two cold-adapted master donor viruses, A/Ann Arbor/6/60 (H2N2) for influenza A vaccines (MDV-A) and B/Ann Arbor/1/66 for influenza B vaccines (MDV-B). Each donor virus donates the cold adapted (*ca*), temperature sensitive (*ts*), and attenuated (*att*) phenotype to the 6:2 reassortant vaccine viruses that contain six internal protein gene segments of MDV and the HA and NA surface proteins of the wild-type (*wt*) influenza virus. Both MDV-A and MDV-B were developed by Dr. John Maassab at the University of Michigan in the 1960s (Maassab 1967). Influenza A/Ann Arbor/6/60 was subjected to serial in vitro passage at gradually reduced temperature in primary chicken kidney cells (PCKC), 2 passages (2x) at 36–37 °C, 7x at 33 °C, 7x at 30 °C, 7x at 25 °C, 6x plaquing at 25 °C and 3x amplification in embryonated chicken eggs. Influenza B/Ann/Arbor/1/66 was passaged less extensively, two passages (2x) at 36–37 °C, 2x at 33 °C, 5x at 27 °C, 6x at 25 °C, 7x plaquing at 25 °C, and 3x amplification in eggs. During cold passage, the MDV-A and MDV-B acquired a number of genetic changes in multiple gene segments, which confer the *ca*, *ts*, and *att* phenotypes that can be imparted to 6:2 reassortant vaccine strains. The *ca* phenotype reflects efficient viral replication at a lower temperature of 25 °C, while most *wt* influenza viruses do not replicate well at this temperature. The *ts* phenotype reflects restricted replication at a higher temperature at which most *wt* viruses can replicate well. The shut-off temperature of MDV-A and MDV-B is different: 39 °C for MDV-A and 37 °C for MDV-B. The *att* phenotype can be measured in the ferret model, viral replication is detected in the nasal tissues but not in the lungs of ferrets intranasally infected with the vaccine virus. The *ca/ts/att* phenotypes provide safety features of the reassortant vaccine strains that can replicate in the cooler nasal tissues but not at the higher core body temperature of the lungs.

3 Genetic Basis of *ca/ts/att* Phenotypes of the Vaccine Donor Viruses

3.1 MDV-A

By comparing viral genomic sequences between the *wt* and *ca* A/Ann Arbor/6/60 strains and introduction of each of the mutations individually and combination, the amino acids that confer the *ts* phenotype have been precisely mapped to three residues (E391, G581, T661) in PB1, one residue (S265) in PB2 and one residue in NP (G34) proteins (Table 1) (Jin et al. 2003). These five loci in the PB1, PB2, and NP genes also confer the *att* phenotype (Jin et al. 2004). The *ca* phenotype of MDV-A could not be experimentally mapped as the available *wt* A/Ann Arbor/6/60 strain had been passaged extensively in tissue culture and also grows well at 25 °C. Since the *ts* and *att* phenotypes are specified by five residues in three gene segments, the chance for the vaccine virus to revert to *wt* phenotype is extremely low, explaining genetic stability of the vaccine strains.

Limited studies have been conducted to understand the molecular mechanism of these loci in specifying viral phenotypes. By minigenome analysis, the five loci have been shown to greatly reduce viral RNA-dependent polymerase activity of AA *ca* at the nonpermissive temperature of 39 °C (Jin et al. 2004). During viral infection in vitro, the vaccine virus can initiate single cycle replication, but multicycle viral replication at 39 °C is significantly reduced. vRNA synthesis and translocation of viral RNP from nucleus to cytoplasm are reduced. In addition, incorporation of the M1 protein into virions is significantly reduced, resulting in irregular viral morphology (Chan et al. 2008).

3.2 MDV-B

The *ca/ts/att* phenotypes of MDV-B have been mapped by reverse genetics (RG) (Chen et al. 2008; Hoffmann et al. 2005). The *ts* loci are specified by three amino acids in the PA and NP proteins: M431 in the PA, A114, and H410 in the NP (Table 1). These three residues and Q159 and V183 residues in the M gene segment contribute to the *att* phenotype. Five residues in three segments confer the *ca* phenotype: R630 in PB2, M431 in the PA, A114, H410, and T509 in the NP. A total of seven loci distributed in four gene segments of MDV-B control the *ca/ts/att* phenotypes, making the vaccine donor genetically stable. These loci not only reduce viral polymerase function but also affect virus assembly and release at the restricted temperature (Chan et al. 2008).

Table 1 Genetic loci of MDV-A and MDV-B

Segment	MDV-A		MDV-B	
	Amino acid	Phenotype	Amino acid	Phenotype
PB2	S265	*ts/att*	R630	*ca*
PB1	E391 G581 T661	*ts/att*	–	–
PA	–	–	M431	*ca/ts/att*
NP	G34	*ts/att*	A114 H410 T509	*ca/ts/att* *ca/ts/att* *ca*
M	–	–	N159 V183	*att*
NS	–	–	–	–

-: No role in the *ca/ts/att* phenotypes

4 LAIV by Reverse Genetics and Yearly LAIV Production Process

LAIV is manufactured in specific pathogen free (SPF) embryonated chicken eggs. Human influenza viruses normally do not replicate well in eggs and viral replication in eggs often results in mutations in the HA receptor binding region. The quasi-species of HA sequence variations from egg adaptation have different abundance and biological impact. While certain changes improve viral growth in eggs without affecting viral antigenicity and immunogenicity, other changes are not suitable for a vaccine. It is therefore critical to evaluate multiple candidate vaccines in order to select an appropriate HA variant for vaccine production. The application of reverse genetics (RG) technology to the production of 6:2 reassortant vaccine viruses has revolutionized the vaccine seed production process. Traditional classical reassortment, which is a very time consuming and unpredictable method, has been replaced by the use of RG for LAIV production since the 2008–2009 influenza season. The 6:2 reassortant vaccine virus contains six internal protein gene segments from MDV-A or MDV-B and the surface HA and NA glycoprotein gene segments of a *wt* virus (Fig. 1).

During vaccine seed production, each candidate vaccine variant is evaluated for yield in eggs, antigenicity is assessed by reactivity with a reference antiserum from ferrets immunized with *wt* virus, and immunogenicity is assessed by examining serum antibody levels achieved in ferrets following intranasal administration of vaccine virus variants. Table 2 summarizes the amino acid sequence changes that have been frequently detected in the HA and their impact on viral biological activities (for a recent review, please see Jin and Chen 2014). Most of the changes do not affect viral antigenicity and immunogenicity, however, several changes

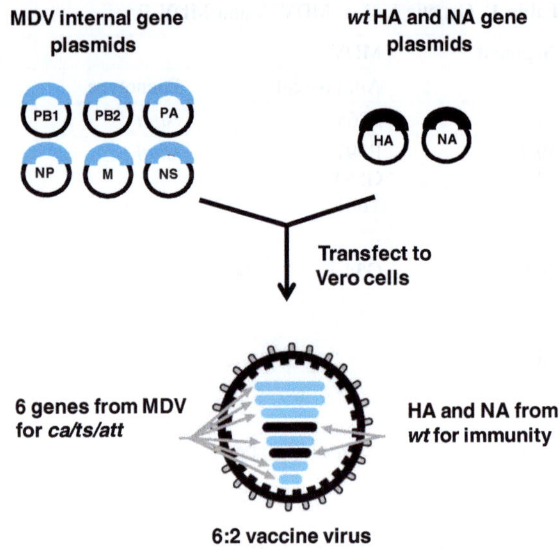

Fig. 1 Generation of reassortant LAIV by RG. The six plasmids of the internal protein gene segments of MDV and two plasmids encoding *wt* HA and NA gene segments are electroporated into Vero cells. Virus recovered from the transfected cells is amplified in embryonated chicken eggs

Table 2 Common egg adaptation sites in the HA of egg-grown influenza viruses

Influenza viruses	HA amino acid[a]	Comments related to residues in bold
H1N1	119, 125, 127, **153–155**, 186, 209, 222, 223	153–155 residues alter viral antigenicity
H3N2	138, **156**, 183, 186, 189, 190, 193, **194**, 195, 196, 219, 226	156 is a major antigenic site 194 affects viral replication in ferrets
B-Vic	197, 199	Glycosylation site
B-Yam	196, 198	Glycosylation site

[a] Amino acid numbering based on HA sequence of each subtype

identified in the HA have been shown to reduce viral antigenicity or to render vaccine virus less immunogenic (Chen et al. 2010a, b).

Once a LAIV seed is selected, the vaccine virus is purified by one round of limited dilution in eggs to produce a Master Virus Seed (MVS) that is used for bulk production of monovalent vaccine. Each vaccine lot is subjected to a lot release test to ensure that no adventitious agents are present. The four vaccine viruses, H1N1, H3N2, B-Yamagata, and B-Victoria, are formulated to contain $10^{7.0\pm0.5}$ FFU (fluorescent focus units)/strain in 0.2-mL in a nasal sprayer. If a new vaccine virus component is incorporated into the annual seasonal vaccine, the vaccine is tested in a small-scale safety trial prior to final release of the vaccine for widespread use.

5 Preclinical Studies of LAIV

Extensive studies have been performed to evaluate vaccine viruses for their attenuated replication, immunogenicity, and protection against *wt* influenza virus challenge infection in the ferret model. Vaccine viruses have been shown to be able to replicate in the nasal turbinates (NT) but not in the lungs of vaccinated ferrets. Although vaccine strains in general elicit hemagglutination inhibition (HAI) antibodies at levels lower than that induced by homologous *wt* virus (MedImmune data), they provide significant protection against replication of homologous challenge virus in the upper and lower respiratory tract (LRT) of ferrets.

Ferret studies have been conducted to compare T/LAIV with Q/LAIV in protection against *wt* challenge infection to address vaccine interference (Bandell et al. 2011). Q/LAIV is comparable to T/LAIV in vaccine-induced protective immune responses against *wt* virus replication in the upper and LRT of vaccinated ferrets (Fig. 2). The vaccine strains A/California/7/2009 (A/CA/09, H1N1), A/Perth/16/2009 (A/Perth/09, H3N2), B/Brisbane/60/2008 (B/Bris/08, Victoria lineage), and B/Wisconsin/1/2010 (B/Wis/10, B/Yamagata lineage) had comparable immunogenicity given in either Q/LAIV or T/LAIV formulation, elicited robust antibody responses to each vaccine component and fully protected ferrets from *wt* virus challenge in the lungs after two doses of vaccine. Each vaccine strain also offered significant protection from *wt* virus replication in the NT. These studies indicate that LAIV strains in multivalent vaccine formulations do not demonstrate evidence of viral or immune interference affecting efficacy of each vaccine component.

6 Clinical Studies of LAIV

Clinical studies of Ann Arbor (AA) *ca*-based LAIV strains in the USA include monovalent, bivalent including two type A strains, trivalent including H1N1, H3N2 and a B strain, and quadrivalent including two type A and two B strains (for review see Murphy and Coelingh 2002). T/LAIV has been evaluated in more than 73 clinical research trials completed worldwide in >141,000 people ranging in age from 6 weeks to >90 years. Approximately 80 million doses have been distributed for commercial use since the initial US licensure in 2003 up through March 2014 (LAIV Scientific Product Monograph 2013–2014, MedImmune, Gaithersburg, MD).

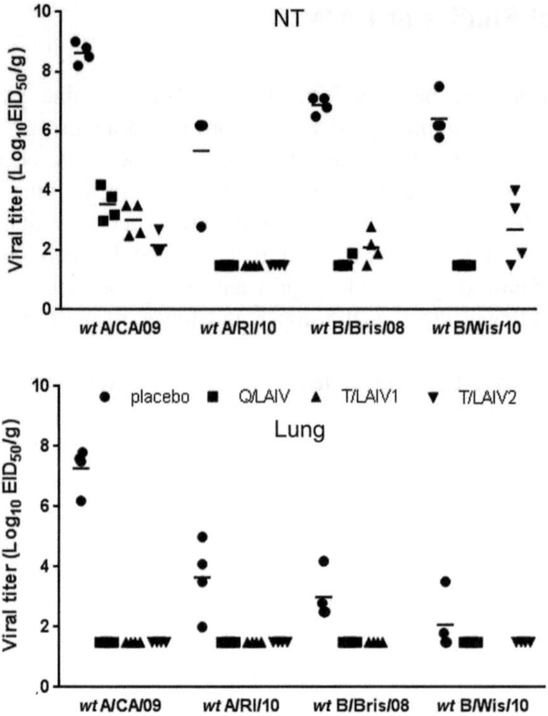

Fig. 2 Challenge virus titers in NT and lung of ferrets vaccinated with Q/LAIV or T/LAIV. Ferrets were vaccinated with sucrose phosphate (SP) buffer, T/LAIV1 (A/CA/09, A/Perth/09, B/Bris/08), T/LAIV2 (A/CA/09, A/Perth/09, B/Wis/10), or Q/LAIV (A/CA/09, A/Perth/09, B/Bris/08 and B/Wis/10) in two doses one month apart. The ferrets were challenged with indicated honologous *wt* viruses with the exception of the H3N2 A/Rhode Island/2010 strain as *wt* A/Perth/09 did not replicate well in ferret lungs. Viral titers in the NT and lung tissues were determined by 50 % egg infectious dose (EID50) assay. The limit of detection of the assay was 1.5 $log_{10}EID_{50}/g$

6.1 Safety

LAIV is generally well tolerated and safe (reviewed by Ambrose et al. 2011). The vaccine viruses infect and replicate in cells lining the nasopharynx of the recipient to induce immunity, but are not able to replicate in the LRT due to their *ts* and *att* phenotypes. The most common solicited adverse reactions are runny nose or nasal congestion (ages 2 to 49 years), fever >100 °F (ages 2–6 years), and sore throat (18–49 years). The rate of headache and tiredness in LAIV recipients is higher than in a placebo control group but is similar to TIV recipients (Baxter et al. 2012a, b; Toback et al. 2013). One study showed that LAIV was associated with an increased rate of all-cause hospitalization among children aged 6–11 months and an increased rate of medically attended wheezing in children aged 6–23 months (Belshe et al. 2007). For this reason, LAIV is not approved for children younger than 24 months of age.

6.2 Transmission and Genetic Stability

Vaccine viruses can be cultured from nasal secretions in the first few days after vaccination. The relationship of viral replication in a vaccine recipient to transmission of vaccine viruses to other individuals has not been well established. LAIV is poorly transmissible because most infection is not symptomatic and this decreases the likelihood of viral spread via cough or sneezing. In addition, levels of vaccine virus replication in nasal tissues are much lower than *wt* virus even in seronegative children making its spread to contacts very inefficiently (Murphy and Coelingh 2002). In studies performed to date, viruses shed from vaccine recipients have been consistently phenotypically and genotypically stable, maintaining the *ca*, *ts*, and *att* phenotypes (Cha et al. 2000; Vesikari et al. 2006). LAIV has been shown to be poorly transmissible to spouses, roommates, and household members under a variety of circumstances in small clinical trials (Murphy and Coelingh 2002). Eighty percent of trivalent LAIV recipients who were 6–36 month old children in a day care setting, shed at least one vaccine strain, with a mean duration of shedding of 7.6 days ranging from 1 to 21 days (Vesikari et al. 2006). Transmission of vaccine viruses from vaccine recipients to placebo subjects was a rare event. The *ca* and *ts* phenotypes were preserved in all recovered viruses tested ($n = 135$ tested of 250 strains isolated at the local laboratory). The probability of a young child acquiring vaccine virus after close contact with a single trivalent LAIV vaccinee in a day care setting was 0.58 % (95 % CI: 0, 1.7) based on the Reed Frost model (Longini et al. 1982). With documented transmission of type B virus in one placebo subject and possible transmission of type A virus in four placebo subjects, the maximum probability of acquiring a transmitted vaccine virus was estimated to be 2.4 %.

6.3 Efficacy

The efficacy and effectiveness of an influenza vaccine can be evaluated by three criteria: (1) comparison of culture-positive influenza infection rates, which are most feasible in young children because they readily shed influenza virus (i.e., vaccine efficacy); (2) a 4-fold antibody increase from baseline levels, which is subject to inherent bias from prior vaccine or natural disease exposure, and therefore is a method of limited value; or (3) observations of clinical events or "medically attended acute respiratory illness" (MAARI) which is a less specific endpoint than culture-confirmed influenza illness, and results in effectiveness point estimates that are significantly lower than efficacy estimates. Adults shed virus in low quantity and for a short duration and thus clinical trials in adults are more commonly conducted using clinical endpoints (Belshe et al. 2004). LAIV efficacy trials in the pediatric population consist of nine controlled studies comprising over 20,000 infants and toddlers, children, and adolescents, during seven influenza seasons (summarized in LAIV Scientific Product Monograph 2013–2014, MedImmune, Gaithersburg, MD). Four placebo-controlled studies were conducted to include revaccination in a second season. Overall, LAIV has an efficacy of 62–93 % against antigenically matched strains and 49–93 % against all strains in children 15–71 months of age. LAIV has demonstrated superiority compared to TIV in 3 active-controlled studies in children. LAIV is about 44 % (range 34.7–52.7 %) better than TIV for matched strains and 31.9–54.9 % better than TIV for all strains. In one of the largest field efficacy trials (MI-CP111), LAIV was shown to be more efficacious than inactivated TIV in children 6–59 months of age (Belshe et al. 2007). Because of the higher efficacy of LAIV in children, LAIV is preferentially recommended in the UK, Germany, Israel, Canada, and Sweden for children of various age groups (Ambrose et al. 2012), and recently for 2–8 year old children in the USA.

LAIV efficacy in adults has been demonstrated in two efficacy trials (Nichol et al. 1999b; Treanor et al. 2000). In the first trial, LAIV was shown to reduce laboratory-documented influenza illness by 85 % compared to TIV in a challenge study conducted in healthy adults 18–41 years of age who were presumed to be susceptible to at least one strain included in the vaccine based on prevaccination antibody titers (Treanor et al. 2000). In the second, larger trial, LAIV recipients exhibited significant reduction in days of febrile illness, missed work, health care provider visits, and antibiotic usage. The efficacy of LAIV and TIV can be affected by a number of factors, such as the age and health of the vaccine recipients and the extent of antigenic similarity between the vaccine strains and circulating strains. In a study conducted by Monto et al. (Monto et al. 2009), LAIV was 50 % less efficacious than TIV in reduction of laboratory-confirmed influenza during the 2008–2009 influenza season when an H3N2 virus was the predominant circulating strain. Based on a subgroup analysis of subjects 50–64 years of age in the study by Nichol et al. (1999a), LAIV was not approved for this age group in the USA. A later study showed that LAIV offered statistically significant protection against culture-confirmed influenza in adults $\geq$60 years of age (De Villiers et al. 2009).

6.4 Immunogenicity

The immunogenicity of 19 different LAIV strains was studied over a period of 25 years at various locations and in different populations (Murphy and Coelingh 2002), and annual commercial vaccines have been evaluated over the past 10 years. Protection against influenza generally correlates with serum IgG hemagglutination-inhibiting antibodies (HAI), especially in seronegative children. After two doses of LAIV, children who were presumed to be susceptible to at least one strain included in the vaccine based on prevaccination antibody titers, mounted an adequate HAI response (>90 % seroconverted to type A/H3 and B strains, and 60–90 % to type A/H1 strain) (Belshe et al. 1998, 2000; Zangwill 2003). Antibodies persisted for 5–8 months after vaccination with LAIV, and protection generally persisted for at least 1 year (Zangwill 2003). In a study of young children, protective efficacy lasted for the duration of the influenza season and as late as 5.5–13 months after the second dose (Ambrose et al. 2008; Tam et al. 2007). In adults, the serologic response has been less robust (<35 % for A/H3 and B and 60–90 % for A/H1), and the correlates of immunity may be related to other immune responses (Gorse et al. 1995; Tomoda et al. 1995; Zangwill 2003). LAIV may be more effective than IIV in inducing a nasal IgA response that is important for viral clearance and recovery, whereas IIV vaccine more consistently elicits serum HA antibodies in adults (Beyer et al. 2002; Cox et al. 2004; Renegar et al. 2004). The role of cell-mediated immune responses in the protection of young children against influenza was studied in a large randomized, double-blind, placebo-controlled dose-ranging efficacy trial with 2,172 children of 6 to <36 months old in Philippines and Thailand (Forrest et al. 2008). LAIV was found to elicit substantial CMI responses as measured by interferon-gamma ELISPOT assay that correlated with protection. Another study conducted in children showed that LAIV induced cell-mediated responses including CD4(+), CD8(+), and $\gamma\delta$ T cells that are relevant for broadly protective heterosubtypic immunity (Hoft et al. 2011). In a study conducted in young adults, although TIV induced higher levels of vaccine-specific plasmablasts and plasmablast-derived polyclonal antibodies (PPAb) than LAIV, LAIV induced a greater vaccine-specific IgA plasmablast response as well as a greater plasmablast response to the conserved influenza nucleoprotein and better cross-reactivity to heterologous strains than TIV (Sasaki et al. 2014).

7 Pandemic LAIV

There are 18 known HA and 11 known NA subtypes of influenza A viruses in nature; 16 HA and 9 NA subtypes have been isolated from waterfowl and shorebirds, and a variety of subtypes have been isolated from other animal species including pigs, horses, and dogs. Animal influenza viruses are the source from which novel HA and NA subtypes are introduced into the human population, by reassortment with other animal or human influenza viruses or direct infection of humans. In the last century, influenza pandemics occurred in 1918, 1957, and 1968 and the first pandemic of this century occurred in 2009. Each of these pandemics was associated with significant morbidity and mortality. Since 1997, animal H5N1, H6N1, H7N7, H7N3, H7N9, H9N2, and H10N8 viruses have caused human infections but have not spread efficiently from person to person. The pandemics and the sporadic emergence of animal viruses into humans underline the need for the generation of pandemic influenza vaccines and their evaluation in humans. The criteria for licensure of currently licensed inactivated influenza vaccines are protective antibodies directed primarily against the HA, the major protective antigen of the virus that induces neutralizing antibody and/or demonstrated efficacy.

LAIV have several attributes related to safety, immunogenicity, cross-protection against antigenic drift strains, high yield, and needle-free administration that make them attractive candidates for control of pandemic influenza. LAIV generally induce broadly cross-reactive protection (Coelingh et al. 2014; Murphy and Coelingh 2002), which may be a useful feature in the event of a pandemic if a vaccine generated from the emerging pandemic strain is not immediately available. Importantly, the infrastructure for manufacture and distribution of a LAIV exists. Therefore, the United States NIH and MedImmune undertook a joint effort to develop and evaluate LAIV bearing the HA and NA genes from animal influenza viruses on the MDV-A backbone as pandemic LAIV (pLAIV) candidates. Our approach includes: (1) generation of a pLAIV bearing an HA and appropriate NA from an animal influenza virus on the attenuated MDV-A background; (2) evaluation of the attenuation, immunogenicity, and protective efficacy of the candidate vaccine in animal models; (3) preparation and qualification of a clinical lot of each pandemic vaccine candidate; (4) evaluation of the safety, infectivity, and immunogenicity of each candidate in humans; (5) storage of human sera obtained from vaccinees to determine cross-reactivity with the newly emerged pandemic viruses; and (6) storage of seed viruses for use in the manufacture of vaccine to prevent disease caused by related pandemic viruses that do emerge such that vaccine manufacture can be initiated with pretested vaccines without delay.

A theoretical concern associated with the use of a pLAIV bearing genes derived from an animal influenza virus is the risk of reassortment of the vaccine virus with a circulating influenza virus, resulting in a novel subtype of influenza that could spread in the human population. Although such a reassortment event may not be of great significance in the face of widespread disease caused by a pandemic influenza strain, it would be an unfavorable outcome if the threatened pandemic did not materialize. This risk would be carefully considered by public health authorities before a decision is made to introduce a live attenuated vaccine in a threatened pandemic. With the exception of one H9N2 *ca* virus, the pLAIV viruses were generated by RG. The HAs of highly pathogenic avian influenza (HPAI) H5 and H7 viruses were modified to remove the multibasic amino acid cleavage motif that is a known virulence determinant for poultry.

7.1 Preclinical Studies

We have developed pLAIV candidates against 6 different subtypes (H1, H2, H5, H6, H7, and H9) (Chen et al. 2003, 2009a, b, 2011b, 2014; Joseph et al. 2008; Min et al. 2010; Suguitan et al. 2006). The genetic loci responsible for the *ts* and *att* phenotypes associated with the MDV-A were confirmed in each of the pLAIV viruses. The replication of the pLAIV viruses was evaluated in the respiratory tract of ferrets 3 days following intranasal administration of 10^7 $TCID_{50}$ of viruses. As discussed previously, highly restricted replication in the LRT of ferrets defines the *att* phenotype of the pLAIV strains (Table 3). Some pLAIV viruses (H2, H5, and H7N3)

Table 3 Replication of intranasally administered pLAIV in the respiratory tract of ferrets and mice

Subtype/Vaccine virus	Virus titer ($\log_{10}TCID_{50}/g$) in the respiratory tract of indicated species			
	Ferrets[a]		Mice (peak titer)[b]	
	URT	LRT	URT	LRT
pH1N1 CA/7/2009 (Chen et al. 2011b)	3.4	1.7	2.0	1.8
H2N2 Ann Arbor/6/60 (Chen et al. 2009a)	5.9	≤1.5[c]	5.0	4.3
H2N3 swine/MO/2006 (Chen et al. 2014)	5.0	≤1.5[c]	4.3	3.1
H5N1 VN/1203/2004 (Suguitan et al. 2006)	4.1	≤1.5[c]	2.6	4.1
H5N1 HK/213/2003	4.5	≤1.5[c]	2.5	5.1
H6N1 teal/HK/W312/97 (Chen et al. 2009b)	2.1*	≤1.5[c]	nd	nd
H7N3 BC/CN-6/2004 (Joseph et al. 2008)	4.7	≤1.5[c]	4.4	2.4
H7N7 NL/219/2003 (Min et al. 2010)	2.8	≤1.5[c]	3.3	3.3
H9N2 ck/HK/G9/1997 (Chen et al. 2003)	2.3	≤1.5[c]	1.4**	≤1.5[c]

[a] Lightly anesthetized ferrets received intranasal administration of 10^7 $TCID_{50}$ (or fluorescent forming units) of virus and virus titers in the upper and lower respiratory tract were determined 3 days later

[b] Lightly anesthetized mice received intranasal administration of 10^6 $TCID_{50}$ of virus and virus titers in the upper and lower respiratory tract were determined at serial time points 2, 3, and 4 days later. The peak titer achieved is indicated

[c] Below the lower limit of detection

nd Not done, *pfu/g, **$TCID_{50}$/ml

replicated to high titer in the upper respiratory tract (URT) of ferrets, while others such as the H6N1, H7N7, and H9N2 vaccine viruses were restricted in replication in the URT. The pLAIV were also evaluated for replication in mice 2, 3, and 4 days following intranasal administration of 10^6 $TCID_{50}$ of virus (Table 3). The body temperature of mice is 37 °C, which is below the shut-off temperature of the ca viruses. Therefore, although the replication of the pLAIV viruses in mice is restricted compared to the corresponding *wt* viruses, they are not as restricted in replication in mice as they are in ferrets that have a core body temperature of ~39 °C.

The immunogenicity of the pLAIV was evaluated in mice and ferrets by measuring the serum antibody response by HAI and/or microneutralization (MN) assays against homologous and heterologous viruses following intranasal administration of one or two doses of pLAIV; neutralizing antibody (MN) titers are reported in Tables 4 and 5. The pH1N1 LAIV that was used for vaccine production incorporated two mutations in the HA gene that improved the yield in eggs and immunogenicity in ferrets (Chen et al. 2010a). The homologous antibody response to one dose of vaccine in mice and ferrets ranged from poor (VN04 H5N1 and H7N7 vaccines) to robust (H6N1 and H9N2 vaccines) (Tables 4 and 5) but a correlation between the magnitude of the antibody response and replication of the pLAIV in mice or ferrets was not apparent (Tables 3, 4 and 5). Notably, in all cases, a second dose of vaccine boosted serum antibody responses against homologous and heterologous viruses.

Table 4 Immunogenicity and efficacy of one or two doses of pLAIV in mice, evaluated against homologous and heterologous viruses of the same subtype

Subtype and vaccine virus	Immunogenicity[a] by MN (GMT)				Efficacy[b] against challenge infection							
	1 dose		2 doses		1 dose				2 doses			
	Homologous	Heterologous	Homologous	Heterologous	Homologous		Heterologous[c]		Homologous		Heterologous[c]	
					URT	LRT	URT	LRT	URT	LRT	URT	LRT
pH1N1 CA/7/2009 (Chen et al. 2011b)	53	nd	595	nd	4+	2+	nd	nd	5+	5+	nd	nd
H2N2 Ann Arbor/6/60 (Chen et al. 2009a, 2014)	nd	nd	80	14–17	5+	5+	2+ to 3+	2+ to 3+	5+	5+	nd	nd
H2N3 swine/MO/2006 (Chen et al. 2014)	57	10–19	2,874	55–941	5+	4+	5+	3+ to 5+	5+	5+	5+	5+
H5N1 VN/1203/2004 (Suguitan et al. 2006)	14	11–15	388	160–528	2+	2+	+ to 5+	+ to 5+	5+	5+	5+	5+
H5N1 HK/213/2003	59	10	1,056	19–61	5+	5+	3+ to 5+	2+	5+	5+	5+	5+
H6N1 teal/HK/W312/97 (Chen et al. 2009b)	94	10–86	543	15–388	5+	5+	5+	5+	5+	5+	5+	5+
H7N3 BC CN-6/2004 (Joseph et al. 2008)	87	<20	470	39–60	5+	5+	2+ to 5+	3+ to 5+	5+	5+	5+	5+
H7N7 NL/219/2003 (Min et al. 2010)	14	21–24	191	153–285	2+	+ to 3+	3+ to 5+	+ to 3+	4+	5+	5+	5+
H9N2 ck/HK/G9/1997 (Chen et al. 2003)	320[d]	340[d]	nd	nd	5+	5+	5+	5+	nd	nd	nd	nd

[a] Serum neutralizing antibody titer measured in a microneutralization (MN) assay

[b] Efficacy was assessed by reduction of replication of wild-type challenge virus compared to mock-vaccinated animals. – <10-fold reduction, + 10 to 99-fold reduction, 2+ 100 to 999-fold reduction, 3+ 1000 to 9999-fold reduction, 4+ >10,000-fold reduction, 5+ complete protection from replication

[c] Heterologous challenge viruses for H2 vaccines: Japan/57 (H2N2); swine/MO/06 (H2N3); for H5 vaccines: HK/491/97, HK/213/2003; Vietnam/1203/2004, Indonesia/5/2005; for H6 vaccines: dk/HK/77, mallard/Alberta/85; for H7 vaccines: turkey/VA/55/02 (H7N2), turkey/UT/24721-10/95 (H7N3); chicken/BC/04 (H7N3), Netherlands/219/03 (H7N7), tk/Italy/99 (H7N1), turkey/England/63 (H7N3); for H9 vaccines: HK/1073/99

[d] HAI titer

nd Not done

Table 5 Immunogenicity and efficacy of pLAIV in ferrets, evaluated against homologous and heterologous viruses of the same subtype

Subtype and vaccine virus [a]	Immunogenicity[b] by MN (GMT)				Efficacy[c] against challenge infection							
	1 dose		2 doses		1 dose				2 doses			
	Homologous	Heterologous	Homologous	Heterologous	Homologous		Heterologous[d]		Homologous		Heterologous[d]	
					URT	LRT	URT	LRT	URT	LRT	URT	LRT
pH1N1 CA/7/2009 (Chen et al. 2011b)	854	nd	2,428	nd	5+	5+	nd	nd	5+	5+	nd	nd
H2N2 Ann Arbor/6/60 (Chen et al. 2009a, 2014)	120	25–45	nd	nd	5+	5+	+ to 3+	5+	nd	nd	nd	nd
H2N3 swine/MO/2006 (Chen et al. 2014)	64	24–86	nd	nd	2+	5+	2+ to 5+	5+	nd	nd	nd	nd
H5N1 VN/1203/2004 (Suguitan et al. 2006)	12	14	15	10–12	3+	+	-	+	4+	5+	+	5+
H5N1 HK/213/2003	466	10	1,955	14–24	5+	5+	–	5+	5+	5+	2+ to 3+	5+
H6N1 teal/HK/W312/97 (Chen et al. 2009b)	269	20–57	nd	nd	3+	5+	– to +	5+	nd	nd	nd	nd
H7N3 BC CN-6/2004 (Joseph et al. 2008)	160	11	264	10	3+	5+	3+	2+	3+	5+	4+	2+
H7N7 NL/219/2003 (Min et al. 2010)	12	10–15	41	54–80	2+	5+	2+ to 3+	5+	3+	5+	4+	5+

[a] The H9N2 ck/HK/G9/97 vaccine virus was not evaluated in ferrets

[b] Serum neutralizing antibody titer measured in a microneutralization (MN) assay

[c] Efficacy was assessed by reduction of replication of wild-type challenge virus compared to mock-vaccinated animals. <10-fold reduction, + 10 to 99-fold reduction, 2+ 100 to 999-fold reduction, 3+ 1,000 to 9,999-fold reduction, 4+ >10,000-fold reduction, 5+ complete protection from replication

[d] Heterologous challenge viruses for H2 vaccines: Japan/57 (H2N2); swine/MO/06 (H2N3); for H5 vaccines: HK/491/97, HK/213/2003; Vietnam/1203/2004, Indonesia/5/2005; for H6 vaccines: Dk/HK/77, mallard/Alberta/85; for H7 vaccines: turkey/VA/55/02 (H7N2), turkey/UT/24721-10/95 (H7N3); chicken/BC/04 (H7N3), Netherlands/219/03 (H7N7), tk/Italy/99 (H7N1), turkey/England/63 (H7N3); for H9 vaccines: HK/1073/99

nd Not done

Protective efficacy of pLAIVs was assessed by determining the ability of one or two doses of intranasally administered vaccine to protect mice from lethal challenge with *wt* virus or to prevent replication of *wt* challenge virus in the URT and LRT of mice and ferrets (Tables 4 and 5). Even vaccines that were poorly immunogenic (e.g., VN04 H5N1 and H7N7 vaccines) provided complete protection from lethal challenge following one dose of vaccine (Min et al. 2010; Suguitan et al. 2006). Two doses of the pLAIVs provided complete protection from replication of homologous *wt* challenge viruses in the URT and LRT of mice and LRT of ferrets; challenge virus titers in the URT of ferrets were reduced compared to mock-immunized animals but protection in the URT was not always complete (Tables 4 and 5). A single dose of vaccine conferred partial to complete protection from challenge virus replication; higher serum antibody titers (MN >80 and HAI of 320) were associated with complete protection. The VN04 H5N1 and H7N7 vaccines that failed to induce a robust antibody response conferred only partial protection following a single dose of vaccine, with a reduction in titer of challenge virus in the range of 40 to 1500-fold compared to mock-immunized animals (Min et al. 2010; Suguitan et al. 2006).

Because it is not possible to predict which strain within a subtype will cause a pandemic and influenza viruses continue to evolve in nature, we evaluated the antibody response and protection from challenge with heterologous viruses. In fact, the data confirmed our hypothesis that a pLAIV would elicit a cross-reactive antibody response against other strains from the same subtype. Two doses of pLAIV elicited cross-reactive antibodies and provided near complete protection from replication of heterologous *wt* viruses in the URT and LRT of mice and LRT of ferrets (Tables 4 and 5).

Another important caveat of preclinical evaluation of pLAIVs is that the studies are generally carried out in influenza-naïve unprimed animals while humans with a prior history of influenza infection or vaccination are immunologically primed. This difference was striking in the H1N1 pandemic in 2009: although people younger than 60 years of age were seronegative to the H1N1pdm virus, all but the youngest children responded to a single dose of inactivated H1N1pdm vaccine while unprimed animals required two doses of inactivated vaccine. We investigated the ability of *wt* seasonal H1N1 virus, seasonal H1N1 LAIV and seasonal TIV to prime mice for an antibody and cellular immune response to a single dose of H1N1pdm LAIV (Chen et al. 2011a) and found that prior exposure to live seasonal H1N1 virus, *wt,* or LAIV, primed mice but seasonal TIV did not. While two doses of H1N1pdm LAIV induced a robust neutralizing serum antibody response, mice that were primed with seasonal H1N1 infection or seasonal LAIV followed by one dose of H1N1pdm LAIV were equally well protected from challenge, in the absence of neutralizing serum antibody (Chen et al. 2011a). Cheng et al. compared TIV and LAIV in ferrets and found that LAIV was superior to TIV in inducing influenza-specific immunity in naïve ferrets (Cheng et al. 2013). Although both types of vaccines induced comparable humoral immune responses in previously primed ferrets, only LAIV provided partial protection from heterologous seasonal H1N1 virus challenge (Cheng et al. 2013). The findings in LAIV-immunized naïve ferrets may explain the efficacy of LAIV in young children.

7.2 Clinical Studies

The pLAIVs described above have been evaluated in phase I clinical trials in small cohorts of healthy adults younger than 50 years of age (Karron et al. 2009a, b; Talaat et al. 2009, 2011, 2012). In order to minimize the risk of reassortment between a pLAIV bearing novel HA and NA genes and circulating human influenza viruses, the clinical trials are conducted in an inpatient unit during months when seasonal influenza activity is not detected, typically between April and December. Vaccine recipients are admitted to the inpatient unit a day prior to vaccine administration in case they are incubating an intercurrent respiratory virus infection and also to determine whether they can adjust to a 9–10 day stay in the inpatient unit. The studies are conducted as open-label inpatient trials with all participants receiving vaccine. Vaccine is administered intranasally as a nasal spray except for the H9N2 ca vaccine that was administered as nose drops. Participants are examined daily while on the inpatient unit by a health care provider. After discharge from the inpatient unit, vaccinees are asked to return to the outpatient clinic. At each visit, staff obtain vital signs, review interim histories, and obtain blood and nasal wash (NW) samples for antibody testing (Coelingh et al. 2014).

Vaccine safety is assessed through daily examinations and infectivity is assessed by viral culture and by realtime reverse transcription-polymerase chain reaction testing of NW specimens. Immunogenicity is assessed by measuring HAI antibodies, neutralizing antibodies, and IgG or IgA antibodies to recombinant HA in serum or NW. As reviewed by Coelingh et al. (2014), the pLAIVs were restricted in replication and were variably and generally not immunogenic in terms of antibody responses in humans. These findings were unexpected because it was anticipated that adults receiving pLAIVs bearing novel HA and NA proteins would respond to the vaccines like children receiving seasonal LAIV, shedding vaccine virus for several days, and developing serum and/or NW antibody responses. However, the H5N1 pLAIV appears to have established long term immune memory because when H5N1 pLAIV vaccine recipients were re-called and given a dose of unadjuvanted inactivated subunit vaccine, a rapid robust and high quality antibody response was detected (Talaat et al. 2014). This observation is being explored further in a series of ongoing clinical trials that will provide insights into the durability of pLAIV-mediated immune memory by determining the optimal interval between the LAIV and inactivated vaccine.

8 Mediators and Correlates of Protection

While serum HAI antibody is a correlate of protection for inactivated influenza virus vaccines, it is not an absolute correlate of protection for LAIV. In addition to serum antibody responses, seasonal LAIVs induce mucosal and cell-mediated immunity (Hoft et al. 2011). Although protective efficacy and effectiveness of seasonal LAIV have been repeatedly demonstrated in preclinical and clinical studies, an immune correlate of protection has not been identified. As reviewed by Bandell et al. (2011), seasonal LAIV was efficacious even in the absence of a rise in serum HAI antibody.

8.1 Studies in Animal Models

The role of humoral and cellular immune mediators and distribution of immune effectors induced by eight different LAIVs at mucosal and systemic sites were evaluated in mice (Lau et al. 2011). All LAIVs tested induced robust systemic immune responses but variable pulmonary immunity. The magnitude of lung immunity, including pulmonary IgA antibody and memory CD8+ T lymphocytes, induced by the vaccines depended on the replication efficiency of the LAIVs and the induction of cytokines/chemokines in the lungs. Both cellular and humoral immunity contribute to the protection provided by LAIV; the relative contribution of the two effector arms in viral clearance depends on the location and the rate of replication of a particular vaccine virus. The relevance of these findings for the human experience was not clear because LAIVs do not replicate in the LRT of humans. Therefore, an upper respiratory tract immunization (URTI) model was developed in mice to mimic the human situation. This permitted assessment of the protective efficacy of an H5N1 LAIV against highly pathogenic H5N1 virus challenge in the absence of significant pulmonary immunity (Lau et al. 2012). The experiments demonstrated that cellular immunity in the lungs is essential for protection against lethal wild-type H5N1 challenge, whereas influenza-specific serum ELISA antibodies and splenic influenza-specific CD8+ CTLs made little contribution to this protection. Optimal protection against wild-type virus challenge requires maturation of humoral responses, with the development of neutralizing activity. Passive transfer of postvaccination serum to naïve mice demonstrated that the magnitude of the humoral response and access of antibodies to the respiratory tract are equally important determinants of protection (Lau et al. 2012).

In a recent study comparing LAIV and TIV in ferrets, while TIV only induced immune responses in primed ferrets, LAIV induced influenza-specific antibody and T cell responses in both naïve and primed ferrets (Cheng et al. 2013). In addition to influenza-specific serum IgA and IgG antibodies, CD4+ and CD8+ T cells were demonstrated in the circulation and in paratracheal lymph nodes and the latter correlated with protection from challenge virus replication in the URT (Cheng et al. 2013).

8.2 Studies in Humans

Immunity to influenza A viruses in humans is conferred primarily by antibodies directed at the HA and NA glycoproteins. Both serum IgG and mucosal IgA antibodies can independently contribute to resistance to influenza virus in humans

(Clements et al. 1986), with serum IgG antibodies providing protection primarily to the LRT and IgA antibodies providing protection primarily to the URT (reviewed in Murphy and Coelingh 2002). Inactivated influenza vaccines induce higher titers of serum antibodies than LAIV in primed individuals, but LAIV are more efficient in inducing mucosal IgA antibody responses (Clements et al. 1986). Thus, serum HAI antibody is not an absolute correlate of protection for LAIV (Ambrose et al. 2008; Edwards et al. 1994; Treanor et al. 1999). Instead, NW IgA induced by LAIV or natural infection is associated with resistance to reinfection. LAIV viruses are shed for a longer duration and to higher titers in immunologically naive, seronegative children than in seronegative adults who have previous experience with homotypic influenza viruses (Murphy and Coelingh 2002). Homotypic immunity induced by prior infection with a drift variant restricts replication of LAIVs in seronegative adults or children to lower titer and for a shorter duration (reviewed in Murphy and Coelingh 2002). In seropositive adults and children, generally only the subset of vaccinees with low preexisting nasal HA-specific IgA antibody titer become infected and they shed a very small quantity of virus.

Although the contribution of CD8+ T cells to protection from influenza virus infection in humans is less clear than in mice and ferrets, the induction of influenza-specific CD4+, CD8+, and $\gamma\delta$ T cells by LAIVs has been demonstrated in children (He et al. 2006; Hoft et al. 2011). In a large field study of seasonal LAIV administered to children, >100 spot forming cells in an interferon-gamma (IFN-γ) ELIspot assay was associated with vaccine efficacy (Forrest et al. 2008). In a prospective study in the UK during the 2009 pandemic, Sridhar et al. found that in the absence of cross-reactive neutralizing antibodies, CD8+ T cells specific to conserved viral epitopes correlated with cross-protection against symptomatic influenza. Higher frequencies of preexisting T cells to conserved CD8 epitopes were found in individuals who developed less severe illness, with total symptom score having the strongest inverse correlation with the frequency of IFN-γ+ interleukin-2- CD8+ T cells (Sridhar et al. 2013).

A robust Type I (IFNγ) memory response was observed including production of cytokines (GM-CSF, IL-1β, IFNα, IL-6) and chemokines (CCL5 and CXCL8 early and CCL2 and CXCL10 late) involved in T cell activation and recruitment, when peripheral blood mononuclear cells from LAIV recipients were cultured with LAIV (Lanthier et al. 2011). Influenza and respiratory syncytial virus infections have been shown to elicit different innate immune signatures by microarray and transcriptomics studies (Herberg et al. 2013), suggesting that LAIVs may also be associated with an innate immune signature. LAIV induced higher expression of type I IFN and interferon stimulated genes (ISGs) than TIV in young children where their genome-wide transcript profiles in whole blood were compared at 7 days following vaccination with LAIV or TIV (Zhu et al. 2010); some of these changes may serve as biomarkers of early responses to LAIV.

9 Future Directions

Live attenuated influenza vaccines are important public health tools for the prevention of seasonal and pandemic influenza. The ability to rapidly produce a vaccine for use in the event of a pandemic requires appropriate infrastructure and capacity that are built on experience with seasonal influenza vaccine. For both seasonal LAIV and pLAIV, the identification of a biomarker that is a reliable immune correlate of protection is a high priority, because this will allow a vaccine against a novel influenza virus to be licensed rapidly in the event of a pandemic threat. The observation that pLAIVs induce long-term immune memory requires further investigation and the feasibility of implementing this immunization strategy needs to be assessed.

Acknowledgments The seasonal influenza vaccine seed development program was conducted by the strain variant team of MedImmune at California. The pandemic vaccine program was conducted under a Cooperative Research and Development Agreement between MedImmune and NIH and was supported in part by the Division of Intramural Research, National Institute of Allergy and Infectious Diseases, NIH. We thank Dr. Zhongying Chen for providing data for Fig. 2 and Drs. Raburn Mallory and Kathy Coelingh for suggestions and comments.

References

Ambrose CS, Luke C, Coelingh K (2008) Current status of live attenuated influenza vaccine in the United States for seasonal and pandemic influenza. Influenza Other Respir Viruses 2:193–202

Ambrose CS, Wu X, Knuf M, Wutzler P (2012) The efficacy of intranasal live attenuated influenza vaccine in children 2 through 17 years of age: a meta-analysis of 8 randomized controlled studies. Vaccine 30:886–892

Ambrose CS, Yi T, Falloon J (2011) An integrated, multistudy analysis of the safety of Ann Arbor strain live attenuated influenza vaccine in children aged 2–17 years. Influenza Other Respir Viruses 5:389–397

Bandell A, Woo J, Coelingh K (2011) Protective efficacy of live-attenuated influenza vaccine (multivalent, Ann Arbor strain): a literature review addressing interference. Expert Rev Vaccines 10:1131–1141

Baxter R, Toback SL, Sifakis F, Hansen J, Bartlett J, Aukes L, Lewis N, Wu X, Ambrose CS (2012a) A postmarketing evaluation of the safety of Ann Arbor strain live attenuated influenza vaccine in adults 18–49 years of age. Vaccine 30:3053–3060

Baxter R, Toback SL, Sifakis F, Hansen J, Bartlett J, Aukes L, Lewis N, Wu X, Ambrose CS (2012b) A postmarketing evaluation of the safety of Ann Arbor strain live attenuated influenza vaccine in children 5 through 17 years of age. Vaccine 30:2989–2998

Belshe RB, Edwards KM, Vesikari T, Black SV, Walker RE, Hultquist M, Kemble G, Connor EM (2007) Live attenuated versus inactivated influenza vaccine in infants and young children. N Engl J Med 356:685–696

Belshe RB, Gruber WC, Mendelman PM, Cho I, Reisinger K, Block SL, Wittes J, Iacuzio D, Piedra P, Treanor J, King J, Kotloff K, Bernstein DI, Hayden FG, Zangwill K, Yan L, Wolff M (2000) Efficacy of vaccination with live attenuated, cold-adapted, trivalent, intranasal influenza virus vaccine against a variant (A/Sydney) not contained in the vaccine. J Pediatr 136:168–175

Belshe RB, Mendelman PM, Treanor J, King J, Gruber WC, Piedra P, Bernstein DI, Hayden FG, Kotloff K, Zangwill K, Iacuzio D, Wolff M (1998) The efficacy of live attenuated, cold-adapted, trivalent, intranasal influenzavirus vaccine in children. N Engl J Med 338:1405–1412

Belshe RB, Nichol KL, Black SB, Shinefield H, Cordova J, Walker R, Hessel C, Cho I, Mendelman PM (2004) Safety, efficacy, and effectiveness of live, attenuated, cold-adapted influenza vaccine in an indicated population aged 5–49 years. Clin Infect Dis. 39:920–927

Beyer WE, Palache AM, de Jong JC, Osterhaus AD (2002) Cold-adapted live influenza vaccine versus inactivated vaccine: systemic vaccine reactions, local and systemic antibody response, and vaccine efficacy. A meta-analysis. Vaccine 20:1340–1353

Cha TA, Kao K, Zhao J, Fast PE, Mendelman PM, Arvin A (2000) Genotypic stability of cold-adapted influenza virus vaccine in an efficacy clinical trial. J Clin Microbiol 38:839–845

Chan W, Zhou H, Kemble G, Jin H (2008) The cold adapted and temperature sensitive influenza A/Ann Arbor/6/60 virus, the master donor virus for live attenuated influenza vaccines, has multiple defects in replication at the restrictive temperature. Virology 380:304–311

Chen GL, Lamirande EW, Cheng X, Torres-Velez F, Orandle M, Jin H, Kemble G, Subbarao K (2014) Evaluation of three live attenuated h2 pandemic influenza vaccine candidates in mice and ferrets. J Virol 88:2867–2876

Chen GL, Lamirande EW, Jin H, Kemble G, Subbarao K (2009a) Safety, immunogencity, and efficacy of a cold-adapted A/Ann Arbor/6/60 (H2N2) vaccine in mice and ferrets. Virology 398:109–114

Chen Z, Santos C, Aspelund A, Gillim-Ross L, Jin H, Kemble G, Subbarao K (2009b) Evaluation of live attenuated influenza a virus H6 vaccines in mice and ferrets. J Virol 83:65–72

Chen GL, Lau YF, Lamirande EW, McCall AW, Subbarao K (2011a) Seasonal influenza infection and live vaccine prime for a response to the 2009 pandemic H1N1 vaccine. Proc Natl Acad Sci USA 108:1140–1145

Chen GL, Min JY, Lamirande EW, Santos C, Jin H, Kemble G, Subbarao K (2011b) Comparison of a live attenuated 2009 H1N1 vaccine with seasonal influenza vaccines against 2009 pandemic H1N1 virus infection in mice and ferrets. J Infect Dis 203:930–936

Chen H, Matsuoka Y, Swayne D, Chen Q, Cox NJ, Murphy BR, Subbarao K (2003) Generation and characterization of a cold-adapted influenza A H9N2 reassortant as a live pandemic influenza virus vaccine candidate. Vaccine 21:4430–4436

Chen Z, Aspelund A, Kemble G, Jin H (2008) Molecular studies of temperature-sensitive replication of the cold-adapted B/Ann Arbor/1/66, the master donor virus for live attenuated influenza FluMist vaccines. Virology 380:354–362

Chen Z, Wang W, Zhou H, Suguitan AL Jr, Shambaugh C, Kim L, Zhao J, Kemble G, Jin H (2010a) Generation of live attenuated novel influenza virus A/California/7/09 (H1N1) vaccines with high yield in embryonated chicken eggs. J Virol 84:44–51

Chen Z, Zhou H, Jin H (2010b) The impact of key amino acid substitutions in the hemagglutinin of influenza A (H3N2) viruses on vaccine production and antibody response. Vaccine 28:4079–4085

Cheng X, Zengel JR, Suguitan AL Jr, Xu Q, Wang W, Lin J, Jin H (2013) Evaluation of the humoral and cellular immune responses elicited by the live attenuated and inactivated influenza vaccines and their roles in heterologous protection in ferrets. J Infect Dis 208:594–602

Clements ML, Betts RF, Tierney EL, Murphy BR (1986) Serum and nasal wash antibodies associated with resistance to experimental challenge with influenza A wild-type virus. J Clin Microbiol 24:157–160

Coelingh K, Talaat KR, Luke CJ, Jin H, Karron RA (2014) Development of live attenuated influenza vaccines against pandemic influenza strains. Expert Rev Vaccines 7:855–871

Cox RJ, Brokstad KA, Ogra P (2004) Influenza virus: immunity and vaccination strategies. Comparison of the immune response to inactivated and live, attenuated influenza vaccines. Scand J Immunol 59:1–15

De Villiers PJ, Steele AD, Hiemstra LA, Rappaport R, Dunning AJ, Gruber WC, Forrest BD, Network LEST (2009) Efficacy and safety of a live attenuated influenza vaccine in adults 60 years of age and older. Vaccine 28:228–234

Edwards KM, Dupont WD, Westrich MK, Plummer WD Jr, Palmer PS, Wright PF (1994) A randomized controlled trial of cold-adapted and inactivated vaccines for the prevention of influenza A disease. J Infect Dis 169:68–76

Forrest BD, Pride MW, Dunning AJ, Capeding MR, Chotpitayasunondh T, Tam JS, Rappaport R, Eldridge JH, Gruber WC (2008) Correlation of cellular immune responses with protection against culture-confirmed influenza virus in young children. Clin Vaccine Immunol 15:1042–1053

Gorse GJ, Campbell MJ, Otto EE, Powers DC, Chambers GW, Newman FK (1995) Increased anti-influenza A virus cytotoxic T cell activity following vaccination of the chronically ill elderly with live attenuated or inactivated influenza virus vaccine. J Infect Dis 172:1–10

Grabenstein JD, Pittman PR, Greenwood JT, Engler RJ (2006) Immunization to protect the US Armed Forces: heritage, current practice, and prospects. Epidemiol Rev 28:3–26

He XS, Holmes TH, Zhang C, Mahmood K, Kemble GW, Lewis DB, Dekker CL, Greenberg HB, Arvin AM (2006) Cellular immune responses in children and adults receiving inactivated or live attenuated influenza vaccines. J Virol 80:11756–11766

Herberg JA, Kaforou M, Gormley S, Sumner ER, Patel S, Jones KD, Paulus S, Fink C, Martinon-Torres F, Montana G, Wright VJ, Levin M (2013) Transcriptomic profiling in childhood H1N1/09 influenza reveals reduced expression of protein synthesis genes. J Infect Dis 208:1664–1668

Hoffmann E, Mahmood K, Chen Z, Yang CF, Spaete J, Greenberg HB, Herlocher ML, Jin H, Kemble G (2005) Multiple gene segments control the temperature sensitivity and attenuation phenotypes of ca B/Ann Arbor/1/66. J Virol 79:11014–11021

Hoft DF, Babusis E, Worku S, Spencer CT, Lottenbach K, Truscott SM, Abate G, Sakala IG, Edwards KM, Creech CB, Gerber MA, Bernstein DI, Newman F, Graham I, Anderson EL, Belshe RB (2011) Live and inactivated influenza vaccines induce similar humoral responses, but only live vaccines induce diverse T-cell responses in young children. J Infect Dis 204:845–853

Jin H, Chen Z (2014) Production of live attenuated influenza vaccines against seasonal and pandemic influenza viruses. Curr Opin Virol 6:34–39

Jin H, Lu B, Zhou H, Kemble G (2004) Genetic studies of FluMist influenza vaccines derived from cold adapted A/Ann Arbor/6/60, options for the control of inluenza V. Elsevier, Okinawa. In: Kawaoka Y (ed), Int Congr Ser 1263, pp 153–156

Jin H, Lu B, Zhou H, Ma C, Zhao J, Yang CF, Kemble G, Greenberg H (2003) Multiple amino acid residues confer temperature sensitivity to human influenza virus vaccine strains (FluMist) derived from cold-adapted A/Ann Arbor/6/60. Virology 306:18–24

Joseph T, McAuliffe J, Lu B, Vogel L, Swayne D, Jin H, Kemble G, Subbarao K (2008) A live attenuated cold-adapted influenza A H7N3 virus vaccine provides protection against homologous and heterologous H7 viruses in mice and ferrets. Virology 378:123–132

Karron RA, Callahan K, Luke C, Thumar B, McAuliffe J, Schappell E, Joseph T, Coelingh K, Jin H, Kemble G, Murphy BR, Subbarao K (2009a) A live attenuated H9N2 influenza vaccine is well tolerated and immunogenic in healthy adults. J Infect Dis 199:711–716

Karron RA, Talaat K, Luke C, Callahan K, Thumar B, Dilorenzo S, McAuliffe J, Schappell E, Suguitan A, Mills K, Chen G, Lamirande E, Coelingh K, Jin H, Murphy BR, Kemble G, Subbarao K (2009b) Evaluation of two live attenuated cold-adapted H5N1 influenza virus vaccines in healthy adults. Vaccine 27:4953–4960

Lanthier PA, Huston GE, Moquin A, Eaton SM, Szaba FM, Kummer LW, Tighe MP, Kohlmeier JE, Blair PJ, Broderick M, Smiley ST, Haynes L (2011) Live attenuated influenza vaccine (LAIV) impacts innate and adaptive immune responses. Vaccine 29:7849–7856

Lau YF, Santos C, Torres-Velez FJ, Subbarao K (2011) The magnitude of local immunity in the lungs of mice induced by live attenuated influenza vaccines is determined by local viral replication and induction of cytokines. J Virol 85:76–85

Lau YF, Wright AR, Subbarao K (2012) The contribution of systemic and pulmonary immune effectors to vaccine-induced protection from H5N1 influenza virus infection. J Virol 86:5089–5098

Longini IM Jr, Koopman JS, Monto AS, Fox JP (1982) Estimating household and community transmission parameters for influenza. Am J Epidemiol 115:736–751

Maassab HF (1967) Adaptation and growth characteristics of influenza virus at 25 degrees C. Nature 213:612–614

Min JY, Vogel L, Matsuoka Y, Lu B, Swayne D, Jin H, Kemble G, Subbarao K (2010) A live attenuated H7N7 candidate vaccine virus induces neutralizing antibody that confers protection from challenge in mice, ferrets, and monkeys. J Virol 84:11950–11960

Monto AS, Ohmit SE, Petrie JG, Johnson E, Truscon R, Teich E, Rotthoff J, Boulton M, Victor JC (2009) Comparative efficacy of inactivated and live attenuated influenza vaccines. N Engl J Med 361:1260–1267

Murphy BR, Coelingh K (2002) Principles underlying the development and use of live attenuated cold-adapted influenza A and B virus vaccines. Viral Immunol 15:295–323

Nichol KL, Mendelman PM, Mallon KP, Jackson LA, Gorse GJ, Belshe RB, Glezen WP, Wittes J (1999a) Effectiveness of live, attenuated intranasal influenza virus vaccine in healthy, working adults: a randomized controlled trial. JAMA 282:137–144

Nichol KL, Mendelman PM, Mallon KP, Jackson LA, Gorse GJ, Belshe RB, Glezen WP, Wittes J (1999b) Effectiveness of live, attenuated intranasal influenza virus vaccine in healthy, working adults: a randomized controlled trial [in process citation]. JAMA 282:137–144

Renegar KB, Small PA Jr, Boykins LG, Wright PF (2004) Role of IgA versus IgG in the control of influenza viral infection in the murine respiratory tract. J Immunol 173:1978–1986

Rota P, Wallis TR, Harmon MW, Rota JS, Kendal AP, Nerome K (1990) Cocirculation of two distinct evolutionary lineages of influenza type B virus since 1983. Virology 175:59–68

Sasaki S, Holmes TH, Albrecht RA, Garcia-Sastre A, Dekker CL, He XS, Greenberg HB (2014) Distinct cross-reactive B-cell responses to live attenuated and inactivated influenza vaccines. JID. doi:10.1093/infdis/jiu190

Sridhar S, Begom S, Bermingham A, Hoschler K, Adamson W, Carman W, Bean T, Barclay W, Deeks JJ, Lalvani A (2013) Cellular immune correlates of protection against symptomatic pandemic influenza. Nat Med 19:1305–1312

Suguitan AL Jr, McAuliffe J, Mills KL, Jin H, Duke G, Lu B, Luke CJ, Murphy B, Swayne DE, Kemble G, Subbarao K (2006) Live, attenuated influenza A H5N1 candidate vaccines provide broad cross-protection in mice and ferrets. PLoS Med 3:e360

Talaat KR, Karron RA, Callahan KA, Luke CJ, DiLorenzo SC, Chen GL, Lamirande EW, Jin H, Coelingh KL, Murphy BR, Kemble G, Subbarao K (2009) A live attenuated H7N3 influenza virus vaccine is well tolerated and immunogenic in a Phase I trial in healthy adults. Vaccine 27:3744–3753

Talaat KR, Karron RA, Liang PH, McMahon BA, Luke CJ, Thumar B, Chen GL, Min JY, Lamirande EW, Jin H, Coelingh KL, Kemble GW, Subbarao K (2012) An open-label phase I trial of a live attenuated H2N2 influenza virus vaccine in healthy adults. Influenza Other Respir Viruses 7:66–73

Talaat KR, Karron RA, Luke CJ, Thumar B, McMahon BA, Chen GL, Lamirande EW, Jin H, Coelingh KL, Kemble G, Subbarao K (2011) An open label Phase I trial of a live attenuated H6N1 influenza virus vaccine in healthy adults. Vaccine 29:3144–3148

Talaat KR, Luke CJ, Khurana J et al (2014) A live attenuated H5N1 vaccine induces long-term immunity in the absence of a primary antibody response. J Infect Dis 209(12):1860–1869. doi:10.1093/infdis/jiu123

Tam JS, Capeding MR, Lum LC, Chotpitayasunondh T, Jiang Z, Huang LM, Lee BW, Qian Y, Samakoses R, Lolekha S, Rajamohanan KP, Narayanan SN, Kirubakaran C, Rappaport R, Razmpour A, Gruber WC, Forrest BD, Pan-Asian C-TPETN (2007) Efficacy and safety of a live attenuated, cold-adapted influenza vaccine, trivalent against culture-confirmed influenza in young children in Asia. Pediatr Infect Dis J 26:619–628

Thompson WW, Shay DK, Weintraub E, Brammer L, Cox N, Anderson LJ, Fukuda K (2003) Mortality associated with influenza and respiratory syncytial virus in the United States. JAMA 289:179–186

Toback SL, Ambrose CS, Eaton A, Hansen J, Aukes L, Lewis N, Wu X, Baxter R (2013) A postlicensure evaluation of the safety of Ann Arbor strain live attenuated influenza vaccine in children 24–59 months of age. Vaccine 31:1812–1818

Tomoda T, Morita H, Kurashige T, Maassab HF (1995) Prevention of influenza by the intranasal administration of cold-recombinant, live-attenuated influenza virus vaccine: importance of interferon-gamma production and local IgA response. Vaccine 13:185–190

Treanor JJ, Hayden FG, Vrooman PS, Barbarash R, Bettis R, Riff D, Singh S, Kinnersley N, Ward P, Mills RG (2000) Efficacy and safety of the oral neuraminidase inhibitor oseltamivir in treating acute influenza: a randomized controlled trial. US Oral Neuraminidase Study Group. JAMA 283:1016–1024

Treanor JJ, Kotloff K, Betts RF, Belshe R, Newman F, Iacuzio D, Wittes J, Bryant M (1999) Evaluation of trivalent, live, cold-adapted (CAIV-T) and inactivated (TIV) influenza vaccines in prevention of virus infection and illness following challenge of adults with wild-type influenza A (H1N1), A (H3N2), and B viruses. Vaccine 18:899–906

Vesikari T, Karvonen A, Korhonen T, Edelman K, Vainionpaa R, Salmi A, Saville MK, Cho I, Razmpour A, Rappaport R, O'Neill R, Georgiu A, Gruber W, Mendelman PM, Forrest B (2006) A randomized, double-blind study of the safety, transmissibility and phenotypic and genotypic stability of cold-adapted influenza virus vaccine. Pediatr Infect Dis J 25:590–595

Zangwill KM (2003) Cold-adapted, live attenuated intranasal influenza virus vaccine. Pediatr Infect Dis J 22:273–274

Zhu W, Higgs BW, Morehouse C, Streicher K, Ambrose CS, Woo J, Kemble GW, Jallal B, Yao Y (2010) A whole genome transcriptional analysis of the early immune response induced by live attenuated and inactivated influenza vaccines in young children. Vaccine 28:2865–2876

Design of Alternative Live Attenuated Influenza Virus Vaccines

Courtney Finch, Weizhong Li and Daniel R. Perez

Abstract Each year due to the ever-evolving nature of influenza, new influenza vaccines must be produced to provide protection against the influenza viruses in circulation. Currently, there are two mainstream strategies to generate seasonal influenza vaccines: inactivated and live-attenuated. Inactivated vaccines are non-replicating forms of whole influenza virus, while live-attenuated vaccines are viruses modified to be replication impaired. Although it is widely believed that by inducing both mucosal and humoral immune responses the live-attenuated vaccine provides better protection than that of the inactivated vaccine, there are large populations of individuals who cannot safely receive the LAIV vaccine. Thus, safer LAIV vaccines are needed to provide adequate protection to these populations. Improvement is also needed in the area of vaccine production. Current strategies relying on traditional tissue culture-based and egg-based methods are slow and delay production time. This chapter describes experimental vaccine generation and production strategies that address the deficiencies in current methods for potential human and agricultural use.

Abbreviations

EID_{50}	Egg Infectious Dose 50
IRES	Internal Ribosome Entry Site
KO	Knockout
LAIV	Live attenuated influenza vaccine
MDCK	Madin-Darby Canine Kindey Cell
MLD_{50}	Mouse Lethal Dose 50
nts	Nucleotides
Pfu	Plaque Forming Units

C. Finch · W. Li · D. R. Perez (✉)
Department of Veterinary Medicine,
College Park and Virginia-Maryland Regional College of Veterinary Medicine,
University of Maryland, College Park, MD, USA
e-mail: avianflu@me.com

Current Topics in Microbiology and Immunology (2015) 386: 205–235

DOI: 10.1007/82_2014_404

Published Online: 9 July 2014

PSI Packaging Signal
UTR Untranslated Region
RG Reverse Genetics
RISC RNA-induced Silencing Complex
WT Wild-Type

Contents

1 Introduction

Influenza virus is an eight-segmented, negative-sense, single-stranded RNA virus in the family *Orthomyxoviridae*. It infects a wide host range including avian, aquatic, and terrestrial species. There are three types of influenza viruses known to infect humans: A, B, and C. Influenza A is capable of infecting the broadest host range of the three influenza types, while influenza B is thought to be a primarily human pathogen. Influenza C is also known to infect humans but infects primarily infants and young children (Calvo et al. 2013, 2006). Each winter, vaccines, both inactivated and live-attenuated, are produced for protection against influenza A and B. The need for seasonal influenza vaccines is a product of the error prone viral polymerase as well as the host's immunological pressure. Since the viral polymerase lacks the ability to correct mistakes made during replication, mutations accumulate causing a phenomenon known as antigenic drift—a gradual change in antigenicity through the accumulation of mutations (Taubenberger and Kash 2010). The segmented nature of the influenza genome allows it to undergo more drastic changes through another process as well: antigenic shift. This is the product of influenza viruses co-infecting the same cell and swapping segments. This can cause a more dramatic change in antigenicity than is caused by antigenic drift (Taubenberger and Kash 2010).

Influenza epidemics and pandemics are the result of the introduction of a novel influenza virus into a population. Influenza surveillance dictates which viruses to include in each year's vaccine. Currently, the seasonal vaccine includes two strains of influenza A and one strain of influenza B; however, recently, a tetravalent vaccine was approved which contains two strains of influenza A and two strains of influenza B. The 2013–2014's influenza season will see the first approved tetravalent vaccines; both live-attenuated and inactivated available for market consumption. Although including a second strain of influenza B will no doubt improve the coverage and protection conferred by the seasonal vaccine, problems remain, and there is room for significant improvement, both in production time and protection. Currently in the US, the live-attenuated, cold adapted A/Ann Arbor/6/60 and B/Ann Arbor/1/66 backbone vaccine is not licensed for the elderly, women who are pregnant, those who are immunocompromised, or those with pre-existing conditions, like asthma (Alexandrova et al. 1990; DeBorde et al. 1987, 1988; Maassab 1967; Maassab and Bryant 1999; Maassab et al. 1969; Monto and Maassab 1977).

As influenza A virus infects a wide variety of host species, it is, in addition to being a significant human pathogen, a significant pathogen in many agricultural species such as chicken and swine. Improved LAIV vaccines are needed for agricultural animals as well, as influenza can have a devastating economic impact on the agricultural industry and the food supply (Leibler et al. 2009). Although there are many alternative vectors and other genetic approaches that have been tested experimentally as platforms for influenza vaccines, this chapter will exclusively focus on novel methods for the generation and production of live-attenuated influenza virus vaccines. These strategies are aimed at accelerating vaccine efficacy or production by manipulation of the influenza genome via mutations, deletions, insertions, and rearrangement.

2 Production of LAIV Vaccines

2.1 *Alternative Strategies to Generate Influenza Virus Vaccines*

The emergence of pandemic and epidemic influenza virus strains such as the pandemic H1N1 virus in 2009 as well as various avian influenza viruses with the ability to cause disease and death in humans has prompted the renewal of efforts to develop alternative or modified virus-generating systems as well as improve virus rescue efficiency to enable a quicker response to outbreaks of novel viruses (Kadota 2013; Schnitzler and Schnitzler 2009).

2.2 Adoption of Universal or Species-Specific Pol I Promoter for Virus Vaccine Generation

The traditional DNA-based reverse genetics (RG) system allows for the production of vaccine seed strains of influenza virus via the co-transfection of 8 (or 12 or 17) plasmids into appropriate cells (Fodor et al. 1999; Hoffmann et al. 2000; Neumann et al. 1999). The more common eight plasmid system (Fig. 1a, left and top right panels) is based on a bidirectional transcription vector, which employs an RNA polymerase II (pol II) promoter to synthesize positive-sense mRNA and an RNA polymerase I (pol I) promoter to transcribe negative-sense viral RNA (vRNA) from the same viral cDNA template (Hoffmann et al. 2000). The pol I promoter

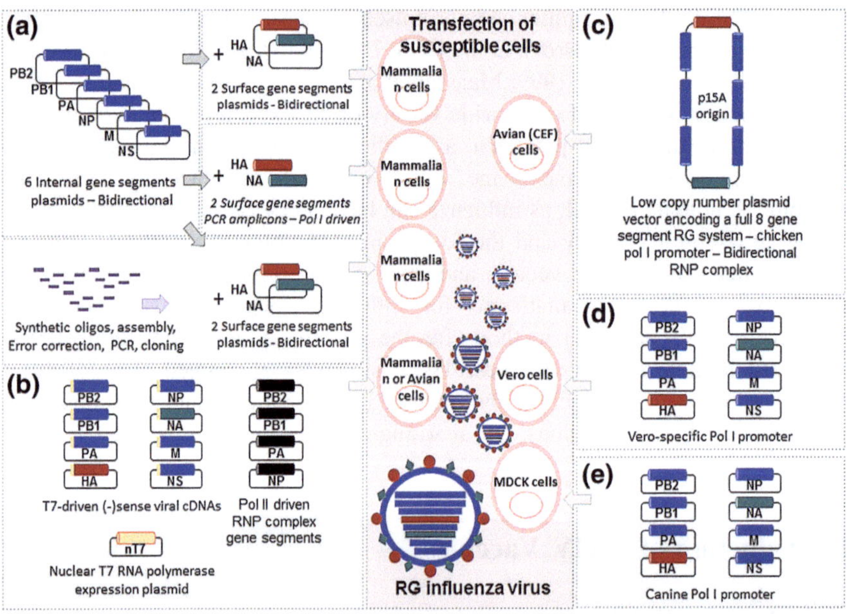

Fig. 1 Variations in reverse genetics systems for influenza virus. Reverse genetics systems and the cells lines required for use of the respective systems are shown. **a** depicts methods to expedite the generation of vaccine seed strains. **b** shows a T7 RNA polymerase reverse genetics system, which can generate virus from cells of multiple origins in the presence of a *nuclear T7 RNA polymerase expression plasmid*. **c–e** show alternative reverse genetics systems which are specific to a cell type/species [Based on (Chen et al. 2012; de Wit et al. 2007; Dormitzer et al. 2013; Massin et al. 2005; Murakami et al. 2008; Wang and Duke 2007; Wood and Robertson 2004)]

ensures the generation of vRNA with accurate 3′ ends, whereas a terminator sequence from pol I (tI) or a hepatitis delta virus ribozyme sequence ensures accurate 5′ ends (Fodor et al. 1999; Hoffmann et al. 2000). In contrast to pol II, transcription driven by pol I exhibits stringent species specificity (Heix and Grummt 1995). For example, RG plasmids harboring human pol I promoters work well in primate-origin cells (e.g, 293T cells) but behave less efficiently in cell lines of canine-origin (Madin-Darby Canine Kidney, MDCK) or porcine-origin (PK15) or not at all in cell lines derived from avian species (Murakami et al. 2008; Wang and Duke 2007). Thus, virus rescue by RG in different cell types may require a distinct set of expression plasmids.

In the past decade, numerous strategies have been exploited to resolve this problem. An RG vector containing a universal RNA polymerase promoter (T7 pol I) has been shown to generate recombinant influenza virus from human-origin (293T), avian-origin (QT6) and MDCK cells (Fig. 1b) (de Wit et al. 2007). Since the T7 RNA polymerase does not exist in animal cells, it is necessary to introduce an extra T7 polymerase expression plasmid with a nuclear localization sequence into the same cells (Fig. 1b) (de Wit et al. 2007). Alternatively, species-specific promoters may be used in order to transfect a single cell type (Fig. 1c–d). For instance, transfection of chicken RNA pol I promoter-based plasmids has been shown to result in virus rescue, although the virus titer is relatively low (Fig. 1c) (Massin et al. 2005; Zhang et al. 2009). Likewise, an alternative 8 plasmid RG system using canine RNA pol I promoter was developed for virus rescue in MDCK cells (Murakami et al. 2008; Wang and Duke 2007), a vaccine approved cell line (Fig. 1e) (Brands et al. 1999; Palache et al. 1999). Finally, efficient virus rescue has been shown in African green monkey kidney epithelial (Vero) cells (Wood and Robertson 2004), with the transfection of plasmids carrying Vero pol I promoters (Fig. 1d) (Song et al. 2013).

2.3 *Improving the Transfection Efficiency of the RG System in Vaccine-Producing Cells*

An important factor affecting vaccine manufacture using RG is transfection efficiency. Although 293T cells are easily transfected with plasmid DNA, they are not yet licensed for use in the vaccine industry. Alternatively, Vero cells are approved for vaccine production (Kistner et al. 1998; Wood and Robertson 2004), but the low-transfection efficacy poses a barrier to robust vaccine production (Kistner et al. 1998, 1999). In order to overcome this, one possible solution is to reduce the number of plasmids required for virus generation. To this end, Neumann et al. placed eight-unidirectional pol I driven vRNA transcription cassettes into one vector. Each cassette corresponded to one of the 8 segments of influenza virus (Fig. 2a). Additionally, three pol II driven transcription cassettes carrying the viral polymerase genes (PB2, PB1 and PA) were cloned into another vector (Neumann

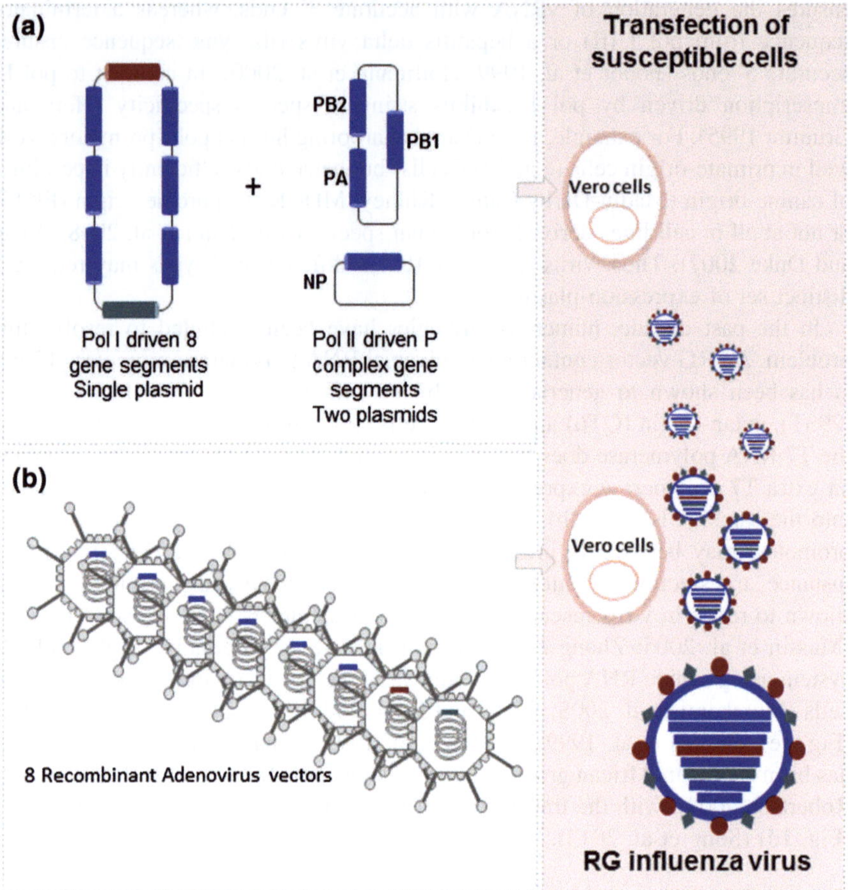

Fig. 2 Variations in reverse genetics systems for influenza virus. Reverse genetics systems designed to increase transfection efficiency of influenza gene segments in Vero cells are shown. **a** depicts a 3-plasmid strategy. **b** describes an adenovirus vector strategy. Each adenovirus is shown carrying 1 segment of influenza virus. Based on (Neumann et al. 2005; Ozawa et al. 2007)

et al. 2005). High titer virus was obtained when these 2 plasmids together with an NP-expression plasmid (3-plasmid system) were transfected into Vero cells (Neumann et al. 2005).

In a separate study, a single plasmid containing all 8 influenza gene segments was constructed, achieving high virus yield in chicken embryo fibroblast (CEF) cells (Fig. 1c) (Zhang et al. 2009). A major challenge inherent to this technology is determining how best to prevent intra-plasmid recombination while maintaining the stability of the construct. In order to address this challenge, the authors used a low-copy-number vector (approximately 15 copies per bacterial cell), minimized the number of CMV promoters (4 CMV promoters were used to initiate the synthesis of the viral RNP complex), and shortened the length of homologous sequences (Zhang et al. 2009). This novel one-plasmid system can produce the vRNA polymerase complex (PB2, PB1, PA, and NP) and 8 vRNA segments upon transfection of cells, generating recombinant virus.

Compared with DNA vectors, the gene transfer efficiency of viral vectors is generally several orders of magnitude higher. An adenovirus vector-mediated RG system was designed (Ozawa et al. 2007) using the bidirectional transcription cassette for each vRNA segment of influenza virus inserted into a replication-incompetent adenovirus vector (AdV) lacking E1 and E3 genes (Fig. 2b). Eight recombinant AdVs were produced. After 3 days co-infection of these viruses in Vero cells, the amount of influenza virus obtained from AdV-infected cells was about 10,000 fold higher than those cells transfected with 12-plasmids (Ozawa et al. 2007).

2.4 Strategies to Accelerate Vaccine Seed Stock Preparation

During influenza pandemics, a rate-limiting step in vaccine production is the generation of vaccine seed strains. The traditional RG system takes time because it relies on a cloning step to generate plasmids expressing hemagglutinin (HA) and neuraminidase (NA) surface gene segments and a clone identification step done by sequencing. To hasten this process, a partial and full PCR-based RG strategy was designed (Chen et al. 2012). Using overlapping PCR, a pol I promoter sequence and a tI termination signal were incorporated into the 5′ and 3′ ends of cDNA copies of each individual gene of influenza A virus to produce a full set of influenza PCR amplicons (Fig. 1a left and middle right panels). When two PCR amplicons encoding the HA and NA gene segments were transfected into 293T/MDCK cells together with six bidirectional RG plasmids, RG influenza viruses were rescued with efficiencies similar to those of the eight plasmids system. Alternatively, when the eight PCR amplicons were introduced into 293T/MDCK cells together with four helper plasmids (expressing vRNA polymerase and NP protein) or four PCR amplicons harboring the PB2, PB1, PA, and NP genes flanked by CMV promoter and bovine growth hormone (bgh) polyadenylation element, the virus was generated successfully. For the first time, this showed that recovery of virus entirely from PCR products is feasible (Chen et al. 2012). This system would eliminate the cloning steps, particularly of HA and NA gene segments, involved in generating a virus vaccine seed stock, which may be crucial in the early stages of vaccine production during a pandemic.

Another option for vaccine generation during an influenza pandemic event is the use of synthetic HA and NA genes generated either by site-directed mutagenesis of DNA encoding closely related virus strains or by chemical synthesis (Verity et al. 2011). This synthetic DNA strategy has one major disadvantage, in that point mutations invariably appear, especially in the long segments like HA (1.8 kb) and NA (1.6 kb). Thus, this strategy requires correction, delaying vaccine production. Most recently, a new method was developed by Dormitzer et al. to eliminate this hindrance (Dormitzer et al. 2013) (Fig. 1a left and bottom panels). Hundreds of overlapping oligonucleotides (about 60 bases in length per segment) were synthesized, assembled together, and mismatched bases removed by a commercially available error-correcting enzyme (ErrASE). Following ErrASE, a PCR amplification procedure was employed to generate the full-length HA and NA genes, which were subsequently ligated into a linearized plasmid such that a CMV promoter and pol I terminator flanked one end of the influenza gene and a pol I promoter and a pol II polyadenylation signal flanked the other end. After another round of high-fidelity PCR amplification with primers corresponding to the transcriptional control regions, HA and NA amplicons used for virus rescue were obtained (Fig. 1a). The first seed virus was generated within one week (Dormitzer et al. 2013), suggesting this technology could be a viable option for a faster pandemic response.

3 Improving LAIV Vaccines: Attenuation Through the Modification of Gene Segments

3.1 Modifying the NS Gene Segment

3.1.1 NS1 Truncation Mutants

Considerable effort has been placed in modifying the influenza NS gene, segment 8, as a means of creating a safer alternative to the current LAIV vaccine strategy. The NS gene encodes two proteins: NS1 and NS2. NS1, or non-structural protein 1, acts as an IFN antagonist, aiding in viral evasion of the host innate immune response (Fukuyama and Kawaoka 2011). NS2, also known as the nuclear export protein (NEP), is involved in the export of viral mRNAs from the host nucleus (Palese and Shaw 2007). Such crucial roles in the viral life cycle make segment 8 a good target for attenuation.

Studies have shown that influenza A and B viruses possessing truncated NS1 proteins are immunogenic and attenuated in a range of animal models (Fig. 3a): mouse, swine, ferret, chicken, and equine (Chambers et al. 2009; Pica et al. 2012; Solórzano et al. 2005; Steel et al. 2009; Wressnigg et al. 2009). Several NS1 truncations have been described. Each truncation involves the insertion of stop codons at the 3′ end of the NS1 ORF causing premature termination of NS1 translation at the C-terminus. Several truncations have been tested for influenza A: NS1 1–73, NS1 1–99, and NS1 1–126 (number range indicates amino acids expressed). IFN expression upon infection of a host cell with one of these truncated NS1 viruses has been shown to correlate with the length of the truncation (Solorzano et al. 2005). Although all NS1 truncations were shown to attenuate the viruses both in vitro and in the swine model, the NS1 1–73 virus has been shown to be the most attenuated (Solorzano et al. 2005). Of the NS1 truncated viruses, NS1

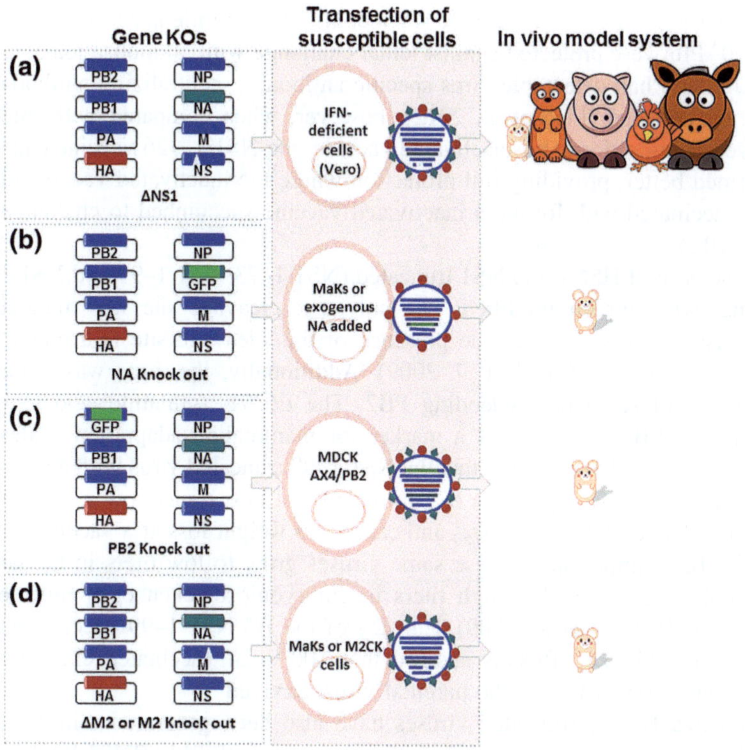

Fig. 3 Live attenuated approaches for influenza viruses—Gene knockout strategies. Four gene knockout strategies are depicted. Cells lines required for growth of the corresponding viruses are also shown as well as the animal models in which each strategy has been tested. **a** describes the NS1 truncation strategy. The *white* Δ in NS denotes the location of the truncation. **b** summarizes the NA knockout strategy. The foreign gene, *GFP*, cloned in placed of NA is shown in *green*. **c** describes the PB2 knockout strategy. As in the NA strategy, the foreign gene, *GFP*, cloned in place of PB2 is shown in *green*. **d** depicts both the M2 truncation and the M2 knockout strategy. As in the NS truncation strategy, the *white* Δ in M denotes the location of the truncation or deletion, in the case of the knockout. Based on (Chambers et al. 2009; Hatta et al. 2011; Pica et al. 2012; Shinya et al. 2004; Solórzano et al. 2005; Steel et al. 2009; Victor et al. 2012; Watanabe et al. 2008, 2009; Wressnigg et al. 2009). Royalty free animal clip art obtained from https://openclipart.org

1–73 is the most deficient in blocking IFN because it contains the longest truncation. However, the NS1 1–99 virus proved more potent from a vaccine efficacy standpoint. Both NS1 1–99 and NS1 1–73 viruses caused significantly fewer lung lesions in swine than did WT virus at the same dose (Solorzano et al. 2005).

The NS1 truncation attenuation strategy has been validated in seasonal viruses as well as highly pathogenic (HP) H5N1 viruses, which have traditionally been a challenge for vaccine developers. Studies have shown that the NS1 1–126 truncation strategy is a potentially excellent LAIV vaccine candidate for high-risk populations unable to receive traditional LAIV vaccines, such as the elderly, based on studies performed in aged mice (Pica et al. 2012). While aged mice vaccinated with 10^3 Pfu were protected against lethal challenge with 50 mouse lethal dose 50 (MLD_{50}) and had detectable virus specific antibodies, neutralizing antibody titers were not detected (Pica et al. 2012); however, when compared with mice that received 50 ng of formalin-inactivated vaccine, the NS1 1–126 vaccine candidates performed better, providing full protection where the inactivated vaccine did not. Mice vaccinated with formalin inactivated vaccine succumbed to challenge (Pica et al. 2012).

In the case of H5N1, the NS1 truncated (NS1 1–73, NS1 1–99 and NS1 1–126) vaccines were further modified. The polybasic cleavage site was mutated to a monobasic cleavage site, as the presence of this cleavage site is a major determinant of virulence (Steel et al. 2009). Additionally, the virus was mutated in codon 627 of segment 1 encoding PB2. The E627K (glutamic acid to lysine) mutation in PB2 is known as a marker for mammalian adaptation (Palese and Shaw 2007). Steel et al. found that the NS1 1–99 truncated virus with a monobasic cleavage site and E at position 627 provided that best protection in mice against lethal challenge of 1,000 MLD_{50} and caused no weight loss at a vaccination dose of 10^6 EID_{50}. Importantly, these same viruses grow to low titers in human lung epithelial cells, A549, but high titers in embryonic chicken eggs (due to E at position 627) (Steel et al. 2009). Efficacy of the H5 NS1 1–99 vaccine was also assessed in chickens. Results showed that 100 % of vaccinated chickens challenged with 100 CLD_{50} of the parental virus survived.

Influenza B NS1 truncated viruses have also been generated. Similar results have been seen in influenza B as in influenza A; even though, BNS1 RNA binding to IFN is not required for IFN antagonism (Donelan et al. 2004). As in influenza A, a series of truncations were made in the C-terminus of NS1: NS1 1–14, NS1 1–38, NS1 1–57 and NS1 1–80 (Wressnigg et al. 2009). These viruses, like those of influenza A, replicate in Vero cells, which do not produce interferons. While all of these truncated viruses are attenuated, the degree of attenuation corresponds to the length of the truncation (Wressnigg et al. 2009). NS1 1–80 is not sufficient to block IFN and induces an IgG response which is greater than that produced by the WT virus (Wressnigg et al. 2009). Mice were fully protected after just one immunization (at 5×10^5 tissue culture infectious dose 50, $TCID_{50}$) of NS1 mutants against 5×10^5 $TCID_{50}$ homologous virus challenge. Viral titers of lung homogenates revealed that none of the mice immunized with an NS1 mutant had detectable virus titers in the lungs after lethal challenge (Wressnigg et al. 2009).

More recently, an NS1 truncation strategy has been tested in human trials. To date, both safety/immunogenicity and heterosubtypic immunity trials have been completed (Morokutti et al. 2014; Wacheck et al. 2010). Referred to as ΔNS1-H1N1, this monovalent vaccine completely lacks the NS1 ORF and carries H1 and N1 surface glycoproteins from A/New Caledonia/20/99 (H1N1). During the safety and immunogenicity trial, 1 of 5 doses of the vaccine was administered intranasally to healthy seronegative adults in spray form. Adverse effects were mild, ranging from headaches to rhinitis. In the highest dose group, 10 of 12 adults seroconverted to the vaccine. Additionally, neutralizing antibodies to heterologous variants were detected (Wacheck et al. 2010). Following a successful safety and immunogenicity study, heterosubtypic immunity induced by this vaccine was evaluated. Seronegative healthy adults were similarly immunized with ΔNS1-H1N1, although at only one high dose. Of those vaccinated 8/12 developed a serum IgG response to the vaccine. Importantly, nasal washes were found to neutralize heterosubtypic H3N2 and H5N1 viruses, and this cross-neutralization generated by the vaccine was determined to be a result of IgA, not IgG.

Manipulation of the NS gene has not been limited to NS1. NEP's open reading frame has also been modified. NEP interacts with M1 to export vRNAs from the nucleus of the infected host cell into the cytoplasm where they are packaged into new influenza virions (Palese and Shaw 2007). Akarsu et al. modified the NEP coding sequence to introduce mutations into the M1 binding region, E67S, E74S, and E75S. Two viruses were generated, E67S/E74S and E67S/E74S/E75S. The introduction of these mutations caused the addition of 7 amino acids at the C-terminus of the protein (Akarsu et al. 2011). Vaccine efficacy of the E67S/E74S virus was tested. E67S/E74S immunized mice challenged with 10 MLD_{50} of the WT (A/WSN/33 (H1N1)) virus saw no weight loss. While a decrease in polymerase activity was detected, peak viral titer of this virus was similar to WT (Akarsu et al. 2011). This is particularly important when considering vaccine development.

3.2 Gene Knockout Strategies

3.2.1 Neuraminidase-Deficient Viruses

Segment 6 of the influenza genome encodes for neuramindase (NA), an enzyme responsible for cleavage of the sialic acids (Palese and Shaw 2007). Neuraminidase allows for release of progeny influenza virion from the host cell (Palese and Shaw 2007). NA is also thought to be involved in reaching the target cell surface by cleaving sialic acids in the mucopolysaccharides covering the surface of the target cell (Cohen et al. 2013). Like segment 8, segment 6 is also a target of manipulation.

Shinya et al. showed that a neuraminidase deficient virus is not only attenuated, but also capable of stably carrying a foreign gene in place of the NA ORF, making this strategy a potential vaccine vector (Shinya et al. 2003). The majority of the NA ORF was replaced ($\sim$1,100 nucleotide deletion) with the green fluorescent protein (GFP) ORF (Fig. 3b). Additionally, 185 nucleotides of NA at the 5′ end of the vRNA and 202 nucleotides (nt) of NA on the 3′ end of the vRNA flanked GFP (Shinya et al. 2004), each region corresponding to packaging signals. Rescue of this virus was achieved through growth in modified MDCK cells (MaKs) that express lower levels of sialic acids (Shinya et al. 2004). In MaKs cells, the NA deficient virus grows to WT titers. Alternatively, NA-deficient viruses can be grown in the presence of exogenous NA added to the cell culture medium. Shinya et al. then demonstrated that, upon vaccination of mice with at least 10^6 Pfu of the NA-deficient virus, complete protection against 100 MLD_{50} of challenge virus was achieved. Seroconversion and neutralizing antibodies were detected at vaccination doses as low as 1.1×10^4 Pfu (Shinya et al. 2004). Additionally, GFP expression was detectable up to five passages in MaKs cells, suggesting that this virus could also be a vaccine vector (Shinya et al. 2004).

3.2.2 PB2-Deficient Viruses

Segment 1 of the influenza genome codes for PB2. The encoded protein interacts with PB1 and PA proteins (encoded by segments 2 and 3, respectively) to form the vRNA-dependent RNA polymerase complex (Palese and Shaw 2007). PB2 binds 5′ cap of the host mRNA, initiating the cap snatching activity of the viral polymerase and allowing for synthesis of viral mRNA (Palese and Shaw 2007). This is a crucial step in the viral life cycle, making PB2 a good target for attenuation.

Like the NA knockout strategy described previously, the PB2 nucleotide sequence of A/WSN/33 (H1N1) (WSN) was deleted, except for the packaging signals. The GFP ORF was cloned in place of the deleted region (Fig. 3c) (Victor et al. 2012). The virus grew to WT levels in AX4/PB2 cells, which have enhanced expression of alpha 2, 6 sialic acid receptors and stably express PB2 (Fig. 3c). A safety profile of the vaccine in mice revealed no weight loss upon vaccination, and tissue collected was virus free. The best protection with this vaccination strategy against a lethal A/Puerto Rico/8/1934 (H1N1) (PR8) challenge of 5 MLD_{50} was seen with 3 doses of the vaccine (at 10^6 Pfu). The best IgG and IgA responses were also seen with 3 immunizations. Post-challenge, no virus was detected in the lungs or nasal turbinates of any mouse that received 2 or 3 doses of the PB2KO vaccine. Interestingly, GFP antibodies were detected in mouse sera suggesting that this strategy may be a viable candidate for a virus vector.

3.3 Viruses Possessing M2 Deletions

Segment 7 of the influenza genome encodes for the M gene. Upon translation in influenza A, it is spliced into M1 and M2. Similarly, segment 7 of influenza B encodes for M gene; however, in the case of influenza B, BM1 and BM2 are derived via a stop–start translation signal separating the ORF of the 2 proteins (Palese and Shaw 2007). M1 is a matrix protein that functions as a structural component of the influenza virion. M2 and BM2 are ion channels that aid in the release of the vRNA into the cytoplasm by facilitating the acidification of the virion (Palese and Shaw 2007). The M2 cytoplasmic tail is also known to be involved in virus assembly and is a determinant of morphology (Palese and Shaw 2007). Viruses possessing deletions of the M2 cytoplasmic tail and complete M2 knockouts have proven to be attenuated in mice in the context of H5N1, pH1N1, and mouse-adapted PR8 (H1N1) viruses (Hatta et al. 2011; Watanabe et al. 2008, 2009).

A series of M2 cytoplasmic tail mutants were created as vaccine possessing deletions of various lengths beginning at the C-terminus in the context of a H5N1 vaccine (Fig. 3d) (Watanabe et al. 2008). Another mutant was constructed which contained a full M2 knockout (Watanabe et al. 2008). Each mutant was constructed by the introduction of premature stop codons in the M2 ORF. Growth kinetics in MDCK cells showed that viruses containing 5 (VN1203M2del5) and 11 (VN1203M2del11) amino acid (aa) deletions grew to similar titers as the WT virus. Titrations of these M2 cytoplasmic tail mutants in mice detected the VN1203M2del5 and VN1203M2del11 viruses in mouse tissues only on day 3 post-infection including lung, nasal turbinates, brain (except for VN1203M2del11), spleen and kidneys, while the longer amino acid deletions of the M2 cytoplasmic tail were undetectable (Watanabe et al. 2008). Both the VN1203M2del5 and VN1203M2del11 viruses were present at lower titers than WT in all tissues assayed.

After modifying the HA cleavage site from a polybasic cleavage site to a monobasic site (ΔHA), the VN1204M2del11 virus was further assessed for protection against WT highly pathogenic A/Vietnam/1203/ 2004 (H5N1) challenge (Watanabe et al. 2008). Mice vaccinated with 100 or 1,000 Pfu of ΔHA VN1203M2del11 virus did not lose weight post-vaccination. Vaccinated mice also showed high levels of IgG in the sera as well as IgG and IgA in lung washes. Little IgA or IgG was found in nasal washes. In each medium, the mice vaccinated with 1,000 Pfu had the highest titers of each immunoglobulin. Viral replication of the vaccine strain was seen in the lungs at both doses and in the nasal turbinate at 1,000 Pfu on day 3 post-vaccination. All vaccinated mice survived challenge of 100 MLD_{50} WT H5N1. None showed weight loss (Watanabe et al. 2008); furthermore, no virus was detected in any immunized mouse tissue at either dose 3 days post-challenge (Watanabe et al. 2008).

Similar findings as those described above in the context of HP H5N1 influenza virus were also found in studies done using the same strategy (11 amino acid deletion in the M2 cytoplasmic tail) with pandemic H1N1 virus, A/California/04/2009 (H1N1) (CA04) (Hatta et al. 2011). As was seen in H5N1, the CA04M2del11 virus grew to WT levels in MDCK cells. Inoculation of mice resulted in little weight loss, although the virus replicated to WT levels in the lungs at 10^4 and 10^5 Pfu. Upon homologous challenge with 10^6 Pfu of WT CA04, none of the CA04M2d3l11 immunized mice lost weight (Hatta et al. 2011). IgG levels in the serum as well as IgG and IgA levels in the nasal wash were comparable to WT; however, IgG and IgA levels in trachea-lung washes were lower than WT levels (Hatta et al. 2011).

Another study analyzed the M2 knockout (M2KO) strategy as an attenuated vaccine in mice in the context of a lethal challenge (100 MLD_{50}) with the A/Puerto Rico/8/1934 (H1N1) virus (Fig. 3d) (Watanabe et al. 2009). Comparable IgG and IgA responses were seen in mice immunized with M2KO virus as those immunized with WT virus. The primary difference between this knockout strategy and the cytoplasmic tail deletion strategy is growth. While the M2 cytoplasmic tail mutations were grown in MDCK cells to near WT levels, the M2KO virus must be grown in M2CK cells, MDCK cells that express M2 (Watanabe et al. 2009).

3.4 Modifications in the HA Cleavage Site

Segment 4 encodes HA. HA protein must be cleaved in order to generate a productive influenza infection (Skehel and Wiley 2000). It is cleaved upon release of the virus from the host cell (Palese and Shaw 2007). The cleavage reaction is the product of an interaction between a host cell protease and the cleavage recognition site of the HA protein. Monobasic cleavage sites are cleaved by trypsin-like proteases present primarily in the upper respiratory tract of humans and many other mammals and the intestinal tract of avian species (Skehel and Wiley 2000), while polybasic cleavage sites are cleaved by furin-like proteases ubiquitously present throughout many cell types. Cleavage by furin-like proteases allows the virus to cause systemic infection in birds or to allow more efficient lower respiratory tract infection in mammals (at least for some strains, like the Asian H5N1 strains) causing a more virulent infection (Palese and Shaw 2007). Thus, altering the enzyme specificity of the cleavage may be a means of attenuating the virus.

Influenza A and influenza B viruses have been engineered to carry the porcine pancreatic elastase cleavage site in the HA gene segment (Fig. 4a). The typical trypsin-like HA cleavage site of A/WSN/33 (H1N1) was altered to recognize elastase by mutating the HA gene segment at nucleotide positions 1,059 and 1,060 from AG to GT. These mutations resulted in an amino acid change of arginine to valine at position 343. In vitro, with the addition of elastase, this virus grew to WT levels in MDCK cells (Stech et al. 2005). The WSN elastase virus (WSN-E) was completely restricted to growth in the presence of elastase, as it does not plaque and cannot be cleaved in the presence of trypsin. The WSN-E virus also showed restricted growth in the mouse model. Mice vaccinated with WSN-E did not exhibit any signs of disease, showed no weight loss after inoculation with 10^6 Pfu of virus, and had no detectable virus in the lung 1 day post-inoculation. In contrast, WT WSN was detected in the lung at each time point assayed. A vaccine study showed that mice inoculated with at least 10^5 Pfu of WSN-E were fully protected from a WT WSN lethal challenge at 10^6 Pfu. Interestingly, all mice immunized with WSN-E formalin inactivated vaccine succumbed to infection after challenge (Stech et al. 2005). Post-challenge, no virus was detected in the lungs of mice immunized with 10^6 Pfu of WSN-E. These mice had IgG and IgA responses similar to mice immunized with 10^3 Pfu of WT WSN (Stech et al. 2005).

The HA cleavage site of influenza B/Lee/40 was similarly modified to recognize elastase; however, in this instance, two viruses were generated after mutating the HA: B/Lee/40-Val (arginine to valine at position 361) and B/Lee/40-Ala (arginine to alanine at 361). In the presence of elastase, each vaccine candidate was shown to grow to WT levels in MDCK cells, although B/Lee/40-Val grew to

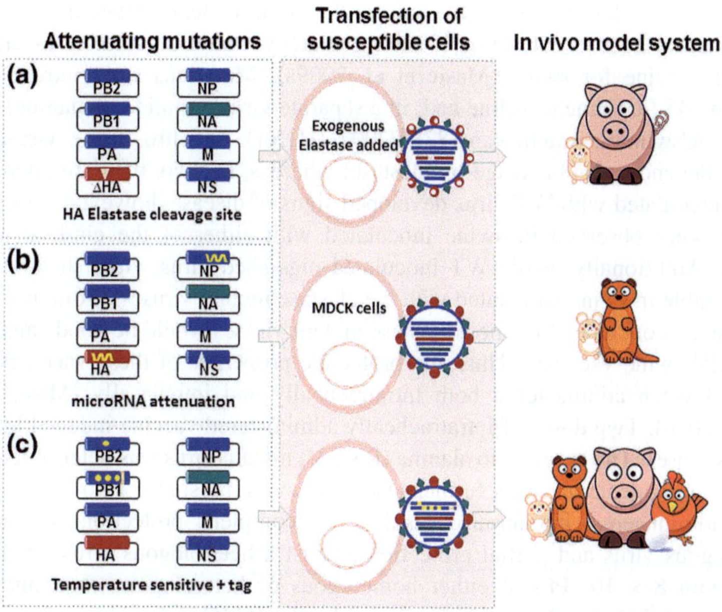

Fig. 4 Live attenuated approaches for influenza viruses—Attenuating mutations. Experimental LAIV strategies based on the mutation of various segments, the cell lines in which the corresponding viruses must be grown, and the animal models in which each strategy has been tested are depicted. **a** describes the elastase HA cleavage site mutation strategy. The *inverted white* Δ represents the mutation site. **b** describes the introduction of microRNAs to attenuate influenza. The sites of microRNA introduction are depicted with a *yellow squiggle line*. **c** illustrates the *temperature sensitive + tag* (*att*) strategy of attenuation. Point mutations are depicted with *yellow dots* in the PB2 and PB1 segments. The HA tag is shown as a *pink rectangle* in PB1. Based on (Babiuk et al. 2011; Cai et al. 2011; Hickman et al. 2008; Langlois et al. 2013; Loving et al. 2013; 2012; Masic et al. 2009b, 2010; Pena et al. 2011; Perez et al. 2009; Solórzano et al. 2010; Song et al. 2007; Stech et al. 2005, 2011)

slightly lower titers. Given this finding, in vivo work was completed using B/Lee/40-Ala, which did not cause weight loss in mice. Post-lethal challenge of WT B/Lee/40 at 10^6 Pfu, no virus was detected in the lungs of mice immunized with at least 10^4 Pfu of B/Lee/40-Ala on day 3 post-challenge. Mice immunized with these doses maintained weight post-challenge and survived. In contrast, mice immunized with B/Lee-40-Ala formalin inactivated vaccine had high viral titers detectable in the lungs on day 3 post-challenge. Weight loss was recorded (Stech et al. 2011). This cleavage modification strategy presents major advantages. Elastase vaccines can be grown to WT levels in approved cell lines while providing adequate protection with just one dose; however, this strategy is prone to reversion. Thus, as the authors suggest, combining this strategy with another, such as the A/Ann Arbor and B/Ann Arbor cold-adapted mutations, may be necessary (Alexandrova et al. 1990; DeBorde et al. 1987, 1988; Maassab 1967; Maassab et al. 1969).

Further work has been done to evaluate the elastase cleavage site in the context of its natural host to determine if such a strategy would be suitable as an agricultural vaccine for swine (Masic et al. 2009a). Mutations were introduced at position 345 (arginine to valine and, in a separate virus, arginine to alanine) in the HA of A/swine/Saskatchewan/18789/2002 (H1N1). In vitro, these viruses are strictly dependent on cleavage by elastase; whereas, in vivo, they are attenuated. Swine inoculated with WT virus developed signs of disease; however, no signs of disease were observed in swine inoculated with either of the elastase mutant viruses. Additionally, while WT inoculated pigs shed virus, virus shedding was undetectable in swine inoculated with the elastase mutant viruses. From this study, Masic et al. concluded that these elastase mutant viruses would be good candidates for LAIV swine vaccines. Thus, the protective properties of these vaccines were assessed when administered both intratracheally and intranasally (Masic et al. 2009b, 2010). Two doses of intratracheally administered vaccine induced IgG and IgA responses. The arginine to alanine (R345V) mutant virus was determined to be more immunogenic and was further tested in a vaccine study. Two doses of this virus administered intranasally resulted in complete protection against the homologous virus and partial protection against a heterologous virus upon challenge with 8×10^5 Pfu of either homologous or heterologous challenge virus (Masic et al. 2009b). Protection conferred by the R345V virus was subsequently evaluated intranasally, as this is a more practical route for vaccine administration. Two intranasal inoculations induced strong IgG and IgA responses as well as a specific IFNγ response. Full protection was achieved against homologous parental challenge as well as a homologous challenge with an antigenic variant. Partial protection was achieved with heterologous challenge (Masic et al. 2010). This strain has been shown to protect against pH1N1 via both routes of administration (Babiuk et al. 2011).

3.5 *Adding Attenuating Features to the Influenza Genome*

3.5.1 MicroRNAs

MicroRNAs (miRNAs) are RNAs generated by RNA polymerase II transcripts of a host cell. Transcripts are cleaved by host endonucleases and used to regulate cell protein expression (tenOever 2013). The miRNA transcripts bind to other host messenger RNA (mRNA) transcripts with partial complementarity and are loaded into the RNA-induced silencing complex (RISC). This process is similar to vRNA silencing (viRNA) in which viRNAs are targeted by the host cell transcripts (with complete complementarity), loaded into RISC, the formation of which is facilitated by DICER (an enzyme that cleaves double stranded RNA), and degraded; however, it is not considered a host defense mechanism. Generally, regulation of protein expression by miRNAs results in a two-fold reduction in protein expression (tenOever 2013). Since vertebrates have miRNAs and there is little reciprocal interaction between RNA viruses and host miRNAs, it is possible to engineer vaccines by manipulating miRNAs (tenOever 2013).

Manipulation of miRNAs to attenuate influenza virus has been shown. Perez et al. demonstrated attenuation of an influenza A virus carrying an miRNA, miRNA 93, which is present in human and murine cells but absent in chicken, hypothesizing that such a modification to the genome would result in attenuation in murine cells but uninhibited replication in eggs (Perez et al. 2009). Segment 5, encoding NP, was mutated in such a way that did not alter the physical properties of the amino acid coding sequence but modified NP such that it contained miRNA response elements, target sites for miRNA (Fig. 4b). Such modifications resulted in the introduction of point mutations. H1N1 and H5N1 viruses generated in this manner were attenuated in mice, reducing mortality by more than 2 logs. Perez et al. proved that this attenuation was directly related to the introduction of miRNA response elements in NP, showing that, when influenza virus carrying miRNA response elements were administered to DICER knockout mice, the viruses grew to WT levels (Perez et al. 2009).

More recently, it was shown that modification of the HA gene through the addition of a series of miRNAs at the C-terminus could also be used to restrict replication and transmission of influenza to species that do not recognize the miRNA present in the virus (Fig. 4b). Studies were aimed at selecting a miRNA that is abundant in human lung A549 cells but absent in ferret lungs and MDCK cells. Langlois et al. hypothesized that such a strategy would not alter the growth or transmission kinetics of the virus in ferrets or MDCK cells. miRNA 192 was identified as a potential candidate. With the incorporation of miRNA 192, HA protein expression was ablated in A549 cells. Additionally, growth of the virus carrying miRNA 192 was uninhibited in MDCK cells, but in MDCK cells engineered to express miRNA, growth was restricted. To demonstrate restriction of the miRNA192 carrying virus in an animal model, mice were infected. These mice saw little change in weight and survived infection, while WT inoculated mice experienced severe weight loss and succumbed to infection (Langlois et al. 2013). Similarly, ferrets were inoculated with a miRNA 192 expressing virus. As expected, transmission was not hindered by the addition of miRNA 192. Virus sequenced from these ferrets revealed the presence of miRNA 192 in the HA, showing stability of this strategy in vivo (Langlois et al. 2013).

Although neither of these strategies was explicitly tested as a vaccine candidate, each could potentially be incorporated into other LAIV strategies to enhance attenuation without losing replication activity. These studies prove that it is possible to engineer a virus that grows to high titers in approved cell lines but is restricted in the species for which the vaccine would be generated. Thus, miRNAs could have implications for influenza vaccines for many species.

3.5.2 Viruses Carrying HA Epitope Tags

Extensive research on another strategy involving the addition of a feature to the influenza genome has been done. Previously, it was found that the temperature sensitive mutations are not always enough to attenuate animal influenza viruses, in particular avian and swine viruses (Song et al. 2007). With the simple addition of the HA tag, the vaccine becomes significantly safer (Song et al. 2007) (Fig. 4c). This strategy was complemented with the introduction of the cold-adapted mutations found in PB2 and PB1 genes of cold-adapted A/Ann Arbor/6/60: K391E, E581G, and S661T in PB1, and N265S in PB2 (DeBorde et al. 1987; Maassab 1967; Maassab et al. 1969; Snyder et al. 1988). The safety and efficacy of this vaccine strategy has been demonstrated in a variety of animal models including: in ovo, mouse, swine, ferret, and chicken (Cai et al. 2011; Hickman et al. 2008; Pena et al. 2011; Solórzano et al. 2010; Song et al. 2007). This strategy has also been shown to be effective in a variety of different backbones against many viruses including H5, H7, and pandemic H1N1 viruses. With each study, this strategy has been shown to complement the attenuation seen with the cold adapted mutations, making an attenuated virus safer and more effective while maintaining a virus that replicates and grows to WT levels (in MDCK cells and in chicken eggs) at low temperatures. Additionally, this strategy also serves as a Differentiating Infected from Vaccinated Animals (DIVA) vaccine, as the HA tag is easily detected and distinguished from WT virus by RT-PCR and western blot. As an added benefit, the tagged virus is stable through at least 10 passages in eggs and tissue culture cells (Cai et al. 2011; Hickman et al. 2008; Pena et al. 2011; Solórzano et al. 2010; Song et al. 2007).

With each backbone that has been modified to carry these mutations and the HA epitope tag (referred to from here on as an *att* backbone) and in every animal model, significant protection against challenge viruses has been shown as well as reduced viral shedding post-vaccination (depending on the dose, no viral shedding), seroconversion, and strong IgA and IgG responses. Studies in swine are particularly pertinent and encouraging when considering improvements to human live-attenuated influenza vaccines and swine vaccines. Swine immunized with an A/turkey/Ohio/313053/2004 (H3N2) modified backbone, ty/04 *att*, and pandemic H1N1surface (A/New York/18/2009 (H1N1)) and challenged with 10^5 $TCID_{50}$ of WT pandemic H1N1 showed IgG responses comparable to swine immunized with an inactivated adjuvanted A/California/2004 (pH1N1) virus (Pena et al. 2011). IgA responses in these groups, however, were significantly different. Swine vaccinated with the ty/04 *att* vaccine had significantly higher IgA antibodies than the group vaccinated with the inactivated virus (Loving et al. 2012, 2013; Pena et al. 2011).

Efficacy of the *att* strategy has also been shown in ovo, the most convenient time to vaccinate poultry, as the process can be automated. At 19 days old, hen eggs were vaccinated with an *att* vaccine possessing an A/chicken/Delaware/VIVA/2004 (H7N2) surface and an A/guinea fowl/Hong Kong/WF10/99 (H9N2) *att* backbone at 10^6 EID_{50}. Results showed a hatchability rate of about 91 % and a protection efficiency of 70–80 % (depending on age at challenge) of chickens subsequently challenged with 500 chicken infectious dose 50 (CID_{50}) of WT H7N2 virus (Cai et al. 2011). Thus, this *att* strategy offers an effective means of vaccinating poultry while reducing labor costs and ensuring uniform vaccination of all eggs.

4 Improving Virus Vaccines: Rearrangement of the Influenza Genome and Use of Viral Vectors

Several lines of evidence have demonstrated that influenza viruses carrying a reorganized or rearranged genome might serve as candidate seed strains for vaccine development. All strategies are based upon our understanding of influenza virus packaging signals. These signals are comprised of the 5′ and 3′ non-coding regions as well as partial coding sequences on the 5′ and 3′ ends. Packaging signals have been shown to be essential for efficient and specific incorporation of each segment into virions (Dos Santos Afonso et al. 2005; Fujii et al. 2005; Liang et al. 2008; Marsh et al. 2007; Muramoto et al. 2006; Watanabe et al. 2003).

4.1 Influenza Viruses Containing an Alternate Number of Gene Segments

Many vaccine strategies have taken advantage of the influenza A packaging signals. One study describes the development of a 9-segment experimental vaccine strategy (Fig. 5a). The PB1 gene of PR8 (H1N1) virus was modified through the replacement of its packaging signals with those of NA (Gao et al. 2010). Synonymous mutations were introduced into the PB1 ORF to delete the original packaging signals while maintaining the amino acid sequence. Thus, in the absence of proper PB1 packaging signals, this chimeric PB1 gene must utilize the NA packaging signals. Then, utilizing the PB1 packaging signals, a ninth gene segment was introduced containing an HA ORF from another virus strain (A/HK/1/68 (H3N2)) flanked by the PB1 packaging signals. A bivalent influenza virus encoding both the H1 HA from PR8 (H1N1) virus and the H3 HA from A/HK/1/68 (H3N2) virus was successfully generated. Notably, this virus was significantly attenuated and exhibited decreased growth in eggs compared to the WT virus. Most importantly, mice inoculated with this virus survived lethal challenge with 100 MLD_{50} of recombinant PR8 virus and 33.3 MLD_{50} of X31 virus carrying A/HK/1/68 (H3N2) HA and NA segments (Gao et al. 2010). Using a similar method, the authors further showed that the ninth segment could also be incorporated into the progeny virus particles by the manipulation of specific packaging signals from PB2 or PA genes (Gao et al. 2010).

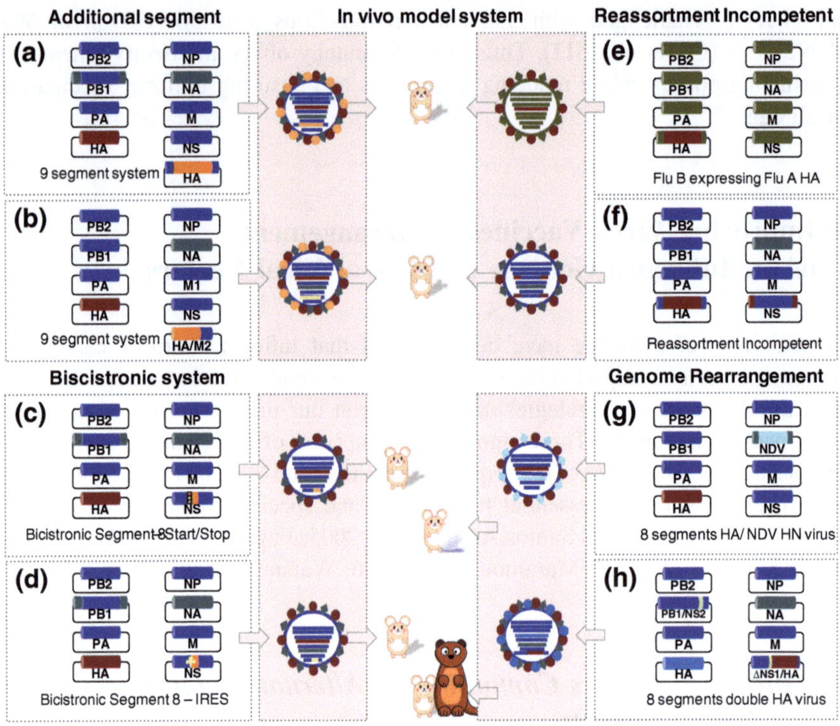

Fig. 5 Live attenuated approaches for influenza viruses—Other strategies. A variety of experimental LAIV strategies and the respective animal models in which each strategy has been evaluated are shown. **a** depicts the 9-segment bivalent strategy in which the PB1 packaging signals were substituted with NA packaging signals. The PB1 packaging signals were then engineered to flank a second HA segment. The second HA segment is shown in *orange*. **b** describes the 9-segment bivalent strategy in which segment 7, M, has been split into 2 plasmids, one carrying *M1* and the other *HA/M2*. **c** illustrates an 8-plasmid bicistronic strategy that makes use of a stop–start element in a truncated NS1 segment, shown as *red, yellow and green dots (stop–start signal)*, and expresses a foreign gene, shown as an *orange rectangle*. **d** shows another bicistronic strategy that utilizes an IRES in the NS segment. **e** represents the influenza A-influenza B HA chimera strategy. The influenza A HA is shown in *dark red*. **f** depicts the reassortment incompetent strategy in which the HA and NS packaging signals have been swapped. **g** illustrates an influenza virus carrying an NDV gene, shown in *light blue*, in place of the NA ectodomain. **h** describes the double HA, bivalent vaccine cloned by rearranging the PB2 and NS segments and introducing a 2A protease. The 2A is depicted as a *white rectangle*. Based on (Gao et al. 2010; Garcia-Sastre et al. 1994a, b; Hai et al. 2011; Kittel et al. 2004, 2005; Pena et al. 2013; Wacheck et al. 2010; Wolschek et al. 2011; Wu et al. 2010)

To construct an H9N2 virus-based bivalent influenza vaccine expressing the HA antigen from two different subtypes, another study employed a different approach. First, M1 and M2 coding regions (A/Chicken/Jiangsu/11/2002 (H9N2)) were cloned separately into RG vector, pHW2000 (Fig. 5b). Subsequently, the extracellular domain of M2 protein (1–24 aa) was substituted with the antigenic sequences of HA1 (1–344 aa) from PR8 (Wu et al. 2010). The recombinant virus produced by the co-transfection of modified M1/M2 constructs and 7 other RG plasmids (2 + 7) was shown to be genetically stable after 10 passages in chicken embryos or MDCK cells. In vivo studies demonstrated that this virus is low pathogenic in mice; furthermore, immunization of mice with this virus conferred complete protection against 100 MLD_{50} H1N1 challenge and 40 MLD_{50} H9N2 challenge.

4.2 Generation Influenza Vaccines Containing Bicistronic Expression Cassettes

Mounting an immune response sufficient to protect against influenza infection has been problematic in the elderly and other high-risk groups. However, the immunogenicity of live attenuated influenza vaccines can be improved through co-administration of biologically active molecules such as cytokines and chemokines (Babai et al. 1999, 2001), especially in the elderly (Mbawuike et al. 1990). This was achieved through the construction of a bicistronic mRNA in an influenza virus segment via multiple approaches, such as the insertion of a stop–start sequence (Kittel et al. 2005; Wolschek et al. 2011), an internal ribosome entry site element (IRES) (Garcia-Sastre et al. 1994a), an internal viral promoter (Machado et al. 2003), and protease cleavage sites (Kittel et al. 2004; Manicassamy et al. 2010; Percy et al. 1994). In most studies, GFP or a reporter (such as luciferase) was used to test the feasibility of the particular strategy.

The stop–start sequence implements an overlapping UAAUG sequence in which the first 3 nt serve as the stop codon terminating translation of the upstream gene while the last 3 nt reinitiate translation of the downstream gene (Fig. 5c). Thus, one mRNA template can produce two separate proteins. Using this method, Kittel et al. rescued a virus encoding truncated NS1 (1–125 aa) and full-length human IL-2 (Kittel et al. 2005). This IL-2 expressing virus was genetically stable in cell culture and the mouse respiratory tract. Additionally, it was safe in mice, despite the high replication capacity, and evoked an enhanced T cell response compared to the control virus (Kittel et al. 2005). This method is especially desirable for the production of immunomodulatory molecules because the expression level of the foreign gene from the stop–start sequence is relatively low. To date, recombinant influenza viruses expressing IL-2, IL-24, and CCL-20 have been successfully rescued (Wolschek et al. 2011). There is precedent for the enhancement of immunity by the co-administration of immunomodulatory molecules. A similar strategy using a DNA based bicistronic plasmid expressing an influenza virus NA protein and IL-2, separated by an internal ribosome entry site (IRES), has been show to enhance protection in mice against PR8 challenge (Henke et al. 2006).

Another approach to introduce exogenous genes into influenza virus involves the application of an IRES, as shown by a study performed by Garcia-Sastre et al.

(Fig. 5d). An IRES from the 5′ noncoding region of the human immunoglobulin heavy-chain-binding protein (BiP) mRNA was employed to promote the translation of foreign polypeptides (GP2 or HGP2) which were fused with an NA segment (Garcia-Sastre et al. 1994a). The major problem limiting the use of an IRES is the highly structured nature of the IRES sequence and size constraints. To date, only short polypeptides (91 and 125 aa) are reported to be expressed by the recombinant influenza virus via this method (Garcia-Sastre et al. 1994a).

Based on the finding that the influenza RNA polymerase is capable of recognizing and binding the internally located 3′ viral promoter (Flick and Hobom 1999), Machado et al. explored the possibility of rescuing a viable influenza virus harboring a dicistronic segment with a heterogenous gene under the control of an internal promoter (Machado et al. 2003). To this end, the authors inserted 19 nt derived from viral 3′ promoter sequence as well as foreign genes (chloramphenicol acetyltransferase (CAT) and VP0, from Mengo virus) between the stop codon and 5′ promoter sequence of the WSN NA segment. The transfected viruses replicated efficiently in MDCK cells and proved stable upon serial passage (Machado et al. 2003); nonetheless, they expressed low levels of foreign gene product (e.g., CAT enzyme), indicating that transcription from the internal promoter is inefficient. In a subsequent study, mice were immunized with these dicistronic viruses. Mice mounted an immune response against both the foreign gene and influenza, suggesting that this strategy may be a good LAIV candidate for a dual vaccine (Vieira Machado et al. 2006).

The introduction of an autocatalytic cleavage site (e.g, 2A protease from enterovirus) between a viral gene product and the desired foreign gene may be a more preferable strategy for construction of a recombinant influenza virus. The 2A strategy has two notable advantages. First, the autocatalytic cleavage site is usually short enough to allow for the insertion of long foreign genes. Second, after self-cleavage of 2A, only 18 additional amino acid residues remain at the C-terminus of first protein and 1 additional residue remains at the N-terminus of the second protein (Percy et al. 1994). These residues are not thought to dramatically affect protein function. To date, a number of publications have described the cloning of foreign genes into the influenza virus genome. GFP (Li et al. 2010) and CAT (Percy et al. 1994) have been cloned into NA. Gluc has been successfully cloned into PB2 (Heaton et al. 2013). The HIV Nef protein (Ferko et al. 2001) has been cloned into NS. Other genes have also been incorporated into the NS segment, such as the early secretory antigenic target protein (ESAT-6) from *M. tuberculosis* (Sereinig et al. 2006) and the H5 antigen from A/Vietnam/1203/04 virus (Pena et al. 2013). All strategies have generated replication competent viruses. In addition to the 2A protease, an even smaller peptide sequence, DIDGGETDG, can be recognized and cut by caspase, a cellular enzyme, and has been shown to provide posttranslational separation of recombinant segments which allows the expression of a foreign gene in its native form (just as 2A does) (Kittel et al. 2004).

4.3 Development of Influenza Vaccines Lacking the Ability to Reassort

In comparison to the inactivated vaccine, the intranasally delivered live-attenuated vaccine efficiently elicits both enhanced mucosal immunity and a broader cellular immune response even at low doses (as the above experiments have shown); nevertheless, concern does exist regarding the risk associated with a possible reassortment (or segment swapping) event between vaccine strain and circulating wild-type virus. This concern is perhaps minor when it comes to humans but it is a major issue that prevents the use of live-attenuated influenza vaccines in livestock and poultry.

Several strategies have been developed to address this safety concern. The first is based on the fact that influenza A and B viruses cannot exchange their genes freely to form a novel progeny virus (Ghate and Air 1999; Kaverin et al. 1983; Tanaka et al. 1984). To generate a reassortment-incompetent influenza vaccine, three different chimeric HA genes were constructed in which the signal peptide sequence, the transmembrane region, and cytoplasmic tail from the B/Yamagata/16/88 virus HA segment were fused to the HA ectodomain from an H1-subtype virus (PR8), an H3-subtype virus (A/Hong Kong/6 8(H3N2)), or an H5-subtype virus (A/Vietnam/1203/04 (H5N1)) (Fig. 5e) (Hai et al. 2011). The chimeric HA gene together with a truncated NS1 gene (1–110 aa) and six other intact genes from B/Yamagata/16/88 virus gave rise to a recombinant influenza B virus expressing influenza A HA protein. These chimeric viruses exhibited an attenuated phenotype both in vitro (small plaque size and reduced virus titer in MDCK cells) and in vivo (2 to 3 logs lower viral replication than wild- type influenza B virus in lungs of mice). The chimeras also retained the ability to induce robust antibody response and protected mice against lethal infection with H1 (challenge dose, 1×10^3 Pfu), H3 (challenge dose, 1×10^6 Pfu) or H5 viruses (challenge dose, 5×10^3 Pfu) (Hai et al. 2011). The major advantage of these influenza B virus-based vaccines against influenza A viruses is that they are unable to donate their HA to wild type influenza A viruses due to the restrictions imposed by the packaging signals.

Another strategy designed to avoid reassortment between vaccines and virulent strains is the application of "swapped" influenza A packaging signals. Packaging signals are specific and unique to each segment, both in length and sequence, as they include 5′ and 3′ noncoding regions as well as partial coding sequences at the 5′ and 3′ ends of each ORF (Goto et al. 2013; Hutchinson et al. 2010). In nature, each packaging signal can be used only once to ensure eight vRNA segments are accurately incorporated into the progeny virions. Thus, rewiring the influenza vRNAs by swapping the packaging signals could be a feasible approach in preventing reassortment of a specific vRNA segment. By cloning the 5′ and 3′ packaging sequences from NS gene onto the 5′ and 3′ ends of HA ORF and eliminating the original packaging elements in HA ORF by synonymous mutations, Gao et al. created a chimeric HA segment which must use the NS packaging signals (Gao and Palese 2009). Conversely, an NS gene flanked by the HA packaging sequence was cloned using the same approach (Fig. 5f). As expected, the recombinant virus encompassing the chimeric HA and NS segments was unable to reassort freely with NS and HA segments from wild-type virus (Gao and Palese 2009). Such a strategy could be expanded to other segments.

Another strategy has shown to be an effective bivalent vaccine against influenza and Newcastle disease virus (NDV), a significant agricultural pathogen in chickens. In two separate studies, Park et al. and Steel et al. modified the NA gene by removing the ectodomain and replacing it with the hemagglutinin-neuraminidase (HN) gene of NDV and H5 avian influenza virus (lacking the polybasic cleavage site) (Park et al. 2006; Steel et al. 2008) (Fig. 5g). HN is the major antigenic protein of NDV. Park et al. demonstrated that the chimeric virus expressed the major antigenic protein of influenza, HA, and of NDV, HN. Additionally, the chimeric virus grew to high titers in eggs. Steel et al. showed efficacy of this vaccine in the mouse model and in ovo. Mice were immunized and boosted with the chimeric virus and challenged with 62.5 MLD_{50} of mouse adapted A/WSN/33 (H1N1) with an H5 surface (lacking the polybasic cleavage site). Post-vaccination, no signs of disease were observed in immunized mice. Post-challenge, all sham-vaccinated mice challenged, succumbed to infection, whereas all vaccinated mice survived with few signs of infection and little weight loss (Steel et al. 2008). The chimeric vaccine was then tested in ovo. Eighteen-day old chicken embryos were vaccinated. Then, at 3-weeks old, these chickens were challenged with either highly virulent NDV AT $10^{5.2}$ EID_{50} or highly pathogenic H5N1 virus at $10^{6.1}$ EID_{50}. Survivability was high for vaccinated chickens challenged with either virus, 80 % for those challenge with H5N1 and 90 % for those challenged with NDV. All sham-vaccinated chickens challenged with either H5N1 or NDV died. Thus, the chimeric virus provided strong protection after in ovo vaccination against lethal challenge (Steel et al. 2008).

Genome rearrangement was used to prevent reassortment and promote attenuation using a bivalent vaccine against both H9 and H5 viruses on an H9N2 backbone (Pena et al. 2013). First, a 2A protease gene and an NS2 gene were cloned at the end of segment 2 (PB1 gene), causing impaired polymerase activity as well as reduced viral replication. Next, a 2A protease gene and an H5 gene were cloned into truncated form of segment 8 (encoding 1–99 aa of NS1 protein) from which the NS2 gene was removed (Fig. 5h). The resulting virus had two HA proteins (H9 and H5) on its envelope. This double HA virus induced protection of mice (after immunization and boost) against lethal H5N1 challenge (Pena et al. 2013). In ferrets, the H5-H9 vaccine (and subsequent boost) provided full protection against H5 challenge (20, 200, and 2,000 MLD_{50}) and significantly reduced viral shedding (Pena et al. 2013). Previous studies showed that NS1 and NS2 are necessary for viral replication. Since these genes are in different segments, any reassortment event will have to encompass both segments (instead of just segments 2 or 8), rendering reassortment less likely. This strategy has the added benefit of being a viral vector. Here, the rearranged H9 virus serves as a vector for the H5

HA surface protein. One can imagine the insertion of other foreign proteins from influenza and other pathogens in this vector, or a similarly constructed vector, to create a dual vaccine.

5 Conclusions and Commentary

As discussed throughout this chapter, there is great need to alternative strategies to the licensed cold adapted, live-attenuated vaccine that provide better protection to all at-risk groups (Alexandrova et al. 1990; DeBorde et al. 1987, 1988; Maassab 1967; Maassab and Bryant 1999; Maassab et al. 1969; Monto and Maassab 1977). There is also great need for better agricultural vaccines and new methods to hasten vaccine production time of a vaccine seed stock during a pandemic. A plethora of candidate strategies exist for both human and agricultural vaccines as well as alternative strategies to the generation of a vaccine seed stock. Many of these strategies show strong efficacy. Indeed, there are many good experimental LAIV candidates when considering both *safety* and *efficacy*. These strategies are numerous but can be summarized into categories: mutations, deletions, insertions, and rearrangement.

Some of these strategies are already being evaluated in clinical trials such as the ΔNS1-H1N1 strategy. Impressively, this monovalent vaccine generated antibody responses, which were cross-reactive with heterosubtypic H3N2, and H5N1 virus. Other strategies, such as the elastase cleavage site strategy and the *att* (HA tag strategy) show great promise for safe and effective agricultural vaccines. Each strategy presents a unique approach to addressing some of the problems that exist in currently licensed vaccines such as immunogenicity in the elderly and the potential for reassortment. The right human strategy must be vetted in many different animal models, be applicable to both influenza A and B, grow to high titers in approved vaccine cell lines, provide safe and efficacious protection to high-risk groups, and be easily grown in large quantities. The right agricultural vaccines must be effective, safe, and most importantly, easy to administer.

Future work should focus on combining LAIV strategies. For example, the microRNA and the *att* strategy could be combined. Combining these strategies would likely enhance stability of the vaccine as well as add a DIVA element to the vaccine without dramatically decreasing replication. Such a vaccine has the potential of being applicable to agricultural animals and humans; furthermore, the selected miRNA could be tailored to the appropriate host without fear of recombination of the vaccine strain with a WT virus in a different host. Research should also be aimed at working within the confines of FDA approved growth medium or closely related growth medium. This will minimize the hurdles involved in seeking FDA approval and will allow manufacturers to use existing vaccine production infrastructure to produce new LAIV vaccines.

Research dollars must also continue to be invested in identifying potential epitopes for incorporation into rearranged genome or bicistronic vaccines in order to more broadly stimulate the immune response to influenza and enhance cross-protection provided by a given vaccine, particularly in the elderly. These epitopes could be influenza derived or simply better stimulate the immune system as in the delivery of immunomodulatory molecules discussed in this chapter.

Again, while there is more research to be done, the field is advancing in such a way that it is only a matter of time before safer, more efficacious LAIV vaccines become available for administration to the public. Likely many of the vaccine strategies discussed in this chapter or some variation of the same themes will, in time, come to market. Meanwhile, the research continues.

References

Akarsu H, Iwatsuki-Horimoto K, Noda T, Kawakami E, Katsura H, Baudin F, Horimoto T, Kawaoka Y (2011) Structure-based design of NS2 mutants for attenuated influenza A virus vaccines. Virus Res 155:240–248. doi:10.1016/j.virusres.2010.10.014

Alexandrova GI, Maassab HF, Kendal AP, Medvedeva TE, Egorov AY, Klimov AI, Cox NJ (1990) Laboratory properties of cold-adapted influenza B live vaccine strains developed in the US and USSR, and their B/Ann Arbor/1/86 cold-adapted reassortant vaccine candidates. Vaccine 8:61–64

Babai I, Barenholz Y, Zakay-Rones Z, Greenbaum E, Samira S, Hayon I, Rochman M, Kedar E (2001) A novel liposomal influenza vaccine (INFLUSOME-VAC) containing hemagglutinin-neuraminidase and IL-2 or GM-CSF induces protective anti-neuraminidase antibodies cross-reacting with a wide spectrum of influenza A viral strains. Vaccine 20:505–515

Babai I, Samira S, Barenholz Y, Zakay-Rones Z, Kedar E (1999) A novel influenza subunit vaccine composed of liposome-encapsulated haemagglutinin/neuraminidase and IL-2 or GM-CSF. II. Induction of TH1 and TH2 responses in mice. Vaccine 17:1239–1250

Babiuk S, Masic A, Graham J, Neufeld J, van der Loop M, Copps J, Berhane Y, Pasick J, Potter A, Babiuk LA, Weingartl H, Zhou Y (2011) An elastase-dependent attenuated heterologous swine influenza virus protects against pandemic H1N1 2009 influenza challenge in swine. Vaccine 29:3118–3123. doi:10.1016/j.vaccine.2011.02.069

Brands R, Visser J, Medema J, Palache AM, van Scharrenburg GJ (1999) Influvac: a safe Madin Darby Canine Kidney (MDCK) cell culture-based influenza vaccine. Dev Biol Stand 98:93–100 (discussion 111)

Cai Y, Song H, Ye J, Shao H, Padmanabhan R, Sutton TC, Perez DR (2011) Improved hatchability and efficient protection after in ovo vaccination with live-attenuated H7N2 and H9N2 avian influenza viruses. Virol J 8:31. doi:10.1186/1743-422X-8-31

Calvo C, García-García ML, Borrell B, Pozo F, Casas I (2013) Prospective study of influenza C in hospitalized children. Pediatr Infect Dis J 32:916–919. doi:10.1097/INF.0b013e31828fca10

Calvo C, García-García ML, Centeno M, Pérez-Breña P, Casas I (2006) Influenza C virus infection in children, Spain. Emerg Infect Dis 12:1621–1622. doi:10.3201/eid1210.051170

Chambers TM, Quinlivan M, Sturgill T, Cullinane A, Horohov DW, Zamarin D, Arkins S, Garcia-Sastre A, Palese P (2009) Influenza A viruses with truncated NS1 as modified live virus vaccines: pilot studies of safety and efficacy in horses. Equine Vet J 41:87–92

Chen H, Ye J, Xu K, Angel M, Shao H, Ferrero A, Sutton T, Perez DR (2012) Partial and full PCR-based reverse genetics strategy for influenza viruses. PLoS One 7:e46378

Cohen M, Zhang XQ, Senaati HP, Chen HW, Varki NM, Schooley RT, Gagneux P (2013) Influenza A penetrates host mucus by cleaving sialic acids with neuraminidase. Virol J 10:321. doi:10.1186/1743-422X-10-321 de Wit E, Spronken MI, Vervaet G, Rimmelzwaan GF, Osterhaus AD, Fouchier RA (2007) A reverse-genetics system for influenza A virus using T7 RNA polymerase. J Gen Virol 88:1281–1287

DeBorde DC, Donabedian AM, Herlocher ML, Naeve CW, Maassab HF (1988) Sequence comparison of wild-type and cold-adapted B/Ann Arbor/1/66 influenza virus genes. Virology 163:429–443

DeBorde DC, Naeve CW, Herlocher ML, Maassab HF (1987) Nucleotide sequences of the PA and PB1 genes of B/Ann Arbor/1/66 virus: comparison with genes of B/Lee/40 and type A influenza viruses. Virus Res 8:33–41

Donelan NR, Dauber B, Wang X, Basler CF, Wolff T, García-Sastre A (2004) The N- and C-terminal domains of the NS1 protein of influenza B virus can independently inhibit IRF-3 and beta interferon promoter activation. J Virol 78:11574–11582. doi:10.1128/JVI.78.21.11574-11582.2004

Dormitzer PR, Suphaphiphat P, Gibson DG, Wentworth DE, Stockwell TB, Algire MA, Alperovich N, Barro M, Brown DM, Craig S, Dattilo BM, Denisova EA, De Souza I, Eickmann M, Dugan VG, Ferrari A, Gomila RC, Han L, Judge C, Mane S, Matrosovich M, Merryman C, Palladino G, Palmer GA, Spencer T, Strecker T, Trusheim H, Uhlendorff J, Wen Y, Yee AC, Zaveri J, Zhou B, Becker S, Donabedian A, Mason PW, Glass JI, Rappuoli R, Venter JC (2013) Synthetic generation of influenza vaccine viruses for rapid response to pandemics. Sci Transl Med 5:185ra68

Dos Santos Afonso E, Escriou N, Leclercq I, van der Werf S, Naffakh N (2005) The generation of recombinant influenza A viruses expressing a PB2 fusion protein requires the conservation of a packaging signal overlapping the coding and noncoding regions at the 5' end of the PB2 segment. Virology 341:34–46

Ferko B, Stasakova J, Sereinig S, Romanova J, Katinger D, Niebler B, Katinger H, Egorov A (2001) Hyperattenuated recombinant influenza A virus nonstructural-protein-encoding vectors induce human immunodeficiency virus type 1 Nef-specific systemic and mucosal immune responses in mice. J Virol 75:8899–8908

Flick R, Hobom G (1999) Transient bicistronic vRNA segments for indirect selection of recombinant influenza viruses. Virology 262:93–103

Fodor E, Devenish L, Engelhardt OG, Palese P, Brownlee GG, Garcia-Sastre A (1999) Rescue of influenza A virus from recombinant DNA. J Virol 73:9679–9682

Fujii K, Fujii Y, Noda T, Muramoto Y, Watanabe T, Takada A, Goto H, Horimoto T, Kawaoka Y (2005) Importance of both the coding and the segment-specific noncoding regions of the influenza A virus NS segment for its efficient incorporation into virions. J Virol 79:3766–3774

Fukuyama S, Kawaoka Y (2011) The pathogenesis of influenza virus infections: the contributions of virus and host factors. Curr Opin Immunol 23:481–486. doi:10.1016/j.coi.2011.07.016

Gao Q, Lowen AC, Wang TT, Palese P (2010) A nine-segment influenza a virus carrying subtype H1 and H3 hemagglutinins. J Virol 84:8062–8071

Gao Q, Palese P (2009) Rewiring the RNAs of influenza virus to prevent reassortment. Proc Natl Acad Sci USA 106:15891–15896

Garcia-Sastre A, Muster T, Barclay WS, Percy N, Palese P (1994a) Use of a mammalian internal ribosomal entry site element for expression of a foreign protein by a transfectant influenza virus. J Virol 68:6254–6261

Garcia-Sastre A, Percy N, Barclay W, Palese P (1994b) Introduction of foreign sequences into the genome of influenza A virus. Dev Biol Stand 82:237–246

Ghate AA, Air GM (1999) Influenza type B neuraminidase can replace the function of type A neuraminidase. Virology 264:265–277

Goto H, Muramoto Y, Noda T, Kawaoka Y (2013) The genome-packaging signal of the influenza A virus genome comprises a genome incorporation signal and a genome-bundling signal. J Virol 87:11316–11322. doi:10.1128/JVI.01301-13

Hai R, Garcia-Sastre A, Swayne DE, Palese P (2011) A reassortment-incompetent live attenuated influenza virus vaccine for protection against pandemic virus strains. J Virol 85:6832–6843

Hatta Y, Hatta M, Bilsel P, Neumann G, Kawaoka Y (2011) An M2 cytoplasmic tail mutant as a live attenuated influenza vaccine against pandemic (H1N1) 2009 influenza virus. Vaccine 29:2308–2312. doi:10.1016/j.vaccine.2011.01.023

Heaton NS, Leyva-Grado VH, Tan GS, Eggink D, Hai R, Palese P (2013) In vivo bioluminescent imaging of influenza a virus infection and characterization of novel cross-protective monoclonal antibodies. J Virol 87:8272–8281

Heix J, Grummt I (1995) Species specificity of transcription by RNA polymerase I. Curr Opin Genet Dev 5:652–656

Henke A, Rohland N, Zell R, Wutzler P (2006) Co-expression of interleukin-2 by a bicistronic plasmid increases the efficacy of DNA immunization to prevent influenza virus infections. Intervirology 49:249–252. doi:10.1159/000092487

Hickman D, Hossain MJ, Song H, Araya Y, Solórzano A, Perez DR (2008) An avian live attenuated master backbone for potential use in epidemic and pandemic influenza vaccines. J Gen Virol 89:2682–2690. doi:10.1099/vir.0.2008/004143-0

Hoffmann E, Neumann G, Kawaoka Y, Hobom G, Webster RG (2000) A DNA transfection system for generation of influenza A virus from eight plasmids. Proc Natl Acad Sci USA 97:6108–6113

Hutchinson EC, von Kirchbach JC, Gog JR, Digard P (2010) Genome packaging in influenza A virus. J Gen Virol 91:313–328. doi:10.1099/vir.0.017608-0

Kadota J (2013) Emergence of a new strain of the avian influenza A (H7N9) virus. Respir Investig 51:49. doi:10.1016/j.resinv.2013.05.001

Kaverin NV, Varich NL, Sklyanskaya EI, Amvrosieva TV, Petrik J, Vovk TC (1983) Studies on heterotypic interference between influenza A and B viruses: a differential inhibition of the synthesis of viral proteins and RNAs. J Gen Virol 64(Pt 10):2139–2146

Kistner O, Barrett PN, Mundt W, Reiter M, Schober-Bendixen S, Dorner F (1998) Development of a mammalian cell (Vero) derived candidate influenza virus vaccine. Vaccine 16:960–968

Kistner O, Barrett PN, Mundt W, Reiter M, Schober-Bendixen S, Eder G, Dorner F (1999) Development of a vero cell-derived influenza whole virus vaccine. Dev Biol Stand 98:101–110 (discussion 111)

Kittel C, Ferko B, Kurz M, Voglauer R, Sereinig S, Romanova J, Stiegler G, Katinger H, Egorov A (2005) Generation of an influenza A virus vector expressing biologically active human interleukin-2 from the NS gene segment. J Virol 79:10672–10677

Kittel C, Sereinig S, Ferko B, Stasakova J, Romanova J, Wolkerstorfer A, Katinger H, Egorov A (2004) Rescue of influenza virus expressing GFP from the NS1 reading frame. Virology 324:67–73

Langlois RA, Albrecht RA, Kimble B, Sutton T, Shapiro JS, Finch C, Angel M, Chua MA, Gonzalez-Reiche AS, Xu K, Perez D, García-Sastre A, Tenoever BR (2013) MicroRNA-based strategy to mitigate the risk of gain-of-function influenza studies. Nat Biotechnol. doi:10.1038/nbt.2666

Leibler JH, Otte J, Roland-Holst D, Pfeiffer DU, Soares Magalhaes R, Rushton J, Graham JP, Silbergeld EK (2009) Industrial food animal production and global health risks: exploring the ecosystems and economics of avian influenza. Ecohealth 6:58–70. doi:10.1007/s10393-009-0226-0

Li F, Feng L, Pan W, Dong Z, Li C, Sun C, Chen L (2010) Generation of replication-competent recombinant influenza A viruses carrying a reporter gene harbored in the neuraminidase segment. J Virol 84:12075–12081

Liang Y, Huang T, Ly H, Parslow TG (2008) Mutational analyses of packaging signals in influenza virus PA, PB1, and PB2 genomic RNA segments. J Virol 82:229–236

Loving CL, Lager KM, Vincent AL, Brockmeier SL, Gauger PC, Anderson TK, Kitikoon P, Perez DR, Kehrli ME Jr (2013) Efficacy in pigs of inactivated and live attenuated influenza virus vaccines against infection and transmission of an emerging H3N2 similar to the 2011–2012 H3N2v. J Virol 87:9895–9903. doi:10.1128/JVI.01038-13

Loving CL, Vincent AL, Pena L, Perez DR (2012) Heightened adaptive immune responses following vaccination with a temperature-sensitive, live-attenuated influenza virus compared to adjuvanted, whole-inactivated virus in pigs. Vaccine 30:5830–5838. doi:10.1016/j.vaccine.2012.07.033

Maassab HF (1967) Adaptation and growth characteristics of influenza virus at 25 °C. Nature 213:612–614

Maassab HF, Bryant ML (1999) The development of live attenuated cold-adapted influenza virus vaccine for humans. Rev Med Virol 9:237–244

Maassab HF, Francis T, Davenport FM, Hennessy AV, Minuse E, Anderson G (1969) Laboratory and clinical characteristics of attenuated strains of influenza virus. Bull World Health Organ 41:589–594

Machado AV, Naffakh N, van der Werf S, Escriou N (2003) Expression of a foreign gene by stable recombinant influenza viruses harboring a dicistronic genomic segment with an internal promoter. Virology 313:235–249

Manicassamy B, Manicassamy S, Belicha-Villanueva A, Pisanelli G, Pulendran B, Garcia-Sastre A (2010) Analysis of in vivo dynamics of influenza virus infection in mice using a GFP reporter virus. Proc Natl Acad Sci USA 107:11531–11536

Marsh GA, Hatami R, Palese P (2007) Specific residues of the influenza A virus hemagglutinin viral RNA are important for efficient packaging into budding virions. J Virol 81:9727–9736

Masic A, Babiuk LA, Zhou Y (2009a) Reverse genetics-generated elastase-dependent swine influenza viruses are attenuated in pigs. J Gen Virol 90:375–385. doi:10.1099/vir.0.005447-0

Masic A, Booth JS, Mutwiri GK, Babiuk LA, Zhou Y (2009b) Elastase-dependent live attenuated swine influenza A viruses are immunogenic and confer protection against swine influenza A virus infection in pigs. J Virol 83:10198–10210. doi:10.1128/JVI.00926-09

Masic A, Lu X, Li J, Mutwiri GK, Babiuk LA, Brown EG, Zhou Y (2010) Immunogenicity and protective efficacy of an elastase-dependent live attenuated swine influenza virus vaccine administered intranasally in pigs. Vaccine 28:7098–7108. doi:10.1016/j.vaccine.2010.08.003

Massin P, Rodrigues P, Marasescu M, van der Werf S, Naffakh N (2005) Cloning of the chicken RNA polymerase I promoter and use for reverse genetics of influenza A viruses in avian cells. J Virol 79:13811–13816

Mbawuike IN, Wyde PR, Anderson PM (1990) Enhancement of the protective efficacy of inactivated influenza A virus vaccine in aged mice by IL-2 liposomes. Vaccine 8:347–352

Monto AS, Maassab HF (1977) Use of influenza vaccine in non-high risk populations. Dev Biol Stand 39:329–335

Morokutti A, Muster T, Ferko B (2014) Intranasal vaccination with a replication-deficient influenza virus induces heterosubtypic neutralising mucosal IgA antibodies in humans. Vaccine. doi:10.1016/j.vaccine.2014.02.009

Murakami S, Horimoto T, Yamada S, Kakugawa S, Goto H, Kawaoka Y (2008) Establishment of canine RNA polymerase I-driven reverse genetics for influenza A virus: its application for H5N1 vaccine production. J Virol 82:1605–1609

Muramoto Y, Takada A, Fujii K, Noda T, Iwatsuki-Horimoto K, Watanabe S, Horimoto T, Kida H, Kawaoka Y (2006) Hierarchy among viral RNA (vRNA) segments in their role in vRNA incorporation into influenza A virions. J Virol 80:2318–2325

Neumann G, Fujii K, Kino Y, Kawaoka Y (2005) An improved reverse genetics system for influenza A virus generation and its implications for vaccine production. Proc Natl Acad Sci USA 102:16825–16829

Neumann G, Watanabe T, Ito H, Watanabe S, Goto H, Gao P, Hughes M, Perez DR, Donis R, Hoffmann E, Hobom G, Kawaoka Y (1999) Generation of influenza A viruses entirely from cloned cDNAs. Proc Nat Acad Sci USA 96:9345–9350

Ozawa M, Goto H, Horimoto T, Kawaoka Y (2007) An adenovirus vector-mediated reverse genetics system for influenza A virus generation. J Virol 81:9556–9559

Palache AM, Scheepers HS, de Regt V, van Ewijk P, Baljet M, Brands R, van Scharrenburg GJ (1999) Safety, reactogenicity and immunogenicity of Madin Darby Canine Kidney cell-derived inactivated influenza subunit vaccine. A meta-analysis of clinical studies. Dev Biol Stand 98:115–125 (discussion 133–4)

Palese P, Shaw ML (2007) Orthomyxoviridae: the viruses and their replication. In: Knipe DM, Howley PM (eds) Fields virology, vol 2, 5th edn. Philadelphia, Lippincott Williams and Wilkins, pp 1647–1689

Park MS, Steel J, Garcia-Sastre A, Swayne D, Palese P (2006) Engineered viral vaccine constructs with dual specificity: avian influenza and Newcastle disease. Proc Natl Acad Sci USA 103:8203–8208. doi:10.1073/pnas.0602566103

Pena L, Sutton T, Chockalingam A, Kumar S, Angel M, Shao H, Chen H, Li W, Perez DR (2013) Influenza viruses with rearranged genomes as live-attenuated vaccines. J Virol 87:5118–5127

Pena L, Vincent AL, Ye J, Ciacci-Zanella JR, Angel M, Lorusso A, Gauger PC, Janke BH, Loving CL, Perez DR (2011) Modifications in the polymerase genes of a swine-like triple-reassortant influenza virus to generate live attenuated vaccines against 2009 pandemic H1N1 viruses. J Virol 85:456–469. doi:10.1128/JVI.01503-10

Percy N, Barclay WS, Garcia-Sastre A, Palese P (1994) Expression of a foreign protein by influenza A virus. J Virol 68:4486–4492

Perez JT, Pham AM, Lorini MH, Chua MA, Steel J, tenOever BR (2009) MicroRNA-mediated species-specific attenuation of influenza A virus. Nat Biotechnol 27:572–576. doi:10.1038/nbt.1542

Pica N, Langlois RA, Krammer F, Margine I, Palese P (2012) NS1-truncated live attenuated virus vaccine provides robust protection to aged mice from viral challenge. J Virol 86:10293–10301. doi:10.1128/JVI.01131-12

Schnitzler SU, Schnitzler P (2009) An update on swine-origin influenza virus A/H1N1: a review. Virus Genes 39:279–292. doi:10.1007/s11262-009-0404-8

Sereinig S, Stukova M, Zabolotnyh N, Ferko B, Kittel C, Romanova J, Vinogradova T, Katinger H, Kiselev O, Egorov A (2006) Influenza virus NS vectors expressing the mycobacterium tuberculosis ESAT-6 protein induce CD4+ Th1 immune response and protect animals against tuberculosis challenge. Clin Vaccine Immunol 13:898–904

Shinya K, Fujii Y, Ito H, Ito T, Kawaoka Y (2004) Characterization of a neuraminidase-deficient influenza a virus as a potential gene delivery vector and a live vaccine. J Virol 78:3083–3088

Skehel JJ, Wiley DC (2000) Receptor binding and membrane fusion in virus entry: the influenza hemagglutinin. Annu Rev Biochem 69:531–569. doi:10.1146/annurev.biochem.69.1.531

Snyder MH, Betts RF, DeBorde D, Tierney EL, Clements ML, Herrington D, Sears SD, Dolin R, Maassab HF, Murphy BR (1988) Four viral genes independently contribute to attenuation of live influenza A/Ann Arbor/6/60 (H2N2) cold-adapted reassortant virus vaccines. J Virol 62:488–495

Solórzano A, Webby RJ, Lager KM, Janke BH, García-Sastre A, Richt JA (2005) Mutations in the NS1 protein of swine influenza virus impair anti-interferon activity and confer attenuation in pigs. J Virol 79:7535–7543. doi:10.1128/JVI.79.12.7535-7543.2005

Solórzano A, Ye J, Pérez DR (2010) Alternative live-attenuated influenza vaccines based on modifications in the polymerase genes protect against epidemic and pandemic flu. J Virol 84:4587–4596. doi:10.1128/JVI.00101-10

Song H, Nieto GR, Perez DR (2007) A new generation of modified live-attenuated avian influenza viruses using a two-strategy combination as potential vaccine candidates. J Virol 81:9238–9248. doi: 10.1128/JVI.00893-07

Song MS, Baek YH, Pascua PN, Kwon HI, Park SJ, Kim EH, Lim GJ, Choi YK (2013) Establishment of Vero cell RNA polymerase I-driven reverse genetics for Influenza A virus and its application for pandemic (H1N1) 2009 influenza virus vaccine production. J Gen Virol 94:1230–1235

Stech J, Garn H, Herwig A, Stech O, Dauber B, Wolff T, Mettenleiter TC, Klenk HD (2011) Influenza B virus with modified hemagglutinin cleavage site as a novel attenuated live vaccine. J Infect Dis 204:1483–1490. doi: 10.1093/infdis/jir613

Stech J, Garn H, Wegmann M, Wagner R, Klenk HD (2005) A new approach to an influenza live vaccine: modification of the cleavage site of hemagglutinin. Nat Med 11:683–689. doi:10.1038/nm1256

Steel J, Burmakina SV, Thomas C, Spackman E, Garcia-Sastre A, Swayne DE, Palese P (2008) A combination in-ovo vaccine for avian influenza virus and Newcastle disease virus. Vaccine 26:522–531. doi:10.1016/j.vaccine.2007.11.032

Steel J, Lowen AC, Pena L, Angel M, Solórzano A, Albrecht R, Perez DR, García-Sastre A, Palese P (2009) Live attenuated influenza viruses containing NS1 truncations as vaccine candidates against H5N1 highly pathogenic avian influenza. J Virol 83:1742–1753. doi:10.1128/JVI.01920-08

Tanaka T, Urabe M, Goto H, Tobita K (1984) Isolation and preliminary characterization of a highly cytolytic influenza B virus variant with an aberrant NS gene. Virology 135:515–523

Taubenberger JK, Kash JC (2010) Influenza virus evolution, host adaptation, and pandemic formation. Cell Host Microbe 7:440–451. doi:10.1016/j.chom.2010.05.009

tenOever BR (2013) RNA viruses and the host microRNA machinery. Nat Rev Microbiol 11:169–180. doi:10.1038/nrmicro2971

Verity EE, Camuglia S, Agius CT, Ong C, Shaw R, Barr I, Middleton D, Rockman S (2011) Rapid generation of pandemic influenza virus vaccine candidate strains using synthetic DNA. Influenza Other Respi Viruses 6:101–109

Victor ST, Watanabe S, Katsura H, Ozawa M, Kawaoka Y (2012) A replication-incompetent PB2-knockout influenza A virus vaccine vector. J Virol 86:4123–4128. doi:10.1128/JVI.06232-11

Vieira Machado A, Naffakh N, Gerbaud S, van der Werf S, Escriou N (2006) Recombinant influenza A viruses harboring optimized dicistronic NA segment with an extended native 5' terminal sequence: induction of heterospecific B and T cell responses in mice. Virology 345:73–87. doi:10.1016/j.virol.2005.09.050

Wacheck V, Egorov A, Groiss F, Pfeiffer A, Fuereder T, Hoeflmayer D, Kundi M, Popow-Kraupp T, Redlberger-Fritz M, Mueller CA, Cinatl J, Michaelis M, Geiler J, Bergmann M, Romanova J, Roethl E, Morokutti A, Wolschek M, Ferko B, Seipelt J, Dick-Gudenus R, Muster T (2010) A novel type of influenza vaccine: safety and immunogenicity of replication-deficient influenza virus created by deletion of the interferon antagonist NS1. J Infect Dis 201:354–362. doi:10.1086/649428

Wang Z, Duke GM (2007) Cloning of the canine RNA polymerase I promoter and establishment of reverse genetics for influenza A and B in MDCK cells. Virol J 4:102

Watanabe S, Imai M, Ohara Y, Odagiri T (2003) Influenza B virus BM2 protein is transported through the trans-Golgi network as an integral membrane protein. J Virol 77:10630–10637

Watanabe S, Watanabe T, Kawaoka Y (2009) Influenza A virus lacking M2 protein as a live attenuated vaccine. J Virol 83:5947–5950. doi:10.1128/JVI.00450-09

Watanabe T, Watanabe S, Kim JH, Hatta M, Kawaoka Y (2008) Novel approach to the development of effective H5N1 influenza A virus vaccines: use of M2 cytoplasmic tail mutants. J Virol 82:2486–2492. doi:10.1128/JVI.01899-07

Wolschek M, Samm E, Seper H, Sturlan S, Kuznetsova I, Schwager C, Khassidov A, Kittel C, Muster T, Egorov A, Bergmann M (2011) Establishment of a chimeric, replication-deficient influenza A virus vector by modulation of splicing efficiency. J Virol 85:2469–2473

Wood JM, Robertson JS (2004) From lethal virus to life-saving vaccine: developing inactivated vaccines for pandemic influenza. Nat Rev Microbiol 2:842–847

Wressnigg N, Shurygina AP, Wolff T, Redlberger-Fritz M, Popow-Kraupp T, Muster T, Egorov A, Kittel C (2009) Influenza B mutant viruses with truncated NS1 proteins grow efficiently in vero cells and are immunogenic in mice. J Gen Virol 90:366–374. doi:10.1099/vir.0.006122-0

Wu R, Guan Y, Yang Z, Chen J, Wang H, Chen Q, Sui Z, Fang F, Chen Z (2010) A live bivalent influenza vaccine based on a H9N2 virus strain. Vaccine 28:673–680

Zhang X, Kong W, Ashraf S, Curtiss R 3rd (2009) A one-plasmid system to generate influenza virus in cultured chicken cells for potential use in influenza vaccine. J Virol 83:9296–9303

Steel J, Burmakina SV, Thomas C, Spackman E, García-Sastre A, Swayne DE, Palese P (2008) A combination in-ovo vaccine for avian influenza virus and Newcastle disease virus. Vaccine 26:522–531. doi:10.1016/j.vaccine.2007.11.032

Steel J, Lowen AC, Pena L, Angel M, Solorzano A, Albrecht R, Perez DR, García-Sastre A, Palese P (2009) Live attenuated influenza viruses containing NS1 truncations as vaccine candidates against H5N1 highly pathogenic avian influenza. J Virol 83:1742–1753. doi:10.1128/JVI.01920-08

Tanaka T, Urabe M, Goto H, Tobita K (1984) Isolation and preliminary characterization of a highly cytolytic influenza B virus variant with an aberrant NS gene. Virology 135:515–523

Taubenberger JK, Kash JC (2010) Influenza virus evolution, host adaptation, and pandemic formation. Cell Host Microbe 7:440–451. doi:10.1016/j.chom.2010.05.009

tenOever BR (2013) RNA viruses and the host microRNA machinery. Nat Rev Microbiol 11:169–180. doi:10.1038/nrmicro2971

Verity EE, Camuglia S, Agius CT, Ong C, Shaw R, Barr I, Middleton D, Rockman S (2011) Rapid generation of pandemic influenza virus vaccine candidate strains using synthetic DNA. [illegible]

[illegible]

Zhang X, Kong W, Ashraf S, Curtiss R 3rd (2009) A one-plasmid system to generate influenza virus in cultured chicken cells for potential use in influenza vaccine. J Virol 83:9[illegible]

Rapid Production of Synthetic Influenza Vaccines

Philip R. Dormitzer

Abstract The strain composition of influenza vaccines must be changed regularly to track influenza virus antigenic evolution. During outbreaks with pandemic potential, strain changes are urgent. The systems for accomplishing vaccine strain changes have required the shipment of viruses and other biological materials around the globe, with delays in vaccine availability, and have used legacy techniques of egg-based virus cultivation, resulting in vaccine mismatches. In collaboration with Synthetic Genomics Vaccines Inc. and the US Biomedical Advanced Research and Development Authority, Novartis has developed a synthetic approach to influenza vaccine virus generation. Synthetic influenza vaccine viruses and mammalian cell culture technology promise influenza vaccines that match circulating influenza strains more closely and are delivered in greater quantities, more rapidly than vaccines produced by conventional technologies. These new technologies could yield an improved influenza vaccine response system in which viral sequence data from many sources are posted on the Internet, are downloaded by vaccine manufacturers, and are used to rescue multiple, attenuated vaccine viruses directly on high yielding backbones. Elements of this system were deployed in the response to the 2013 H7N9 influenza outbreak in China. The result was the production, clinical testing, and stockpiling of an H7N9 vaccine before the second wave of the outbreak struck at the end of 2013. Future directions in synthetic influenza vaccine technology include the automation of influenza virus rescue from sequence data and the merger of synthetic and self-amplifying mRNA vaccine technologies. The result could be a more robust and effective influenza vaccine system.

P. R. Dormitzer (✉)
Novartis Vaccines, 350 Massachusetts Ave., Cambridge, MA 02139, USA
e-mail: philip.dormitzer@novartis.com

Current Topics in Microbiology and Immunology (2015) 386: 237–273
DOI: 10.1007/82_2014_399

Published Online: 5 July 2014

Contents

1 Introduction

The dictum that "good manufacturing is boring" does not apply to influenza vaccines. For almost all other pharmaceuticals, every lot of product, every year, as nearly as possible, is composed of exactly the same materials, manufactured by the exactly same process, and tested by exactly the same assays. To approach this ideal, pharmaceutical manufacturing should be repetitively, monotonously boring. In a singular exception, influenza vaccine manufacturing is consistently exciting, often uncomfortably so, for manufacturers, regulators, and public health officials. For most influenza seasons and during pandemics or outbreaks with pandemic potential, a global network of surveillance laboratories, reference laboratories, and influenza vaccine manufacturers race against the clock to adjust the vaccine to counter the virus' constant antigenic variation (Stohr 2013). If every year's influenza vaccine perfectly matched previous years' vaccines, influenza immunization would soon cease to offer protection, as occurred in 1947, when the first influenza vaccine began to fail, only 4 years after it was first shown to be effective in humans (Francis et al. 1947).

To start a new influenza vaccine manufacturing campaign, a key material, the vaccine seed virus, often must be changed to match circulating strains. Because each new vaccine seed virus may have unique growth and antigen productivity characteristics, the conditions of virus infection often must be optimized. Because the new virus and its proteins will have unique biochemical characteristics, the processes for virus purification, antigen extraction, antigen purification, and vaccine formulation may need to be adjusted. Because the new virus will have unique antigenic characteristics, the strain-specific antigen standards and antisera used to measure antigenic similarity or difference and to assay vaccine antigen content must be re-derived and calibrated. For pandemic strains and novel strains with pandemic potential, the distribution in human populations of pre-existing levels of specific antibodies and T cells may be unknown, creating uncertainty regarding the optimal antigen dose, number of injections, and need for an adjuvant. Therefore, for pandemic or pre-pandemic vaccines, basic immunization parameters may need to be re-established through clinical testing.

Because new influenza variants emerge and spread globally through human populations so rapidly, the global system of laboratories, agencies, and manufacturers, using current techniques, does not always provide new, well-matched influenza vaccines in time (CDC 2004a, b; WHO 2013a). Due in part to antigenic changes that occur during egg adaptation, low strain isolation rates in eggs for H3N2 strains, difficulty in selecting a B strain of the correct lineage, and the six month or greater lag between strain selection and vaccine distribution, seasonal influenza vaccines often include strains that do not accurately match those circulating in humans at the time that the vaccines are distributed (Kishida et al. 2012; Schild et al. 1983; Skowronski et al. 2014; Tricco et al. 2013). During pandemics, little if any vaccine has been available during the initial waves of virus spread (Tizzoni et al. 2012). Recent efforts to improve vaccine responses to the emergence of new influenza variants have included research into universal influenza vaccines, increasing the number of strains in each vaccine, and increasing the speed and accuracy of vaccine strain changes.

A universal flu vaccine would protect against a greater variety of influenza strains over a longer period of time than today's vaccines and would lessen or eliminate the need to change the vaccine to track viral evolution. Adjuvants, such as the oil-in-water emulsion MF59, do increase the breadth of vaccine-elicited immunity but not sufficiently to obviate the need for seasonal vaccine strain changes (Orsi et al. 2013). In recent years, a series of scientific discoveries has invigorated universal flu vaccine development efforts. Yet, even a severe case of naturally acquired influenza does not elicit long-lasting immunity that protects against multiple influenza virus subtypes or even against substantially drifted strains of the same subtype. Therefore, despite exciting science and the long-term promise of universal influenza immunization, in the near future, it is unlikely that a universal flu vaccine will be deployed and eliminate the need for the rapid production of new, strain-specific influenza vaccines.

Including more strains in each vaccine could increase vaccine coverage of antigenic variants. Influenza B viruses belong to two major lineages, Yamagata and Victoria, which have limited antigenic cross-reactivity. Both lineages circulate in human populations. A trivalent seasonal influenza vaccine contains only one B strain. The current strain selection system picked the B lineage that would dominate a new vaccine's influenza season in only five of the 10 years from 2000 to 2011, a success rate no better than random (Ambrose and Levin 2012). In response, quadrivalent vaccines, with two influenza A strains (of the H1N1 and H3N2 subtypes) and two influenza B strains (of the Yamagata and Victoria lineages), have been introduced (ACIP 2013). Quadrivalent vaccines can offer increased coverage in those years in which a significant amount of disease is caused by the B lineage not included in the trivalent vaccine. However, as the number of strains and amount of antigen in each vaccine dose increases, the number of doses that can be produced decreases. The challenge of adding even one new strain to existing influenza vaccines indicates that the degree of multivalency that would be needed to yield universality through the inclusion of multiple strains is not feasible with currently used vaccine technologies, even if one could predict future antigenic variation well enough to know which strains to include. The near impossibility of predicting new pandemic strains with accuracy means that a highly multivalent vaccine could, at best, prime for limited cross-reactivity with pandemic strains but not target them precisely enough to eliminate the need for strain-specific pandemic vaccines.

The challenges facing universal flu vaccine approaches and the limitations to strain prediction and multivalency result in a need to increase the speed and accuracy of influenza vaccine strain changes. Increased accessibility of viral gene sequencing promises a far more widely distributed and rapid ability to detect the emergence and spread of new viral variants. Digital communication via the Internet allows sequence information to be transmitted far more rapidly, reliably, safely, and widely than biological materials (such as respiratory secretions, viruses, and sera) can be shipped through the mail. Synthetic biology now enables digitally transmitted sequences to be converted rapidly into the genes that encode new influenza variants (Dormitzer et al. 2013). Molecular virology techniques readily convert synthesized genes into vaccine viruses, tailored to safe and efficient influenza vaccine manufacturing. Combined, the advances in nucleic acid sequencing, digital communication, synthetic biology, and molecular virology promise simplification of the influenza surveillance and strain selection system, substantial acceleration of vaccine strain changes, and improved match between vaccine antigens and circulating, disease-causing, wild-type influenza virus strains (Table 1).

2 The Current System of Seasonal, Pandemic, and Pre-Pandemic Influenza Surveillance and Vaccine Virus Generation

For influenza vaccines with hemagglutinin (HA) or neuraminidase (NA) antigens that are generated from sources other than synthetic genes [including whole inactivated virus, split, recombinant or nonrecombinant subunit, recombinant virus-like-particle (VLP), and live attenuated vaccines], a circulating wild-type influenza virus from the respiratory secretions of a patient with influenza is an essential starting material. Under the current system, for nonrecombinant influenza vaccines, the wild-type virus must be isolated in eggs, passaged in eggs, and characterized antigenically and genetically to produce a "vaccine prototype virus" [also called a "candidate vaccine virus (CVV)"]. For influenza type A strains, "high growth reassortant (HGR) viruses" are usually produced as an intermediate step between the wild-type virus and the prototype vaccine virus. To make a high growth reassortant, the isolated and passaged wild-type virus descendant is mated in eggs with a donor

Table 1 Opportunities to improve influenza surveillance and strain generation

Current state	Opportunity	Benefits
National Influenza Centers (NICs) ship respiratory samples and influenza virus isolates to World Health Organization Collaborating Centers (WHO CCs) for processing and analysis	NICs conduct direct metagenomic sequencing of respiratory samples and immediately post anonymized HA and NA sequence data in publically accessible databases	No delay due to shipment of samples from NICs to WHO CCs. No loss of viability in shipment. Lower biosafety risk in transit. Greater access of scientific community to data
Influenza surveillance data generation primarily by NICs	Influenza surveillance data generation a by-product of routine metagenomic clinical diagnosis of respiratory infections with continuous bioinformatics analysis of sequence data stream	Greatly expanded influenza surveillance database. New influenza variants detected promptly
Viruses for use in vaccine manufacturing re-isolated from respiratory secretions on eggs at WHO CCs, with accompanying egg-adaptive mutations	Viruses rescued on mammalian cells from genes synthesized based on posted sequences of HA and NA genes in respiratory specimens	No egg-adaptive mutations. More antigenic variants rescued. Better antigenic match of vaccines to wild-type viruses. Potential for improved vaccine efficacy. No introduction of adventitious agents from human respiratory secretions
Isolated viruses reassorted onto attenuated, high growth backbones	Viruses rescued directly from synthesized HA and NA genes on attenuated, high growth backbones	Time savings by generation of HGRs immediately after sequences posted with no intermediate steps. Improved virus rescue success rates. No need to cultivate virulent wild-type viruses
Low throughput vaccine prototype and HGR generation techniques used	Automated, highly parallel production of prototype vaccine viruses	With a greater selection of prototype viruses, higher yielding, better matched vaccine viruses available sooner
Strain selection conducted in closed door meetings with antigenic data released for open scientific review after selection made. Subsequent critiques of strain selection	Antigenic data posted as metadata in publically accessible sequence databases as soon as the data are generated. Open scientific review of data before an open strain selection meeting	Better strain selection, informed by open scientific review. Reduced second-guessing of strain selection after the fact

(continued)

Table 1 (continued)

Current state	Opportunity	Benefits
Activities leading to vaccine seed viruses dispersed between WHO CCs, reassortant laboratories, and manufacturers, with materials shipped between laboratories	All activities to generate a seed virus stock, starting with downloading HA and NA sequences, consolidated in manufacturers' laboratories	Time savings as steps in seed virus generation overlapped, with some steps conducted at risk while analyses of previous step pending. No shipping and fewer permitting delays. No switching between virus growth platforms. Fewer communication gaps. A single quality standard
Separate consideration of human biosafety and poultry or swine biosafety for permitting of shipment or use of new zoonotic influenza strains in the US	Greater integration of CDC and USDA evaluation of new influenza strains	Faster pandemic vaccine response
Predictably attenuated vaccine prototype viruses for high pathogenicity avian strains considered select agents until after a months-long evaluation and exclusion process	Presumptive exclusion from select agent status for vaccine viruses for high pathogenicity avian strains when the HA polybasic cleavage site is removed and an attenuated vaccine backbone is used	Months saved in the vaccine response to a high pathogenicity avian influenza pandemic
Most influenza vaccines produced in eggs	Most vaccine production in cell culture	Together with cell culture-based vaccine seed virus production and surveillance, would eliminate vaccine mismatch due to egg-adaptive mutations. Completely eliminate all traces of egg allergens from vaccines. Eliminate adventitious agents and bioburden originating from chickens. More rapid start of vaccine production under containment in early days of a pandemic. More rapid scale up of antigen production for pandemics. Eliminate chance of vaccine system failure in a pandemic of a strain that is highly virulent for both humans and chickens

(continued)

Table 1 (continued)

Current state	Opportunity	Benefits
Egg-based vaccine potency reagents supplied by Essential Regulatory Laboratories (ERLs) before mammalian cell-based reagents	No preferential provision of egg-based vaccine potency reagents to manufacturers	Eliminate delay in release of mammalian cell-produced influenza vaccines relative to egg-produced vaccines
Single radial immunodiffusion (SRID) used to assay potency for vaccine release, requiring generation of new sheep antiserum for each strain change	Purely biophysical, conformationally-sensitive vaccine potency assay available days after sequence is posted	Eliminate delay in vaccine release due to lack of calibrated potency reagents
After vaccine prototype virus generated, months of additional work to make the first vaccine batch	Fully synthetic SAM® influenza vaccine	First vaccine batch generated approximately one week after sequences posted

strain [such as A/Puerto Rico/8/34 (PR8) for inactivated vaccines or A/Ann Arbor/6/60 or A/Leningrad/134/57 for live attenuated vaccines] to combine the isolate's HA, NA, and potentially other genome segments with a donor genetic backbone with more favorable properties for vaccine production (Ghendon et al. 1984; Kilbourne 1969; Maassab et al. 1969). Even for influenza vaccines and vaccine candidates produced recombinantly, a wild-type virus starting material is needed as the source of the viral RNA used to produce cDNA encoding HA or NA. The cDNA is used to rescue a recombinant influenza virus, baculovirus, or other vector or to produce an influenza antigen-expressing cell line (Fries et al. 2013; Nicolson et al. 2005; Treanor et al. 2011). In all of these variants of non synthetic generation of the genes encoding HA or NA, various physical materials (respiratory secretions, infectious viruses, viral RNA, or cloned virus genes) must be shipped from the site of collection to one or more intermediate processing sites and on to vaccine manufacturers, generally crossing multiple national borders, with potential for loss of biological activity, and (for potential pandemic viruses) often with delays for permitting.

A large and complex network of laboratories and authorities carry out influenza surveillance, strain selection, development of potency reagents, and the initial steps in the generation of vaccine viruses (WHO Writing Group 2012). This network, coordinated by the World Health Organization (WHO) makes up the Global Influenza Surveillance and Response System (GISRS). The first set of laboratories, the globally distributed National Influenza Centres (approximately 141 laboratories at the time of writing), obtain respiratory secretions from patients to isolate wild-type influenza viruses by culture in chicken eggs or, more often, in Madin-Darby canine kidney (MDCK) cells. This continuous cell line is highly sensitive to infection by influenza virus but not by most other viruses (Roth et al. 2012). Influenza-positive specimens of interest are then shipped to one of the second set of laboratories, the six WHO Collaborating Centres (CCs). The WHO

CCs have the expertise and panels of reagents needed to characterize influenza viruses antigenically and often carry out other phenotypic and genetic analyses of new strains to produce vaccine prototype strains. Reassortment of the egg-isolated viruses to make HGRs may take place in a WHO CC or in additional reassortment laboratories, which include an academic laboratory (at New York Medical College, which produces HGRs for inactivated vaccines) and industrial laboratories (at CSL in Australia, which produces HGRs for inactivated vaccines, and at MedImmune, which produces live attenuated vaccine viruses). Shipment of viruses and viral antigen preparations to another set of laboratories, the four Essential Regulatory Laboratories (ERLs), is required to generate the calibrated reagents used to assay HA antigen content for the release of most nonreplicating influenza vaccines.

Based on the analysis of epidemiologic, antigenic, and other phenotypic information from the GISRS and other laboratories, the influenza experts on a WHO Technical Advisory Group issue strain selection recommendations twice a year (once for the northern hemisphere and once for the southern hemisphere), designating "reference viruses" that the viruses used to make vaccine antigens must match antigenically. These recommendations are then reviewed and generally endorsed by national regulatory authorities. The WHO can recommend influenza virus strains for vaccine production, but only national regulatory agencies have the authority to approve or reject influenza vaccines based on their strain composition and other characteristics. For seasonal influenza vaccines, the regulatory mechanisms of control over vaccine content include initial licensure and annual vaccine license updates. For pandemic vaccines, there are additional mechanisms, such as "mock-up file" updates or emergency use authorization to speed vaccine distribution for public health emergencies (FDA 2007; CPMP 2004). Based on the WHO recommendations and often in anticipation of likely recommendations, vaccine prototype viruses and reference viruses are shipped from GISRS laboratories to vaccine manufacturers. Other reagents shipped by the GISRS network to manufacturers include the ferret antisera used to assess antigenic identity, the sheep antisera and calibrated antigen standards used to assess vaccine HA content, and in some cases extracted viral RNA or cloned genes.

Using the vaccine prototype viruses received from the GISRS network, manufacturers make carefully controlled "vaccine seed virus" stocks that meet regulatory requirements for inoculation into eggs or cell culture fermenters for vaccine antigen production under "good manufacturing practice (GMP)" quality systems. The generation of seed virus stocks involves adapting a prototype vaccine virus to the manufacturer's production platform by serial passage in eggs or mammalian cells, as well as adventitious agent testing and additional characterization. An additional cycle of shipping biological materials ensues as the vaccine seed viruses and vaccine bulks are shipped from manufacturers to WHO CCs, ERLs, and national regulatory authorities for testing for antigenic similarity to the reference viruses, for HA content, and for other characteristics.

A primary strength of the GISRS is its long track record of achievement. It is well-established, global in scope, and a repository of expertise in the practice of influenza vaccine generation. Influenza remains the most variable virus for which we can produce effective vaccines, and this achievement is due, in large part, to the functioning of the GISRS. The speed with which new influenza vaccines are produced in response to epidemiologic events is unparalleled for any other mass-distributed pharmaceutical product for human use, and it is extraordinary that such a complex set of activities unfolds twice a year with the success rate that the GISRS has demonstrated.

In response to the threat of a highly pathogenic H5N1 avian influenza pandemic, the GISRS has adopted influenza reverse genetics technology (Nicolson et al. 2005). Influenza reverse genetics refers to the transfection of mammalian cells with cloned and sometimes modified influenza genes to generate infectious influenza viruses (Hoffmann et al. 2000). The technology is needed because wild type, high pathogenicity H5N1 influenza viruses are too hazardous to use as vaccine seed viruses for manufacturing and are inefficient at producing HA and NA antigens, killing chicken embryos before HA accumulates to high levels (Subbarao et al. 2003). Many of the WHO CCs have cloned the HA genes of the high pathogenicity strains, used reverse genetics to eliminate each strain's HA polybasic cleavage site (a key pathogenicity determinant), rescued these attenuated pre-pandemic vaccine viruses in Vero cells on PR8 backbones, and made them available to manufacturers and researchers, but only after passage in chicken eggs (Nicolson et al. 2005; WHO 2014a). The use of reverse genetics technology for vaccine virus generation has not been generalized to GISRS operations for seasonal vaccines.

The GISRS will now have to adapt to newly emerging, revolutionary methods of prototype vaccine virus generation that go beyond the use of reverse genetics for pandemic response. Reliance on legacy technologies may result in now avoidable delays, shipping mishaps, and vaccine mismatches. In a practice for which there are now alternatives, viruses previously isolated from respiratory secretions on mammalian (MDCK) cells are generally re-isolated in eggs from shipped respiratory secretions by the WHO CCs. For pragmatic reasons, the MDCK cell lines and laboratory practices in NICs are standardized for initial virus isolation for surveillance, not for generating virus preparations suitable for use as starting materials to manufacture vaccines under GMP for injection into large populations of humans. Therefore, re-isolation of viruses on eggs at the WHO CCs is always necessary but not always successful, particularly for H3N2 strains. Recent circulating H3N2 strains have had an isolation rate in eggs as much as 30-fold lower than the rate in MDCK cells (Stevens et al. 2010). In some years, such as 2004, no well-matched H3N2 strain could be isolated in eggs in time to produce a seasonal vaccine, resulting in a substantial vaccine mismatch for that subtype, an occurrence associated with decreased vaccine effectiveness (Belongia et al. 2009; Centers for Disease Control and Prevention 2004b; Widjaja et al. 2006).

One major concern with the current system is that, even when viruses do successfully adapt to growth in eggs, adaptation consistently causes mutations in the sialoside binding site of HA, as the virus adapts from recognizing the dominant influenza virus receptors in human respiratory epithelium (α-2,6 sialosides) to recognizing the dominant receptors in the chicken egg allantoic cavity (α-2,3 sialosides) (Katz et al. 1990; Schild et al. 1983; Shinya et al. 2006). Because potent neutralizing antibodies bind near the sialoside binding pocket on the HA head, egg-adaptive genetic changes can alter the antigenicity of the virus, creating a mismatch between vaccine antigens and the antigens of circulating viruses (Kishida et al. 2012; Skowronski et al. 2014).

Egg-adaptive mutations in recent WHO-recommended, egg-isolated A/H3N2 and B Victoria lineage viruses used for vaccine production have heightened concerns and emphasized the need for an improved system of vaccine prototype virus development that does not include virus passage in eggs. For the H3N2 subtype, an antigenic and serologic analysis by a WHO CC of the egg-adapted, A/Perth/16/2009-like, A/Victoria/210/2009-based, X187 reassortant vaccine virus (used for the 2010–2011 and 2011–2012 northern hemisphere campaigns) showed significantly reduced match to circulating influenza strains due to egg adaptive mutations (Kishida et al. 2012). Similar conclusions are reached by antigenic and serologic analyses comparing MDCK-isolated with egg-adapted A/Victoria/361/2011 H3N2 vaccine viruses (used for the 2012–2013 and 2013–2014 northern hemisphere campaigns) and by inspection of antigenic cartographic maps comparing MDCK-isolated with egg-adapted A/Texas/50/2012 H3N2 vaccine viruses (introduced in 2014) (Cox 2013, 2014; Skowronski et al. 2014). Analysis of the B/Brisbane/60/2008 Victoria lineage (the type B lineage chosen for the 2010–2011 and 2011–2012 northern hemisphere trivalent vaccines and for a component of the 2012–2013 and 2013–2014 northern hemisphere quadrivalent vaccines) vaccine virus also shows a mismatch to circulating strains due to egg adaptive mutations (Kishida et al. 2012). Thus, for the 4 years prior to the writing of this paper, the only reliably matched components of the trivalent or quadrivalent influenza vaccines have been the A/California/7/2009-like A/H1N1 strains that were introduced after the 2009 pandemic and, in some years, the B Yamagata lineage component.

Because of incomplete presentation of the cultivation history of strains, it is difficult to determine from publically available literature how commonly significant vaccine mismatch due to egg-adaptation occurred before 2010. Only since 2013 has the antigenic distinction between MDCK cell-isolated and egg-isolated versions of virus strains with the same name been highlighted consistently in WHO and CDC strain selection reports (Cox 2013, 2014; WHO 2013a, 2014c). For the 2013–2014 northern hemisphere season, the WHO advisory panel broke with precedent by specifying that H3N2 vaccine prototype viruses should antigenically match a mammalian cell-adapted A/Victoria/361/2011 strain (WHO 2013a). However, no manufacturer, even those that could produce vaccine antigen in mammalian cells, had the license modifications needed to use vaccine seed viruses isolated on mammalian cells. Therefore, no manufacturer could act on the improved recommendation. As this barrier to the use of vaccine seed viruses with no egg passage history remained (because of the need for time-consuming regulatory adaptations), for the 2014–2015 northern hemisphere campaign the WHO dropped the distinction between egg-adapted and mammalian cell-adapted H3N2 viruses in its recommendation (Cox 2014; WHO 2014c).

For full implementation of completely egg-free production, timely supply of mammalian cell-based potency testing reagents from the ERLs will be required in the future. Such reagents are just now being introduced, but because calibrated egg-based antigen standards and antisera are still made available for vaccine release before mammalian cell-based standards, the release of potentially better-matched mammalian-cell based vaccines is delayed relative to egg-based vaccines.

During the 2013–2014 northern hemisphere campaign, the impact of the H3N2 and B Victoria lineage mismatches was mitigated in the United States by the predominance of H1N1 strains (Cox 2014). However during the 2010–2011, 2011–2012, and 2012–2013 seasons, H3N2 strains dominated in the US (Finelli 2013; Grohskopf 2011, 2012). During the 2012–2013 influenza season, for example, particularly low vaccine effectiveness was documented. Against H3N2 strains, for vaccine recipients in the United States across age groups, vaccine effectiveness was 47 % [95 % confidence interval (CI) 35–58 %], and in those over 65, effectiveness was a mere 9 % (95 % CI -84–55 %) (Centers for Disease Control and Prevention 2013). An analysis of vaccine effectiveness in Canada revealed similar findings (Skowronski et al. 2014).

Introduction of synthetic vaccine prototype virus generation and exclusive use of mammalian cells for vaccine seed stock production and vaccine antigen manufacture could reduce the level of vaccine antigenic mismatch to circulating strains. It remains to be determined how large an improvement in influenza vaccine effectiveness would result from the complete elimination of eggs from all aspects of the influenza vaccine enterprise—isolation of viruses to provide sequence and antigenic data, vaccine virus production, and vaccine antigen production.

3 The 2009 H1N1 Pandemic Response

The 2009 pandemic was caused by a H1N1 influenza variant that was antigenically more distant from the H1N1 strains that were introduced in 1977, most likely through a laboratory release, than from the 1918 pandemic strain (Wei et al. 2010; Zimmer and Burke 2009). The GISRS system provided Novartis Vaccines and other manufacturers with an initial high growth reassortant virus (X179A) approximately six weeks after the outbreak was first recognized to have spread to the United States from Mexico (Centers for Disease Control and Prevention 2009). The vaccine prototype virus was produced by conventional reassortment in eggs of a circulating H1N1 pandemic strain (Robertson et al. 2011). Vaccine seed preparations made from this initial vaccine prototype virus produced about one-third of typical H1N1 HA yields in manufacturing, and a vaccine did not become widely available until after the second pandemic wave had peaked in October and November of 2009 (Tizzoni et al. 2012). A high yielding vaccine virus (NIBRG-121xp), generated by serial passage in eggs of a first generation H1N1 pandemic reverse genetics-derived vaccine virus, was not available until 126 days after the first US cases were identified (Robertson et al. 2011).

Novartis Vaccines responded to the H1N1 outbreak by attempting to generate its own vaccine virus by reverse genetics (Hoffmann et al. 2000). Although this effort did not lead to the vaccine virus that was used to make any of Novartis' three licensed H1N1 pandemic vaccines, the results of the effort led to the plan to develop a system to generate vaccine viruses from synthetic DNA, without needing to receive physical virus isolates, extracted viral RNA, or cloned viral cDNA. In April 2009, Novartis only practiced influenza reverse genetics on a very limited scale, to generate basic research reagents for immunology experiments, had not contemplated making its own vaccine viruses, and had not even cloned the genes encoding the standard PR8 vaccine backbone into a suitable vector. An initial attempt to rescue a H1N1 pandemic vaccine virus using HA and NA genes synthesized by a commercial synthetic DNA provider did not yield a viable virus. However, reverse genetics rescue using HA and NA genes that Novartis cloned from H1N1 viral RNA provided by the US CDC and backbone genes rapidly cloned from PR8 succeeded, resulting in the first H1N1 potential pandemic vaccine virus globally, on May 11, 2009, well before a vaccine virus was available from GISRS (Dormitzer et al. 2013).

Novartis' initial reverse genetics-derived virus could not be used to make vaccines for human use because the virus had been rescued on 293T cells, which were not approved for use in human vaccine production. Therefore, Novartis adapted the reverse genetic rescue process to use its manufacturing MDCK 33016PF cell line and, with academic collaborators at the Phillips-Universität Marburg biosafety level 4 (BSL4) laboratory, reproduced the rescue under highly controlled circumstances (Strecker et al. 2012). The resulting vaccine virus was available 2 days after a vaccine virus was first received at a Novartis manufacturing site from the GISRS. Novartis decided not to use the virus it had rescued for vaccine manufacturing. The regulatory risks of using a vaccine virus generated by a new process were too great, once a vaccine virus produced by the GISRS using the standard processes became available. Had the H1N1 vaccine not been approved for use due to lack of regulatory acceptance of a virus produced by a novel process, there would have been no time to produce a new vaccine, with potentially damaging public health and business consequences.

The speed with which a small group of scientists generated a vaccine virus, refining techniques along the way, signaled that new technologies had the potential to generate vaccine viruses much more rapidly than legacy technologies. Therefore, Novartis partnered with the J. Craig Venter Institute (JCVI), Synthetic Genomics Vaccines Inc. (SGVI), and the US Biomedical Advanced Research and Development Authority (BARDA) to develop a synthetic approach to vaccine virus generation.

4 The Basic Technologies of Synthetic Influenza Vaccine Virus Generation

At the start of the synthetic vaccine virus program, gene synthesis technologies were well advanced. JCVI had synthesized a complete, modified *Mycoplasma mycoides* genome and used that genetic "software" to "reboot" cellular "hardware," to generate a microbe with an entirely synthetic genome (Gibson et al. 2010a). In addition, a complete mouse mitochondrial genome had been synthesized by a technique (Gibson assembly) in which three enzymes (T5 exonuclease, Phusion polymerase, and *Taq* ligase) work together in a single tube, single temperature reaction to stitch together 60 base oligonucleotides, which overlap complementary oligonucleotides by 20 bases to form a gapped double-stranded DNA template (Gibson et al. 2010b). The observation that the mycoplasma genome was assembled from 10 kb synthetic intermediates, each a bit smaller than a 13.5 kb influenza genome, indicated that the synthetic production of influenza genomes for vaccine virus rescue was practical (Gibson et al. 2010a).

Given the success in generating a much larger, fully functional genome, it was somewhat surprising that our initial attempts to generate vaccine viruses quickly using synthetic technology failed. The cause was a high error rate in gene synthesis. The errors originated in oligonucleotide synthesis by phosphoramidite chemistry, which omits a residue approximately once every 500–750 bases due to failure of chemical coupling (Gibson et al. 2010b). The resulting genes contain frame shifts, rendering them unusable. Approximately 3 % of the HA (1.7 kb) and NA (1.5 kb) genes had the intended nucleotide sequence (Dormitzer et al. 2013). During the assembly of the entire 1,080 kb mycoplasma genome, stepwise construction, in which candidate assembly intermediates were cloned, amplified, purified, and sequenced, and those with the correct sequence were selected for the next stage of assembly, followed by repeat cloning, amplification, purification, sequencing, and assembly, overcame the inaccuracy of chemical oligonucleotide synthesis (Gibson et al. 2010a). This process was too slow and labor intensive to make multiple influenza viruses rapidly for vaccine strain changes.

The solution was to eliminate gaps between oligonucleotides, to assemble entire coding sequences in a single step, and to introduce enzymatic error correction (Dormitzer et al. 2013). In a double-stranded DNA molecule, a deletion on one strand kinks the molecule. That deformation can be recognized enzymatically, and the affected DNA cleaved (ErrASE, Novici Biotech). By chemically synthesizing oligonucleotides corresponding to the entirety of each strand of a double-stranded DNA molecule (with staggers between oligonucleotide boundaries on each strand but no gaps between the oligonucleotides that constitute each strand), any deletion in one strand is very unlikely to be matched with a corresponding deletion on the complementary strand. The application of two rounds of enzymatic recognition and cleavage of such kinked molecules followed by amplification results in over 90 % of synthesized HA and NA genes having the intended sequence (Dormitzer et al. 2013).

The remainder of the error correction is provided by biological selection. HA or NA genes with frame shift mutations will rarely allow the rescue of viable viruses.

Because the error rate in viruses rescued from error-corrected genes is so low, it is not necessary to clone and sequence synthetic genes before virus rescue. Rather, oligonucleotide synthesis, gene assembly, enzymatic error correction, and virus rescue are carried out in an unbroken, rapid process. After virus rescue, viral genome sequencing is done in parallel with downstream virus processing activities, such as amplification and phenotypic characterization. Less than a day is needed from downloading a nucleotide sequence of a new influenza virus to the completion of HA and NA linear gene cassettes ready to transfect, complete with dual promoter control sequences for genomic RNA and mRNA expression (Dormitzer et al. 2013). Backbone genes are prepared in advance as aliquoted, highly purified plasmid preparations, ready to use in various combinations with newly synthesized HA and NA linear gene cassettes. Rapidly synthesized genes could be used not only to rescue influenza vaccine viruses but also to make gene constructs for alternative, recombinant influenza vaccine technologies, such as subunit or virus-like particle vaccines expressed from recombinant baculovirus-infected insect cells, and to make other reagents useful for pandemic or outbreak responses, such as defective lentivirus-based pseudoviruses for neutralization assays (Alberini et al. 2009; Dormitzer et al. 2012; Fries et al. 2013; Landry et al. 2010; Treanor et al. 2011).

The cell lines used to make vaccines are scrutinized intensively. Adventitious agent and oncogenic potential, genetic and phenotypic stability, banking procedures, culture conditions, media raw material origins, and documentation are all carefully examined and controlled (FDA 2010). Adapting influenza virus reverse genetic rescue to the same MDCK 33016PF cell line used for vaccine manufacturing allowed a single, well characterized and accepted cell line to be used from vaccine virus generation to vaccine antigen production (Dormitzer et al. 2013). An early report indicated that the DNA-dependent RNA polymerase I (pol I) used to produce negative-strand, genomic RNAs in the ambisense influenza reverse genetics rescue system required a species-specific promoter (Wang and Duke 2007). Therefore, we anticipated that canine pol I promoters would be needed for reverse genetic rescue in MDCK cells. However, unlike the parental MDCK cell line, the suspension and serum-free adapted MDCK 33016PF cell line (which was confirmed to be of canine origin) supported virus rescue using the human pol I promoter, likely due to mutation during adaptation of the cell line to growth in serum-free suspension culture (Suphaphiphat et al. 2010). The use of a synthetic genome and a highly controlled cell line for vaccine virus rescue and that same mammalian cell line for vaccine production allows for a more tightly controlled adventitious agent safety profile.

Two of the starting materials of conventional influenza virus vaccines are not highly controlled or well characterized—the secretions aspirated or swabbed from the upper respiratory tracts of acutely ill humans and the hundreds of millions of fertilized eggs that pass through the cloacae of factory-farmed chickens and are collected for each year's vaccine manufacturing campaign. The manufacturing processes used for conventional influenza vaccine manufacturing have proven sufficient, with rare exceptions, to suppress bioburden during processing until final sterile filtration and to inactivate or otherwise eliminate adventitious agents (Centers for Disease Control and Prevention 2004a). Nevertheless, not introducing human respiratory secretions or chicken cloacal contents, with their flora of bacteria and adventitious viruses, into the manufacturing process in the first place is a superior option, more in conformance with modern hygienic standards for pharmaceutical manufacturing.

The MDCK cell substrate for each batch of cell culture-produced flu vaccine is obtained from sterile, banked aliquots of a single, exhaustively tested preparation of a continuous cell line (Onions et al. 2010). The origin of a synthetic vaccine virus strain from electronically transmitted data completely eliminates the possibility of introducing adventitious agents from the original human respiratory samples into the vaccine manufacturing process. Data transmission over the Internet interposed between the biological sample and the vaccine virus serves as an infallible sterilizing "ultrafilter." Of course, controls for bioburden and adventitious agent introduction and elimination remain in place in synthetic vaccine seed virus generation, bulk antigen manufacturing, and vaccine formulation and filling, but these now function as fail-safe mechanisms, not primary lines of defense.

Synthetic and reverse genetic technologies allow greater control over the vaccine virus generation process. Conventional reassortment is a stochastic process, and a wide variety of genome segment constellations can result (Kilbourne 1969). Isolation, characterization, and selection of individual reassortants are needed and often rate limiting. Synthetic virus rescue allows specification of the starting genomes of the new viruses, with subsequent mutations accumulating during adaptation. The greater efficiency of the synthetic approach allows a set of backbones to be compared for each new HA and NA rather than reliance on a single backbone reassortant partner. Novel backbones for type A viruses that combine PR8 genome segments with genome segments from other nonhigh pathogenicity influenza virus strains increase vaccine virus rescue efficiencies by up to 1000-fold (as measured by infectious titer after transfection) and increase HA yields in mammalian cells (typically 1.3–9.9 times the yield of conventional reference strains) and in eggs (by similar amounts), with variation by strain (Dormitzer et al. 2013). Novel backbones for B strains allow reliable rescue of these viruses without the need to synthesize the entire genome of a new isolate (Dormitzer et al. 2013). By rescuing many potential synthetic vaccine viruses in parallel, the highest yielding strains can be selected early, rather than after many months delay for sequential testing and prolonged adaptation of serially produced reassortants.

Precise specification of the genome of a new vaccine virus is limited by available knowledge of wild-type virus sequences. During the early days of an outbreak, the coding sequences of the HA and NA genome segments of the new strain are often available. However, the sequence of the genome segment ends is often missing in sequence databases or may be misleading, if derived from polymerase chain reaction (PCR) amplification primers rather than the actual influenza genome. Single nucleotide changes in the 3′ and 5′ noncoding regions of influenza virus genome segments can have a large impact on virus rescue efficiency, virus growth, and HA yield (Dormitzer et al. 2013). Therefore, a key task at the start of gene synthesis for vaccine virus rescue is deduction of one or more sets of genome segment ends. This task requires surveying archived data for accurate influenza genome segment sequences with similar coding regions to the new strain, examining the ends of the archived sequences to obtain consensus end sequences, and deciding which observed end variants should be used in the set of HA and NA gene syntheses. Given the variation in coding sequence between isolates during an outbreak (whether natural or as a result of sequencing errors), ambiguity regarding end sequences, and the advantages of testing multiple potential backbones, human judgment is required to determine an initial vaccine virus rescue strategy.

Additional increases in HA yield can be achieved by making chimeric HA and NA genes that encode the antigenically essential regions of a circulating strain and terminal regions from a strain well-adapted to growth in an MDCK cell or egg substrate (Gomila et al. 2013; Harvey et al. 2011). The ability to make informed choices and rescue multiple potential vaccine viruses in parallel is essential for rapid success in generating antigenically well-matched, high-yielding synthetic vaccine seed viruses, optimized for vaccine antigen production.

5 Performance of Synthetic Technology in Vaccine Virus Generation

Synthetic technology has demonstrated its ability to produce a wide variety of high-yielding, attenuated, research grade influenza vaccine viruses rapidly and has led the global response to the H7N9 influenza outbreak by producing a virus that was used to make a vaccine candidate that elicited effective immune responses in a phase I trial and was stockpiled by the US government before the second wave of the outbreak (Bart et al. 2014). The Novartis-SGVI-JCVI synthetic influenza virus team has produced synthetic, research grade viruses for more than 50 strains, including those of the A/H1N1 (pre- and post-2009), A/H3N2, A/H3N2v (swine origin), A/H2N2, A/H2N3, A/H5N1, A/H7N7, A/H7N9, A/H9N2, B/Yamagata, and B/Victoria lineages (unpublished data) (Dormitzer et al. 2013). The BARDA-sponsored project to develop the synthetic vaccine virus system has passed two key milestone tests. The first, administered in 2011, assessed the nascent system's response to a simulated outbreak. The US CDC and BARDA provided the synthesis team with the coding sequences, but not the terminal sequences, of the HA and NA genome segments of an unknown strain. The team found that the HA coding sequences most closely resembled those of a low pathogenicity avian H7N3 strain (A/Canada goose/BC/3752/2007) and the NA coding sequences most closely resembled those of a low pathogenicity avian H10N9 virus (A/king eider/

Alaska/44397-858/2008). Based on available, related H7 and N9 complete genome segment sequences, the team deduced potential terminal sequences for virus synthesis. From the start of gene synthesis until verification of potential vaccine virus recovery, 4 days and 4 h elapsed, including the time needed to ship the synthetic HA and NA gene cassettes from a synthesis laboratory in California to a virus rescue laboratory in Massachusetts (Dormitzer et al. 2013).

The second milestone test required the synthetic vaccine virus team to anticipate the southern hemisphere strain selection for 2013. By the time of the WHO Technical Advisory Group's strain selection announcement in September, 2012, the team was to have synthesized a set of strains that included viruses that match each of the WHO-selected reference strains by hemagglutination inhibition (HI) testing and produce more HA in laboratory scale cultures than any vaccine prototype virus made available by the GISRS. The synthetic system exceeded expectations, yet also stumbled over the mismatches of the current egg-based vaccine virus generation system.

The anticipation of the WHO strain selection was straightforward, as there were no strain changes between the 2012–2013 northern hemisphere influenza season and the 2013 southern hemisphere season (WHO 2012). The joint Novartis-JCVI-SGVI team analyzed publically available sequence and antigenic data on the strains that were circulating in humans using bioinformatics tools developed at JCVI and also tracked information on strain selection made available by the WHO CCs. By the time of the strain selection, the team had synthesized 6 A/H1N1 viruses, 14 A/H3N2 viruses, 2 B Victoria lineage viruses, and 5 B Yamagata lineage viruses on multiple backbones and had characterized the strains for genetic identity, growth in MDCK cells, and HA yield, with antigenic testing done for selected strains. All of the synthetic strains had complete HA and NA sequence identity to the intended sequences. The synthesized viruses included strains selected because they matched circulating strains well or because they matched strains likely to be selected by the WHO Technical Advisory group. For each component of WHO recommendation for 2013 southern hemisphere trivalent vaccines, at least one synthetic virus that was antigenically "like" the recommended reference virus had equivalent or superior growth and HA yield relative to the reference strain and to the corresponding seed virus being used by Novartis for vaccine production.

For the additional strain included in quadrivalent vaccines, a strain of the B Victoria lineage, the team synthesized a virus, B/Brisbane/60/2008, that matched those circulating in humans antigenically and produced approximately triple the HA yield of the reference strain from the GISRS. The B/Brisbane/60/2008 HA and NA sequences used by the team for synthesis came from an MDCK-isolate. However, as detailed above (Sect. 2) the WHO Technical Advisory Group maintained its previous selection of a B/Victoria lineage reference virus, also named B/Brisbane/60/2008, that had an egg-adaptive mutation that altered it antigenically so that it no longer matched the B Victoria lineage viruses circulating in humans (Kishida et al. 2012). The team had not appreciated that the MDCK-isolated B/Brisbane/60/2010 sequence that it had used to generate the synthetic virus was not the same as the egg-adapted B/Brisbane/60/2010 reference strain sequence. Therefore, HI testing showed that the synthetic, MDCK-adapted B/Brisbane/60/2008 had more than a four fold HI difference from the egg-adapted WHO B/Brisbane/60/2008 reference strain, and the assignment from BARDA to synthesize a virus that anticipated the strain selection by the Technical Advisory Group was, technically, not fulfilled. (Within 8 days of recognizing the antigenic difference between the two B/Brisbane/60/2008 viruses, the team synthesized a synthetic B/Brisbane/60/2008 with the egg-adaptive mutation and confirmed its antigenic identity to the reference virus.) In a more fundamental sense, the synthetic system exceeded expectations by surpassing the GISRS in matching the strains that caused disease in humans that year because, unlike the GISRS, the synthetic system was not reliant on legacy, egg-based technology.

As described in Sect. 2, data released from GISRS five months after the second milestone test and independent analyses showed that egg-adapted strains of the H3N2 reference virus selected by the WHO Technical Advisory Group (A/Victoria/361/2011) also failed to match circulating strains due to egg-adaptive mutations (Cox 2013; Skowronski et al. 2014). The synthetic vaccine virus team had synthetized several alternative A/Victoria/361/2011 H3N2 strains based on sequences from either egg-adapted or MDCK-adapted viruses. The synthetic H3N2 virus fully characterized for the milestone test, although passaged exclusively in mammalian cells, was generated based on the egg-adapted viral sequence, and it therefore shared the mismatch of the H3N2 reference virus with circulating H3N2 strains and met the criterion of matching the egg-adapted reference strain antigenically.

The experience demonstrates how the synthetic seed virus system could help overcome one of the major issues inherent in the current system: the possibility that egg-adaptive antigenic changes to a vaccine prototype virus make it sufficiently different from its wild-type ancestor that vaccine effectiveness may be reduced (Kishida et al. 2012; Skowronski et al. 2014). A condition for this improvement is that the GISRS abandons the use of legacy, egg-based technology to generate sequences, reference strains, and strain recommendations or that national regulatory authorities overrule WHO Technical Working Group recommendations for viruses that do not match circulating, wild-type strains. Adjustments to vaccine licenses to allow production of vaccines using prototype viruses that have never been passaged in eggs are necessary so that WHO recommendations for better matched virus strains can be followed by the production of better matched vaccines by non-egg-based vaccine manufacturers.

The nascent synthetic vaccine prototype virus system has been tested by a real world outbreak with pandemic potential (Bart et al. 2014). On March 31, 2013 (Easter Sunday), the China CDC announced an outbreak of H7N9 influenza in humans in Shanghai (Gao et al. 2013). In a far-sighted action, Chinese public health authorities immediately posted the HA and NA gene coding sequences in the publically accessible Global Initiative on Sharing All Influenza Data (GISAID) database. Although the synthetic vaccine virus system was still in the research stage, the synthetic virus team responded by starting gene synthesis at SGVI in La Jolla, California, on the morning of Monday, April 1. Gene synthesis was completed on Tuesday, April 2. Virus rescue using the synthesized genes started at

Novartis in Cambridge, Massachusetts on Wednesday, April 3 and was completed on Saturday, April 6 with sequence confirmation obtained on Monday, April 8. On April 3, the synthetic genes were provided to the US CDC with no restrictions on further distribution. The US CDC first received the wild-type virus from the China CDC on April 11, allowing the start of vaccine virus generation using nonsynthetic technology. As of February 13, 2014, there were eight attenuated vaccine viruses available from WHO CCs, all produced by reverse genetics (WHO 2014d). Four had been rescued using the synthetic HA and NA genes provided by the synthetic vaccine virus team and four using cDNA. None of the available H7N9 vaccine viruses had been produced by conventional, egg-based reassortment technology.

After further processing at the Philipps-Universität Marburg BSL4 laboratory and the Novartis Marburg influenza seed virus laboratory, one of the synthetic H7N9 vaccine viruses was used in the MDCK-based vaccine manufacturing process to produce phase I clinical trial material. On November 14, 2013, Novartis announced interim results of the phase I trial. The trial showed that, with two 15 μg doses, each adjuvanted with MF59, neutralization titers greater than 1:40 against the H7N9 strain were achieved in healthy adults (Bart et al. 2014). Vaccine lots were stockpiled by the US government in December, 2013. Synthetic vaccine viruses and MDCK-based vaccine technology allowed the production and stockpiling of a clinically tested pre-pandemic H7N9 vaccine before the start of the second wave of the outbreak at the end of 2013 (WHO 2014b).

6 Supporting Technologies for Optimal Implementation

Several supporting technologies would allow the benefits of synthetic vaccine viruses to be fully realized. These technologies include those used to sequence viral genomes in respiratory specimens, distribute the data, analyze the data, and assay vaccine antigens. Currently, viral sequence data are rarely obtained directly from respiratory samples at the NICs at the time of collection. Rather, sequences are obtained from viruses that have been cultured from the respiratory secretions in eggs or MDCK cells. In many cases, sequencing is only done after respiratory secretion or viral samples have been shipped from a NIC to a remote WHO CC, and there is a further delay before sequences, sometimes degraded by egg adaptive mutations, are posted on publically accessible databases.

Advances in metagenomic detection of viruses could synergize with synthetic seed virus generation by greatly accelerating and expanding the real-time surveillance and sequence information available for vaccine virus synthesis. Second generation sequencing techniques and bioinformatics processing enable sequencing and analysis of viral genomes in complex mixtures without the need for sequence-specific primers. With metagenomic techniques, influenza gene sequences can be obtained directly from nasal swabs (Yongfeng et al. 2011). Metagenomic analysis is a potentially disruptive technology because it could provide a universal, culture-free tool for microbiological diagnosis, detecting essentially any pathogen in almost any clinical specimen, and replacing existing methods of microbiologic diagnosis. This promise and the rapid and continuing advancement of the underlying technologies suggest that metagenomic pathogen detection is likely to become increasingly capable, accessible, and widespread in the coming years (Bibby 2013).

With implementation of metagenomics for routine clinical diagnosis, influenza surveillance could expand far beyond the roughly 140 NICs. Rather, influenza surveillance could become a byproduct of clinical care, distributed among many thousands of clinics, which would generate viral sequence data for routine primary diagnosis of respiratory illnesses and also post real-time, anonymized viral sequence data to web-based databases. More sophisticated centers could provide more specialized data, including deep sequencing results. Once today's ubiquitous availability of the infrastructure for electronic data sharing is matched by widespread implementation of the emerging technologies for direct, rapid virus sequencing in clinical specimens and synthetic vaccine prototype virus generation, virus isolation and shipment of viruses and respiratory specimens to WHO CCs would no longer be needed. By eliminating the mutations that result from viral adaptation to growth in eggs, direct sequencing of viral genomes in respiratory secretions would provide data that better represent disease-causing strains. Real time uploading of sequences could be followed by immediate rescue at remote locations of potential vaccine viruses with optimized backbones in mammalian cells (Fig. 1). Vaccine prototype virus production and antigenic testing using banked ferret sera against previous strains would take place simultaneously at the sites of virus synthesis, followed by generation of ferret antisera against the new strains for confirmatory, two-way antigenic testing. The result would be the generation of potential high-yielding vaccine viruses within days of a new disease-causing influenza variant first appearing in the human population.

The bioinformatics infrastructure to support this effort is partly in place. GISAID provides rapid, searchable, broad-based access to posted influenza sequence data in a standardized format (www.gisaid.org) (Bogner et al. 2006). To the degree that sequences accompanied by relevant metadata about location, time, sequencing technique, disease severity, drug sensitivity, and antigenic characterization are made rapidly and widely available, synthetic technology can provide more rapid and accurate vaccine responses.

Analyzing the stream of influenza sequence data to select the strains to synthesize is enabled by sophisticated bioinformatics. In the GISRS, sequence analysis of influenza viruses is a relatively recent addition to antigenic characterization, which is carried out by generating post-infection ferret antisera and using those sera to inhibit the agglutination of red blood cells by influenza viruses (HI) (Committee on Standard Serological Procedures in Influenza Studies 1950). HI data are generated using poorly characterized, complex, and heterogeneous reagents (red blood cells, influenza virus preparations, and polyclonal antisera) giving the assay high intrinsic variability (Ndifon et al. 2009). Although it cannot overcome the inherent limitations of the HI assay, "antigenic cartography," a mathematical technique that reduces the multidimensional space generated by a

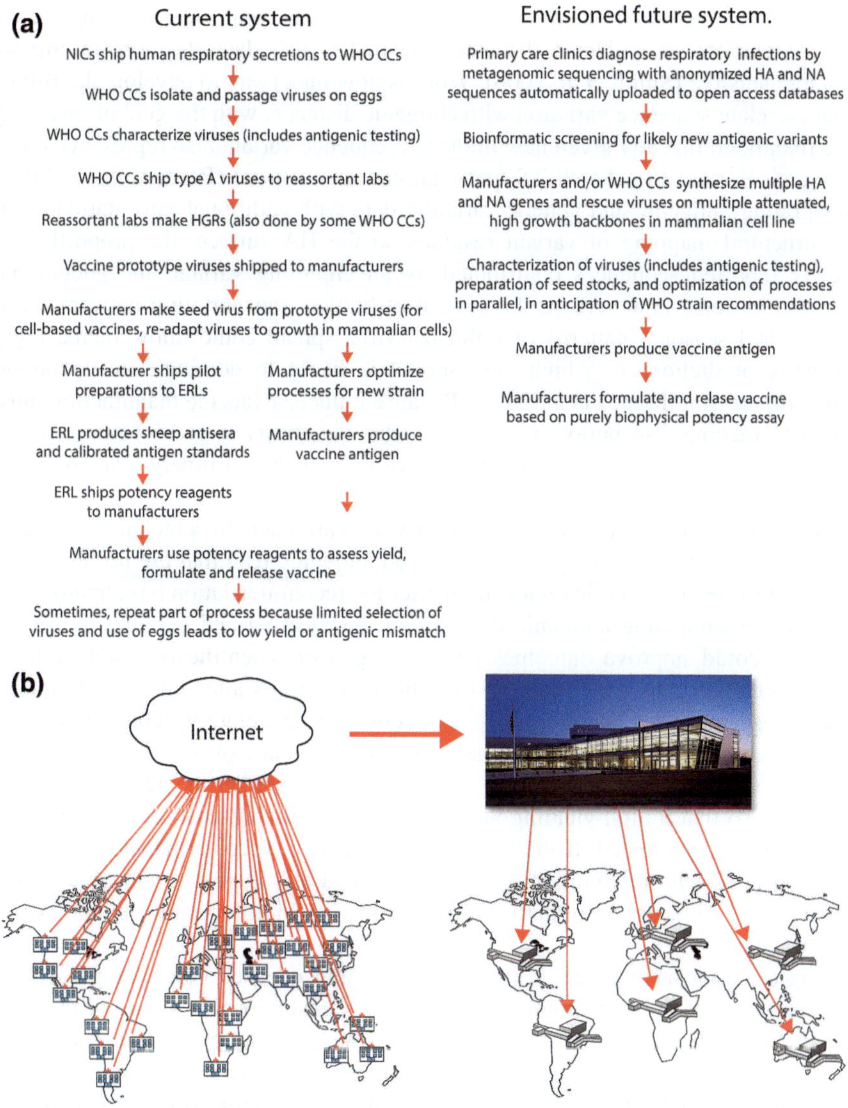

Fig. 1 **a** Comparison of current and envisioned influenza surveillance, vaccine virus generation, and vaccine production system. **b** Vision for future system. NICs and clinical laboratories sequence flu genes directly from respiratory secretions. Sequence data are posted on the web with open access and are continuously monitored by algorithms that detect sequences suggestive of new antigenic variants. Potential vaccine viruses with synthesized HA and NA genes are rescued in mammalian cells qualified for vaccine manufacture and on high growth backbones and are tested as potential vaccine prototype viruses. Seed viruses are shipped to additional manufacturing sites. When the technology matures, this shipment can be replaced by electronic transfer and local synthesis

network of cross-HI comparisons to two-dimensional, visually appealing approximations of antigenic distance, can make such datasets more intuitively comprehensible (Smith et al. 2004). Work is now underway to develop algorithms that correlate sequence variation with antigenic distance, with the goal of assessing the likelihood that any given new influenza sequence variant also represents a new antigenic variant (Stockwell TS, personal communication) (Bedford et al. 2014). Integrating antigenic and genetic variation data with additional information, such as structural mapping of variant residues on the HA surface, the proportion of newly reported sequences contributed by an emerging variant, the geographic distribution of a new variant, the pattern of human transportation networks, and established seasonal patterns of influenza virus spread could allow increasingly accurate predictions of which new variant is likely to dominate an upcoming influenza season (Lemey et al. 2014). Because influenza vaccine manufacture must precede vaccine distribution by many months, the ability to predict future dominant strains more accurately would improve the match and timely availability of influenza vaccines.

In the current GISRS system, strain selections are made by a technical advisory group in closed-door deliberations, based on antigenic data that are not generally released for open scientific review until after the recommendation has already been issued. Disseminating antigenic data before the meeting and opening the deliberations could improve outcomes by allowing open scientific review to inform strain selection rather than merely to critique selections after the fact. Synthetic technology increases the ability of manufacturers to generate vaccine viruses and adapt manufacturing protocols to new strains in advance of WHO strain recommendations, using any information that is gleaned to predict the advisory group's decision, so that a high-yielding vaccine virus is available as soon as the recommendation is announced. If the flow of information to vaccine manufacturers and the general scientific community can be hastened and increased though a diversification of sequence information sources and with bioinformatics, public health could benefit.

Once a vaccine is made, it must be tested and released before it is used for clinical testing or mass immunization. Like conventional vaccine seed virus generation, influenza vaccine potency testing requires the generation and distribution of strain-specific reagents. For most licensed influenza vaccines, SRID is the test that determines how much immunologically active (that is, capable of eliciting functional antibodies in a vaccine recipient) HA is present in the vaccine. In this modified Ouchterlony test, the new vaccine antigen (or a control antigen preparation) is placed in a well cut into an agarose gel suffused with a sheep antiserum generated against HA cleaved by bromelain from the surface of inactivated influenza virions (Schild et al. 1975). As the antigen diffuses into the gel, antigen-antibody complexes form an immunoprecipitin ring, and the diameter of that ring is taken to be proportional to the amount of immunologically active HA.

The technique has numerous deficiencies. The properties of the sheep antiserum depend on the quality of the bromelain-cleaved HA antigen used to immunize the sheep. The antigen standards (which are inactivated viruses that may perform differently in the assay than the HA in the vaccine) are calibrated based on relative intensity of bands on an SDS-PAGE gel, effectively negating the purported ability of the assay to discriminate based on HA conformation. Most importantly for the implementation of synthetic influenza vaccine virus technology, the process of generating the sheep antiserum and calibrated antigen standards can take months. Indeed, influenza vaccine bulks can sit in warehouses, with formulation and release delayed until calibrated potency testing reagents arrive. For example, during the H1N1 pandemic response and H7N9 outbreak response, reagents were not available in time for clinical trials of the vaccines, and the trials were started at risk based on vaccine formulation with surrogate assays (Bart et al. 2014; Clark et al. 2009b).

As vaccine bulks are produced more rapidly using synthetic technology, the delays in release could have greater impact. The problem is now widely recognized by regulators and manufacturers alike, and a variety of new influenza vaccine potency assays are under development (Dormitzer et al. 2012). In a parallel to synthetic vaccine seeds, some of these new potency assays deploy new technologies that could eliminate the need for any strain-specific reagent that cannot be generated rapidly based on sequence data (Williams et al. 2008). Meanwhile, the earlier availability of synthetic vaccine viruses, from which HA can be cleaved by bromelain to immunize sheep, can speed the initiation of the process of generating calibrated sets of antigen standards and antisera.

7 Quality, Regulatory, Safety, Security, Intellectual Property, Economic, and Diplomatic Aspects of Synthetic Vaccine Virus Generation

Simplifying vaccine virus generation would accelerate vaccine responses. Currently, vaccine virus generation activities are dispersed between institutions (Fig. 1). Under ordinary circumstances, a WHO CC or reassortant laboratory will only release a vaccine prototype virus to manufacturers after it has completed (or nearly completed) thorough characterization. Therefore, the manufacturer cannot start producing the seed virus stock and adjusting vaccine manufacturing processes to the virus' unique characteristics at risk while vaccine prototype virus characterization is underway. If all steps of synthetic vaccine virus generation occurred within a vaccine manufacturing facility on the substrate used for vaccine production, virus generation, adaptation, characterization, and manufacturing adjustment activities could overlap more extensively, with savings in time.

The scientific aspects of synthetic vaccine virus technology are sufficiently well understood for routine use of the technology in influenza vaccine manufacturing. The key areas of focus to advance the technology are nonscientific. For example, implementation of robust quality systems is needed. To limit the amount of post-rescue processing and testing needed before use of synthetic viruses to produce a vaccine for human injection, all animal-sourced materials are being eliminated from the synthetic vaccine virus generation process. Systems of raw material and supplier management, standards of practice, validated assays, and rigorous documentation are being put in place to make newly rescued viruses suitable for immediate use in GMP influenza vaccine manufacturing. Despite these controls, the complicated decision-making around the selection of HA and NA genes to synthesize, the reconstruction of genome segment ends, and the adjustment of processes and assays to account for the biological variation between influenza virus strains will make vaccine virus synthesis, like many other aspects of influenza vaccine manufacturing, inevitably nonroutine. Collaboration between epidemiologists, bioinformaticians, virologists, engineers, and quality experts will be needed to carry out vaccine virus generation reliably in a manufacturing context.

A regulatory path for full implementation of synthetic vaccine virus seeds for pre-pandemic, pandemic, and seasonal vaccine manufacture must be established. The completion of the first clinical trial using a synthetic H7N9 vaccine seed virus under an Investigational New Drug application with the US Food and Drug Administration (FDA) has initiated the process (Bart et al. 2014). The mechanisms already in place to update existing influenza vaccine licenses for strain changes should facilitate the implementation of synthetic seed virus generation technology.

Biosafety and biosecurity issues involved in vaccine virus generation necessitate compliance with a complex web of regulation. In addition to regulation from national drug licensing authorities such as the FDA and European Medicines Agency (EMA), synthetic vaccine virus generation requires compliance with institutional biosafety rules, municipal public health regulations, recombinant DNA regulations, select agent regulations, dual use guidance, US Department of Agriculture (USDA) permitting, genetically modified organism regulations (in the EU), and regulations for shipping infectious agents internationally.

In the response to the H7N9 outbreak, delays in permitting by the US Department of Agriculture (USDA) forced much of the work to be done outside the US. The wild-type virus, which had caused severe human disease in China, was not pathogenic in birds (Abdelwhab et al. 2014). Nevertheless, its avian origin necessitated USDA permitting before the Novartis Holly Springs, North Carolina influenza cell culture manufacturing facility could receive the attenuated vaccine virus from the Novartis Cambridge, Massachusetts research facility. The permit could not be obtained in time for the outbreak response. Fortunately, it was possible to ship the vaccine virus from the Novartis Cambridge Research facility to Phillips-Universität in Marburg, Germany (with a delay while the virus was held in customs in Frankfurt), to transfer the virus from the University BSL4 laboratory to the Novartis Marburg vaccine manufacturing facility after additional processing and testing was completed, and finally to ship the manufactured vaccine back to the United States for clinical testing and for supply to the US government's pre-pandemic vaccine stockpile. In addition to demonstrating the need for regulatory changes to make the system more conducive to protecting human health from zoonotic disease, this example also highlights the anticipated advantages of consolidating all functions, from gene synthesis to vaccine release, at a single facility and replacing the shipment of viruses with the emailing of gene sequences.

The 2009 H1N1 and 2013 H7N9 responses also highlight the important role of biosafety considerations in determining the pace of pandemic and outbreak responses. In 2009, mammalian cell culture technology allowed Novartis to be the first western vaccine manufacturer to launch clinical trials of a pandemic vaccine (Clark et al. 2009a). Clinical trial material was produced at biosafety level (BSL) three in the Marburg influenza cell culture manufacturing facility using a conventional vaccine virus [not considered a genetically modified organism (GMO)], while egg-based manufacturing facilities sat idle, waiting for authorities to downgrade the containment level for the H1N1 pandemic strain, which was not highly pathogenic. The open nature of egg-based manufacturing processes precluded vaccine production under BSL3 for most influenza vaccine manufacturers.

In the 2013 response to the H7N9 outbreak, just as USDA permitting in the US blocked early work on a vaccine at the Novartis Holly Springs influenza cell culture manufacturing facility, GMO regulations in Germany blocked manufacturing using the highest yielding H7N9 vaccine viruses at the Marburg manufacturing facility. The synthetic viruses were considered GMOs. The highest yielding virus, which had an alternative backbone, was judged a BSL3 agent by German authorities. Under existing permits, only BSL2 GMOs could be handled in the Novartis Marburg facility. As a result, a lower-yielding H7N9 vaccine virus that had a PR8 backbone and was considered a BSL2 agent was used to produce the vaccine. The downgrading of new potential pandemic viruses from BSL3 to BSL2 generally requires pathogenicity testing in ferrets (WHO 2013b). The availability of influenza seronegative ferrets of the recommended age is limited, particularly in outbreak situations, when there is high demand for the animals. Currently, pathogenicity testing requires a wild-type virus comparator that has been dose titrated in the animals and time-consuming pathologic examination of and virus isolation from harvested tissues. Thus, biosafety testing can cause considerable delays unless one is able to carry out vaccine virus generation and vaccine manufacturing in high containment facilities.

Biosecurity regulations in the US pose a risk to public health through their potential to block effective and timely outbreak and pandemic responses. In contrast to biosafety measures, which are intended to prevent unintended harm from exposure to or release of pathogens, biosecurity measures are intended to prevent the intentional misuse of highly pathogenic agents by individuals with malicious intent. Fortunately, the H1N1 and H7N9 viruses were not classified as highly pathogenic avian influenza (HPAI) strains. Had they been classified as HPAI, not only the virulent wild-type viruses, but also the highly attenuated vaccine viruses would initially have been classified as Select Agents, imposing extensive biosecurity requirements on the facilities, processes, and personnel practices needed for vaccine development and production (HHS and USDA 2012a, b, c).

Extensive experience has shown that reliably attenuated vaccine viruses targeting H5N1 HPAI can be made by removing the HA polybasic cleavage site and placing the NA and modified HA genes on vaccine genetic backbones (Steinhauer 1999). As of February 2014, 23 H5N1 vaccine viruses attenuated in this way were available for distribution from WHO CCs, and more such strains are being prepared to track the ongoing diversification of the subtype (WHO 2014a). With current regulations, vaccine viruses for HPAI can be excluded from select agent status after they are demonstrated to be attenuated through a series of tests, including pathogenicity testing in chickens (USDA 2004). However, for each new HPAI variant, the first vaccine virus generated is designated a select agent until attenuation for poultry is demonstrated experimentally and an administrative exemption is granted by the USDA. These steps can take months and delay vaccine development against high pathogenicity avian influenza strains with human pathogenic potential.

Any vaccine development or production using an attenuated vaccine virus for an HPAI strain that is conducted before a select agent exemption is granted must take place in a facility that meets biocontainment and biosecurity standards that are intended to safeguard against far more pathogenic infectious agents than any actually used in influenza vaccine production. The cost of implementing select agent standards for pre-pandemic or pandemic vaccine production would make production of seasonal vaccines in the same facility prohibitively expensive. Production of seasonal vaccines in the facilities that make pre-pandemic or pandemic influenza vaccines is necessary to maintain the facilities' readiness and economic viability. Therefore, changes in biosecurity regulations to allow presumptive exclusion from select agent status of influenza vaccine viruses with predictably attenuating modifications would increase pandemic preparedness.

To optimally protect human populations, biosecurity and rapid, effective vaccine responses are both necessary. The synthetic creation of viruses with pathogenic potential does, indeed, raise biosecurity issues and must be practiced responsibly within a framework of appropriate governance, compliance and transparency (Garfinkel et al. 2007). Controversial experiments that increased transmissibility between ferrets of H5N1 influenza viruses were not based on synthetic techniques but nevertheless increased concerns around the potential for harmful consequences from the generation of influenza viruses in the laboratory (Berns et al. 2012; Herfst et al. 2012; Imai et al. 2012). Although synthetic vaccine virus generation does not enable the creation of viruses that are fundamentally different from viruses that could be created with nonsynthetic reverse genetic technology, more virus variants can be created more quickly using gene synthesis. The increased speed and diversity possible through the application of synthetic techniques provide an advantage to those who seek to protect health by quickly developing countermeasures against natural or man-made, newly emerged biological threats. Those with malicious intent need not rush, as a perpetrator can choose the time of attack. It is, therefore, in the public interest that biosecurity regulations be crafted carefully to avoid unintended consequences that degrade our capability to respond rapidly to natural or human-made infectious diseases with countermeasures, such as vaccines, disproportionately to their degradation of the capabilities of bioterrorists.

Intellectual property and economic considerations are superimposed upon the quality, regulatory, biosafety, and biosecurity aspects of implementing synthetic vaccine virus technology. The intellectual property landscape for influenza reverse genetics is complex and raises economic barriers to the implementation of synthetic technologies (Marsh and Tannock 2005). Much of the underlying research to develop influenza reverse genetics was funded by the US government. Therefore, provision of reverse genetics-based products, such as pre-pandemic or pandemic vaccines, to the US government raises few intellectual property issues. However, seasonal influenza vaccines are primarily sold to non-US government entities, and intellectual property considerations and the commodity nature of the seasonal vaccine market create disincentives to make the investments needed to apply reverse-genetics technology, including synthetic technology, to the manufacture of these products. To be implemented rapidly, reliably, and at sufficient scale in an emergency, pandemic vaccine responses must be grounded in the processes and infrastructure of seasonal vaccine production (Rappuoli and Dormitzer 2012). Thus, intellectual property barriers to the implementation of new technologies for seasonal vaccine production also jeopardize their implementation for pandemic vaccine responses.

The use of synthetic vaccine viruses has raised a particularly complex set of issues regarding the implementation of the Pandemic Influenza Preparedness (PIP) Framework. Some nations have sought to control access to viruses isolated in their territories, asserting the sovereignty over biological resources recognized in the Convention on Biological Diversity (Fidler 2008). Influenza immunization is practiced almost exclusively in wealthy nations, leaving poorer nations with little direct benefit from openly sharing with the global community influenza viruses isolated in their territories (Stohr 2014). On May 24, 2011, lengthy multilateral talks to address the public health interests in open virus sharing and in distributing the benefits of pandemic influenza immunization more broadly resulted in the adoption of the PIP Framework by the World Health Assembly (WHO 2011). Under the PIP Framework, pre-pandemic or pandemic viruses and other biological materials are shared with vaccine manufacturers in exchange for manufacturers providing pandemic vaccines and other benefits to developing countries. As a probably unanticipated consequence, the PIP Framework has, in effect, changed the free exchange of vaccine viruses for public health purposes to a highly regulated market for pandemic and pre-pandemic vaccine viruses.

In the World Health Assembly deliberations, agreement was not reached on how the PIP Framework would apply to the sharing of influenza genetic sequence data. Because synthetic technology eliminates the need to share influenza viruses to make pandemic or other influenza vaccines, it challenges the assumptions that underlie the PIP Framework. Synthetic vaccine virus technology raises the question, for example, of whether PIP Framework requirements for benefit sharing should be triggered by manufacturers' use of gene sequences posted by the GISRS in publically accessible databases. On the one hand, if pandemic vaccine benefits are not shared with nations whose laboratories post influenza sequence data, some countries may refuse to share such data, impeding pandemic responses. On the other hand, claims of ownership over unmodified gene sequences found in nature are increasingly rejected by courts; establishing the origin of gene sequences freely exchanged over the Internet is impractical; and attempts to regulate or monitor the electronic flow of scientific communication could impose burdens that would inhibit basic research and vaccine development activities that are in the public interest (World Intellectual Property Organization 2007). The viability of the GISRS could even be affected by the outcome of the deliberations. As routine clinical diagnosis of respiratory infections shifts to more general sequence-based diagnostics that do not require pathogen isolation, the generation of influenza genetic sequence data is likely to shift from the GISRS to a more dispersed and heterogeneous set of laboratories (Sect. 6). If application of the PIP Framework to sequence data creates an incentive to delay the start of synthetic vaccine virus generation until relevant influenza sequences are available from sources other than the GISRS, the development of essential vaccines will be slowed. Creating disincentives to using influenza sequences from the GISRS but not from other sources could diminish the role of the GISRS and the level of support that it currently enjoys. The humanitarian and practical arguments for broadening the distribution of the benefits of immunization against pandemic and other influenza strains are compelling. Synthetic vaccine technology may necessitate that future benefit sharing regimens be based on the social responsibilities of nations and institutions rather than on an exchange of viruses for vaccines and other benefits.

8 Emerging Synthetic Influenza Vaccine Technologies

Automation of vaccine virus synthesis and the development of fully synthetic vaccines could further accelerate vaccine production. The chemical synthesis of oligonucleotides is already automated. Assembly of synthetic genes from oligonucleotides involves only a few basic operations—micro-pipetting, mixing, and incubation. These steps are highly amenable to robotic automation. This potential has inspired the concept of the digital-biological converter (DBC), a device that combines electronic data manipulation, oligonucleotide synthesis, and enzymatic gene assembly (Venter 2013). Digital-biological converters could greatly increase throughput by synthesizing many genes in parallel. They could increase accuracy by eliminating sources of human error. They could increase the accessibility of synthetic technology through the distribution of integrated units that are programmed remotely and need only be stocked with raw materials so that they can be operated by workers who, although well trained in biosafety procedures, need not be highly specialized scientists.

The next step of synthetic vaccine virus generation, transfection of HA and NA gene cassettes and backbone genes on plasmids, requires mammalian cell culture. Robotic, high throughput devices have been developed that transfect mammalian cells, harvest viruses, and analyze expressed proteins (Chung et al. 2008; Elsliger et al. 2010; Rines et al. 2006). Thus, the entire synthetic influenza vaccine virus generation process, from oligonucleotide synthesis to virus recovery from transfected cells, is amenable to automation. As new strains appear in the global stream of sequence information and are analyzed by bioinformatics algorithms for likelihood of antigenic change and increasing epidemiologic importance, DBCs can generate multiple coding sequence and genome segment terminal variants on multiple alternative vaccine backbones. The goal is to have already generated high-yielding vaccine viruses by the time that the importance of a new strain is recognized. The most challenging aspects of automated vaccine virus generation are likely to be the development of automated assays to select the most suitable viruses and the integration of quality control measures and robust documentation into the devices' operation.

The current use of synthetic technology for influenza vaccines is to create vaccine viruses, a key starting material for vaccine manufacturing but not vaccines themselves. A new vaccine technology in development, the SAM® vaccine technology, promises fully synthetic vaccines (Geall et al. 2012). The platform combines self-amplifying mRNA and a synthetic, liposomal, nonviral delivery system. SAM RNA is produced from a cell-free enzymatic transcription reaction, and it encodes the antigen of interest and an RNA-dependent RNA polymerase. The lipid delivery system provides efficient delivery of the RNA cargo to muscle cells at the site of injection and protection of the RNA from enzymatic degradation during delivery. After delivery, the mRNA directs the expression of the polymerase, which amplifies the RNA intra-cytoplasmically and launches expression of a subgenomic message that directs high-level target antigen expression. The replicating RNA appears to the innate immune system like a virus, triggering a robust adaptive immune response (Deering et al. 2014). The lack of any genes that encode a viral entry apparatus or capsid precludes efficient cell-to-cell-spread. The result is a vaccine that has the potent immunogenicity of viral vectored vaccines, without the risk of generating infectious virus during manufacturing, and also has the plug-and-play facility of a DNA vaccine, without the risk of genome integration after injection. In experimental animals, SAM vaccines are much more potent than DNA vaccines or nonamplifying RNA vaccines, eliciting seroconversion against a respiratory syncytial virus F glycoprotein antigen with as little as 10 ng of RNA (Geall et al. 2012). If SAM vaccines prove successful in human trials, they could be ideally suited to influenza immunization, facilitating rapid strain change without the process adjustments required to accommodate the differing characteristics of each new virus and HA.

Novartis and SGVI deployed this technology in the H7N9 response (Hekele et al. 2013). The synthetic HA and NA genes assembled two days after the H7N9 HA and NA gene coding sequences were posted on GISAID were used not only as substrates for vaccine virus rescue (Sect. 5) but also as substrates for SAM vaccine generation. A formulated SAM vaccine was generated eight days after the gene sequences were posted. The vaccine was used to immunize mice, generating an antiserum that confirmed expression of the H7 HA from MDCK cells infected with the synthetic vaccine virus. Although the synthetic vaccine virus and the synthetic SAM vaccine were generated at a similar pace, the production of the conventional vaccine required many more steps over the course of the next months, while the experimental SAM vaccine was ready for injection into laboratory animals.

The production of a SAM vaccine from a synthetic gene cassette simply requires additional enzymatic reactions and encapsulation in a lipid delivery system. No mammalian cell culture is required, eliminating the biological materials and processes in vaccine manufacturing that are most complex and difficult to control. Thus, the generation of SAM vaccine candidates could be fully automated and conducted in a highly parallelized manner. SAM vaccine production also promises to have a remarkably small physical footprint. Thus, if SAM technology proves itself in the clinic, the concept of the DBC can be extended to a mobile vaccine manufacturing unit, small enough to fit in a shipping container, remotely programmable, and capable of very rapid vaccine responses.

9 Conclusions

Combining direct metagenomic sequencing of respiratory specimens, digital sequence data transmission and analysis, chemical oligonucleotide synthesis, enzymatic gene assembly and error correction, reverse genetics influenza virus rescue, and purely biophysical vaccine potency release assays promises a radical simplification, acceleration, and improved targeting of conventional influenza vaccine manufacture (Table 1, Fig. 1). From the stream of influenza virus sequences, transmitted globally and analyzed continuously, vaccine viruses on high growth, attenuated backbones could be synthesized by DBCs. Rescued viruses could simultaneously be analyzed for antigenic identity with panels of ferret sera against pre-existing strains and evaluated for vaccine manufacturing suitability. Antigenic mismatches due to egg adaptive mutations, risk of adventitious agents from human respiratory secretions or chicken cloacal contents, and delays in transfer of viruses between institutions could be eliminated. Rather, high growth vaccine viruses could be available in advance of confirmation that a new strain is posing a global public health threat. With the development of DBCs, transfers of vaccine viruses between manufacturing sites could even be conducted electronically, with re-rescue at each site. If SAM technology fulfills its promise, pandemic vaccine batches could be produced from portable manufacturing devices deployed globally, based on electronic information transmitted from a synthetic virus reference laboratory. In combination, these technologies could greatly improve our ability to respond effectively to the continuous variation of influenza viruses and the consequent seasonal and pandemic disease threats. The new technologies will not make influenza vaccine manufacturing properly boring, but they could make it considerably more effective at protecting the human population.

Acknowledgments I thank the synthetic influenza vaccine virus, medical countermeasures, and SAM vaccine teams: P. Suphaphiphat, D. G. Gibson, D. E. Wentworth, T. B. Stockwell, M. A. Algire, N. Alperovich, M. Barro, D. M. Brown, S. Craig, B. M. Dattilo, E. A. Denisova, I. De Souza, M. Eickmann, V. G. Dugan, Hekele, A., S. Bertholet, J. Archer, G. Palladino, L. A. Brito, G. R. Otten, M. Brazzoli, S. Buccato, A. Bonci, D. Casini:, D. Maione, Z.-Q. Qi, J. E. Gill, N. C. Caiazza, J. Urano, B. Hubby, G. F. Gao, Y. Shu, E. De Gregorio, C. W. Mandl, E. C. Settembre, J. B. Ulmer, A. Verma, C. A. Shaw, A. Heckle, K. Banerjee, E. McGurrin, K. Lee, D. Hering, R. Deck, C. Salisbury, M. Mansoura, G. Bodle, L. Solon, M. Hohenboken, N. Kanesa-thasan, S. Fekete, R. May, J. Klock, S. Jauch, O. Brahim, J. Girompini, A. Rak, R. Orlandi, F. Porter, J. Chapman, Y. Cu, C. W. Beard, T. Krucker, D. T. O'Hagan, M. Singh, N. M. Valiante, S. W. Barnett, A. Ferrari, R. C. Gomila, L. Han, C. Judge, S. Mane, M. Matrosovich, C. Merryman, G. A. Palmer, T. Spencer, T. Strecker, H. Trusheim, J. Uhlendorff, Y. Wen, A. C. Yee, J. Zaveri, B. Zhou, S. Becker, A. Donabedian, P. W. Mason, J. I. Glass, A. J. Geall, R. Rappuoli, J. C. Venter. I thank K. Stohr for his careful review of the manuscript and insightful recommendations.

Funding

The work reviewed in this paper was supported in part by BARDA contract HHSO100201000061C and by funds from the Novartis Foundation.

Disclosure

PRD is a Novartis Vaccines employee and a Novartis shareholder.

References

Abdelwhab EM, Veits J, Mettenleiter TC (2014) Prevalence and control of H7 avian influenza viruses in birds and humans. Epidemiol Infect 142:896–920. doi:10.1017/S0950268813003324

Advisory Committee on Immunization Practices (2013) Prevention and control of influenza with vaccines: interim recommendations of the Advisory Committee on Immunization Practices (ACIP), 2013. MMWR Morb Mortal Wkly Rep 62:356

Alberini I, Del Tordello E, Fasolo A, Temperton NJ, Galli G, Gentile C, Montomoli E, Hilbert AK, Banzhoff A, Del Giudice G, Donnelly JJ, Rappuoli R, Capecchi B (2009) Pseudoparticle neutralization is a reliable assay to measure immunity and cross-reactivity to H5N1 influenza viruses. Vaccine 27:5998–6003. doi:10.1016/j.vaccine.2009.07.079

Ambrose CS, Levin MJ (2012) The rationale for quadrivalent influenza vaccines. Hum Vaccin Immunother 8:81–88. doi:10.4161/hv.8.1.17623

Bart SA, Hohenboken M, Della Cioppa G, Narasimhan V, Dormitzer PR, Kanesa-thasan N (2014) A cell culture-derived MF59 adjuvanted pandemic A/H7N9 vaccine is immunogenic in adults. Sci Transl Med 6:234ra55. doi:10.1126/scitranslmed.3008761

Bedford T, Suchard MA, Lemey P, Dudas G, Gregory V, Hay AJ, McCauley JW, Russell CA, Smith DJ, Rambaut A (2014) Integrating influenza antigenic dynamics with molecular evolution. Elife 3: e01914. doi: 10.7554/eLife.01914

Belongia EA, Kieke BA, Donahue JG, Greenlee RT, Balish A, Foust A, Lindstrom S, Shay DK, Marshfield Influenza Study Group (2009) Effectiveness of inactivated influenza vaccines varied substantially with antigenic match from the 2004-2005 season to the 2006-2007 season. J Infect Dis 199:159–167. doi: 10.1086/595861

Berns KI, Casadevall A, Cohen ML, Ehrlich SA, Enquist LW, Fitch JP, Franz DR, Fraser-Liggett CM, Grant CM, Imperiale MJ, Kanabrocki J, Keim PS, Lemon SM, Levy SB, Lumpkin JR, Miller JF, Murch R, Nance ME, Osterholm MT, Relman DA, Roth JA, Vidaver AK (2012) Policy: adaptations of avian flu virus are a cause for concern. Nature 482:153–154. doi:10.1038/482153a

Bibby K (2013) Metagenomic identification of viral pathogens. Trends Biotechnol 31:275–279. doi:10.1016/j.tibtech.2013.01.016

Bogner P, Capua I, Cox NJ, Lipman DJ (2006) A global initiative on sharing avian flu data. Nature 442:981–981. doi:10.1038/442981a

Centers for Disease Control and Prevention (2004a) Updated interim influenza vaccination recommendations–2004–05 influenza season. MMWR Morb Mortal Wkly Rep 53:1183–1184

Centers for Disease Control and Prevention (2004b) Preliminary assessment of the effectiveness of the 2003–04 inactivated influenza vaccine–Colorado, December 2003. MMWR Morb Mortal Wkly Rep 53:8–11

Centers for Disease Control and Prevention (2009) Swine influenza A (H1N1) infection in two children–Southern California, March–April 2009. MMWR Morb Mortal Wkly Rep 58:400–402

Centers for Disease Control and Prevention (2013) Interim adjusted estimates of seasonal influenza vaccine effectiveness—United States, Feb 2013. MMWR Morb Mortal Wkly Rep 62:119–123

Chung N, Locco L, Huff KW, Bartz S, Linsley PS, Ferrer M, Strulovici B (2008) An efficient and fully automated high-throughput transfection method for genome-scale siRNA screens. J Biomol Screen 13:142–148. doi:10.1177/1087057107312032

Clark TW, Pareek M, Hoschler K, Dillon H, Nicholson KG, Groth N, Stephenson I (2009a) Trial of 2009 influenza A (H1N1) monovalent MF59-adjuvanted vaccine. N Engl J Med 361:2424–2435. doi:10.1056/NEJMoa0907650

Clark TW, Pareek M, Hoschler K, Dillon H, Nicholson KG, Groth N, Stephenson I (2009b) Trial of influenza A (H1N1) 2009 monovalent MF59-adjuvanted vaccine—preliminary report. N Engl J Med 361. doi:10.1056/NEJMoa0907650

Committee for Proprietary Medicinal Products (2004) Guideline on submission of marketing authorization for pandemic influenza vaccines through the centralized procedure. http://www.ema.europa.eu/docs/en_GB/document_library/Scientific_guideline/2009/09/WC500003815.pdf

Committee on Standard Serological Procedures in Influenza Studies (1950) Agglutination-inhibition test proposed as a standard of reference in influenza diagnostic studies. J Immunol 65:347–353

Cox NJ (2013) Information for the vaccines and related biological products advisory committee, CBER, FDA. http://www.fda.gov/downloads/AdvisoryCommittees/CommitteesMeetingMaterials/BloodVaccinesandOtherBiologics/VaccinesandRelatedBiologicalProductsAdvisoryCommittee/UCM343326.pptx

Cox NJ (2014) Information for the vaccines and related biological products Advisory Committee, CBER, FDA. http://www.fda.gov/downloads/AdvisoryCommittees/CommitteesMeetingMaterials/BloodVaccinesandOtherBiologics/VaccinesandRelatedBiologicalProductsAdvisoryCommittee/UCM390700.pptx

Deering RP, Kommareddy S, Ulmer JB, Brito LA, Geall AJ (2014) Nucleic acid vaccines: prospects for non-viral delivery of mRNA vaccines. Expert Opin Drug Deliv 11:885–899. doi:10.1517/17425247.2014.901308

Dormitzer PR, Tsai TF, Del Giudice G (2012) New technologies for influenza vaccines. Hum Vaccin Immunother 8:45–58. doi:10.4161/hv.8.1.18859

Dormitzer PR, Suphaphiphat P, Gibson DG, Wentworth DE, Stockwell TB, Algire MA, Alperovich N, Barro M, Brown DM, Craig S, Dattilo BM, Denisova EA, De Souza I, Eickmann M, Dugan VG, Ferrari A, Gomila RC, Han L, Judge C, Mane S, Matrosovich M, Merryman C, Palladino G, Palmer GA, Spencer T, Strecker T, Trusheim H, Uhlendorff J, Wen Y, Yee AC, Zaveri J, Zhou B, Becker S, Donabedian A, Mason PW, Glass JI, Rappuoli R, Venter JC (2013) Synthetic generation of influenza vaccine viruses for rapid response to pandemics. Sci Transl Med 5:185ra68. doi:10.1126/scitranslmed.3006368

Elsliger MA, Deacon AM, Godzik A, Lesley SA, Wooley J, Wuthrich K, Wilson IA (2010) The JCSG high-throughput structural biology pipeline. Acta Crystallogr Sect F Struct Biol Cryst Commun 66:1137–1142. doi:10.1107/S1744309110038212

FDA, CBER (2010) Guidance for industry. Characterization and qualification of cell substrates and other biological materials used in the production of viral vaccines for infectious disease indications. http://www.fda.gov/downloads/BiologicsBloodVaccines/GuidanceCompliance RegulatoryInformation/Guidances/Vaccines/UCM202439.pdf

Fidler DP (2008) Influenza virus samples, international law, and global health diplomacy. Emerg Infect Dis 14:88–94. doi:10.3201/eid1401.070700

Finelli L (2013) Influenza activity update. http://www.fda.gov/downloads/AdvisoryCommittees/CommitteesMeetingMaterials/BloodVaccinesandOtherBiologics/VaccinesandRelatedBiologicalProductsAdvisoryCommittee/UCM343328.pptx

Francis T, Salk JE, Quilligan JJ (1947) Experience with vaccination against influenza in the spring of 1947: a preliminary report. Am J Public Health Nations Health 37:1013–1016

Fries LF, Smith GE, Glenn GM (2013) A recombinant virus-like particle influenza A (H7N9) vaccine. N Engl J Med 369:2564–2566. doi:10.1056/NEJMc1313186

Gao R, Cao B, Hu Y, Feng Z, Wang D, Hu W, Chen J, Jie Z, Qiu H, Xu K, Xu X, Lu H, Zhu W, Gao Z, Xiang N, Shen Y, He Z, Gu Y, Zhang Z, Yang Y, Zhao X, Zhou L, Li X, Zou S, Zhang Y, Yang L, Guo J, Dong J, Li Q, Dong L, Zhu Y, Bai T, Wang S, Hao P, Yang W, Han J, Yu H, Li D, Gao GF, Wu G, Wang Y, Yuan Z, Shu Y (2013) Human infection with a novel avian-origin influenza A (H7N9) virus. N Engl J Med 368:1888–1897. doi:10.1056/NEJMoa1304459

Garfinkel MS, Endy D, Epstein GL, Friedman RM (2007) Synthetic genomics options for governance. Biosecur Bioterror 5:359–362. doi:10.1089/bsp.2007.0923

Geall AJ, Verma A, Otten GR, Shaw CA, Hekele A, Banerjee K, Cu Y, Beard CW, Brito LA, Krucker T, O'Hagan DT, Singh M, Mason PW, Valiante NM, Dormitzer PR, Barnett SW, Rappuoli R, Ulmer JB, Mandl CW (2012) Nonviral delivery of self-amplifying RNA vaccines. Proc Natl Acad Sci USA 109:14604–14609. doi:10.1073/pnas.1209367109

Ghendon YZ, Polezhaev FI, Lisovskaya KV, Medvedeva TE, Alexandrova GI, Klimov AI (1984) Recombinant cold-adapted attenuated influenza A vaccines for use in children: molecular genetic analysis of the cold-adapted donor and recombinants. Infect Immun 44:730–733

Gibson DG, Glass JI, Lartigue C, Noskov VN, Chuang RY, Algire MA, Benders GA, Montague MG, Ma L, Moodie MM, Merryman C, Vashee S, Krishnakumar R, Assad-Garcia N, Andrews-Pfannkoch C, Denisova EA, Young L, Qi ZQ, Segall-Shapiro TH, Calvey CH, Parmar PP, Hutchison CA 3rd, Smith HO, Venter JC (2010a) Creation of a bacterial cell controlled by a chemically synthesized genome. Science 329:52–56. doi:10.1126/science.1190719

Gibson DG, Smith HO, Hutchison CA 3rd, Venter JC, Merryman C (2010b) Chemical synthesis of the mouse mitochondrial genome. Nat Methods 7:901–903. doi:10.1038/nmeth.1515

Gomila RC, Suphaphiphat P, Judge C, Spencer T, Ferrari A, Wen Y, Palladino G, Dormitzer PR, Mason PW (2013) Improving influenza virus backbones by including terminal regions of MDCK-adapted strains on hemagglutinin and neuraminidase gene segments. Vaccine 31:4736–4743. doi:10.1016/j.vaccine.2013.08.026

Grohskopf L (2011) U.S. influenza surveillance, VRBPAC meeting. http://www.fda.gov/downloads/AdvisoryCommittees/CommitteesMeetingMaterials/BloodVaccinesandOtherBiologics/VaccinesandRelatedBiologicalProductsAdvisoryCommittee/UCM246396.pptx

Grohskopf L (2012) U.S. Influenza surveillance, 2011–2012 season. http://www.fda.gov/downloads/AdvisoryCommittees/CommitteesMeetingMaterials/BloodVaccinesandOtherBiologics/VaccinesandRelatedBiologicalProductsAdvisoryCommittee/UCM297004.pptx

Harvey R, Guilfoyle KA, Roseby S, Robertson JS, Engelhardt OG (2011) Improved antigen yield in pandemic H1N1 (2009) candidate vaccine viruses with chimeric hemagglutinin molecules. J Virol 85:6086–6090. doi:10.1128/JVI.00096-11

Hekele A, Bertholet S, Archer J, Gibson DG, Palladino G, Brito LA, Otten GR, Brazzoli M, Buccato S, Bonci A, Casini: D, Maione D, Qi Z-Q, Gill JE, Caiazza NC, Urano J, Hubby B, Gao GF, Shu Y, De Gregorio E, Mandl CW, Mason PW, Settembre EC, Ulmer JB, Venter JC, Dormitzer PR, Rappuoli R, Geall AJ (2013) Rapidly produced SAM® vaccine against H7N9 influenza is immunogenic in mice. Emerg Microb Infect 2:e52

Herfst S, Schrauwen EJ, Linster M, Chutinimitkul S, de Wit E, Munster VJ, Sorrell EM, Bestebroer TM, Burke DF, Smith DJ, Rimmelzwaan GF, Osterhaus AD, Fouchier RA (2012) Airborne transmission of influenza A/H5N1 virus between ferrets. Science 336:1534–1541. doi:10.1126/science.1213362

HHS, USDA (2012a) Title 7: Agriculture. Part 331—possession, use, and transfer of select agents and toxins. In: US Departments of Health and Human Services (HHS) and Agriculture (USDA) 7 C.F.R part 331

HHS, USDA (2012b) Title 9: animals and animal products. Part 121—possession, use, and transfer of select agents and toxins. In: US Departments of Health and Human Services (HHS) and Agriculture (USDA) 9 C.F.R part 121

HHS, USDA (2012c) Title 42: public health. Part 73—select agents and toxins. In: US Departments of Health and Human Services (HHS) and Agriculture (USDA) 42 C.F.R part 73

Hoffmann E, Neumann G, Kawaoka Y, Hobom G, Webster RG (2000) A DNA transfection system for generation of influenza A virus from eight plasmids. Proc Natl Acad Sci USA 97:6108–6113. doi:10.1073/pnas.100133697

Imai M, Watanabe T, Hatta M, Das SC, Ozawa M, Shinya K, Zhong G, Hanson A, Katsura H, Watanabe S, Li C, Kawakami E, Yamada S, Kiso M, Suzuki Y, Maher EA, Neumann G, Kawaoka Y (2012) Experimental adaptation of an influenza H5 HA confers respiratory droplet transmission to a reassortant H5 HA/H1N1 virus in ferrets. Nature 486:420–428. doi:10.1038/nature10831

Katz JM, Wang M, Webster RG (1990) Direct sequencing of the HA gene of influenza (H3N2) virus in original clinical samples reveals sequence identity with mammalian cell-grown virus. J Virol 64:1808–1811

Kilbourne ED (1969) Future influenza vaccines and the use of genetic recombinants. Bull World Health Organ 41:643–645

Kishida N, Fujisaki S, Yokoyama M, Sato H, Saito R, Ikematsu H, Xu H, Takashita E, Tashiro M, Takao S, Yano T, Suga T, Kawakami C, Yamamoto M, Kajiyama K, Saito H, Shimada S, Watanabe S, Aoki S, Taira K, Kon M, Lin JH, Odagiri T (2012) Evaluation of influenza virus A/H3N2 and B vaccines on the basis of cross-reactivity of postvaccination human serum antibodies against influenza viruses A/H3N2 and B isolated in MDCK cells and embryonated hen eggs. Clin Vaccine Immunol 19:897–908. doi:10.1128/CVI.05726-11

Landry N, Ward BJ, Trepanier S, Montomoli E, Dargis M, Lapini G, Vezina LP (2010) Preclinical and clinical development of plant-made virus-like particle vaccine against avian H5N1 influenza. PLoS One 5:e15559. doi:10.1371/journal.pone.0015559

Lemey P, Rambaut A, Bedford T, Faria N, Bielejec F, Baele G, Russell CA, Smith DJ, Pybus OG, Brockmann D, Suchard MA (2014) Unifying viral genetics and human transportation data to predict the global transmission dynamics of human influenza H3N2. PLoS Pathog 10:e1003932. doi:10.1371/journal.ppat.1003932

Maassab HF, Francis T Jr, Davenport FM, Hennessy AV, Minuse E, Anderson G (1969) Laboratory and clinical characteristics of attenuated strains of influenza virus. Bull World Health Organ 41:589–594

Marsh GA, Tannock GA (2005) The role of reverse genetics in the development of vaccines against respiratory viruses. Expert Opin Biol Ther 5:369–380. doi:10.1517/14712598.5.3.369

Ndifon W, Dushoff J, Levin SA (2009) On the use of hemagglutination-inhibition for influenza surveillance: surveillance data are predictive of influenza vaccine effectiveness. Vaccine 27:2447–2452. doi:10.1016/j.vaccine.2009.02.047

Nicolson C, Major D, Wood JM, Robertson JS (2005) Generation of influenza vaccine viruses on Vero cells by reverse genetics: an H5N1 candidate vaccine strain produced under a quality system. Vaccine 23:2943–2952. doi:10.1016/j.vaccine.2004.08.054

Onions D, Egan W, Jarrett R, Novicki D, Gregersen JP (2010) Validation of the safety of MDCK cells as a substrate for the production of a cell-derived influenza vaccine. Biologicals 38:544–551. doi:10.1016/j.biologicals.2010.04.003

Orsi A, Ansaldi F, de Florentiis D, Ceravolo A, Parodi V, Canepa P, Coppelli M, Icardi G, Durando P (2013) Cross-protection against drifted influenza viruses: options offered by adjuvanted and intradermal vaccines. Hum Vaccin Immunother 9:582–590

Rappuoli R, Dormitzer PR (2012) Influenza: options to improve pandemic preparation. Science 336:1531–1533. doi:10.1126/science.1221466

Rines DR, Tu B, Miraglia L, Welch GL, Zhang J, Hull MV, Orth AP, Chanda SK (2006) High-content screening of functional genomic libraries. Methods Enzymol 414:530–565. doi:10.1016/S0076-6879(06)14028-8

Robertson JS, Nicolson C, Harvey R, Johnson R, Major D, Guilfoyle K, Roseby S, Newman R, Collin R, Wallis C, Engelhardt OG, Wood JM, Le J, Manojkumar R, Pokorny BA, Silverman J, Devis R, Bucher D, Verity E, Agius C, Camuglia S, Ong C, Rockman S, Curtis A, Schoofs P, Zoueva O, Xie H, Li X, Lin Z, Ye Z, Chen LM, O'Neill E, Balish A, Lipatov AS, Guo Z, Isakova I, Davis CT, Rivailler P, Gustin KM, Belser JA, Maines TR, Tumpey TM, Xu X, Katz JM, Klimov A, Cox NJ, Donis RO (2011) The development of vaccine viruses against pandemic A(H1N1) influenza. Vaccine 29:1836–1843. doi:10.1016/j.vaccine.2010.12.044

Roth B, Mohr H, Enders M, Garten W, Gregersen JP (2012) Isolation of influenza viruses in MDCK 33016PF cells and clearance of contaminating respiratory viruses. Vaccine 30:517–522. doi:10.1016/j.vaccine.2011.11.063

Schild GC, Wood JM, Newman RW (1975) A single-radial-immunodiffusion technique for the assay of influenza haemagglutinin antigen. Proposals for an assay method for the haemagglutinin content of influenza vaccines. Bull World Health Organ 52:223–231

Schild GC, Oxford JS, de Jong JC, Webster RG (1983) Evidence for host-cell selection of influenza virus antigenic variants. Nature 303:706–709

Shinya K, Ebina M, Yamada S, Ono M, Kasai N, Kawaoka Y (2006) Avian flu: influenza virus receptors in the human airway. Nature 440:435–436

Skowronski DM, Janjua NZ, De Serres G, Sabaiduc S, Eshaghi A, Dickinson JA, Fonseca K, Winter AL, Gubbay JB, Krajden M, Petric M, Charest H, Bastien N, Kwindt TL, Mahmud SM, Van Caeseele P, Li Y (2014) Low 2012–13 influenza vaccine effectiveness associated with mutation in the egg-adapted H3N2 vaccine strain not antigenic drift in circulating viruses. PLoS One 9:e92153. doi:10.1371/journal.pone.0092153

Smith DJ, Lapedes AS, de Jong JC, Bestebroer TM, Rimmelzwaan GF, Osterhaus AD, Fouchier RA (2004) Mapping the antigenic and genetic evolution of influenza virus. Science 305:371–376. doi:10.1126/science.1097211

Steinhauer DA (1999) Role of hemagglutinin cleavage for the pathogenicity of influenza virus. Virology 258:1–20. doi:10.1006/viro.1999.9716

Stevens J, Chen LM, Carney PJ, Garten R, Foust A, Le J, Pokorny BA, Manojkumar R, Silverman J, Devis R, Rhea K, Xu X, Bucher DJ, Paulson JC, Cox NJ, Klimov A, Donis RO (2010) Receptor specificity of influenza A H3N2 viruses isolated in mammalian cells and embryonated chicken eggs. J Virol 84:8287–8299. doi:10.1128/JVI.00058-10

Stohr K (2013) Influenza vaccine production. In: Webster RG, Monto AS, Braciale TJ, Lamb RA (eds) Textbook of influenza, 2nd edn. Wiley, West Sussex, pp 352–372

Stohr K (2014) Perspective: Ill prepared for a pandemic. Nature 507:S20–S21

Strecker T, Uhlendorff J, Diederich S, Lenz-Bauer C, Trusheim H, Roth B, Kolesnikova L, Aepinus C, Dornow R, Gerlach J, Matrosovich M, Valley U, Eickmann M, Becker S (2012) Exploring synergies between academia and vaccine manufacturers: a pilot study on how to rapidly produce vaccines to combat emerging pathogens. Clin Chem Lab Med 50:1275–1279. doi:10.1515/cclm-2011-0650

Subbarao K, Chen H, Swayne D, Mingay L, Fodor E, Brownlee G, Xu X, Lu X, Katz J, Cox N, Matsuoka Y (2003) Evaluation of a genetically modified reassortant H5N1 influenza A virus vaccine candidate generated by plasmid-based reverse genetics. Virology 305:192–200

Suphaphiphat P, Keiner B, Trusheim H, Crotta S, Tuccino AB, Zhang P, Dormitzer PR, Mason PW, Franti M (2010) Human RNA polymerase I-driven reverse genetics for influenza a virus in canine cells. J Virol 84:3721–3725. doi:10.1128/JVI.01925-09

Tizzoni M, Bajardi P, Poletto C, Ramasco JJ, Balcan D, Goncalves B, Perra N, Colizza V, Vespignani A (2012) Real-time numerical forecast of global epidemic spreading: case study of 2009 A/H1N1pdm. BMC Med 10:165. doi:10.1186/1741-7015-10-165

Treanor JJ, El Sahly H, King J, Graham I, Izikson R, Kohberger R, Patriarca P, Cox M (2011) Protective efficacy of a trivalent recombinant hemagglutinin protein vaccine (FluBlok(R)) against influenza in healthy adults: a randomized, placebo-controlled trial. Vaccine 29:7733–7739. doi:10.1016/j.vaccine.2011.07.128

Tricco AC, Chit A, Soobiah C, Hallett D, Meier G, Chen MH, Tashkandi M, Bauch CT, Loeb M (2013) Comparing influenza vaccine efficacy against mismatched and matched strains: a systematic review and meta-analysis. BMC Med 11:153. doi:10.1186/1741-7015-11-153

US Food and Drug Administration (2007) Guidance—emergency use authorization of medical products. http://www.fda.gov/RegulatoryInformation/Guidances/ucm125127.htm

USDA (2004) Data necessary to consider select agent exclusion requests attenuated strains of highly pathogenic avian influenza (HPAI) viruses. http://www.selectagents.gov/resources/DataRequirementsforExclusionConsideration.pdf

Venter JC (2013) Life at the speed of light. Viking, The Penguin Group, New York

Wang Z, Duke GM (2007) Cloning of the canine RNA polymerase I promoter and establishment of reverse genetics for influenza A and B in MDCK cells. Virol J 4:102. doi:10.1186/1743-422X-4-102

Wei CJ, Boyington JC, Dai K, Houser KV, Pearce MB, Kong WP, Yang ZY, Tumpey TM, Nabel GJ (2010) Cross-neutralization of 1918 and 2009 influenza viruses: role of glycans in viral evolution and vaccine design. Sci Transl Med 2:24ra21

WHO (2011) Pandemic influenza preparedness framework for the sharing of influenza viruses and access to vaccine and other benefits. http://whqlibdoc.who.int/publications/2011/9789241503082_eng.pdf

WHO (2012) Recommended composition of influenza virus vaccines for use in the 2013 southern hemisphere influenza season. http://www.who.int/influenza/vaccines/virus/recommendations/201209recommendation.pdf

WHO (2013a) Recommended composition of influenza virus vaccines for use in the 2013–2014 northern hemisphere influenza season. http://www.who.int/influenza/vaccines/virus/recommendations/201302_recommendation.pdf

WHO (2013b) Update of WHO biosafety risk assessment and guidelines for the production and quality control of human influenza vaccines against avian influenza A(H7N9) virus. As of 23 May 2013 (replaces version of 10 May 2013). http://www.who.int/biologicals/BIOSAFETY_RISK_ASSESSMENT_21_MAY_2013.pdf

WHO (2014a) Antigenic and genetic characteristics of zoonotic influenza viruses and development of candidate vaccine viruses for pandemic preparedness. http://www.who.int/influenza/vaccines/virus/201402_h5h7h9h10_vaccinevirusupdate.pdf

WHO (2014b) Confirmed human cases of avian influenza A(H7N9) reported to WHO. Report 15—data in WHO/HQ as of 11 March 2014 17:00 GMT+1. http://www.who.int/influenza/human_animal_interface/influenza_h7n9/15_ReportWebH7N9Number_20140311.pdf?ua=1

WHO (2014c) Recommended composition of influenza virus vaccines for use in the 2014–2015 northern hemisphere influenza season. http://www.who.int/influenza/vaccines/virus/recommendations/201402recommendation.pdf?ua=1

WHO (2014d) Summary of status of development and availability of avian influenza A(H7N9) candidate vaccine viruses and potency testing reagents. http://www.who.int/influenza/vaccines/virus/candidates_reagents/summary_a_h7n9_cvv_20140213.pdf?ua=1

WHO Writing Group, Ampofo WK, Baylor N, Cobey S, Cox NJ, Daves S, Edwards S, Ferguson N, Grohmann G, Hay A, Katz J, Kullabutr K, Lambert L, Levandowski R, Mishra AC, Monto A, Siqueira M, Tashiro M, Waddell AL, Wairagkar N, Wood J, Zambon M, Zhang W (2012) Improving influenza vaccine virus selection: report of a WHO informal consultation held at WHO headquarters, Geneva, Switzerland, 14–16 June 2010. Influenza Respir Viruses 6:142–152, e1–5. doi:10.1111/j.1750-2659.2011.00277.x

Widjaja L, Ilyushina N, Webster RG, Webby RJ (2006) Molecular changes associated with adaptation of human influenza A virus in embryonated chicken eggs. Virology 350:137–145

Williams TL, Luna L, Guo Z, Cox NJ, Pirkle JL, Donis RO, Barr JR (2008) Quantification of influenza virus hemagglutinins in complex mixtures using isotope dilution tandem mass spectrometry. Vaccine 26:2510–2520

World Intellectual Property Organization (2007) Working paper—patent issues related to influenza viruses and their genes. http://www.wipo.int/export/sites/www/policy/en/global_health/pdf/influenza.pdf

Yongfeng H, Fan Y, Jie D, Jian Y, Ting Z, Lilian S, Jin Q (2011) Direct pathogen detection from swab samples using a new high-throughput sequencing technology. Clin Microbiol Infect 17:241–244. doi:10.1111/j.1469-0691.2010.03246.x

Zimmer SM, Burke DS (2009) Historical perspective–emergence of influenza A (H1N1) viruses. N Engl J Med 361:279–285. doi:10.1056/NEJMra0904322

Influenza Neuraminidase as a Vaccine Antigen

Maryna C. Eichelberger and Hongquan Wan

Abstract Neuraminidase (NA) is the second most abundant influenza surface glycoprotein and contributes to virus replication in several ways, most notably by removing sialic acids from the host and viral glycoproteins, releasing newly formed virus particles from infected cells. Antibodies that block this enzyme activity restrict virus replication in vitro. This chapter describes foundational epidemiologic and human influenza challenge studies that provide evidence of an association between NA inhibiting antibodies and resistance to disease. Mouse challenge studies show that while NA immunity is infection-permissive, NA-specific antibodies attenuate infection and prevent severe disease. NA immunity is most effective against homologous viruses but there is substantial protection against viruses with a heterologous NA (different lineage within a NA subtype). Monoclonal antibodies specific for conserved antigenic domains of subtype N1 protect against seasonal and pandemic H1N1 as well as H5N1 virus challenge. Clinical studies demonstrate that licensed seasonal vaccines contain immunogenic amounts of NA, but the contribution of this immunity to vaccine efficacy is currently not known. New types of influenza vaccines could be designed to elicit NA immunity. Because NA induces heterologous immunity, it could be an important constituent of universal influenza vaccines that aim to protect against unexpected emerging viruses.

Abbreviations

ELISA	Enzyme-linked immunosorbent assay
ELLA	Enzyme-linked lectin assay
HA	Hemagglutinin

M.C. Eichelberger (✉) · H. Wan
Division of Viral Products, Office of Vaccine Research and Review,
Center for Biologics Research and Regulation, US Food and Drug Administration,
HFM445, Silver Spring, MD 20892, USA
e-mail: Maryna.Eichelberger@fda.hhs.gov

H. Wan
e-mail: Hongquan.Wan@fda.hhs.gov

Current Topics in Microbiology and Immunology (2015) 386: 275–299
DOI: 10.1007/82_2014_398

Published Online: 18 July 2014

HI	Hemagglutination inhibition
NA	Neuraminidase
NI	Neuraminidase inhibition/inhibiting
TBA	Thiobarbituric acid
VLP	Virus-like particle

Contents

1 Introduction

Past studies have demonstrated an impact of neuraminidase (NA)-specific antibodies on resistance to influenza and urged consideration of NA as a vaccine antigen. Studies conducted shortly after the 1968 pandemic in which the circulating H2N2 virus was replaced by an H3N2 virus showed that NA inhibiting (NI) antibodies were associated with resistance against disease (Monto and Kendal 1973; Murphy et al. 1972). While it was clear that these antibodies did not inhibit virus attachment and entry, Kilbourne and Couch recognized the potential benefit of non-neutralizing immunity that would be provided by a NA vaccine, explaining that although infection would not be prevented, the antibodies elicited to NA would attenuate virus replication, resulting in mild disease symptoms which would in turn allow induction of a robust durable strain-specific immune response (Couch et al. 1974; Kilbourne 1972).

Monto and Kendal advised that induction of anti-NA antibodies by influenza vaccines would maximize protection against clinical disease (Monto and Kendal 1973). They pointed out the genetic independence of HA and NA, noting that this may provide the means to induce protection against emerging pandemic strains that share the same NA subtype as the previously circulating virus. The breadth of this protection was addressed in murine studies performed by Schulman and Kilbourne—effective NA immunity was observed against viruses with the homologous NA antigen, and in addition, there was significant protection against influenza strains that had a heterologous NA antigen (Schulman et al. 1968).

Recent appreciation for the broad immunity offered by NA-specific antibodies stems from the need to develop vaccines against avian influenza H5N1 viruses (Gillim-Ross and Subbarao 2007). The demonstration that NA-specific antibodies against seasonal H1N1 viruses provide some protection against lethal H5N1 challenge in mice (Sandbulte et al. 2007) provides evidence that induction of NA immunity may be a good pandemic vaccine strategy. Although progress has been made toward developing a vaccine with standardized amounts of NA, several obstacles still need to be overcome. For example, a practical assay for routine measurement of serologic responses to NA can be used to assess the immunogenicity of NA in investigational vaccines, but the significance of these data cannot be interpreted because the titer that correlates with protection against disease has not been determined.

This chapter focuses on NA-specific immunity mediated by antibodies and will only briefly mention the potential contribution of NA-specific T cells to immunity. The following sections describe the role that NA plays in viral replication, the antigenic structure of NA, early studies showing an association between NA immunity and resistance against disease, and more recent studies showing protection against seasonal and pandemic viruses by NI antibodies. The NA content of experimental and licensed vaccines is addressed and the progress that has been made to support further development of NA-based vaccines is described throughout the text.

2 NA Structure and Function

NA is present on virions and the infected cell surface as a homotetramer, with each subunit containing an enzyme active site. The native tetramer is required for enzyme activity and it is this native form of NA that induces enzyme-inhibiting antibodies—NI antibodies are not elicited to denatured molecules. Since only the NA tetramer exhibits enzyme activity, this functional property correlates with immunogenicity (Brett and Johansson 2006; Sultana et al. 2011). Enzyme activity itself, however, is not required for induction of an antibody response as robust NI titers can be induced in the presence of antivirals that inhibit enzyme activity (Sultana et al. 2011). It may be difficult to produce monomers or even dimers of NA with native antigenic structure and enzyme activity because of the multiple inter-subunit interactions (Ca^{2+} (Brett and Johansson 2006; Chong et al. 1991; Johansson and Brett 2003), a salt bridge (Colacino et al. 1997), disulfide bonds (Saito et al. 1995) and carbohydrate groups (Wu et al. 2009)) that stabilize the quaternary structure.

NA structure has been defined at a molecular level for many different subtypes—N1 of 1918 H1N1 (Xu et al. 2008), 2009 H1N1 pandemic (Li et al. 2010), and H5N1 (Russell et al. 2006) viruses, N2 (Varghese and Colman 1991), N4 (Russell et al. 2006), N5 (Wang et al. 2011), N6 (Russell et al. 2006), N8 (Russell et al. 2006), N9 (Tulip et al. 1991), and N10 (Li et al. 2012; Zhu et al. 2012) as well as influenza B (Burmeister et al. 1992). NAs of influenza A and B share the same structural and enzyme active site elements—each monomer is composed of a 6-bladed propeller structure with each blade composed of four antiparallel beta sheets stabilized by disulfide bonds and connected by flexible loops. The enzyme active site is a cavity comprised of highly conserved amino acids, some of which contact substrate while others hold these contact amino acids in a fairly rigid structure. The structural domains of NA, including the enzyme active site and antigenic epitopes, are reviewed and illustrated in Air (2012).

There is less NA than HA on the surface of influenza virus particles, however the proportion is virus-specific. Most viruses have an HA:NA ratio of ~5:1, but this ratio is ~2:1 in the 2009 H1N1pdm virus (Getie-Kebtie et al. 2013). NA activity is essential for virus replication, playing a role at several different points of the virus life cycle (Fig. 1). NA facilitates access to respiratory tract epithelial cells by allowing release of virions from decoy receptors present on mucins (Matrosovich et al. 2004). This receptor-destroying activity most likely does not prevent HA binding and infection because the small amount of NA appears to be segregated from HA on the virus surface (Calder et al. 2010). NA is essential for release of nascent virus particles, with inadequate enzyme activity resulting in reduced plaque size due to inefficient cell-to-cell spread (Kilbourne et al. 1968). This activity also prevents aggregation of virions by removing sialic acids (receptors) from its own glycoproteins (Palese et al. 1974). This may explain the association between NA activity and transmissibility (Lakdawala et al. 2011; Yen et al. 2011) since non-aggregated virions are more likely to be transmitted in small aerosol droplets that are inhaled into the lower respiratory tract.

3 Antigenic Domains of NA

The NA antigens of influenza A and B viruses are genetically and serologically distinct. NA subtypes of influenza A viruses can also be distinguished by sequence or antigenic analysis. Within each NA subtype there are genetically different heterologous lineages that are serologically distinct. For example, the NA of seasonal H1N1, 2009 H1N1pdm, and H5N1 viruses differ in reactivity with ferret antisera against each virus—however, there is a small but measurable degree of

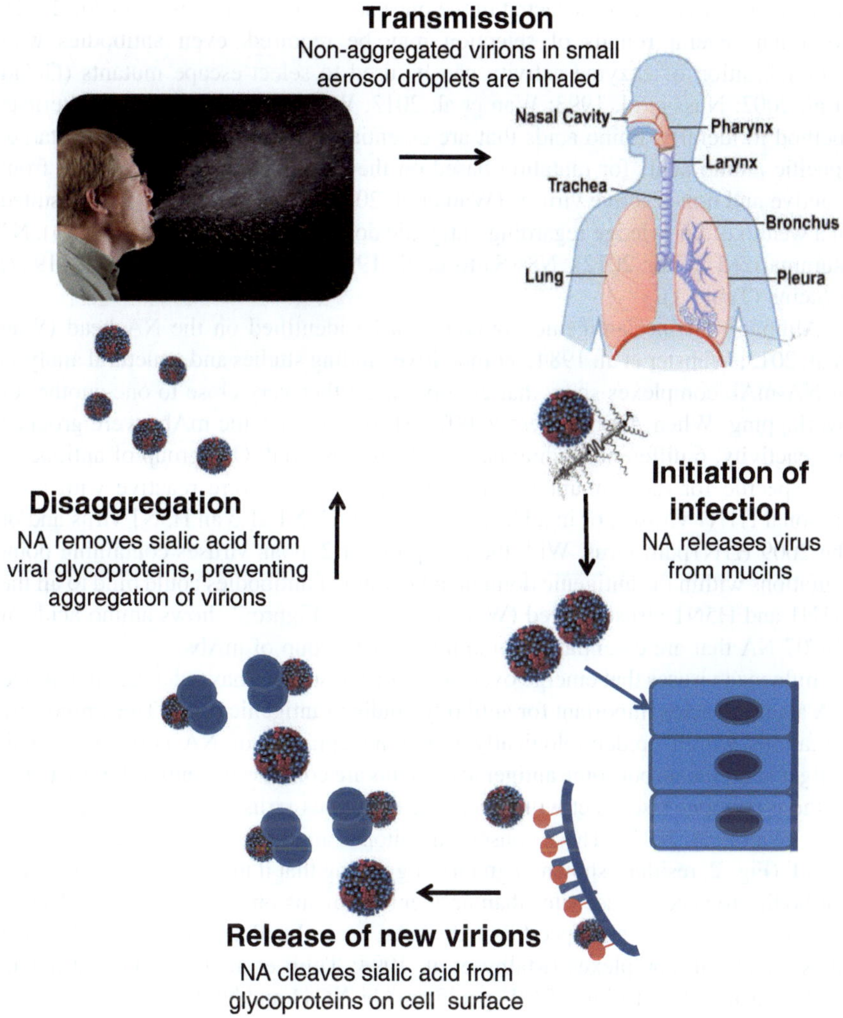

Fig. 1 NA plays a role at different points of the influenza virus life cycle (1) initiation of infection by releasing virions from decoy receptors on mucins; (2) release of newly formed virions from infected cells by cleaving sialic acids from the cell surface; (3) disaggregation or preventing aggregation of virus particles by removing sialic acids from viral glycoproteins; (4) preventing formation of aggregates also increases the opportunity for aerosol transmission

cross-reactivity (Chen et al. 2012). Analyses with polyclonal sera therefore suggest that NA contains immunodominant strain-specific epitopes in addition to some conserved epitopes to which broadly reactive antibodies can bind.

Antibodies that inhibit NA activity efficiently bind to conformational epitopes on the 'head' of each monomer. Amino acids that are critical for binding of monoclonal antibodies (mAbs) that inhibit enzyme activity have been identified by sequencing virus variants selected in the presence of mAbs (reviewed in Air 2012). Although several rounds of selection may be required, even antibodies with poor inhibition of enzyme activity can be used to select escape mutants (Gulati et al. 2002; Nuss et al. 1993; Wan et al. 2013; Webster et al. 1984). An alternate method to identify amino acids that are essential for antibody binding is to target specific amino acids for mutation based on the alignment of NA sequences from reactive and non-reactive viruses (Wan et al. 2013). These strategies have resulted in a wealth of knowledge regarding antigenic domains of N1 (Wan et al. 2013), N2 (summarized in Air 2012), N8 (Saito et al. 1994) and N9 (Webster et al. 1987) proteins (Table 1).

Although distinct antigenic domains can be identified on the NA head (Wan et al. 2013; Webster et al. 1984), competitive binding studies and structural analysis of NA-mAb complexes show that epitopes are either very close to one another or overlapping. When A/Brisbane/59/2007 (BR/07) N1-specific mAbs were grouped by reactivity, 6 different binding patterns were observed. One group of antibodies was specific for the immunizing antigen, other groups were reactive with most seasonal H1N1 viruses, or in addition to seasonal H1N1 also an H5N1 virus and/or the 2009 H1N1pdm virus. With the exception of 2 avian viruses containing point mutations within the antigenic domain, one group of antibodies could bind to all the H1N1 and H5N1 viruses tested (Wan et al. 2013). Figure 2 shows amino acids of BR/07 NA that are essential for binding of each group of mAbs.

Influenza viruses that emerge over the course of seasons have changes in HA and NA at amino acids important for antibody binding (antigenic drift). The amino acid mutations within epidemiologically important epitopes of NA correspond with antigenic domains, but some antigenic domains are conserved—antibodies that bind to these epitopes also react with distant heterologous viruses within the same subtype (Wan et al. 2013). These conserved epitopes are on the lateral face of the NA 'head' (Fig. 2, residues shown in green), suggesting that it may be more difficult for antibodies to access these sites than antigenic domains on the top of the molecule.

The epitopes of 3 NA-specific mAbs have been elucidated by x-ray diffraction of NA and Fab complexes (Malby et al. 1994; Tulip et al. 1992; Venkatramani et al. 2006). The footprints of N9-specific mAbs NC41 and NC10 show that a large overlapping surface area of NA is buried when these antibodies bind, but the molecular interactions between antigen and antibody in each case is distinct. The epitope of a N2-specific antibody shows an expansive discontinuous footprint with a network of water molecules mediating H-bonds that stabilize the interaction. Interestingly, the single amino acid at position 199 that is essential for antibody binding forms a direct H-bond with CDR3 of the antibody heavy chain. The structure of the antigen in complex with antibody is not significantly altered and in all cases it appears that antibodies inhibit enzyme activity by steric hindrance, reducing access of the large natural substrate to the active site.

Further studies of antibody-NA complexes to define the specificities and binding avidities of antibodies that inhibit enzyme activity are warranted as the information can be used to facilitate the design and evaluation of NA-containing vaccines.

Table 1 Amino acids essential for mAb binding to NA

Amino acid[a]	NA subtype and the antigen (virus) used as immunogen[b]					
	N1	N2			N8	N9
	BR/07	RI/57	TOK/67	MEM/98	Dk/UK/63	Tern/AU/75
150		+[c]			+	
198				+		
199				+	+	
220				+		+
221			+	+		
246 (248)	+					
247 (249)	+					
248 (250)	+					
253			+			
271 (273)	+					
284					+	
307 (309)	+					
329		+				+
334		+				
337 (338)	+					
338 (339)	+					
340 (341)	+					
342 (343)	+	+	+		+	
346					+	
367					+	+
368		+	+			+
369						+
370		+				+
372					+	+
398 (396)	+					
399 (397)	+					
400					+	+
403		+				
458 (456)	+					

This table is an update of NA residues previously reported (Air 2012).

[a] Amino acids residue numbers follows N2 numbering with N1 numbering shown in parentheses

[b] The amino acids critical for antibody binding were originally reported for BR/07 (Wan et al. 2013), RI/57 (Webster et al. 1984), TOK/67 (Lentz et al. 1984), MEM/98 (Gulati et al. 2002), Dk/UK/63 (Saito et al. 1994), and Tern/AU/75 (Air et al. 1990; Tulip et al. 1992).

[c] "+" identifies the position of the amino acid that is essential for monoclonal antibody binding using N2 numbering. The corresponding N1 numbering is shown in parentheses where relevant. Amino acids of N1 subtype that are conserved in both avian and human viruses are shown in bold.

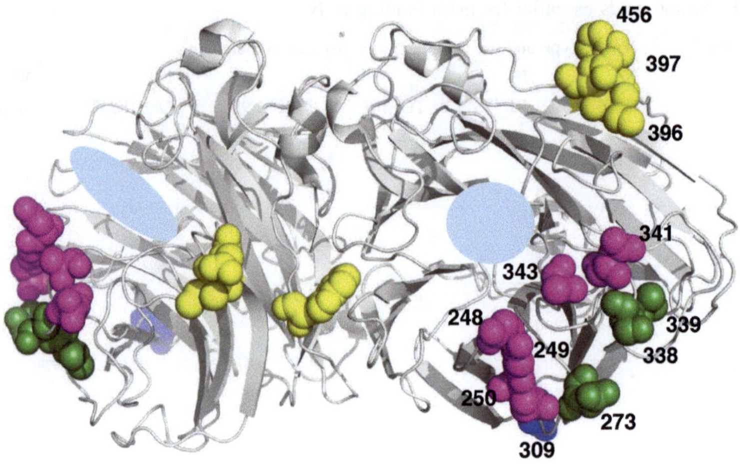

Fig. 2 Residues of NA (subtype N1) essential for binding mAbs specific for BR/07 shown on the head region (*top view*) of a monomer (PDB code 3NSS, generated with Pymol software, Delano Scientific), with the location of the enzyme active site circled in *blue*. Amino acids 248, 249, 250, 341 and 343 (shown in *pink*) are essential for binding a group of mAbs specific for NA of BR/07 and closely-related seasonal H1N1 viruses; amino acids 273, 338 and 339 (shown in *green*) are essential for binding a group of mAbs that are broadly reactive against seasonal H1N1, 1918 and 2009 pandemic H1N1 and H5N1 viruses. These amino acids are conserved in almost all strains within these lineages; amino acids 396, 397 and 456 (shown in *yellow*) are conserved in seasonal H1N1 and H5N1 viruses only; amino acid 309 is on the bottom of the NA head and hardly visible in this view

4 Evidence of NA-Mediated Immunity

4.1 Antigenic Drift

Changes in amino acid sequence within antigenic domains of NA suggest that these sites have been subject to antibody pressure, providing indirect evidence that NA antibodies play an important role in limiting virus replication. Although not all amino acid changes result in loss of polyclonal antibody binding, studies with mAbs suggest that these residues are indeed the targets of the humoral response (Venkatramani et al. 2006; Wan et al. 2013). Interestingly, the loss of reactivity with polyclonal antisera can result from a single amino acid change within an immunodominant epitope. For example, the introduction of a single amino acid change in the NA of A/Solomon Islands/3/2006 (SI/06) at position 329 resulted in reduced enzyme inhibition by ferret and human anti-SI/06 sera (Fig. 3) (Sandbulte et al. 2011).

The ability to predict amino acid changes that result in the loss of antibody binding to antigens of emerging seasonal influenza viruses would allow early selection of virus strains for vaccine manufacture. Recent studies show that very few amino acids within a single epitope are responsible for antigenic drift of HA

(a)

	Ferret antiserum against			
NA source	**TX/91**	**NC/99**	**SI/06**	**BR/07**
TX/91	**320**	2560	1280	320
NC/99	160	**1280**	1280	160
SI/06	160	1280	**1280**	160
BR/07	<5	80	80	**640**

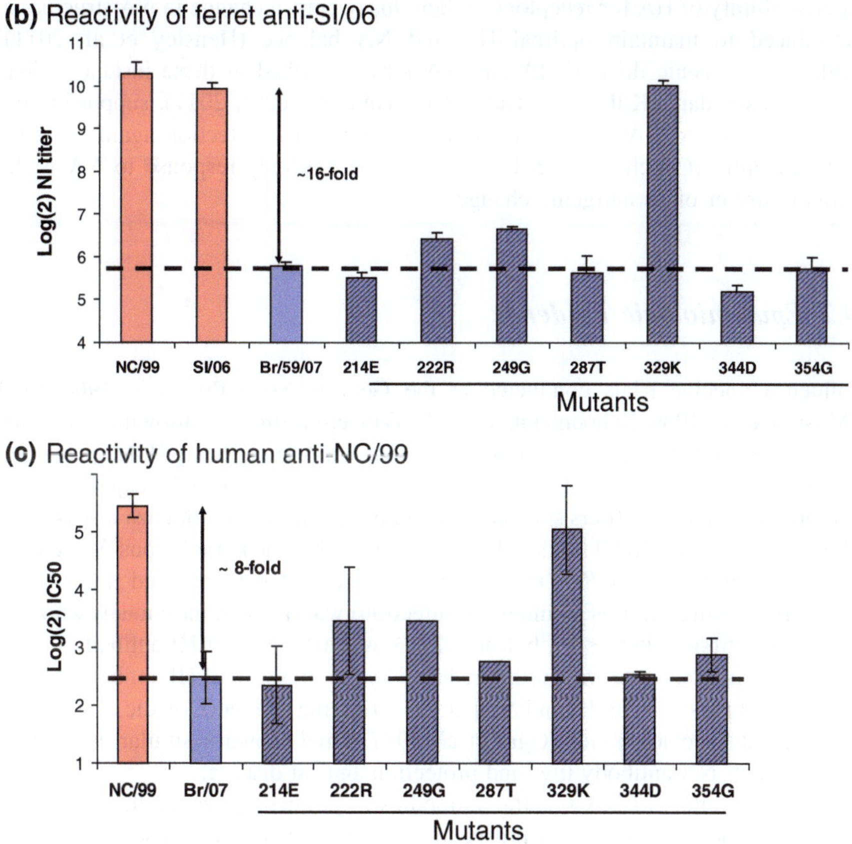

Fig. 3 A single amino acid mutation in the NA of BR/07 results in reduced reactivity with ferret and human antisera. **a** Antigenic analysis of NA from H1N1 seasonal viruses; **b** and **c**: Binding of antiserum to the NA of BR/07 is restored when variants contain a single point mutation at residue 329. Reassortant mutant BR/07 viruses were generated by reverse genetics using plasmids that contained changes introduced by site-directed mutagenesis. Only the change at residue 329 restored binding of (**b**) ferret anti-SI/06, and (**c**) human antiserum to NA of BR/07

(Koel et al. 2013), suggesting that it may be possible to predict changes that are epidemiologically important for this antigen. Interestingly, while NA amino acid 329 was identified as critical for binding of polyclonal antisera to the seasonal virus SI/06 (H1N1) and this position is also recognized by N2 and N9-specific mAbs (Table 1), amino acid 329 was not essential for binding of any of the 25 mAbs with reactivity to the NA of A/Brisbane/59/2007 (H1N1) (Wan et al. 2013). This suggests that antigenic drift of seasonal SI/06-like H1N1 viruses resulted in a change in the immunodominance of NA epitopes in H1N1 viruses isolated in 2007. Since there are currently no criteria for predicting which NA epitopes are immunodominant, antigenic drift is defined by NI analysis using ferret antisera. There is evidence that antigenic drift of HA can occur in association with an altered affinity of HA for receptors—when this occurs, a change in NA structure is introduced to maintain optimal HA and NA balance (Hensley et al. 2011). Although antigenic drift of HA and NA may be linked in these instances, it is usually discordant (Kilbourne et al. 1990; Sandbulte et al. 2011), supporting the idea that HA and NA-specific immunity contribute to protection against disease independently (Couch et al. 2013) and that the antibody response to NA is the primary driver of its antigenic change.

4.2 Epidemiologic Evidence

Influenza vaccine trials conducted at the Georgia State Prison in 1968–1969 (Mostow et al. 1969; Schoenbaum et al. 1969) were fortuitous, allowing correlates of vaccine efficacy against the subsequent influenza A/Hong Kong H3N2 pandemic outbreak to be examined (Dowdle et al. 1973). Evaluation of hemagglutination inhibition (HI) and NI titers showed that while prevention of influenza disease was significantly related to HI titers, NI titers against either the homologous A/Aichi/68 or heterologous A/Japan/62 (H2N2) strains correlated with reduced illness. The attack rate (using fever as an index for infection) was 45 % in individuals who had HI or NI antibody titers $\leq$10, but only 24 % when NI but not HI antibodies were present. This attack rate was further reduced by the presence of HI antibodies, with only 7 % of persons with HI and NI titers >160 having a fever (Dowdle et al. 1973). Subsequent vaccine studies (Ogra et al. 1977) have shown a similar correlation between anti-NA antibody titer and protection against disease.

A similar effect of NA-specific antibodies in protecting against the 1968 pandemic was demonstrated in a prospective study of respiratory disease in Tecumseh, Michigan (Monto and Kendal 1973). In this study, the number of adults infected with the H3N2 virus during the 1968–1969 winter (as measured by either clinical illness or increased HI titers against H3N2) was inversely proportional to the serum anti-NA titer prior to the influenza outbreak. These results suggest that the relatively mild H3N2 pandemic in 1968 was indeed the result of pre-existing NA-specific antibodies.

NI antibody titers against the 2009 H1N1 virus are evident in the sera of older individuals following vaccination with seasonal inactivated trivalent vaccine (Marcelin et al. 2010), possibly explaining the low incidence of H1N1 pandemic disease in the elderly (Khandaker et al. 2011). Indeed the importance of NA immunity against naturally occurring influenza was demonstrated by evaluating HI and NI antibody titers in a study conducted during 2009–2011 (Couch et al. 2013); serum HI and NI titers correlated with reduced infection and increased NI titers were associated with reduced illness. Importantly, this study showed that HI and NI antibody titers are independent predictors of immunity and therefore induction of NA immunity is beneficial to public health.

4.3 Clinical Challenge Studies

The H3N2 pandemic of 1968 provided an opportunity to evaluate whether antibody responses against the NA of the previously circulating H2N2 virus were associated with resistance to the newly emerging pandemic virus. Volunteers that had no pre-existing H3-specific antibodies and a range of NI antibody titers were challenged with the newly emerging H3N2 virus (Murphy et al. 1972). Even though there was evidence of infection (virus recovered in nasal wash), the severity of disease caused by the H3N2 challenge and the duration of virus shedding depended on the level of NA antibodies in serum.

Another clinical challenge study was performed to compare immunologic markers of protection in volunteers previously infected with wild-type virus and those vaccinated with licensed split, inactivated trivalent (H1N1, H3N2 and B components) or live, attenuated bivalent (H1N1 and H3N2) influenza vaccines (Clements et al. 1986). Pre-existing serum NI titers correlated inversely with clinical symptoms, peak virus titers, and duration of virus shedding in all study groups, suggesting NA-specific antibodies correlate with efficacy of both vaccine types. Interestingly, serum HI titers correlated with resistance to disease in recipients of inactivated but not live, attenuated vaccine suggesting that other mechanisms induced by live, attenuated vaccines contribute to immunity – in addition to NI antibodies, this could include γ-interferon (IFN)-secreting T cells (Forrest et al. 2008) and mucosal HA-specific IgA (Clements et al. 1986).

4.4 Mouse Challenge Studies

Animal models have been used to directly demonstrate the impact of NA-specific antibodies on virus replication and disease. Immunization of mice with NA purified from an N2-containing reassortant virus X7(F1) resulted in a reduction of lung virus titers and lung pathology when the mice were challenged with virus containing the homologous NA (Schulman et al. 1968). To demonstrate that protection was mediated by antibodies, serum transfer studies were conducted. The results showed that passive transfer of anti-NA antibodies to naïve mice reduced the replication of challenge viruses containing either the homologous or heterologous NA (same subtype but different species origin).

More recent studies similarly demonstrate broad protection by NA-specific immunity; these studies are important because they show the potential benefit of NA-specific antibodies against pandemic viruses. Immunization with the NA of a seasonal H1N1 virus provides substantial protection against heterologous 2009 H1N1pdm virus challenge (Marcelin et al. 2011). Broad protection against H5N1 infection is also observed in a large proportion of mice vaccinated with the NA of seasonal H1N1 viruses—both DNA (Sandbulte et al. 2007) and VLP (Easterbrook et al. 2012) vaccines induced such heterologous immunity. This broad NA-based immunity is not intuitive from serologic analyses that show large differences in antigenic structure of NA of seasonal H1N1, 2009 H1N1pdm, and H5N1 viruses. However, a low level of reproducible cross-reactivity is present (Chen et al. 2012) which points to the presence of conserved epitopes. Conserved amino acids that are required for binding broadly-reactive mAbs were recently identified (Wan et al. 2013) and are shown in Table 1.

Mice treated prophylactically with a mAb specific for a seasonal H1N1 virus were protected against this strain only, while mice treated with mAbs that bind to a conserved antigenic domain of N1 were protected against challenge with lethal doses of seasonal H1N1 and 2009 H1N1 pdm viruses and have substantial resistance against H5N1 infection (Fig. 4) (Wan et al. 2013). These data suggest that antibodies against conserved epitopes are likely to be important contributors to the heterologous protection induced by NA immunization.

A report of NA-specific heterosubtypic immunity (Quan et al. 2012) is substantiated by demonstration of protection by antibodies specific for a peptide that is universally conserved with influenza A NAs (Doyle et al. 2013), however high antibody concentrations are required for protection, making this an unlikely goal of NA-based vaccines.

5 Immunogenicity of NA

A colorimetric assay developed to quantify free sialic acid was originally used to measure functional NA-specific antibody titers in serum (Webster and Laver 1967). This method was based on the assays of Warren (1959) and Aminoff (1959) that quantified free sialic acid using thiobarbituric acid (TBA) and additional chemical reactions. While the assay is specific, it is cumbersome to perform and not suitable for determining NA antibody titers in large numbers of samples. Alternative assays that are more practical include a miniaturized TBA method (Sandbulte et al. 2009) and an assay that quantifies enzyme activity by measuring the amount of galactose that becomes available following release of sialic acid (Lambre et al. 1990). This latter assay is performed in a 96-well plate format and

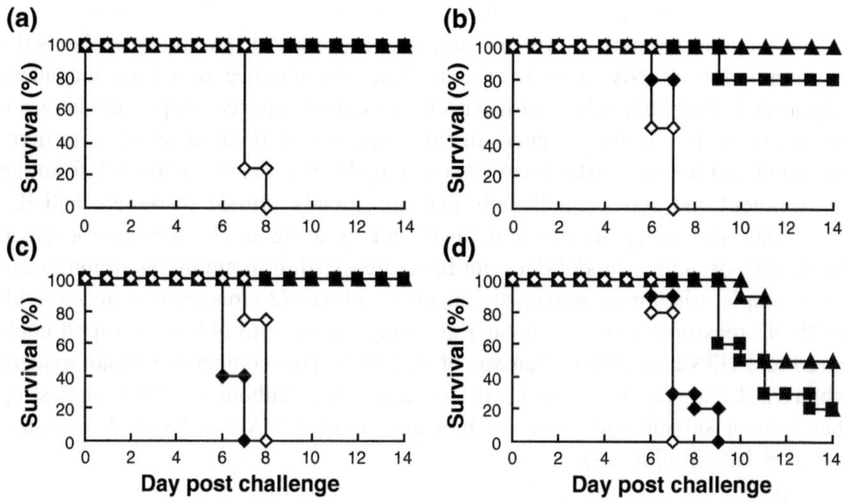

Fig. 4 Mice treated prophylactically with NA-inhibiting antibodies are protected against homologous and heterologous lethal virus challenge. DBA/2 mice treated with BR/07 strain-specific mAb 3A2 (◆) and broadly-reactive 1H5 (▲) or 3H10 (■) 12 h before virus challenge in addition to control mice treated with PBS (◇) were challenged with 10 MLD_{50} of **a** seasonal H1N1 BR/07, **b** 2009 H1N1pdm CA/09-X179A, **c** attenuated VN/04 (H5N1) virus or **d** 20LD_{50} of wild-type VN/04. Experimental details and a full set of results have been published (Wan et al. 2013)

uses peroxidase conjugated to peanut agglutinin, a lectin specific for galactose, to quantify NA activity. It is relatively easy to test large numbers of serum samples in this enzyme-linked lectin assay (ELLA), and is therefore the method of choice for measuring NA-specific antibody responses in animal as well as human studies (Cate et al. 2010; Couch et al. 2013; Fries et al. 2012, 2013; Sultana et al. 2011). Alternatively, an ELISA can be used to quantify NA-specific antibody titers (Khan et al. 1982), however the purified NA needed as antigen in the assay is often not available.

NA must be in its native form to induce functional NI antibodies. Since enzyme activity requires an intact tetramer, it can be used as a measure of this antigen's native form and immunogenicity. Enzyme activity per se is not required for immunogenicity (Sultana et al. 2011) and therefore there is some concern that enzyme activity is not necessarily the best way to measure NA potency. Besides, enzyme activity is not strain-specific and so it is not possible to quantify the activity of each NA subtype in seasonal trivalent and quadrivalent vaccines. ELISA has been used to quantify NA and may be a suitable platform to measure NA potency.

Immunization with the same amount of purified HA and NA results in similar increases in antibody titers to each of these antigens, demonstrating that these antigens have similar immunogenicity (Johansson et al. 1989). However, the antibody responses to NA can be less than anticipated, particularly when whole virus vaccines are used to boost the response (Kilbourne 1976; Kilbourne et al. 1987). This discrepancy in primary antibody responses to HA and NA reflects the lower amounts of NA in each vaccine dose; the absence of robust secondary responses to NA when whole virus vaccines are used reflects competition between the antigens. HA is the 'winner' in this competition because anti-HA is more prevalent and therefore whole virus is taken up by B cells, removing NA from the environment and activating B cells that are already primed to secrete anti-HA antibodies. This competition can be overcome by using an HA subtype for which the human or animal model does not have pre-existing immunity as immunogen. For example, when mice previously infected with H3N2 virus are immunized with an H7N2 reassortant virus, a greater antibody response to NA is measured compared to a H3N2 vaccine (Johansson et al. 1987). This competition is not evident when viral antigens are dissociated (Johansson and Kilbourne 1993), suggesting that split or subunit influenza vaccines and purified NA can be used to induce effective NA-specific responses.

Antigenic sin is a concept that was termed to describe recall responses to HA, with secondary exposure to a drift variant resulting in an increase in the quantity and avidity of antibodies to the original immunogen (Fazekas de St and Webster 1966; Webster 1966). Antigenic sin is also evident in NA-specific antibody responses. As described earlier in this Chapter, NA contains both strain-specific and conserved antigenic domains. Sera of individuals recently infected with 2009 H1N1pdm virus have increased NI titers against the otherwise antigenically-distinct NA of seasonal H1N1 virus. While this could provide some benefit in that the increase in antibodies against conserved epitopes would result in immunity against potential pandemic strains, it should be kept in mind that the most effective NA immunity is afforded by a homologous vaccine.

6 Mechanism of Action

Reduced virus replication in the presence of NA-specific antibodies in vitro is largely due to inhibition of enzyme activity. Inhibition of enzyme activity is usually the result of steric hindrance, with antibody binding to the NA head preventing large sialylated glycans from entering the enzyme active pocket. Antibodies that bind very close to the enzyme active pocket can inhibit access of small substrates to the enzyme active site (Webster et al. 1987), but since the natural substrate is large, even antibodies that bind some distance from the enzyme active pocket can inhibit cleavage of sialic acid. This inhibition of substrate cleavage limits virus replication by preventing release of newly formed virus particles from the host cell surface. Without removal of sialic acid from the viral glycoproteins, spread of virus particles from cell to cell as well as transmission as an aerosol is impeded due to virus aggregation. Inhibition of NA activity can also impact initiation of infection. While NA-specific antibodies do not inhibit virus binding or infection of cells, in vitro studies show that NA activity facilitates the initiation of infection of epithelial cells (Matrosovich et al. 2004; Ohuchi et al. 2006), probably by releasing virus particles from decoy receptors present on mucins or possibly affecting virus entry in ways currently not understood. Antibodies that inhibit NA activity may therefore reduce the number of cells infected. This may explain why NI titers correlate with reduced infectivity in clinical studies (Couch et al. 2013).

Although the most effective response to NA in vivo is likely to be one that includes high avidity enzyme-inhibiting antibodies, other mechanisms may contribute to immunity. For example, antibodies that bind without inhibiting NA activity may bind to infected cells thereby providing a target for FcR-positive natural killer cells or complement.

In addition to antibody-mediated mechanisms that contribute to NA immunity, it is important to note that NA contains epitopes recognized by $CD4^+$ and $CD8^+$ T cells (De Groot et al. 2009; Jameson et al. 1998; Moise et al. 2013). When NA-specific $CD4^+$ T cells are primed following immunization they not only provide essential help to activation and maturation of B cells secreting antibodies to NA, they can also provide help for antibody responses to other vaccine antigens, including HA. In addition, both $CD4^+$ and $CD8^+$ T cells can contribute to immunity through secretion of antiviral cytokines and/or perforins (Brown et al. 2012; McKinstry et al. 2012). Reducing virus load by clearance of infected cells in this way could result in a mild course of disease.

Besides categorizing NA as an antigen, the enzyme activity of NA can modulate the magnitude and type of T cell response by promoting contact between antigen presenting cells and antigen-specific T cells (Oh and Eichelberger 1999, 2000). Serum antibody responses to HA were increased in mice immunized with a H1N1 vaccine supplemented with NA (Johansson et al. 1998), suggesting NA provides adjuvant activity. However, further studies that compare the magnitude of the influenza-specific antibody and T cell response to vaccines formulated with active and inactive NA are needed to conclusively demonstrate that NA does indeed contribute to immunity by influencing initiation of the response to vaccine antigens.

7 NA Content of Vaccines

7.1 Human Experimental NA-Based Vaccine Studies

NA-based vaccines have been clinically tested and shown to be effective in small studies. Early studies of vaccines designed to induce NA-specific antibodies were whole inactivated virus preparations. To avoid recall responses to HA, inactivated reassortant virus, X-32, that had a mismatched HA of an equine virus (H7) and the

NA of a 1968 seasonal H3N2 virus was used as vaccine in a clinical study conducted in incarcerated adults (Couch et al. 1974). All volunteers were negative for antibodies to HA of either the circulating H3N2 virus or H7N2 vaccine. Serum NI antibody titers measured 5 weeks post-vaccination were significantly increased (>4-fold) in almost all volunteers, including a small group of volunteers that had pre-existing NI antibodies. All volunteers were subsequently challenged with a wild-type H3N2 virus containing the homologous NA. Clinical symptoms and viral titers in nasal wash samples were compared in the H7N2 and control influenza B-vaccinated groups. While the frequency of infection was not statistically different between the groups, clinical illness was observed in fewer H7N2-vaccinated individuals and virus titers in the nasal wash were significantly less than in the control group. The reduction in virus titer correlated with increased NI titers measured in either serum or nasal wash.

A subsequent study compared the ability of reassortant viruses X-37 that has both HA and NA of A/England/43/72 (H3N2), and X-38 that has a mismatched HA (H7) and the homologous NA, to induce N2-specific antibodies (Kilbourne 1976). A significant increase in NI titer was observed in 69 % of individuals vaccinated with the H7N2 virus, but only 25 % of those vaccinated with the H3N2 virus; in addition, the mean NI titer of the H7N2 vaccinees was twice that of the H3N2-vaccinated group. These results are a demonstration of antigenic competition between HA and NA when there is pre-existing immunity against both antigens and whole virus is used as immunogen. As in the previous study, during a natural outbreak of H3N2 in this latter population, the H7N2 vaccine and placebo recipients were infected at approximately the same rate, however vaccination protected against illness, with absence of clinical signs correlating with anti-NA antibody titers.

The safety and immunogenicity of a purified NA vaccine has also been tested in the clinic (Kilbourne et al. 1995). No severe adverse events were reported. Mild local reactions at the site of injection were reported with the highest dose of purified NA (69.6 μg). These reactions were similar to those of the trivalent inactivated vaccine comparator. Antibody responses to NA were dependent on dose, with a 2.6 μg dose resulting in 2.5-fold increases in NI antibody titer in 40 % of subjects while a 69.6 μg dose resulted in an 8.6-fold increase in 90 % of the subjects.

These clinical studies support the use of split, inactivated virus or purified NA to induce NI antibodies. Challenge studies performed several decades ago suggest that very low NI titers protect against disease (Clements et al. 1986; Murphy et al. 1972). The traditional TBA assay was used in these instances for serology. While antibody titers measured by ELLA are proportional to those measured by TBA, they can be somewhat higher (Fritz et al. 2012) and therefore additional clinical studies are needed to establish an NI titer that correlates with protection against disease. Such a correlate would be helpful for interpretation of immunogenicity data and for establishing the dose of NA needed to elicit effective NA immunity.

7.2 *Licensed Influenza Vaccines*

Current influenza vaccines are standardized for HA content: the potency of licensed seasonal vaccines is measured by single radical immunodiffusion assay which quantifies the antigenic form of HA based on reactivity with HA-specific sheep antiserum. Standardization of the NA content of split, inactivated vaccines is difficult because the ratio of HA:NA is strain-specific (Gerentes et al. 1999) and the stability of NA in split, inactivated vaccines has not been established. It is not easy to quantify the antigenic form of NA corresponding to each component (influenza A subtypes and influenza B lineages) in trivalent or quadrivalent vaccine formulations—even though enzyme activity correlates with the amount of immunogenic tetramers, this assay is not strain specific. Even so, clinical immunogenicity studies show that in most years the quantities of NA in these vaccines are sufficient to increase NI antibody titers in young, healthy adults (Couch et al. 2012).

Antibody responses are substantially diminished in the elderly. A high-dose split, inactivated vaccine (Fluzone, High Dose, 60 μg HA of each virus strain/dose) is available for persons ≥65 years old and compared to the standard vaccine dose (Fluzone, 15 μg HA) was shown to result in increased antibody responses to both HA (Couch et al. 2007) and NA (Cate et al. 2010) in this age group. One approach to reduce the amount of antigen per dose and yet retain immunogenicity is to administer the vaccine intradermally. Such a vaccine (Fluzone Intradermal, Sanofi) containing 9 μg HA/strain has been approved for use in persons 18–64 years old with clinical data to show that HA-specific antibody responses are similar to those of the standard vaccine administered intramuscularly (Gorse et al. 2013). NI antibody titers following intradermal vaccination have not been reported.

The potency of live, attenuated influenza vaccines is based on their infectivity. Since infection results in expression of NA on the host cell surface, even if spread of new virus particles is limited by pre-existing NA immunity, it is likely that a live, attenuated vaccine will initiate and/or boost a NA-specific response. Indeed, increased NA antibody titers have been demonstrated after live, attenuated influenza vaccination although seroconversion rates are sometimes less than after immunization with inactivated vaccine (Couch et al. 2012; Hassantoufighi et al. 2010). Nevertheless, increased NI antibody titers in children vaccinated with live, attenuated influenza vaccine were associated with decreased clinical disease in virus challenge studies (Clements et al. 1986). It should be kept in mind that NI antibodies are not the only potential mediator of immunity induced by live, attenuated vaccines—γ-IFN-secreting T cells, (Forrest et al. 2008) and mucosal HA-specific IgA (Clements et al. 1986) also correlate with reduced disease and it is therefore likely that live, attenuated vaccine efficacy reflects the sum of a number of different humoral and cell-mediated responses.

7.3 Development of New Vaccine Types

The need to design influenza vaccines that are readily available at the onset of a pandemic has resulted in development of new vaccine strategies. Some of these next generation vaccines, particularly those that utilize recombinant proteins or virus-like particles (VLPs), have the potential to incorporate consistent amounts of NA. The immunogenicity of NA in many of these approaches has recently been reviewed (Johansson and Cox 2011). Vaccines formulated with adjuvant could increase antibody responses to both HA and NA. Indeed, examination of the specificity and avidity of antibodies elicited in the presence of adjuvant shows increased avidity and broadening of the antibody response to both HA and NA (Khurana et al. 2010), making it feasible to induce effective NA immunity with smaller amounts of antigen.

Both H5N1 and H7N9 viruses have pandemic potential. The immunogenicity of NA in a non-adjuvanted Vero-cell produced whole virus inactivated H5N1 vaccine was demonstrated in a clinical study (Fritz et al. 2012), but it is not known whether the NI titers achieved are sufficient to protect against disease. A recent clinical study demonstrated that the immunogenicity of a H7N9 VLP vaccine was increased by the addition of ISCOMATRIX, resulting in increased seroconversion rates and antibody titers to NA (Fries et al. 2013). Interestingly, a booster dose increased both HI and NI antibody titers, suggesting that the antigenic competition observed in responses to whole virus vaccines may not be an issue with a VLP vaccine platform.

A clear benefit of NA immunity is its breadth of protection due to the presence of conserved antigenic domains within each NA subtype. This makes NA an attractive antigen to include as a component of a universal vaccine or even to consider as a stand-alone pandemic vaccine containing equivalent doses of each targeted NA subtype. In 1971 Kilbourne proposed that a vaccine containing a mixture of NA subtypes would protect against emerging unexpected viruses. Since it would not be possible to demonstrate effectiveness of such a vaccine prior to a pandemic, it would be extremely helpful to identify the NI antibody titer that is associated with protection against clinical disease and to define the vaccine dose needed to induce the seroprotective titer.

For vaccines that are dependent on inducing responses to NA, the vaccine dose will need to be measured by quantifying the amount of NA with native structure. As discussed earlier, enzyme activity provides a useful tool to quantify the native NA tetramer in vaccine intermediates or monovalent vaccines, but is not suitable to measure NA content of polyvalent vaccines. We are currently evaluating ELISA for its ability to quantify the native form of NA using mAbs that bind to conformation-dependent epitopes and that discriminate between NA types/subtypes.

8 Conclusions and Future Perspectives

Effective influenza vaccines that are based on NA content undoubtedly require a good understanding of the antigenic structure of NA, its stability, immunogenicity, and dose needed for clinical effectiveness. While animal and clinical studies consistently demonstrate the benefit of NA-specific antibodies, there is a need for additional information and tools to support the development of either a stand-alone NA vaccine or an inactivated split or recombinant protein vaccine that contains a specified amount of NA. For example, it would be helpful to establish the NI antibody titer associated with resistance against disease, to identify the NA dose that induces this titer in humans, and to have an in vitro method to measure the potency of NA in multivalent vaccines.

Since stand-alone NA vaccines and vaccines that contain standardized amounts of both NA and HA differ in the kind of immunity generated, the type of vaccine developed would depend on the targeted clinical end-point. For example, a vaccine without HA (either recombinant NAs or reassortant viruses with mismatched HAs from avian viruses) would result in an immune response that is infection-permissive, allowing subsequent infection with the circulating seasonal or pandemic virus and the induction of long-term protective immunity, whereas a vaccine that includes both HA and NA components of the targeted infecting virus would induce antibodies that neutralize HA-matched virus infectivity. In the latter case, infection may be prevented and a full spectrum of antibody and T cell responses, including high avidity strain-specific antibodies and broadly-reactive $CD8^+$ T cells, may not be activated.

Influenza vaccines that induce broadly reactive cell-mediated immunity or antibodies to M2 have a similar impact as NA immunity in that infection is permitted but replication is attenuated (Price et al. 2010). This heterosubtypic immunity is critical for protection against a novel challenge strain (Bodewes et al. 2009a) and consequently infection-permissive immunity can be viewed as beneficial (Bodewes et al. 2009b), with models predicting the long-term benefit of immunity established as a result of infection (Carrat et al. 2006).

Since the world-wide population is primed against N1 and N2 antigens, the severity of pandemic H5N1, H2N2, and H7N2 virus outbreaks may be limited by pre-existing NA immunity. In the absence of NA-immunity, novel viruses such as H7N9 that have HA and NA subtypes unique to the human population, may be a far greater global threat. The most effective means to avert or limit such a pandemic would be through vaccination. A vaccine that includes induction of N9-specific immunity would be of great benefit, especially if the emerging virus has a HA that is antigenically-distinct from the vaccine strain.

Both animal and human studies provide evidence of heterologous protection associated with NA-specific antibodies. However, NA immunity is most effective against viruses with an antigenically-matched NA and therefore it is desirable to select viruses for vaccine production that have both the HA and NA antigenically matched to the circulating (or potential pandemic) influenza virus. This has generally been the case for viruses selected for seasonal vaccine production, although there are instances when prior knowledge of NA antigenic structure may have facilitated selection of a better matched strain (Sandbulte et al. 2011).

In 1972 Walter Dowdle wrote in response to the finding that NA-specific antibodies are associated with resistance to disease (Murphy et al. 1972): "We can no longer ignore a major antigenic constituent (NA) of the influenza virion. Surveillance of influenza viruses must be concerned with antigenic changes in both the HA and the NA. All vaccines, live or inactivated, must be formulated and evaluated on the relevancy and potency of both antigens" (Dowdle 1972). More than four decades later, it is hoped that the progress made toward routine measurement of NI antibody titers, better understanding of NA antigenic structure and drift, and the development of ways to measure NA immunogenicity will facilitate consideration of NA content in next generation influenza vaccines.

Acknowledgments The authors thank Suzanne Epstein, Jerry Weir, and Hana Golding for critical reading of this chapter and are indebted to Gillian Air, Bob Couch, Bert Johansson, Arnold Monto, Jeff Taubenberger, and Rob Webster for past discussions and their research programs that have provided invaluable tools and information toward understanding NA immunity. Work in the authors' laboratory is supported by intramural CBER Panflu funds.

References

Air GM (2012) Influenza neuraminidase. Influenza Other Respir Viruses 6(4):245–256. doi:10.1111/j.1750-2659.2011.00304.x

Air GM, Laver WG, Webster RG (1990) Mechanism of antigenic variation in an individual epitope on influenza virus N9 neuraminidase. J Virol 64(12):5797–5803

Aminoff D (1959) The determination of free sialic acid in the presence of the bound compound. Virology 7(3):355–357

Bodewes R, Kreijtz JH, Baas C, Geelhoed-Mieras MM, de Mutsert G, van Amerongen G, van den Brand JM, Fouchier RA, Osterhaus AD, Rimmelzwaan GF (2009a) Vaccination against human influenza A/H3N2 virus prevents the induction of heterosubtypic immunity against lethal infection with avian influenza A/H5N1 virus. PLoS ONE 4(5):e5538. doi:10.1371/journal.pone.0005538

Bodewes R, Kreijtz JH, Rimmelzwaan GF (2009b) Yearly influenza vaccinations: a double-edged sword? Lancet Infect Dis 9(12):784–788. doi:10.1016/S1473-3099(09)70263-4

Brett IC, Johansson BE (2006) Variation in the divalent cation requirements of influenza A virus N1 neuraminidases. J Biochem 139(3):439–447. doi:10.1093/jb/mvj051

Brown DM, Lee S, Garcia-Hernandez Mde L, Swain SL (2012) Multifunctional CD4 cells expressing gamma interferon and perforin mediate protection against lethal influenza virus infection. J Virol 86(12):6792–6803. doi:10.1128/JVI.07172-11

Burmeister WP, Ruigrok RW, Cusack S (1992) The 2.2 A resolution crystal structure of influenza B neuraminidase and its complex with sialic acid. EMBO J 11(1):49–56

Calder LJ, Wasilewski S, Berriman JA, Rosenthal PB (2010) Structural organization of a filamentous influenza A virus. Proc Natl Acad Sci USA 107(23):10685–10690. doi:10.1073/pnas.1002123107

Carrat F, Lavenu A, Cauchemez S, Deleger S (2006) Repeated influenza vaccination of healthy children and adults: borrow now, pay later? Epidemiol Infect 134(1):63–70. doi:10.1017/S0950268805005479

Cate TR, Rayford Y, Nino D, Winokur P, Brady R, Belshe R, Chen W, Atmar RL, Couch RB (2010) A high dosage influenza vaccine induced significantly more neuraminidase antibody than standard vaccine among elderly subjects. Vaccine 28(9):2076–2079

Chen Z, Kim L, Subbarao K, Jin H (2012) The 2009 pandemic H1N1 virus induces anti-neuraminidase (NA) antibodies that cross-react with the NA of H5N1 viruses in ferrets. Vaccine 30(15):2516–2522. doi:10.1016/j.vaccine.2012.01.090

Chong AK, Pegg MS, von Itzstein M (1991) Influenza virus sialidase: effect of calcium on steady-state kinetic parameters. Biochim Biophys Acta 1077(1):65–71

Clements ML, Betts RF, Tierney EL, Murphy BR (1986) Serum and nasal wash antibodies associated with resistance to experimental challenge with influenza A wild-type virus. J Clin Microbiol 24(1):157–160

Colacino JM, Chirgadze NY, Garman E, Murti KG, Loncharich RJ, Baxter AJ, Staschke KA, Laver WG (1997) A single sequence change destabilizes the influenza virus neuraminidase tetramer. Virology 236(1):66–75. doi:10.1006/viro.1997.8709

Couch RB, Atmar RL, Franco LM, Quarles JM, Wells J, Arden N, Nino D, Belmont JW (2013) Antibody correlates and predictors of immunity to naturally occurring influenza in humans and the importance of antibody to the neuraminidase. J Infect Dis 207(6):974–981

Couch RB, Atmar RL, Keitel WA, Quarles JM, Wells J, Arden N, Nino D (2012) Randomized comparative study of the serum antihemagglutinin and antineuraminidase antibody responses to six licensed trivalent influenza vaccines. Vaccine 31(1):190–195

Couch RB, Kasel JA, Gerin JL, Schulman JL, Kilbourne ED (1974) Induction of partial immunity to influenza by a neuraminidase-specific vaccine. J Infect Dis 129(4):411–420

Couch RB, Winokur P, Brady R, Belshe R, Chen WH, Cate TR, Sigurdardottir B, Hoeper A, Graham IL, Edelman R, He F, Nino D, Capellan J, Ruben FL (2007) Safety and immunogenicity of a high dosage trivalent influenza vaccine among elderly subjects. Vaccine 25(44):7656–7663. doi:10.1016/j.vaccine.2007.08.042

De Groot AS, Ardito M, McClaine EM, Moise L, Martin WD (2009) Immunoinformatic comparison of T cell epitopes contained in novel swine origin influenza A (H1N1) virus with epitopes in 2008–2009 conventional influenza vaccine. Vaccine 27(42):5740–5747. doi:10.1016/j.vaccine.2009.07.040

Dowdle WR (1972) Influenza anti-neuraminidase: the second best antibody. N Engl J Med 286(25):1360–1361. doi:10.1056/NEJM197206222862511

Dowdle WR, Coleman MT, Mostow SR, Kaye HS, Schoenbaum SC (1973) Inactivated influenza vaccines. 2. Laboratory indices of protection. Postgrad Med J 49(569):159–163

Doyle TM, Hashem AM, Li C, Van Domselaar G, Larocque L, Wang J, Smith D, Cyr T, Farnsworth A, He R, Hurt AC, Brown EG, Li X (2013) Universal anti-neuraminidase antibody inhibiting all influenza A subtypes. Antiviral Res 100(2):567–574. doi:10.1016/j.antiviral.2013.09.018

Easterbrook JD, Schwartzman LM, Gao J, Kash JC, Morens DM, Couzens L, Wan H, Eichelberger MC, Taubenberger JK (2012) Protection against a lethal H5N1 influenza challenge by intranasal immunization with virus-like particles containing 2009 pandemic H1N1 neuraminidase in mice. Virology 432(1):39–44. doi:10.1016/j.virol.2012.06.003

Fazekas de St G, Webster RG (1966) Disquisitions of original antigenic sin. I. evidence in man. J Exp Med 124(3):331–345

Forrest BD, Pride MW, Dunning AJ, Capeding MR, Chotpitayasunondh T, Tam JS, Rappaport R, Eldridge JH, Gruber WC (2008) Correlation of cellular immune responses with protection against culture-confirmed influenza virus in young children. Clin Vaccine Immunol 15(7):1042–1053. doi:10.1128/CVI.00397-07

Fries LF, Smith GE, Glenn GM (2013) A recombinant viruslike particle influenza A (H7N9) vaccine. N Engl J Med 369(26):2564–2566. doi:10.1056/NEJMc1313186

Fritz R, Sabarth N, Kiermayr S, Hohenadl C, Howard MK, Ilk R, Kistner O, Ehrlich HJ, Barrett PN, Kreil TR (2012) A vero cell-derived whole-virus H5N1 vaccine effectively induces neuraminidase-inhibiting antibodies. J Infect Dis 205(1):28–34. doi:10.1093/infdis/jir711

Gerentes L, Kessler N, Aymard M (1999) Difficulties in standardizing the neuraminidase content of influenza vaccines. Dev Biol Stand 98:189–196; discussion 197

Getie-Kebtie M, Sultana I, Eichelberger M, Alterman M (2013) Label-free mass spectrometry-based quantification of hemagglutinin and neuraminidase in influenza virus preparations and vaccines. Influenza Other Respir Viruses 7(4):521–530. doi:10.1111/irv.12001

Gillim-Ross L, Subbarao K (2007) Can immunity induced by the human influenza virus N1 neuraminidase provide some protection from avian influenza H5N1 viruses? PLoS medicine 4(2):e91. doi:10.1371/journal.pmed.0040091

Gorse GJ, Falsey AR, Fling JA, Poling TL, Strout CB, Tsang PH (2013) Intradermally-administered influenza virus vaccine is safe and immunogenic in healthy adults 18–64 years of age. Vaccine 31(19):2358–2365. doi:10.1016/j.vaccine.2013.03.008

Gulati U, Hwang CC, Venkatramani L, Gulati S, Stray SJ, Lee JT, Laver WG, Bochkarev A, Zlotnick A, Air GM (2002) Antibody epitopes on the neuraminidase of a recent H3N2 influenza virus (A/Memphis/31/98). J Virol 76(23):12274–12280

Hassantoufighi A, Zhang H, Sandbulte M, Gao J, Manischewitz J, King L, Golding H, Straight TM, Eichelberger MC (2010) A practical influenza neutralization assay to simultaneously quantify hemagglutinin and neuraminidase-inhibiting antibody responses. Vaccine 28(3):790–797

Hensley SE, Das SR, Gibbs JS, Bailey AL, Schmidt LM, Bennink JR, Yewdell JW (2011) Influenza A virus hemagglutinin antibody escape promotes neuraminidase antigenic variation and drug resistance. PLoS ONE 6(2):e15190. doi:10.1371/journal.pone.0015190

Jameson J, Cruz J, Ennis FA (1998) Human cytotoxic T-lymphocyte repertoire to influenza A viruses. J Virol 72(11):8682–8689

Johansson BE, Brett IC (2003) Variation in the divalent cation requirements of influenza a virus N2 neuraminidases. J Biochem 134(3):345–352

Johansson BE, Bucher DJ, Kilbourne ED (1989) Purified influenza virus hemagglutinin and neuraminidase are equivalent in stimulation of antibody response but induce contrasting types of immunity to infection. J Virol 63(3):1239–1246

Johansson BE, Cox MM (2011) Influenza viral neuraminidase: the forgotten antigen. Expert Rev Vaccines 10(12):1683–1695. doi:10.1586/erv.11.130

Johansson BE, Kilbourne ED (1993) Dissociation of influenza virus hemagglutinin and neuraminidase eliminates their intravirionic antigenic competition. J Virol 67(10):5721–5723

Johansson BE, Matthews JT, Kilbourne ED (1998) Supplementation of conventional influenza A vaccine with purified viral neuraminidase results in a balanced and broadened immune response. Vaccine 16(9–10):1009–1015

Johansson BE, Moran TM, Bona CA, Popple SW, Kilbourne ED (1987) Immunologic response to influenza virus neuraminidase is influenced by prior experience with the associated viral hemagglutinin. II. Sequential infection of mice simulates human experience. J Immunol 139(6):2010–2014

Khan MW, Gallagher M, Bucher D, Cerini CP, Kilbourne ED (1982) Detection of influenza virus neuraminidase-specific antibodies by an enzyme-linked immunosorbent assay. J Clin Microbiol 16(1):115–122

Khandaker G, Dierig A, Rashid H, King C, Heron L, Booy R (2011) Systematic review of clinical and epidemiological features of the pandemic influenza A (H1N1) 2009. Influenza Other Respir Viruses 5(3):148–156. doi:10.1111/j.1750-2659.2011.00199.x

Khurana S, Chearwae W, Castellino F, Manischewitz J, King LR, Honorkiewicz A, Rock MT, Edwards KM, Del Giudice G, Rappuoli R, Golding H (2010) Vaccines with MF59 adjuvant expand the antibody repertoire to target protective sites of pandemic avian H5N1 influenza virus. Sci Transl Med 2(15):15ra5. doi:10.1126/scitranslmed.3000624

Kilbourne ED (1972) Orthomyxoviruses and paramyxoviruses. In: Melnick JL (ed) International virology, 2nd edn. Karger, Basel, Switzerland, pp 121–137

Kilbourne ED (1976) Comparative efficacy of neuraminidase-specific and conventional influenza virus vaccines in induction of antibody to neuraminidase in humans. J Infect Dis 134(4):384–394

Kilbourne ED, Cerini CP, Khan MW, Mitchell JW Jr, Ogra PL (1987) Immunologic response to the influenza virus neuraminidase is influenced by prior experience with the associated viral hemagglutinin. I. Studies in human vaccinees. J Immunol 138(9):3010–3013

Kilbourne ED, Couch RB, Kasel JA, Keitel WA, Cate TR, Quarles JH, Grajower B, Pokorny BA, Johansson BE (1995) Purified influenza A virus N2 neuraminidase vaccine is immunogenic and non-toxic in humans. Vaccine 13(18):1799–1803

Kilbourne ED, Johansson BE, Grajower B (1990) Independent and disparate evolution in nature of influenza A virus hemagglutinin and neuraminidase glycoproteins. Proc Natl Acad Sci USA 87(2):786–790

Kilbourne ED, Laver WG, Schulman JL, Webster RG (1968) Antiviral activity of antiserum specific for an influenza virus neuraminidase. J Virol 2(4):281–288

Koel BF, Burke DF, Bestebroer TM, van der Vliet S, Zondag GC, Vervaet G, Skepner E, Lewis NS, Spronken MI, Russell CA, Eropkin MY, Hurt AC, Barr IG, de Jong JC, Rimmelzwaan GF, Osterhaus AD, Fouchier RA, Smith DJ (2013) Substitutions near the receptor binding site determine major antigenic change during influenza virus evolution. Science 342(6161):976–979. doi:10.1126/science.1244730

Lakdawala SS, Lamirande EW, Suguitan AL Jr, Wang W, Santos CP, Vogel L, Matsuoka Y, Lindsley WG, Jin H, Subbarao K (2011) Eurasian-origin gene segments contribute to the transmissibility, aerosol release, and morphology of the 2009 pandemic H1N1 influenza virus. PLoS Pathog 7(12):e1002443. doi:10.1371/journal.ppat.1002443

Lambre CR, Terzidis H, Greffard A, Webster RG (1990) Measurement of anti-influenza neuraminidase antibody using a peroxidase-linked lectin and microtitre plates coated with natural substrates. J Immunol Methods 135(1–2):49–57

Lentz MR, Air GM, Laver WG, Webster RG (1984) Sequence of the neuraminidase gene of influenza virus A/Tokyo/3/67 and previously uncharacterized monoclonal variants. Virology 135(1):257–265

Li Q, Qi J, Zhang W, Vavricka CJ, Shi Y, Wei J, Feng E, Shen J, Chen J, Liu D, He J, Yan J, Liu H, Jiang H, Teng M, Li X, Gao GF (2010) The 2009 pandemic H1N1 neuraminidase N1 lacks the 150-cavity in its active site. Nat Struct Mol Biol 17(10):1266–1268. doi:10.1038/nsmb.1909

Li Q, Sun X, Li Z, Liu Y, Vavricka CJ, Qi J, Gao GF (2012) Structural and functional characterization of neuraminidase-like molecule N10 derived from bat influenza A virus. Proc Natl Acad Sci USA 109(46):18897–18902. doi:10.1073/pnas.1211037109

Malby RL, Tulip WR, Harley VR, McKimm-Breschkin JL, Laver WG, Webster RG, Colman PM (1994) The structure of a complex between the NC10 antibody and influenza virus neuraminidase and comparison with the overlapping binding site of the NC41 antibody. Structure 2(8):733–746

Marcelin G, Bland HM, Negovetich NJ, Sandbulte MR, Ellebedy AH, Webb AD, Griffin YS, DeBeauchamp JL, McElhaney JE, Webby RJ (2010) Inactivated seasonal influenza vaccines increase serum antibodies to the neuraminidase of pandemic influenza A(H1N1) 2009 virus in an age-dependent manner. J Infect Dis 202(11):1634–1638. doi:10.1086/657084

Marcelin G, DuBois R, Rubrum A, Russell CJ, McElhaney JE, Webby RJ (2011) A contributing role for anti-neuraminidase antibodies on immunity to pandemic H1N1 2009 influenza A virus. PLoS ONE 6(10):e26335. doi:10.1371/journal.pone.0026335

Matrosovich MN, Matrosovich TY, Gray T, Roberts NA, Klenk HD (2004) Neuraminidase is important for the initiation of influenza virus infection in human airway epithelium. J Virol 78(22):12665–12667. doi:10.1128/JVI.78.22.12665-12667.2004

McKinstry KK, Strutt TM, Kuang Y, Brown DM, Sell S, Dutton RW, Swain SL (2012) Memory CD4+ T cells protect against influenza through multiple synergizing mechanisms. J Clin Investig 122(8):2847–2856. doi:10.1172/JCI63689

Moise L, Tassone R, Latimer H, Terry F, Levitz L, Haran JP, Ross TM, Boyle CM, Martin WD, De Groot AS (2013) Immunization with cross-conserved H1N1 influenza CD4 T-cell epitopes

lowers viral burden in HLA DR3 transgenic mice. Hum Vaccines Immunotherapeutics 9(10):2060–2068
Monto AS, Kendal AP (1973) Effect of neuraminidase antibody on Hong Kong influenza. Lancet 1(7804):623–625
Mostow SR, Schoenbaum SC, Dowdle WR, Coleman MT, Kaye HS (1969) Studies with inactivated influenza vaccines purified by zonal centrifugation. 1. Adverse reactions and serological responses. Bull World Health Organ 41(3):525–530
Murphy BR, Kasel JA, Chanock RM (1972) Association of serum anti-neuraminidase antibody with resistance to influenza in man. N Engl J Med 286(25):1329–1332. doi:10.1056/NEJM197206222862502
Nuss JM, Whitaker PB, Air GM (1993) Identification of critical contact residues in the NC41 epitope of a subtype N9 influenza virus neuraminidase. Proteins 15(2):121–132. doi:10.1002/prot.340150204
Ogra PL, Chow T, Beutner KR, Rubi E, Strussenberg J, DeMello S, Rizzone C (1977) Clinical and immunologic evaluation of neuraminidase-specific influenza A virus vaccine in humans. J Infect Dis 135(4):499–506
Oh S, Eichelberger MC (1999) Influenza virus neuraminidase alters allogeneic T cell proliferation. Virology 264(2):427–435. doi:10.1006/viro.1999.0019
Oh S, Eichelberger MC (2000) Polarization of allogeneic T-cell responses by influenza virus-infected dendritic cells. J Virol 74(17):7738–7744
Ohuchi M, Asaoka N, Sakai T, Ohuchi R (2006) Roles of neuraminidase in the initial stage of influenza virus infection. Microbes Infect/Institut Pasteur 8(5):1287–1293. doi:10.1016/j.micinf.2005.12.008
Palese P, Tobita K, Ueda M, Compans RW (1974) Characterization of temperature sensitive influenza virus mutants defective in neuraminidase. Virology 61(2):397–410
Price GE, Soboleski MR, Lo CY, Misplon JA, Quirion MR, Houser KV, Pearce MB, Pappas C, Tumpey TM, Epstein SL (2010) Single-dose mucosal immunization with a candidate universal influenza vaccine provides rapid protection from virulent H5N1, H3N2 and H1N1 viruses. PLoS ONE 5(10):e13162. doi:10.1371/journal.pone.0013162
Quan FS, Kim MC, Lee BJ, Song JM, Compans RW, Kang SM (2012) Influenza M1 VLPs containing neuraminidase induce heterosubtypic cross-protection. Virology 430(2):127–135. doi:10.1016/j.virol.2012.05.006
Russell RJ, Haire LF, Stevens DJ, Collins PJ, Lin YP, Blackburn GM, Hay AJ, Gamblin SJ, Skehel JJ (2006) The structure of H5N1 avian influenza neuraminidase suggests new opportunities for drug design. Nature 443(7107):45–49. doi:10.1038/nature05114
Saito T, Taylor G, Laver WG, Kawaoka Y, Webster RG (1994) Antigenicity of the N8 influenza A virus neuraminidase: existence of an epitope at the subunit interface of the neuraminidase. J Virol 68(3):1790–1796
Saito T, Taylor G, Webster RG (1995) Steps in maturation of influenza A virus neuraminidase. J Virol 69(8):5011–5017
Sandbulte MR, Gao J, Straight TM, Eichelberger MC (2009) A miniaturized assay for influenza neuraminidase-inhibiting antibodies utilizing reverse genetics-derived antigens. Influenza Other Respir Viruses 3(5):233–240
Sandbulte MR, Jimenez GS, Boon AC, Smith LR, Treanor JJ, Webby RJ (2007) Cross-reactive neuraminidase antibodies afford partial protection against H5N1 in mice and are present in unexposed humans. PLoS Med 4(2):e59. doi:10.1371/journal.pmed.0040059
Sandbulte MR, Westgeest KB, Gao J, Xu X, Klimov AI, Russell CA, Burke DF, Smith DJ, Fouchier RA, Eichelberger MC (2011) Discordant antigenic drift of neuraminidase and hemagglutinin in H1N1 and H3N2 influenza viruses. Proc Natl Acad Sci USA 108(51):20748–20753
Schoenbaum SC, Mostow SR, Dowdle WR, Coleman MT, Kaye HS (1969) Studies with inactivated influenza vaccines purified by zonal centrifugation. 2. Efficacy. Bull World Health Organ 41(3):531–535

Schulman JL, Khakpour M, Kilbourne ED (1968) Protective effects of specific immunity to viral neuraminidase on influenza virus infection of mice. J Virol 2(8):778–786

Sultana I, Gao J, Markoff L, Eichelberger MC (2011) Influenza neuraminidase-inhibiting antibodies are induced in the presence of zanamivir. Vaccine 29(14):2601–2606. doi:10.1016/j.vaccine.2011.01.047

Tulip WR, Varghese JN, Baker AT, van Donkelaar A, Laver WG, Webster RG, Colman PM (1991) Refined atomic structures of N9 subtype influenza virus neuraminidase and escape mutants. J Mol Biol 221(2):487–497

Tulip WR, Varghese JN, Laver WG, Webster RG, Colman PM (1992) Refined crystal structure of the influenza virus N9 neuraminidase-NC41 Fab complex. J Mol Biol 227(1):122–148

Varghese JN, Colman PM (1991) Three-dimensional structure of the neuraminidase of influenza virus A/Tokyo/3/67 at 2.2 A resolution. J Mol Biol 221(2):473–486

Venkatramani L, Bochkareva E, Lee JT, Gulati U, Graeme Laver W, Bochkarev A, Air GM (2006) An epidemiologically significant epitope of a 1998 human influenza virus neuraminidase forms a highly hydrated interface in the NA-antibody complex. J Mol Biol 356(3):651–663. doi:10.1016/j.jmb.2005.11.061

Wan H, Gao J, Xu K, Chen H, Couzens LK, Rivers KH, Easterbrook JD, Yang K, Zhong L, Rajabi M, Ye J, Sultana I, Wan XF, Liu X, Perez DR, Taubenberger JK, Eichelberger MC (2013) Molecular basis for broad neuraminidase immunity: conserved epitopes in seasonal and pandemic H1N1 as well as H5N1 influenza viruses. J Virol 87(16):9290–9300. doi:10.1128/JVI.01203-13

Wang M, Qi J, Liu Y, Vavricka CJ, Wu Y, Li Q, Gao GF (2011) Influenza A virus N5 neuraminidase has an extended 150-cavity. J Virol 85(16):8431–8435. doi:10.1128/JVI.00638-11

Warren L (1959) The thiobarbituric acid assay of sialic acids. J Biol Chem 234(8):1971–1975

Webster RG (1966) Original antigenic sin in ferrets: the response to sequential infections with influenza viruses. J Immunol 97(2):177–183

Webster RG, Air GM, Metzger DW, Colman PM, Varghese JN, Baker AT, Laver WG (1987) Antigenic structure and variation in an influenza virus N9 neuraminidase. J Virol 61(9):2910–2916

Webster RG, Brown LE, Laver WG (1984) Antigenic and biological characterization of influenza virus neuraminidase (N2) with monoclonal antibodies. Virology 135(1):30–42

Webster RG, Laver WG (1967) Preparation and properties of antibody directed specifically against the neuraminidase of influenza virus. J Immunol 99(1):49–55

Wu ZL, Ethen C, Hickey GE, Jiang W (2009) Active 1918 pandemic flu viral neuraminidase has distinct N-glycan profile and is resistant to trypsin digestion. Biochem Biophys Res Commun 379(3):749–753. doi:10.1016/j.bbrc.2008.12.139

Xu X, Zhu X, Dwek RA, Stevens J, Wilson IA (2008) Structural characterization of the 1918 influenza virus H1N1 neuraminidase. J Virol 82(21):10493–10501. doi:10.1128/JVI.00959-08

Yen HL, Liang CH, Wu CY, Forrest HL, Ferguson A, Choy KT, Jones J, Wong DD, Cheung PP, Hsu CH, Li OT, Yuen KM, Chan RW, Poon LL, Chan MC, Nicholls JM, Krauss S, Wong CH, Guan Y, Webster RG, Webby RJ, Peiris M (2011) Hemagglutinin-neuraminidase balance confers respiratory-droplet transmissibility of the pandemic H1N1 influenza virus in ferrets. Proc Natl Acad Sci USA 108(34):14264–14269. doi:10.1073/pnas.1111000108

Zhu X, Yang H, Guo Z, Yu W, Carney PJ, Li Y, Chen LM, Paulson JC, Donis RO, Tong S, Stevens J, Wilson IA (2012) Crystal structures of two subtype N10 neuraminidase-like proteins from bat influenza A viruses reveal a diverged putative active site. Proc Natl Acad Sci USA 109(46):18903–18908. doi:10.1073/pnas.1212579109

Advances in Universal Influenza Virus Vaccine Design and Antibody Mediated Therapies Based on Conserved Regions of the Hemagglutinin

Florian Krammer, Peter Palese and John Steel

Abstract The threat of novel influenza viruses emerging into the human population from animal reservoirs, as well as the short duration of protection conferred by licensed vaccines against human seasonal strains has spurred research efforts to improve upon current vaccines and develop novel therapeutics against influenza viruses. In recent years these efforts have resulted in the identification of novel, highly conserved epitopes for neutralizing antibodies on the influenza virus hemagglutinin protein, which are present in both the stalk and globular head domains of the molecule. The existence of such epitopes may allow for generation of novel therapeutic antibodies, in addition to serving as attractive targets of novel vaccine design. The aims of developing improved vaccines include eliciting broader protection from drifted strains, inducing long-lived immunity against seasonal strains, and allowing for the rational design of vaccines that can be stockpiled for use as pre-pandemic vaccines. In addition, an increased focus on influenza virus vaccine research has prompted an improved understanding of how the immune system responds to influenza virus infection.

Abbreviations

bnAb	Broadly neutralizing antibody
CDR	Complementarity determining region
DTT	Dithiothreitol
H1, H2, H3, etc	Hemagglutinin subtype 1, 2, 3, etc
HA	Hemagglutinin
HA1	Hemagglutinin subunit 1
HA2	Hemaggltinin subunit 2

F. Krammer · P. Palese
Department of Microbiology, Icahn School of Medicine at Mount Sinai, New York, USA

J. Steel (✉)
Department of Microbiology and Immunology, Emory University School of Medicine, Atlanta, Georgia, USA
e-mail: john.steel@emory.edu

Current Topics in Microbiology and Immunology (2015) 386: 301–321
DOI: 10.1007/82_2014_408

Published Online: 10 July 2014

HAI	Hemagglutination inhibition
mAb	Monoclonal antibody
N1, N2, etc	Neuraminidase subtype 1, 2, etc
nAb	Neutralizing antibody
pH1N1	2009 pandemic H1N1
RBS	Receptor binding site
sH1N1	Seasonal H1N1

Contents

1 Introduction

Influenza A viruses circulate annually among human populations and are a source of significant morbidity and mortality. It is estimated that 10–20 % of the US population is infected with influenza viruses Influenzaeach year, and as many as 49,000 associated deaths occur annually (Glezen and Couch 1978; Fox et al. 1982; Thompson et al. 2004; CDC 2010). Correspondingly, a recent study indicated that approximately 20 % of the UK population may be infected annually (Hayward et al. 2014). In addition to the disease burden caused by seasonal human influenza virus lineages, zoonotic infections, against which there is an absence of immunity in the human population, occasionally result in the emergence of pandemic strains (Neumann et al. 2009). The emergence of the (pandemic) H1N1 subtype influenza virus from the swine reservoir in 2009 (Itoh et al. 2009) and human infections by the avian H5N1 and H7N9 viruses further highlight the potential risk posed by animal reservoirs of influenza A viruses.

Although a limited number of therapeutic drugs are available to combat influenza (Muthuri et al. 2014), they are typically costly, and public health measures that rely on single drug therapy suffer from the potential emergence of drug resistant strains of influenza viruses Influenza (Hayden and Hay 1992; Samson et al. 2013). Thus, the development of multiple therapeutic drugs, especially those that target distinct aspects of the viral lifecycle, are of critical importance.

The most cost-effective strategy to protect against influenza-related disease is vaccination. Current vaccination approaches are effective (Tricco et al. 2013; McNeil et al. 2014), particularly among healthy adult individuals and children (Osterholm et al. 2012), but are hampered by the need to achieve a close match between circulating strains and those included in the vaccine. Due to the rapid and unpredictable antigenic drift of seasonal influenza viruses, such a match is often difficult to attain. The possibility of a zoonotic influenza A virus entering the human population and establishing a novel human lineage represents a further challenge to current vaccination strategies. Since it is impossible to predict which subtype and which strain will cause the next influenza pandemic, current strain-specific approaches will fall short in a pandemic setting. Moreover, current influenza vaccines are recognized to be less effective in high-risk groups, such as the elderly, the very young, and the immune-compromised (Osterholm et al. 2012; Beyer et al. 2013).

Rational attempts to improve influenza vaccines would benefit from a better understanding of the immunological correlates of protection from influenza disease, and the mechanisms underlying such protection. The detailed mechanisms by which the immune system responds to influenza viruses Influenza infection, or vaccination, are remarkably poorly understood and most likely vary depending upon how viral antigen is presented to immune cells (Bucasas et al. 2011; Li et al. 2013).

The best-established correlate of protection from disease following inactivated influenza virus vaccination measures serum-mediated viral hemagglutination inhibition (HAI) of red blood cells: an HAI titer of approximately 1/40 correlates well with protection from disease in humans (Ellebedy and Webby 2009; Katz et al. 2011). Although the HAI assay detects classical neutralizing antibodies that block receptor binding, several alternative immune mechanisms that interfere with influenza virus replication have been described. These include antibodies that inhibit viral fusion with the cellular membrane (Ekiert et al. 2009; Wang et al. 2010b; Tan et al. 2012; Brandenburg et al. 2013), mucosal antibodies (Renegar and Small 1991; Seibert et al. 2013), complement pathways (Terajima et al. 2011; Co et al. 2012; Dilillo et al. 2014), and antibody dependent cellular cytotoxicity (Jegaskanda et al. 2013; Dilillo et al. 2014). The correlation between these alternative modes of in vitro neutralization and protection from disease in vivo are not well studied. This raises the possibility that vaccination strategies may be developed to exploit previously unappreciated protection modalities. To this end, advances in the characterization of novel conserved and protective epitopes present in the hemagglutinin protein have provoked interest in the field. This chapter focuses on studies examining neutralizing antibodies directed against conserved regions of the influenza viruses Influenza, and approaches designed to utilize these epitopes in novel vaccination strategies. If successful, such vaccines stand to increase protection from drifted strains, thereby reducing the need for annual vaccination. Moreover, broadly protective vaccines would prove highly valuable against pandemic strains.

2 Neutralizing Antibodies Directed Against Conserved Regions of the influenza viruses HA

The development of multiple broadly neutralizing monoclonal therapeutic vaccineantibodies (bnAbs) targeting the influenza hemagglutinin is desirable for two reasons. Firstly, such drugs may be used as therapeutic agents, which could be administered singly, or as cocktails of multiple antibodies and/or other therapeutic drugs, potentially providing effective clinical protection from influenza. Secondly, the use of drug cocktails may prevent, or limit the emergence of drug resistant strains of virus into human populations. Two main classes of broadly neutralizing antibodies against conserved regions of the HA have been described: those directed against the conserved, membrane proximal stalk (or stem) domain of the HA, and those directed against the membrane distal receptor binding site (RBS).

2.1 Stalk-Reactive Neutralizing Monoclonal Antibodies

The earliest reports of hemagglutinin stalk-reactive antibodies relied on a sensitive radioimmunoprecipitation assay to identify antibodies present in rabbit immune sera, which mapped to the hemagglutinin HA2 domain, (Polakova et al. 1978; Russ et al. 1978a, b). In 1983, Graves and colleagues characterized immune sera obtained from mice vaccinated with inactivated whole influenza virus which had been acid- and DTT-treated to remove the globular head of the HA (Graves et al. 1983). While data from this study demonstrated that antigenic epitopes were preserved in the hemagglutinin in the absence of the globular head domain, virus-neutralizing activity was not observed, possibly due to the loss of conformation of the immunizing antigen.

The first virus neutralizing stalk-reactive monoclonal antibody (mAb) was isolated from a mouse using traditional hybridoma technology in 1993 by Okuno et al. (1993). This antibody, C179, has fusion inhibiting activity and is able to bind and neutralize a broad range of group 1 HA encoding viruses, including H1, H2, H5, and H6 subtype strains (Okuno et al. 1994; Smirnov et al. 1999). Development of powerful new technologies such as plasmablast sorting followed by single cell PCR, phage display libraries for antibody screening, and divergent technologies to recover antibody coding sequences from memory B-cells has aided in the isolation of more of these relatively rare antibodies. The first examples of bnAbs isolated using phage display screening and specific to the hemagglutinin of influenza virus were reported in 2008 (Kashyap et al. 2008). These recombinant antibodies were constructed from individual heavy and light chain sequences derived from B-cells of individuals who had survived infection with H5N1 virus. They were identified using a phage display screen that enriched for antibodies specific for influenza H5 subtype HA. One such bnAb (A06) exhibited in vitro neutralization of H5N1 and seasonal H1N1 subtype influenza viruses Influenza at concentrations of antibody as low as 1–10 ug/ml (Kashyap et al. 2008). Clone A06 was also effective in vivo against the H1N1 subtype 2009 pandemic influenza virus, conferring protection from death in mice treated either prophylactically, or therapeutically up to 3 days post infection (Kashyap et al. 2010).

Two further, well-characterized human mAbs also isolated using phage technology, CR6261 and F10, were described in 2008 and 2009, respectively (Throsby et al. 2008; Sui et al. 2009). Both mAbs neutralize a broad range of group 1 HAs. Structural characterizations revealed that the footprints of both antibodies localize to the stalk domain and overlap that of the murine mAb C179 (Ekiert et al. 2009; Sui et al. 2009; Dreyfus et al. 2013). The activity of a distinct broadly neutralizing Ab, 12D1, targets a micro-conformational epitope on the long alpha helix of the H3 stalk domain, demonstrating that stalk-reactive antibodies also exist for group 2 HAs (Wang et al. 2010b). Clone 12D1 was isolated from mice sequentially vaccinated with divergent H3 HAs that share conserved epitopes, an approach that was subsequently used to generate the pan-H1 stalk-reactive antibody 6F12 (Tan et al. 2012). A third, more membrane proximal epitope on the stalk domain was defined by the pan-group 2 antibody CR8020 (Ekiert et al. 2011). To date, stalk-reactive antibodies can be grouped into three categories: antibodies that broadly neutralize within a specific subtype, including 12D1 and 6F12; antibodies that broadly neutralize strains within group 1 (CR6261, F10 etc.) or group 2 (CR8020, CR8043 etc. Friesen et al. (2014)); and antibodies that are pan-HA reactive. The last group is currently limited to three characterized members, FI6 and 39.29, which exhibit binding to cross-group HAs of type A influenza viruses (Corti et al. 2011; Nakamura et al. 2013), and CR9114, which is reactive against HAs of both influenza A and B viruses (Dreyfus et al. 2012). However, the number of stalk-reactive antibodies described is growing rapidly. Several laboratories, including that of Patrick Wilson's at the University of Chicago, have isolated, but not yet fully characterized, large numbers of antibodies belonging to each of the aforementioned categories (Corti et al. 2010; Wrammert et al. 2011; Li et al. 2012; Thomson et al. 2012; Nakamura et al. 2013; Whittle et al. 2014).

In contrast to canonical neutralizing HAI active antibodies that function by blocking the interactions between the RBS and the host receptor, stalk-reactive antibodies work through a plethora of mechanisms downstream of the initial binding event. First and foremost, stalk-reactive antibodies prevent fusion of the viral and endosomal membranes during acidification of the endosome (Ekiert et al. 2009; Wang et al. 2010b; Tan et al. 2012; Brandenburg et al. 2013). Antibodies bind to the HA outside of the cell and are then (likely) imported into the endosome together with the virus. To allow progression of the viral lifecycle, the HA must undergo a conformational change that triggers membrane fusion, upon acidification of the endosome. Stalk-reactive antibodies prevent this conformational step by locking the HA in the pre-fusion conformation. It has been shown that C179 interacts with about 70 % of the HA trimers of an influenza virion at neutralizing concentrations of as low as 25 μg/ml (Okuno et al. 1994). In addition, stalk-reactive antibodies are also able to inhibit viral egress and cleavage of HA by blocking access to the proteolytic cleavage site between HA1 and HA2 (Ekiert et al. 2009, 2011; Krammer and Palese 2013;

Friesen et al. 2014). Finally, stalk-targeting antibodies can limit viral spread through complement dependent lysis and antibody-dependent cell mediated cytotoxicity (Terajima et al. 2011; Dilillo et al. 2014). Typically, such antibodies interact with antigen by binding to accessible hydrophobic pockets located within the HA stalk. Notably, a large majority of the stalk binding antibodies employ a heavy chain-directed interaction with HA in which hydrophobic residues present in an extended heavy chain complementarity determining region (HCDR) (typically, but not exclusively HCDR2 or 3) interact with hydrophobic residues present in the HA to fill a hydrophobic pocket (Table 1). Correct positioning of the extended loop is supported by further mutations present in the same and other CDRs. The germline heavy chain gene Vh1-69 appears to be frequently employed in the generation of antibodies that interact with epitopes in the HA stem, possibly due to the presence of several hydrophobic residues encoded in this gene. Since stalk-reactive antibodies have very broad therapeutic activity, they are currently being considered and tested as anti-viral therapeutics in humans. Furthermore, they serve as important tools for antibody-guided universal vaccine approaches (see Sect. 4 below).

2.2 *Receptor Binding Site-Reactive Neutralizing Monoclonal Antibodies*

The globular head region of HA is considered to be hypervariable at multiple sites (Gerhard et al. 1981; Caton et al. 1982; Brown et al. 1990), resulting in the antigenic drift that is responsible for the narrow strain specificity of currently licensed influenza vaccines. However, due to functional constraints associated with HA binding to the sialic acid receptor, there is a highly conserved region of the HA globular head which encompasses the RBS (Wilson et al. 1981; Weis et al. 1988). Advances in cloning and screening technologies have permitted the identification of increasing numbers of neutralizing monoclonal therapeutic vaccine antibodies specific to HA including a small number of broadly neutralizing antibodies that map to a previously unappreciated epitope close to and overlapping with the RBS of the protein (Ekiert et al. 2009; Yoshida et al. 2009; Krause et al. 2011; Ohshima et al. 2011; Whittle et al. 2011; Lee et al. 2012; Xu et al. 2013) (Table 1). These newly isolated antibodies may be of therapeutic interest, as they may confer significantly broader protection from influenza viruses Influenza infection and disease than -specific antibodies that interact with the conventional antigenic sites. These RBS-directed antibodies may also be refractory to virus-mediated escape from protection. Of further interest, such antibodies appear to possess several common features that may be associated with their reactivity. Several RBS-specific antibodies bind antigen predominantly through heavy chain directed interactions, and have unusually long, somatically hypermutated CDRs. Additionally, multiple studies have indicated that avidity may be an important mechanism that increases the neutralizing breadth of at least some of these antibodies (Ekiert et al. 2012; Lee et al. 2012).

Table 1 Characteristics of select broadly neutralizing influenza hemagglutinin-specific monoclonal antibodies

Antibody	Host	Extent of subtype reactivity	Germline gene restriction	Predominant mediators of interaction with antigen	Reference
Receptor binding site (RBS) specific antibodies					
2G1, 8M2	Human	H2	V_h1-69	HCDR 2	Xu et al. (2013)
8M2	Human	H2, H3	V_h1-69	HCDR 2, 3	Xu et al. (2013)
8F8	Human	Pan-H2	V_h3-33	HCDR 3	Xu et al. (2013)
C05	Human	H1, H2, H3, H9	V_h3-23	HCDR 3	Ekiert et al. (2012)
S139/1	Mouse	H1, H2, H3, H13, H16	J551.17	HCDR 2	Lee et al. (2012)
5J8	Human	H1	V_h4-b	unknown	Krause et al. (2011)
CH65	Human	H1	V_h1-2	HCDR 1, 2, 3 and LCDR 1	Whittle et al. (2011)
F045-092; F026-427	Human	H1, H2, H3, H5	V_h1-69	Unknown	Ohshima et al. (2011)
Stem specific antibodies					
C179	Mouse	H1, H2, H5, H6, H9	unknown	HCDR 1, 3, LCDR 1	Okuno et al. (1993), Dreyfus et al. (2013)
A06	Human	H1, H5	V_h1-e	HCDR 2	Kashyap et al. (2008)
CR6261	Human	H1, other group 1	V_h1-69	HCDR 1, 2	Throsby et al. (2008)
F10	Human	H1, other group 1	V_h1-69	HCDR 1, 2	Sui et al. (2009)
12D1	Mouse	H3, H5	unknown	unknown	Wang et al. (2010b)
6F12	Mouse	Pan-H1	unknown	unknown	Tan et al. (2012)
CR9114	Human	Pan influenza type A and B	V_h1-69	HCDR 1, 2, 3	Dreyfus et al. (2012)
FI6	Human	Pan-type A	V_h3-30	HCDR 3	Corti et al. (2011)
CR8043	Human	H3, H10	V_h1-3	HCDR 1, 3	Friesen et al. (2014)

The epitope(s) recognized by several RBS-targeting bnAbs include(s) a strictly conserved hydrophobic tryptophan residue within the floor of the RBS groove, at HA1 position 153. This amino acid residue appears critical in the binding of several of the recently described bnAbs to the HA protein.

One recent study has demonstrated that three human mAbs conferring atypically broad, pan-H2 subtype neutralization activity (Xu et al. 2013) similarly exploit aromatic residues in the CDRs of their respective heavy chains. These antibodies utilize the presence of other supporting changes from germline sequences in order to interact with the receptor binding pocket of the HA. The interactions are characterized by the extension of the heavy chain into the RBS pocket, resulting in an antibody–antigen interaction footprint of approximately 200 Å^2 or more, out of a total antibody-antigen interaction of approximately 800 Å^2. The hydrophobic residues on antibody and antigen interact by π-π stacking to fill a hydrophobic cavity in the RBS. Intriguingly, this raises the possibility that by focusing the interaction between HA and mAb on a few critical, highly conserved residues thus limiting the contribution of supporting interactions surrounding the RBS, such RBS-directed antibodies may limit the loss of binding upon subsequent genetic drift in the hypervariable antigenic sites of the HA. The downstream consequence of such binding would be greater broadly neutralizing activity. Antibody CO5, which binds and neutralizes multiple strains belonging to group one and two subtypes (Kashyap et al. 2008, 2010) has been shown to interact with the influenza HA via π-π stacking of HA1 TRP 153 with a hydrophobic residue in a CDR of the antibody heavy chain (Ekiert et al. 2012; Xu et al. 2013). mAbs CO5, 2G1, 8M2, 8F8, S139/1, CH65, and likely F045-092 and F026-427 (Ohshima et al. 2011; Whittle et al. 2011; Ekiert et al. 2012; Lee et al. 2012; Xu et al. 2013), (Table 1), also possess residues in the HCDR domains which interact with the RBS of hemagglutinin.

The germline gene V_h1-69, which encodes the variable heavy region of human immunoglobulin genes, partially encodes three out of nine of these broadly neutralizing mAbs. The repeated use of the V_h1-69 gene may be due to the unique presence among variable heavy genes of two hydrophobic residues encoded in this germline sequence (Ile 53 and Phe 54). These hydrophobic residues may give V_h1-69 encoded mAbs a selective advantage in terms of initiating and subsequently increasing the strength of interactions with the hydrophobic pocket of the HA RBS through somatic hypermutation. However, it is important to keep in mind that alternative germline genes, for example V_h3-33 and V_h3-23, can also encode RBS-specific bnAbs. Such antibodies function, at least in some cases, through a mechanism similar to that of 2G1, except that the antigen-interacting hydrophobic residues present in their CDR domains are obtained through somatic hypermutation, as opposed to being encoded in the germline. The ability to generate bnAbs from multiple germline alleles is an important consideration when developing broadly protective vaccines, as a critical criterion for such strategies will be the ability to elicit neutralizing responses from a genetically diverse population.

2.3 Vestigial Esterase Domain-Reactive Neutralizing Monoclonal Antibodies

A third non-conventional, conserved neutralizing epitope in the influenza viruses Influenza H5 hemagglutinin and a cognate antibody were identified in 2013. The neutralizing mAb (H5M9) was crystallized in association with the HA, and the structure demonstrated that the antibody does not interfere with receptor binding. Instead H5M9 recognizes an epitope that includes amino acids 273–278 in the conserved vestigial esterase domain, as well as residues 53–62, 78–83a, and 117–119 of the HA molecule (Zhu et al. 2013). A second antibody (HA-7) generated against the H5 HA from A/Anhui/1/2005, that is specific for a putative overlapping epitope including HA residue E83a, was independently reported (Du et al. 2013). One possible explanation for the observed broadly neutralizing activity of these mAbs is that they inhibit the conformational rearrangement of the HA.

3 Induction of Stalk-Reactive Antibodies by Natural Infection and Standard Vaccination

Until recently, quantitative data about the frequency of stalk-reactive antibodies in serum was unavailable. Qualitative studies analyzing plasmablast and memory B-cells indicated that stalk-reactive antibodies could be found only occasionally in humans exposed to seasonal influenza viruses by vaccination, or in one cited study, infection (Throsby et al. 2008; Wrammert et al. 2008; Corti et al. 2010; Moody et al. 2011). However, a higher frequency of these antibodies was found after infection or vaccination with pandemic H1N1 (Wrammert et al. 2011; Li et al. 2012; Thomson et al. 2012). The first quantitative approach to measure stalk-reactive antibodies in human sera was made by Sui and colleagues using a competition-based assay involving the stalk-reactive antibody F10. These authors found a wide prevalence of F10-like antibodies in human sera, yet such antibodies exist at low levels. It is estimated that they account for approximately 0.001 % of total antibody (Sui et al. 2011). Using chimeric HAs that consisted of group 1 or group 2 stalks (H1 and H3 subtype respectively) and exotic head domains (Fig. 1) to which humans are naïve, stalk-reactive antibodies in sera were detected directly (Hai et al. 2012). Assays for detection of stalk-binding antibodies have been reported that use recombinant cHA in ELISA or other immuno-based assays (Tan et al. 2012) or by using cHA-expressing viruses that have irrelevant neuraminidases (usually N3) in neutralization assays. Using cHAs as substrate, Pica and colleagues demonstrated that individuals infected with pandemic H1N1 developed a strong response to the HA stalk domain (Pica et al. 2012). These data are consistent with studies performed in the Wilson and Schrader laboratories (Wrammert et al. 2011; Li et al. 2012; Thomson et al. 2012), which found that stalk-reactive antibodies represented an estimated 7 % of the total serum IgG of human individuals and also reported strong cross-reactivity

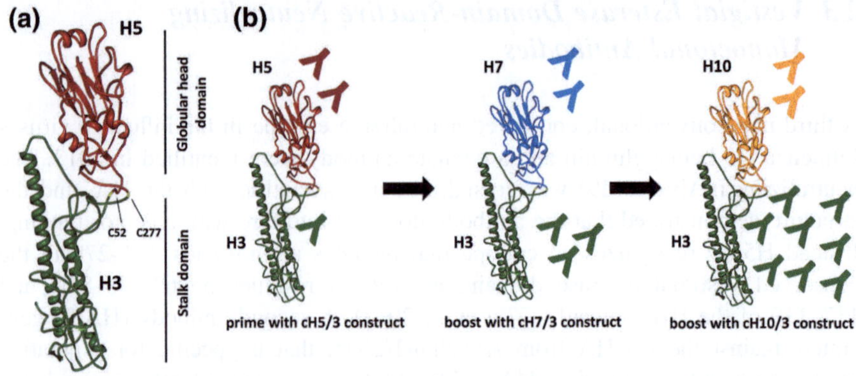

Fig. 1 Schematic of a chimeric HA-based vaccination strategy. **a** Chimeric HAs are combinations of heterosubtypic head domains with stalk domains of H1 (Group 1) or H3 (Group 2) HAs. Here we show a chimeric H5/H3 HA which consists of the membrane distal head domain of H5 HA (*red*) and the membrane proximal stalk domain of H3 HA (*green*). A disulfide linkage between cysteines 52 and 277 (indicated in *yellow*) serves to demarcate the stalk and head domains. **b** Vaccination regimen based on chimeric HAs. Vaccination with chimeric H5/H3 HA induces a primary response against the H5 head and an almost undetectable response against the immunosubdominant H3 stalk domain. Upon sequential boosting with chimeric H7/H3 HA (H7 head (*blue*) on top of H3 stalk (*green*)) and chimeric H10/H3 HA (H10 head domain (*golden*) on top of an H3 stalk domain (*green*)), only a primary response is mounted against the heterosubtypic head domains but antibody titers against conserved epitopes in the H3 stalk domain are boosted. All structures are based on PDB# 1RU7 and were visualized in Protein Workshop. Modified from Krammer et al. (2014b)

to H5 HA. Since earlier qualitative studies found no or very low levels of stalk-reactive antibodies in individuals exposed to seasonal influenza viruses (Wrammert et al. 2008; Corti et al. 2010; Moody et al. 2011) (by vaccination and/or infection) it has been suggested that the unique combination of a conserved stalk to which people were already primed and a new head domain to which people were naive (the head domain of pH1N1 and sH1N1 share less than 70 % amino acid identity) specifically boosted stalk-reactive antibodies (Pica et al. 2012). The same phenomenon was also observed in the mouse model, where animals sequentially infected with two drifted sH1N1 strains developed significantly lower levels of stalk-reactive antibodies than animals sequentially infected with sH1N1 and pH1N1 strains (Krammer et al. 2012). Moreover, individuals exposed to the A/New Jersey/76 H1N1 swine influenza virus vaccine (in which the HA is only distantly related to seasonal H1N1 HA) showed higher levels of stalk-reactive antibodies than unvaccinated individuals (Miller et al. 2013b). In a longitudinal study that examined immunity to influenza virus in a sub-cohort of the Framingham heart study, researchers found that people exposed to H2N2 virus had higher group I stalk titers than individuals who had no HI antibodies against this virus subtype (Miller et al. 2013a). Since the stalk domain is relatively conserved among all group 1 HAs (H1, H5, H6, H8, H9, H11, H12, H13, H16, H17, and H18), it is likely that exposure to H2—which has a completely different head but a conserved stalk—boosted stalk-reactive antibody titers. The same study also reported that group 1 stalk-reactive antibodies are in general present at higher titers in humans than group 2 stalk-reactive antibodies (Miller et al. 2013a). This makes sense considering group 1 HA viruses have circulated as drifted strains of multiple subtypes in the human population during the last 100 years, with varying globular heads but relatively conserved stalk domains. In contrast, a single subtype of group 2 HA virus, H3N2, has circulated in humans over the same period of time (Fig. 2). However, there is also evidence that group 2 stalk-reactive antibodies, mainly induced by natural infection, are present at low levels in the population (Margine et al. 2013a). In a recent study it was shown that individuals infected with H7N9 virus—which has a conserved group 2 stalk but a head domain that is quite divergent from H3—had elevated levels of group 2 cross-reactivity likely based on stalk-reactive antibodies (Guo et al. 2014). Similarly, group 1 stalk-reactive antibodies could be isolated from humans infected with H5N1 influenza viruses Influenzaor vaccinated with H5N1 hemagglutinin (Kashyap et al. 2008; Whittle et al. 2014). Based on these data it has been hypothesized that baseline levels of stalk-reactive antibodies are induced in the population primarily by natural infection, and that these antibodies can then be boosted by exposure to divergent HAs that share a conserved stalk domain with the priming virus. Such events have occurred in 1957, when people primed by H1N1 were subsequently exposed to H2N2 and again in 2009 when people primed by sH1N1 (and H2N2) were exposed to pH1N1 (Palese and Wang 2011). In each case, the virus circulating before the introduction of the novel pandemic virus disappeared, suggesting that elevated stalk-reactive antibody levels might play an important role in the elimination of seasonal influenza viruses from the human population (Palese and Wang 2011). The extinction of H2N2 in 1968 provides an exceptional case as its disappearance was likely caused by the induction of cross-reactive N2 NA antibodies by H3N2. Stalk-reactive antibodies are unlikely to be responsible for elimination of the preceding virus lineage in this example, since H2 and H3 belong to different HA groups and antibodies cross-reactive against group 1 and group 2 are extremely rare.

4 Stalk-Based Universal Influenza Virus Constructs

4.1 Stalk-Based Vaccine Constructs Lacking the Hemagglutinin Globular Head

As the globular head domain of the influenza HA possesses the immunodominant epitopes of the protein, early attempts to induce antibodies specific for the stalk domain focused on generating antigens in which the globular head domain was absent. Graves and colleagues used a whole influenza virus which had been chemically treated to remove the globular head of the HA as an immunogen in mice. This strategy succeeded in eliciting serum antibodies directed towards the stem domain (Graves et al. 1983). In 1993, Okuno et al. (1993) identified a mAb

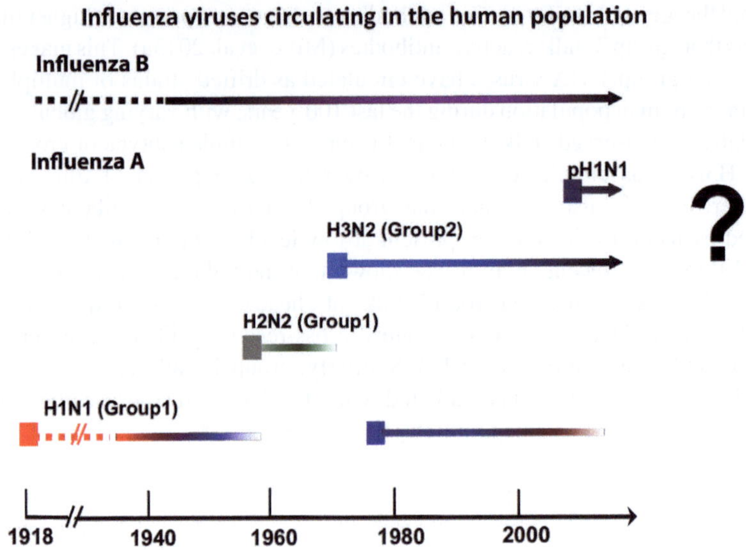

Fig. 2 Circulation of influenza virus strains in the human population since 1918. Influenza A and B viruses have circulated in humans continuously throughout the twentieth and twenty-first centuries. Multiple influenza A virus lineages have circulated during the same time period. H1N1 was introduced into the human population in 1918 and induced a baseline level of anti-group 1 stalk (Anti-G1 stalk) and anti-N1 NA antibody titers. Titers likely remained stable in the population till 1957 when H2N2 crossed the species barrier into humans. H1 and H2 HAs belong to group 1, with highly similar stalk domains but more divergent globular head domains. The introduction of H2N2 might therefore have boosted antibodies against conserved epitopes in the stalk domain which in turn contributed to the extinction of H1N1 in humans in 1957. Furthermore, the introduction of H2N2 would have induced baseline titers of anti-N2 NA antibodies in the population. H2N2 circulated from 1957 till 1968 when H3N2 was introduced. H3 HA is a group 2 HA, divergent from group 1 H2 HA, but the NA is highly related to the N2 of H2N2. The combination of novel HA with an NA for which humans were already primed might have boosted anti-N2 NA titers, facilitating the elimination of H2N2 from the population. After 1968 N2 NA titers may have declined to 1957–1968 levels due to population turnover. Also, introduction of H3N2 would have induced baseline antibody titers against the stalk of group 2 HA (anti-G2 stalk). N1 titers probably started to decline after 1957 due to population turnover but were brought back to baseline in 1977 when H1N1 was re-introduced. Similarly, anti-group 1 HA stalk titers probably started to decline on a population level back to the 1918–1957 baseline until 2009 when they were boosted by the 2009 pH1N1 virus

(C179) which was directed against the stalk region of the HA and conferred protection from challenge with an H1 subtype influenza virus in mice (Okuno et al. 1994). Sagawa et al. (1996) transfected a headless construct of an H2 HA into cells and when these same transfected cells were used to immunize mice partial protection following viral challenge with an H1N1 virus was observed. Similarly, a headless HA construct based on the A/PR/8/34 HA generated stalk-specific sera possessing pan-H1 subtype cross-reactivity in ELISA assays. Immunization with such constructs protected mice from lethal challenge (Steel et al. 2010).

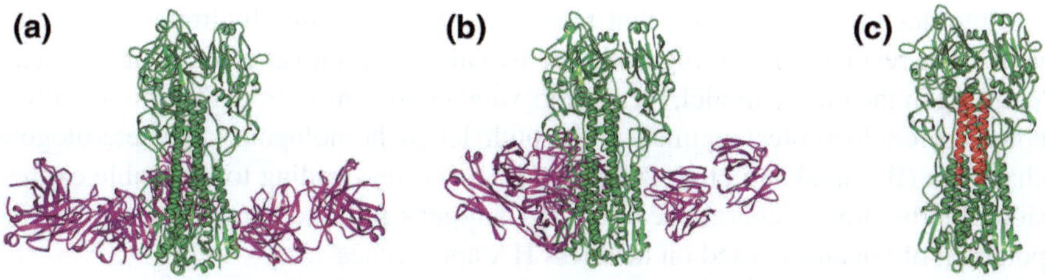

Fig. 3 The three main epitopes on the HA stalk domain. **a** shows the structure of H3 HA (*green*) in combination with mAb CR8020 (Fab, *purple*). The footprint of CR8020 represents so far the most membrane proximal epitope on the stalk and is shared with CR8043. **b** The structure of H3 HA (*green*) with mAb CR9114 (Fab, *purple*). CR9114 uses a footprint that overlaps with most isolated stalk-reactive antibodies including CR6261, F10, FI6, and C179. **c** The epitope of mAb 12D1 (in *red*, here shown on an H3 HA) is so far the most membrane distal epitope on the stalk domain. Structures are based on PDB# 3SDY (**a**, **c**) and 4FQY (**b**) and were visualized in Protein Workshop

Interestingly, although ELISA titers to the homologous protein (PR8) were higher in animals vaccinated with full length hemagglutinin than those who received headless HA, the antibody titers to heterologous and heterosubtypic HA protein in ELISA assay were lower in those mice vaccinated with full length hemagglutinin (Steel et al. 2010).

A neutralizing epitope present in the alpha-helical portion of the influenza hemagglutinin HA2 domain (amino acids 76–130 (HA2)) and recognized by the neutralizing mAb 12D1 (Fig. 3) has been identified by Wang et al. (2010b). When this epitope was used to immunize mice, animals were protected from lethal challenge with either H3N2 or H5N1 subtype influenza viruses (Wang et al. 2010a). Two distinct epitopes in the hemagglutinin stem domain have additionally been identified through crystallographic studies that employed stem-directed mAbs in complex with the hemagglutinin molecule (Fig. 3) (Corti and Lanzavecchia 2013; Subbarao and Matsuoka 2013).

While it has been established that headless HA vaccination strategies can lead to the generation of higher levels of cross-reactive serum antibodies than identical vaccination regimens using full length HA antigen (Steel et al. 2010), headless hemagglutinin based approaches suffer considerably from inaccurate protein folding and poor antigen expression (Steel et al. 2010). In this regard, recent studies from Lu et al. (2014) and Bommakanti et al. (2010, 2012) aimed to improve the expression of the HA2 domain. Experiments by Lu et al demonstrated that a rationally engineered headless HA molecule that retains the antigenically conserved sites on the HA stalk can be expressed at very high concentration and be recognized by conformationally dependent stem-specific antibodies. The HA antigen has amino acid changes introduced into the construct, which alter intramolecular electrostatic interactions and reorganize intramolecular disulfide bonds, leading to expression of a stabilized protein (Lu et al. 2014). Bommakanti and colleagues similarly demonstrated stabilization of the stem domains of both group 1 and group 2 HA molecules through the introduction of mutations that replaced solvent exposed hydrophobic patches with polar residues. These regions were revealed by removal of the globular head. Working in the mouse model, the authors went on to demonstrate that this stabilized construct could protect animals from both lethal homologous and heterologous challenge (Bommakanti et al. 2010, 2012). Advances leading to the stable expression of structurally accurate headless HA antigens stand to increase the protective potential of vaccines based on headless HA approaches.

4.2 Chimeric Hemagglutinin-Based Vaccine Constructs

An alternative strategy to induce stalk-reactive antibodies is based on the observation that sequential exposure to influenza viruses with divergent head but conserved stalk domains refocuses the immune response to the usually subdominant stalk. Vaccination with chimeric HAs exploits this approach. Chimeric HAs consist of H1 (group 1) or H3 (group 2) stalk domains combined with 'exotic' head domains, usually of avian origin (Hai et al. 2012). A conserved disulfide bond between cysteines 52 and 277 is used to demarcate the head and stalk domains. The region between these amino acids represents the head domain while the rest of the HA ectodomain is comprised of the stalk domain (N- and C-terminus of the HA1 and the ectodomain of HA2). The use of a heterologous head domain stabilizes structural epitopes in the stalk domain. Importantly, the stalk, in contrast to many headless HA approaches, is correctly folded and fully functional. In fact, influenza viruses Influenza expressing cHAs can be rescued and grown to titers comparable to wild type in embryonated eggs and cell culture (Hai et al. 2012). It was subsequently shown that sequential vaccination with different cHAs that have the same stalk but divergent heads induces high titers of stalk-reactive antibodies in mice and ferrets and broadly protects from lethal challenge with divergent group 1 and group 2 viruses including H5N1 and H7N9 viruses (Krammer and Palese 2013, 2014; Krammer et al. 2013, 2014a, b; Margine et al. 2013b). However, it is important to note that to date no cross-group protection has been observed (Krammer et al. 2013). Animals vaccinated with group 1 constructs failed to mount titers against the group 2 stalk and were not protected from group 2 (H3N2) virus challenge. This indicates that a successful cHA-based vaccine should minimally include three components: a group 1, a group 2 and an influenza B cHA (Krammer and Palese 2014). Chimeric HA based vaccine approaches have been successfully applied in the form of DNA vaccines, recombinant protein vaccines and viral vectors as well as in combination with several experimental adjuvants including oil-in water emulsions similar to the ones licensed for use in humans (Goff et al. 2013; Krammer and Palese 2013, 2014; Krammer et al. 2013, 2014a, b; Margine et al. 2013b). Vaccination with viruses expressing cHAs with exotic heads and N1 or N2 NAs may also enhance the immune response to the relatively conserved NAs. The resulting immune response, based on stalk-specific as well as

NA-specific conserved epitopes may afford the cross protective responses necessary for a universal influenza virus vaccine.

4.3 Other Approaches

In addition to headless and chimeric HA constructs, a number of other strategies have been attempted to induce neutralizing antibodies to the HA stem. A vaccine based on the completely conserved fusion peptide was able to provide protection against homologous and heterosubtypic challenge (Janulíková et al. 2012). Furthermore, rationally designed nanoparticles based on the Flock House virus capsid have been used to elicit CR6261-like antibodies (Schneemann et al. 2012). A bacterial ferritin nanoparticle displaying HA trimers on its surface was also able to induce broadly reactive antibodies against both the head as well as the stalk domain of H1 and protected ferrets from heterologous H1N1 challenge (Kanekiyo et al. 2013). However, this approach was unable to elicit significant amounts of heterosubtypic immunity (Kanekiyo et al. 2013). Finally regimens using DNA or live virus priming followed by inactivated virus boosts are currently being investigated as novel strategies to increase broadly neutralizing antibody responses (Wei et al. 2010; Talaat et al. 2014).

5 Conclusions and Future Perspective

Recent developments in technologies that allow screening for and isolation of Abs derived from humans and animals exposed to influenza viruses Influenza antigens have expanded the extent of our knowledge on the repertoire of antibodies that are generated in response to influenza viruses. Examples of relatively rare, or previously unrecognized, classes of broadly neutralizing antibody have been identified, and common themes are emerging in relation to the mechanisms of neutralization of these antibodies. Biochemical, virological, as well as crystallography-based studies have allowed the detailed characterization of these novel antibodies, which map to conserved epitopes on group I or group II HA proteins (stem or globular head domains). These antibodies neutralize virus through distinct mechanisms, such as inhibition of receptor binding or fusion of the viral and cellular membranes. The availability of multiple classes of antibodies that neutralize virus through different mechanisms, as well as antibodies that function through a single mechanism but bind to the viral antigen using differing fine specificities, provide opportunities to develop multi-drug cocktails for use in humans.

Furthermore, the recent surge of interest in bnAbs, especially those antibodies that recognize the stalk domain of the hemagglutinin molecule, have stimulated research into the development of alternative influenza virus vaccines and vaccine regimens, in order to elicit greater cross protective responses to influenza virus.

Considerable progress has been made towards demonstrating the potential utility of headless and chimeric hemagglutinin-based antigens, but further research is needed to understand how best to direct the antibody response to conserved epitopes and how to optimally elicit potent antibodies specific to such conserved epitopes. Efforts towards improved influenza vaccines designed to induce the broadest and most potently protective responses would greatly benefit from a better understanding of the immunological correlates of protection from disease. Taken together, the data reviewed here highlight the exciting advances being made to fulfill the vital and unmet need for improved influenza vaccines and vaccination practices.

Acknowledgments PP and FK are supported, in part, by NIH P01 AI097092, U19 AI109946, and HHSN272201400008C. JS is supported in part by HHSN272201400004C. We very much thank Caitlin Mullarkey for helpful discussions and editorial review.

References

Beyer WE, McElhaney J, Smith DJ, Monto AS, Nguyen-Van-Tam JS, Osterhaus AD (2013) Cochrane re-arranged: support for policies to vaccinate elderly people against influenza. Vaccine 31:6030–6033. doi:S0264-410X(13)01339-X, 10.1016/j.vaccine.2013.09.063

Bommakanti G, Citron MP, Hepler RW et al (2010) Design of an HA2-based Escherichia coli expressed influenza immunogen that protects mice from pathogenic challenge. Proc Natl Acad Sci USA 107:13701–13706. doi:10.1073/pnas.1007465107

Bommakanti G, Lu X, Citron MP et al (2012) Design of Escherichia coli-expressed stalk domain immunogens of H1N1 hemagglutinin that protect mice from lethal challenge. J Virol 86:13434–13444. doi:10.1128/JVI.01429-12

Brandenburg B, Koudstaal W, Goudsmit J et al (2013) Mechanisms of hemagglutinin targeted influenza virus neutralization. PLoS One 8:e80034. doi:10.1371/journal.pone.0080034

Brown LE, Murray JM, White DO, Jackson DC (1990) An analysis of the properties of monoclonal antibodies directed to epitopes on influenza virus hemagglutinin. Arch Virol 114:1–26

Bucasas KL, Franco LM, Shaw CA et al (2011) Early patterns of gene expression correlate with the humoral immune response to influenza vaccination in humans. J Infect Dis 203:921–929. doi:10.1093/infdis/jiq156

Caton AJ, Brownlee GG, Yewdell JW, Gerhard W (1982) The antigenic structure of the influenza virus A/PR/8/34 hemagglutinin (H1 subtype). Cell 31:417–427. doi:10.1016/0092-8674(82)90135-0

CDC (2010) Estimates of deaths associated with seasonal influenza—United States, 1976–2007. MMWR Morb Mortal Wkly Rep 59:1057–1062.

Co MD, Cruz J, Takeda A, Ennis FA, Terajima M (2012) Comparison of complement dependent lytic, hemagglutination inhibition and microneutralization antibody responses in influenza vaccinated individuals. Hum Vaccin Immunother 8:1218–1222. doi:10.4161/hv.21025

Corti D, Lanzavecchia A (2013) Broadly neutralizing antiviral antibodies. Annu Rev Immunol 31:705–742. doi:10.1146/annurev-immunol-032712-095916

Corti D, Suguitan AL Jr, Pinna D et al (2010) Heterosubtypic neutralizing antibodies are produced by individuals immunized with a seasonal influenza vaccine. J Clin Invest 120:1663–1673. doi:10.1172/JCI41902

Corti D, Voss J, Gamblin SJ et al (2011) A neutralizing antibody selected from plasma cells that binds to group 1 and group 2 influenza A hemagglutinins. Science 333:850–856. doi:10.1126/science.1205669

Dilillo DJ, Tan GS, Palese P, Ravetch JV (2014) Broadly neutralizing hemagglutinin stalk-specific antibodies require FcgammaR interactions for protection against influenza virus in vivo. Nat Med 20:143–151. doi:10.1038/nm.3443

Dreyfus C, Laursen NS, Kwaks T et al (2012) Highly conserved protective epitopes on influenza B viruses. Science 337:1343–1348. doi:10.1126/science.1222908

Dreyfus C, Ekiert DC, Wilson IA (2013) Structure of a classical broadly neutralizing stem antibody in complex with a pandemic H2 influenza virus hemagglutinin. J Virol 87:7149–7154. doi:10.1128/JVI.02975-12

Du L, Jin L, Zhao G et al (2013) Identification and structural characterization of a broadly neutralizing antibody targeting a novel conserved epitope on the influenza virus H5N1 hemagglutinin. J Virol 87:2215–2225. doi:10.1128/JVI.02344-12

Ekiert DC, Bhabha G, Elsliger MA et al (2009) Antibody recognition of a highly conserved influenza virus epitope. Science 324:246–251. doi:10.1126/science.1171491

Ekiert DC, Friesen RH, Bhabha G et al (2011) A highly conserved neutralizing epitope on group 2 influenza A viruses. Science 333:843–850. doi:10.1126/science.1204839

Ekiert DC, Kashyap AK, Steel J et al (2012) Cross-neutralization of influenza A viruses mediated by a single antibody loop. Nature 489:526–532. doi:10.1038/nature11414

Ellebedy AH, Webby RJ (2009) Influenza vaccines. Vaccine 27(Suppl 4):D65–D68. doi:S0264-410X(09)01214-6, 10.1016/j.vaccine.2009.08.038

Fox JP, Cooney MK, Hall CE, Foy HM (1982) Influenzavirus infections in Seattle families, 1975–1979. II. Pattern of infection in invaded households and relation of age and prior antibody to occurrence of infection and related illness. Am J Epidemiol 116:228–242

Friesen RH, Lee PS, Stoop EJ et al (2014) A common solution to group 2 influenza virus neutralization. Proc Natl Acad Sci USA 111:445–450. doi:10.1073/pnas.1319058110

Gerhard W, Yewdell J, Frankel ME, Webster R (1981) Antigenic structure of influenza virus haemagglutinin defined by hybridoma antibodies. Nature 290:713–717

Glezen WP, Couch RB (1978) Interpandemic influenza in the Houston area, 1974–1976. N Engl J Med 298:587–592. doi:10.1056/NEJM197803162981103

Goff PH, Eggink D, Seibert CW, Hai R, Martínez-Gil L, Krammer F, Palese P (2013) Adjuvants and immunization strategies to induce influenza virus hemagglutinin stalk antibodies. PLoS One 8:e79194. doi:10.1371/journal.pone.0079194

Graves PN, Schulman JL, Young JF, Palese P (1983) Preparation of influenza virus subviral particles lacking the HA1 subunit of hemagglutinin: unmasking of cross-reactive HA2 determinants. Virology 126:106–116

Guo L, Zhang X, Ren L et al (2014) Human antibody responses to avian influenza A(H7N9) virus, 2013. Emerg Infect Dis 20:192–200. doi:10.3201/eid2002.131094

Hai R, Krammer F, Tan GS et al (2012) Influenza viruses expressing chimeric hemagglutinins: globular head and stalk domains derived from different subtypes. J Virol 86:5774–5781. doi:10.1128/JVI.00137-12

Hayden FG, Hay AJ (1992) Emergence and transmission of influenza A viruses resistant to amantadine and rimantadine. Curr Top Microbiol Immunol 176:119–130

Hayward AC, Fragaszy EB, Bermingham A et al (2014) Comparative community burden and severity of seasonal and pandemic influenza: results of the Flu Watch cohort study. Lancet Respir Med 2(6):445–454. doi: 10.1016/52213-2600 (14) 70034-7

Itoh Y, Shinya K, Kiso M et al (2009) In vitro and in vivo characterization of new swine-origin H1N1 influenza viruses. Nature 460:1021–1025. doi:10.1038/nature08260

Janulíková J, Staneková Z, Mucha V, Kostolanský F, Varečková E (2012) Two distinct regions of HA2 glycopolypeptide of influenza virus hemagglutinin elicit cross-protective immunity against influenza. Acta Virol 56:169–176

Jegaskanda S, Job ER, Kramski M et al (2013) Cross-reactive influenza-specific antibody-dependent cellular cytotoxicity antibodies in the absence of neutralizing antibodies. J Immunol 190:1837–1848. doi:10.4049/jimmunol.1201574

Kanekiyo M, Wei CJ, Yassine HM et al (2013) Self-assembling influenza nanoparticle vaccines elicit broadly neutralizing H1N1 antibodies. Nature. doi:10.1038/nature12202

Kashyap AK, Steel J, Oner AF et al (2008) Combinatorial antibody libraries from survivors of the Turkish H5N1 avian influenza outbreak reveal virus neutralization strategies. Proc Natl Acad Sci USA 105:5986–5991

Kashyap AK, Steel J, Rubrum A et al (2010) Protection from the 2009 H1N1 pandemic influenza by an antibody from combinatorial survivor-based libraries. PLoS Pathog 6:e1000990. doi:10.1371/journal.ppat.1000990

Katz JM, Hancock K, Xu X (2011) Serologic assays for influenza surveillance, diagnosis and vaccine evaluation. Expert Rev Anti Infect Ther 9:669–683. doi:10.1586/eri.11.51

Krammer F, Palese P (2013) Influenza virus hemagglutinin stalk-based antibodies and vaccines. Curr Opin Virol 3:521–530. doi:10.1016/j.coviro.2013.07.007

Krammer F, Palese P (2014) Universal influenza virus vaccines: need for clinical trials. Nat Immunol 15:3–5. doi:10.1038/ni.2761

Krammer F, Pica N, Hai R, Tan GS, Palese P (2012) Hemagglutinin stalk-reactive antibodies are boosted following sequential infection with seasonal and pandemic H1N1 influenza virus in mice. J Virol 86:10302–10307. doi:10.1128/JVI.01336-12

Krammer F, Pica N, Hai R, Margine I, Palese P (2013) Chimeric hemagglutinin influenza virus vaccine constructs elicit broadly protective stalk-specific antibodies. J Virol 87:6542–6550. doi:10.1128/JVI.00641-13

Krammer F, Hai R, Yondola M et al (2014a) Assessment of influenza virus hemagglutinin stalk-based immunity in ferrets. J Virol 88:3432–3442. doi:10.1128/JVI.03004-13

Krammer F, Margine I, Hai R et al (2014b) H3 Stalk-based chimeric hemagglutinin influenza virus constructs protect mice from H7N9 challenge. J Virol 88:2340–2343. doi:10.1128/JVI.03183-13

Krause JC, Tsibane T, Tumpey TM, Huffman CJ, Basler CF, Crowe JE Jr (2011) A broadly neutralizing human monoclonal antibody that recognizes a conserved, novel epitope on the globular head of the influenza H1N1 virus hemagglutinin. J Virol 85:10905–10908. doi:10.1128/JVI.00700-11

Lee PS, Yoshida R, Ekiert DC, Sakai N, Suzuki Y, Takada A, Wilson IA (2012) Heterosubtypic antibody recognition of the influenza virus hemagglutinin receptor binding site enhanced by avidity. Proc Natl Acad Sci USA 109:17040–17045. doi:10.1073/pnas.1212371109

Li GM, Chiu C, Wrammert J et al (2012) Pandemic H1N1 influenza vaccine induces a recall response in humans that favors broadly cross-reactive memory B cells. Proc Natl Acad Sci USA 109:9047–9052. doi:10.1073/pnas.1118979109

Li S, Nakaya HI, Kazmin DA, Oh JZ, Pulendran B (2013) Systems biological approaches to measure and understand vaccine immunity in humans. Semin Immunol 25:209–218. doi:S1044-5323(13)00032-8, 10.1016/j.smim.2013.05.003

Lu Y, Welsh JP, Swartz JR (2014) Production and stabilization of the trimeric influenza hemagglutinin stem domain for potentially broadly protective influenza vaccines. Proc Natl Acad Sci USA 111:125–130. doi:10.1073/pnas.1308701110

Margine I, Hai R, Albrecht RA et al (2013a) H3N2 influenza virus infection induces broadly reactive hemagglutinin stalk antibodies in humans and mice. J Virol 87:4728–4737. doi:10.1128/JVI.03509-12

Margine I, Krammer F, Hai R et al (2013b) Hemagglutinin stalk-based universal vaccine constructs protect against group 2 influenza A viruses. J Virol 87:10435–10446. doi:10.1128/JVI.01715-13

McNeil S, Shinde V, Andrew M, et al (2014) Interim estimates of 2013/2014 influenza clinical severity and vaccine effectiveness in the prevention of laboratory-confirmed influenza-related hospitalisation. Euro Surveill Mar 6; 19(9). pii 20729.

Miller MS, Gardner TJ, Krammer F, Aguado LC, Tortorella D, Basler CF, Palese P (2013a) Neutralizing antibodies against previously encountered influenza virus strains increase over time: a longitudinal analysis. Sci Transl Med 5:198ra107. doi:10.1126/scitranslmed.3006637

Miller MS, Tsibane T, Krammer F, Hai R, Rahmat S, Basler CF, Palese P (2013b) 1976 and 2009 H1N1 influenza virus vaccines boost anti-hemagglutinin stalk antibodies in humans. J Infect Dis 207:98–105. doi:10.1093/infdis/jis652

Moody MA, Zhang R, Walter EB et al (2011) H3N2 influenza infection elicits more cross-reactive and less clonally expanded anti-hemagglutinin antibodies than influenza vaccination. PLoS One 6:e25797. doi:10.1371/journal.pone.0025797

Muthuri SG, Venkatesan S, Myles PR et al (2014) Effectiveness of neuraminidase inhibitors in reducing mortality in patients admitted to hospital with influenza A H1N1pdm09 virus infection: a meta-analysis of individual participant data. Lancet Respir Med 2(5):395–404. doi: 10.1016/52213-2600 (14) 70041-4

Nakamura G, Chai N, Park S et al (2013) An in vivo human-plasmablast enrichment technique allows rapid identification of therapeutic influenza A antibodies. Cell Host Microbe 14:93–103. doi:10.1016/j.chom.2013.06.004

Neumann G, Noda T, Kawaoka Y (2009) Emergence and pandemic potential of swine-origin H1N1 influenza virus. Nature 459:931–939. doi:10.1038/nature08157

Ohshima N, Iba Y, Kubota-Koketsu R, Asano Y, Okuno Y, Kurosawa Y (2011) Naturally occurring antibodies in humans can neutralize a variety of influenza virus strains, including H3, H1, H2, and H5. J Virol 85:11048–11057. doi:10.1128/JVI.05397-11

Okuno Y, Isegawa Y, Sasao F, Ueda S (1993) A common neutralizing epitope conserved between the hemagglutinins of influenza A virus H1 and H2 strains. J Virol 67:2552–2558

Okuno Y, Matsumoto K, Isegawa Y, Ueda S (1994) Protection against the mouse-adapted A/FM/1/47 strain of influenza A virus in mice by a monoclonal antibody with cross-neutralizing activity among H1 and H2 strains. J Virol 68:517–520

Osterholm MT, Kelley NS, Sommer A, Belongia EA (2012) Efficacy and effectiveness of influenza vaccines: a systematic review and meta-analysis. Lancet Infect Dis 12:36–44. doi:http://dx.doi.org/10.1016/S1473-3099(11)70295-X

Palese P, Wang TT (2011) Why do influenza virus subtypes die out? A hypothesis. MBio 2. doi:10.1128/mBio.00150-11

Pica N, Hai R, Krammer F et al (2012) Hemagglutinin stalk antibodies elicited by the 2009 pandemic influenza virus as a mechanism for the extinction of seasonal H1N1 viruses. Proc Natl Acad Sci USA 109:2573–2578. doi:10.1073/pnas.1200039109

Polakova K, Russ G, Styk B (1978) Antigenic glycopolypeptides HA1 and HA2 of influenza virus haemagglutinin. I. Gel filtration in 6 M guanidine hydrochloride. Acta Virol 22:362–370

Renegar KB, Small PA Jr (1991) Immunoglobulin A mediation of murine nasal anti-influenza virus immunity. J Virol 65:2146–2148

Russ G, Styk B, Polakova K (1978a) Antigenic glycopolypeptides HA1 and HA2 of influenza virus haemagglutinin. II. Reactivity with rabbit sera against intact virus and purified undissociated haemagglutinin. Acta Virol 22:371–382

Russ G, Styk B, Polakova K (1978b) Radioimmunoassay of influenza A virus haemagglutinin. I. Preparation and properties of radioactive 125I-labelled bromelain-released haemagglutinin. Acta Virol 22:1–10

Sagawa H, Ohshima A, Kato I, Okuno Y, Isegawa Y (1996) The immunological activity of a deletion mutant of influenza virus haemagglutinin lacking the globular region. J Gen Virol 77 (Pt 7):1483–1487

Samson M, Pizzorno A, Abed Y, Boivin G (2013) Influenza virus resistance to neuraminidase inhibitors. Antiviral Res 98:174–185. doi:S0166-3542(13)00068-5, 10.1016/j.antiviral.2013.03.014

Schneemann A, Speir JA, Tan GS, Khayat R, Ekiert DC, Matsuoka Y, Wilson IA (2012) A virus-like particle that elicits cross-reactive antibodies to the conserved stem of influenza virus hemagglutinin. J Virol 86:11686–11697. doi:10.1128/JVI.01694-12

Seibert CW, Rahmat S, Krause JC et al (2013) Recombinant IgA is sufficient to prevent influenza virus transmission in guinea pigs. J Virol 87:7793–7804. doi:10.1128/JVI.00979-13

Smirnov YA, Lipatov AS, Gitelman AK, Okuno Y, Van Beek R, Osterhaus AD, Claas EC (1999) An epitope shared by the hemagglutinins of H1, H2, H5, and H6 subtypes of influenza A virus. Acta Virol 43:237–244

Steel J, Lowen AC, Wang TT, et al (2010) Influenza virus vaccine based on the conserved hemagglutinin stalk domain. mBio 1. doi:10.1128/mBio.00018-10

Subbarao K, Matsuoka Y (2013) The prospects and challenges of universal vaccines for influenza. Trends Microbiol 21:350–358. doi:S0966-842X(13)00074-7, 10.1016/j.tim.2013.04.003

Sui J, Hwang WC, Perez S et al (2009) Structural and functional bases for broad-spectrum neutralization of avian and human influenza A viruses. Nat Struct Mol Biol 16:265–273. doi:10.1038/nsmb.1566

Sui J, Sheehan J, Hwang WC et al (2011) Wide prevalence of heterosubtypic broadly neutralizing human anti-influenza a antibodies. Clin Infect Dis 52:1003–1009. doi:10.1093/cid/cir121

Talaat KR, Luke CJ, Khurana S et al (2014) A live attenuated H5N1 vaccine induces long-term immunity in the absence of a primary antibody response. J Infect Dis. doi:10.1093/infdis/jiu123

Tan GS, Krammer F, Eggink D, Kongchanagul A, Moran TM, Palese P (2012) A pan-H1 anti-hemagglutinin monoclonal antibody with potent broad-spectrum efficacy in vivo. J Virol 86:6179–6188. doi:10.1128/JVI.00469-12

Terajima M, Cruz J, Co MD et al (2011) Complement-dependent lysis of influenza a virus-infected cells by broadly cross-reactive human monoclonal antibodies. J Virol 85:13463–13467. doi:10.1128/JVI.05193-11

Thompson WW, Shay DK, Weintraub E, Brammer L, Bridges CB, Cox NJ, Fukuda K (2004) Influenza-associated hospitalizations in the United States. J Am Med Assoc 292:1333–1340. doi:10.1001/jama.292.11.1333

Thomson CA, Wang Y, Jackson LM et al (2012) Pandemic H1N1 influenza infection and vaccination in humans induces cross-protective antibodies that target the hemagglutinin stem. Front Immunol 3:87. doi:10.3389/fimmu.2012.00087

Throsby M, van den Brink E, Jongeneelen M et al (2008) Heterosubtypic neutralizing monoclonal antibodies cross-protective against H5N1 and H1N1 recovered from human IgM+ memory B cells. PLoS ONE 3:e3942

Tricco AC, Chit A, Soobiah C et al (2013) Comparing influenza vaccine efficacy against mismatched and matched strains: a systematic review and meta-analysis. BMC Med 11:153. doi:10.1186/1741-7015-11-153

Wang TT, Tan GS, Hai R et al (2010a) Vaccination with a synthetic peptide from the influenza virus hemagglutinin provides protection against distinct viral subtypes. Proc Nat Acad Sci USA 107:18979–18984. doi:10.1073/pnas.1013387107

Wang TT, Tan GS, Hai R, Pica N, Petersen E, Moran TM, Palese P (2010b) Broadly protective monoclonal antibodies against H3 influenza viruses following sequential immunization with different hemagglutinins. PLoS Pathog 6:e1000796. doi:10.1371/journal.ppat.1000796

Wei CJ, Boyington JC, McTamney PM et al (2010) Induction of broadly neutralizing H1N1 influenza antibodies by vaccination. Science 329:1060–1064. doi:10.1126/science.1192517

Weis W, Brown JH, Cusack S, Paulson JC, Skehel JJ, Wiley DC (1988) Structure of the influenza virus haemagglutinin complexed with its receptor, sialic acid. Nature 333:426–431. doi:10.1038/333426a0

Whittle JR, Zhang R, Khurana S et al (2011) Broadly neutralizing human antibody that recognizes the receptor-binding pocket of influenza virus hemagglutinin. Proc Natl Acad Sci USA 108:14216–14221. doi:10.1073/pnas.1111497108

Whittle JR, Wheatley AK, Wu L et al (2014) Flow cytometry reveals that H5N1 vaccination elicits cross-reactive stem-directed antibodies from multiple Ig heavy chain lineages. J Virol. doi:10.1128/JVI.03422-13

Wilson IA, Skehel JJ, Wiley DC (1981) Structure of the haemagglutinin membrane glycoprotein of influenza virus at 3 A resolution. Nature 289:366–373

Wrammert J, Smith K, Miller J et al (2008) Rapid cloning of high-affinity human monoclonal antibodies against influenza virus. Nature 453:667–671. doi:10.1038/nature06890

Wrammert J, Koutsonanos D, Li GM et al (2011) Broadly cross-reactive antibodies dominate the human B cell response against 2009 pandemic H1N1 influenza virus infection. J Exp Med 208:181–193. doi:10.1084/jem.20101352

Xu R, Krause JC, McBride R, Paulson JC, Crowe JE Jr, Wilson IA (2013) A recurring motif for antibody recognition of the receptor-binding site of influenza hemagglutinin. Nat Struct Mol Biol 20:363–370. doi:10.1038/nsmb.2500

Yoshida R, Igarashi M, Ozaki H et al (2009) Cross-protective potential of a novel monoclonal antibody directed against antigenic site B of the hemagglutinin of influenza A viruses. PLoS Pathog 5:e1000350. doi:10.1371/journal.ppat.1000350

Zhu X, Guo YH, Jiang T et al (2013) A unique and conserved neutralization epitope in H5N1 influenza viruses identified by an antibody against the A/Goose/Guangdong/1/96 hemagglutinin. J Virol 87:12619–12635. doi:10.1128/JVI.01577-13

Structural Characterization of Viral Epitopes Recognized by Broadly Cross-Reactive Antibodies

Peter S. Lee and Ian A. Wilson

Abstract Influenza hemagglutinin (HA) is the major surface glycoprotein on influenza viruses and mediates viral attachment and subsequent fusion with host cells. The HA is the major target of the immune response, but due to its high level of variability, as evidenced by substantial antigenic diversity, it had been historically considered to elicit only a narrow, strain-specific antibody response. However, a recent explosion in the discovery of broadly neutralizing antibodies (bnAbs) to influenza virus has identified two major supersites of vulnerability on the HA through structural characterization of HA-antibody complexes. These commonly targeted epitopes are involved with receptor binding as well as the fusion machinery and, hence, are functionally conserved and less prone to mutation. These bnAbs can neutralize viruses by blocking infection or the spread of infection by preventing progeny release. Structural analyses of these bnAbs show they exhibit striking similarities and trends in recognition of the HA and use recurring recognition motifs, despite substantial differences in their germline genes. This information can be utilized in design of novel therapeutics as well as in immunogens for improved vaccines with greater breadth and efficacy.

Abbreviations

bnAb	Broadly neutralizing antibody
CDR	Complementarity determining region
EM	Electron microscopy
Fab	Fragment antigen binding
HA	Hemagglutinin
IgG	Immunoglobulin G

P. S. Lee · I. A. Wilson (✉)
Department of Integrative Structural and Computational Biology and Skaggs Institute for Chemical Biology, The Scripps Research Institute, 10550 North Torrey Pines Road, La Jolla, CA 92037, USA
e-mail: wilson@scripps.edu

Current Topics in Microbiology and Immunology (2015) 386: 323–341
DOI: 10.1007/82_2014_413

Published Online: 19 July 2014

Contents

1 Introduction

Influenza viruses cause major respiratory disease each year, commonly known as the flu, and are a significant health challenge and economic burden worldwide (Molinari et al. 2007). Several countermeasures are available to combat the flu such as inhibitors against the surface glycoprotein neuraminidase or the M2 proton channel; however, the effectiveness of these antivirals has become severely diminished as viruses evolve to become drug-resistant (Bright et al. 2006; de Jong et al. 2005; Kiso et al. 2004). Vaccinations against the flu, which were first administered in the 1940s, remains the best means of flu control and prevention. However, unlike other infectious diseases with available vaccine regimens, such as for smallpox, polio, and measles, there is currently no "magic bullet" to abolish future flu infections due to the high diversity and ever-changing antigenicity of the influenza viruses. Therefore, design and development of a universal or more long-term flu vaccine would be highly desirable for the elicitation of antibody responses that can accommodate the enormous diversity and continual changes in influenza viruses and which target the highly conserved functional epitopes.

Fortunately, only a few subtypes of influenza viruses have caused human pandemics and these are type A H1N1, H2N2, and H3N2. In fact, H1N1 and H3N2 have dominated the human type A viruses for nearly a century (1918–present) with a brief interlude by H2N2 viruses (1957–1968). Human type B viruses have two lineages but these viruses do not lead to the same mortality rates associated with human A viruses. All of these viruses are under constant surveillance and are closely monitored to follow influenza activity such as illnesses, severity, and to determine what the dominant circulating virus will be in any given year (Salzberg 2008). Vaccines are, therefore, predictions of candidate strains that may circulate in the upcoming season. Currently, two influenza A strains (H1N1 and H3N2) and one or two influenza B strains (Victoria and/or Yamagata lineages) are included in the annual vaccine, as these viruses currently circulate in humans on an annual basis. The vaccines are administered by injection of inactivated virus (the "flu shot") or by an intranasal spray of live, attenuated virus. However, the effectiveness of the vaccine is highly dependent on the match between the strains in its formulation and the dominant circulating virus. This selection process is further complicated by the high mutability rate of influenza viruses and, thus, the vaccine formulations need to be updated accordingly almost every year.

In addition to seasonal flu, unpredictable outbreaks from other hemagglutinin (HA) subtypes can sporadically infect humans and cause severe disease such as H5N1, H7N7, H9N2, as well as the recent H7N9 and H10N8 viruses (Chen et al. 2014; Gao et al. 2013). These viruses have been associated with an devastatingly high mortality rate, which can reach up to ~60 %, compared to ~0.01 % for seasonal viruses (CDC 2010). Fortunately, none of these deadly viruses have been able to spread by sustainable human-to-human transmission. Nonetheless, the unpredictability and pandemic potential of these divergent viruses underscores the need for broader-spectrum therapy and pandemic preparedness.

HA is the major surface glycoprotein on influenza viruses and is the primary target for the humoral immune response to influenza virus. The HA currently has been classified into 18 distinct subtypes (Tong et al. 2013), based on their reactivity to polysera for type A viruses (designated H1–H18), and two lineages for type B viruses (Victoria and Yamagata). Type A HAs can be further classified into two phylogenetic groups; group 1: H1, H2, H5, H6, H8, H9, H11, H12, H13, H16, H17, and H18; and group 2: H3, H4, H7, H10, H14, and H15.

The influenza HA glycoprotein is a class I viral fusion protein and mediates viral entry into host cells. It is synthesized as a precursor polypeptide, termed HA0, and assembles into pre-fusion homotrimers (Wilson et al. 1981). The HA0 trimers are subsequently matured by host proteases, which generate disulfide-linked HA1 and HA2 subunits. In general terms, the HA can structurally be considered to be composed of "head" and "stem" domains (Fig. 1). The globular membrane-distal HA head is composed entirely of HA1 residues, which form the receptor binding pocket (three per HA trimer) that mediate interactions between the virus and host cell sialosides (Weis et al. 1988). Directly below the HA head, the membrane-proximal HA stem contains the fusion machinery. The stem is largely α-helical and is composed primarily of HA2 residues and some ascending and descending HA1 residues. The mature HA (HA1/HA2) is similar in structure to the HA0 precursor except at the cleavage site where the fusion peptide, located at the N-terminus of the HA2 subunit, now inserts deeply into a hydrophobic pocket around the trimer axis. In the HA0 form, the uncleaved fusion peptide forms a loop that protrudes at the HA surface (Chen et al. 1998; Stevens et al. 2004). The pre-fusion mature HA conformation is pH-dependent and metastable, and acidification triggers major conformational changes among the central HA2 helices that lead to the post-fusion state (Bullough et al. 1994; Skehel et al. 1982). Despite the diversity of the HAs, they almost all share the conserved function of host cell binding and membrane fusion, with the exception of the recently

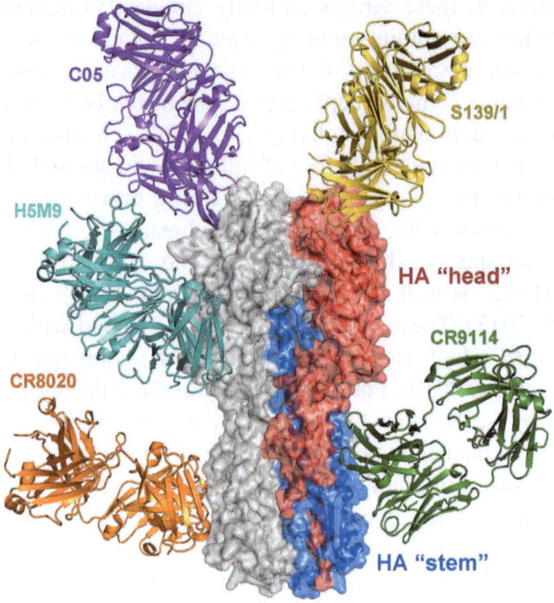

Fig. 1 Structure of the influenza hemagglutinin (*HA*) and broadly neutralizing antibody (bnAb) binding sites. A single protomer of the trimeric HA is *colored* with HA1 and HA2 residues in *red* and *blue*, respectively. The membrane-distal HA "head" contains the receptor binding site (three per HA) and is comprised of HA1 residues. The membrane-proximal HA "stem" contains the fusion machinery and is primarily comprised of HA2 residues. All antibodies (C05, PDB 4FP8; S139/1, PDB 4GMS; H5M9, PDB 4MHH; CR8020, PDB 3SDY; CR9114, PDB 4FQI) have been modeled onto the A/Hong Kong/1/1968 (H3N2) HA (PDB 4FNK)

identified H17 and H18 HAs from bat influenza viruses (Sun et al. 2013; Tong et al. 2013; Zhu et al. 2013b). Therefore, blocking receptor binding or inhibiting the progression of HA maturation and membrane fusion are effective means of preventing or ameliorating HA-mediated virus infection (Brandenburg et al. 2013).

There has been a recent explosion in the discovery of broadly neutralizing antibodies (bnAbs) to human influenza viruses. These bnAbs target conserved sites on the HA head and stem and block influenza infection or its progression at critical HA junctures. These bnAbs have varying levels of cross-reactivity against divergent strains within and across subtypes. Moreover, structural studies by x-ray crystallography and electron microscopy (EM) studies have revealed supersites of vulnerability on the HA that are recognized by bnAbs [see recent reviews (Corti and Lanzavecchia 2013; Ekiert and Wilson 2012; Julien et al. 2012)]. Altogether, analysis of the growing arsenal of these bnAb-HA structures have revealed recurring modes of recognition that are now the main source of inspiration for design of vaccines and antibody-based therapeutics in the form of small molecules, peptides, and designed proteins against the HA.

2 HA Head-Reactive Antibodies

The HA head has long been considered to be able to elicit only a narrow, strain-specific antibody response as it undergoes rapid mutation to change its surface antigenicity by sequence variation and glycan incorporation to evade and escape recognition from our immune system. Accordingly, classical antigenic sites on the HA head have been mapped by tracking patterns of natural amino acid variation, as well as laboratory escape mutants, and these sites have been long considered as hot spots for antigenic drift (Caton et al. 1982; Wiley et al. 1981). These antigenic sites are prone to higher sequence variability and, thus, the cross-reactivity of antibodies to strains other than to the immunizing strain is severely restricted. For example, antibody 2D1, which binds near the top of the HA, recognizes only HAs from the pandemic 1918 and 2009 H1N1 viruses, which are highly antigenically similar at the 2D1 epitope despite being separated by nearly a century (Xu et al. 2010).

However, the notion of strain specificity has been challenged by a recent surge in the isolation and characterization of a number of broader-spectrum antibodies against the HA head. Depending on the sequence conservation of the epitope, the antibodies can have broader reactivity. The epitopes of some of these antibodies are located at various locations on the globular HA head (Fig. 1) (Cho et al. 2014; Dreyfus et al. 2012; Fleury et al. 1999, 2000; Zhu et al. 2013a; Iba et al. 2014). For instance, antibody H5M9 contacts a nearly invariant epitope among H5 HAs at the vestigial esterase domain that is distant from the receptor binding site and somewhat closer to the fusion domain (Zhu et al. 2013a). In addition, antibody CR8071 recognizes an epitope that is highly conserved among nearly all flu type B strains also on the side of the HA head (Dreyfus et al. 2012). Antibodies HC45 and BH151 also bind a similar region on H3 HAs, but their breadth has not been determined (Fleury et al. 1999, 2000). Antibodies GC0757 and GC0857 also target the side of the HA head, but bind a different epitope on the opposite face of the HA (Cho et al. 2014). Yet, the vast majority of the broader-spectrum antibodies against the HA head target the receptor binding site (Barbey-Martin et al. 2002; Ekiert et al. 2012; Fleury et al. 1998; Hong et al. 2013; Lee et al. 2012; Schmidt et al. 2013; Tsibane et al. 2012; Whittle et al. 2011; Xu et al. 2013). Since the receptor binding site is functionally conserved for receptor binding, it has restricted sequence variation compared to the rest of the HA head (Martin et al. 1998), and now appears to be a fascinating and amenable target of bnAbs.

2.1 Receptor Binding Site-Targeted Antibodies

The HA receptor binding site is a broad, shallow pocket located at the apex of the globular HA head. The framework of the receptor binding pocket is formed by the 130 loop, 150 loop, 220 loop, and 190 helix, which are designated by their numbering in the HA sequence (Fig. 2a). To date, 11 receptor binding site-targeted antibodies

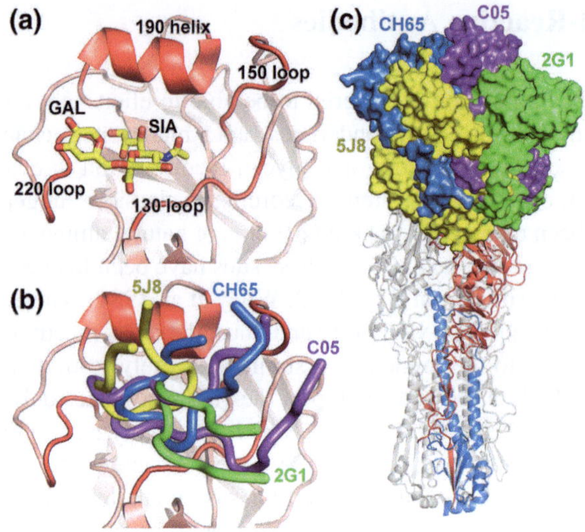

Fig. 2 Recognition of the HA receptor binding site. **a** The receptor binding site of HA is framed by the 130 loop, 150 loop, 190 helix, and the 220 loop (labeled and highlighted in *red*), which binds sialoglycans (PDB 2YP4). **b** Receptor binding site-targeted antibodies 5J8 (*yellow* PDB 4M5Z), CH65 (*blue* PDB 3SM5), 2G1 (*green* PDB 4HG4), and C05 (*purple* PDB 4FP8) insert CDR loops into the binding pocket to compete with the sialoglycan receptor. **c** Superimposition of the receptor binding site-targeted antibodies reveal that they bind the HA using different angles of approach

have been structurally characterized. All the receptor binding site-targeted antibodies commonly insert a complementarity determining region (CDR) loop into the binding pocket and thereby directly block HA from interacting with host cell sialosides (Fig. 2b). However, due to the small footprint of the receptor binding site, most antibodies can only insert a single CDR loop, typically using heavy chain CDR loop 3 (HCDR3) and occasionally HCDR2. Since the receptor binding site is located near the top of the HA, there is substantial conformational freedom of the antibody approach angle to this site (Fig. 2c), which plays a role in their breadth of recognition. The antibodies can be loosely classified as having either greatly expanded individual subtype recognition or an increased level of heterosubtypic recognition, and thus these different bnAbs have quite varying degrees of breadth and potency. Nonetheless, the convergence of interactions at the receptor binding site substantiates the concept that this epitope is a supersite of vulnerability akin to an extensive glycan-dependent site found on the HIV-1 Env trimer (Kong et al. 2013).

2.1.1 Receptor Binding Site Recognition of a Single Subtype

Antibodies CH65 and CH67, which derive from the same B-cell clonal lineage, have been characterized to bind and neutralize seasonal H1 strains that have infected humans since 1986 (Schmidt et al. 2013; Whittle et al. 2011). However, these antibodies have weak to no activity against the 2009 pandemic H1 strain. In contrast, antibody 5J8, which was isolated from a human donor using hybridoma technology, has reactivity against HAs from the 1918 and 2009 pandemic H1N1 viruses as well as other seasonal isolates (Hong et al. 2013; Krause et al. 2011). Crystal structures of CH65, CH67, and 5J8 in complex with the HA reveal that they all recognize an epitope in and around the receptor binding site and all insert their HCDR3 loop into the binding pocket. The pandemic HA strains incorporate an amino acid insertion at position 133a (between residues 133 and 134 in the 130 loop), which changes the local conformation of the loop and is a binding determinant for these antibodies. CH65 and CH67 cannot accommodate the 133a insertion (typically a lysine residue) and are sterically blocked from binding. In contrast, 5J8 accommodates the insertion by using a different angle of approach on the HA, compared with CH65 and CH67, and thus avoids the main-chain bulge due to the 133a insertion. In addition, 5J8 makes favorable electrostatic interactions with the side chain of the 133a residue. As such, these antibodies converge onto the receptor binding site of human H1 isolates, yet use different sets of interactions and angles of approach, and complement one another for coverage of human H1 isolates that have circulated since H1N1 viruses reemerged in humans in 1977.

H2N2 viruses have circulated in humans starting from 1957 but persisted only for 10 years. However, there has been recent concern that H2N2 viruses may reemerge in humans as immunity has dropped in the population (Nabel et al. 2011). Antibodies 2G1, 8F8, and 8M2 were isolated from human donors by the hybridoma technology and were found to recognize and neutralize human H2N2 viruses that spanned from 1957–1963 (Krause et al. 2012; Xu et al. 2013). Just as for the anti-H1 receptor binding site-targeted antibodies, crystal structures of these three antibodies in complex with the HA reveal that these antibodies all reach into the binding pocket. Antibody 8F8 primarily inserts HCDR3, whereas 8M2 and 2G1 use the hydrophobic HCDR2 encoded by the V_H1-69 germline gene. The 8M2 and 2G1 antibodies adopt different orientations ($\sim$180° rotation around V_H/V_L) on the HA to center their HCDR2 in the receptor binding site while their HCDR3s interact on the periphery on opposite ends of the receptor binding site. These studies also isolated escape mutants in and around the receptor binding site. Interestingly, these mutants come at a detrimental fitness cost to the virus such that the receptor binding properties of the HA have diminished. This finding substantiates the notion of limited mutability of the receptor binding site due to the conservation of function.

2.1.2 Heterosubtypic Recognition of the Receptor Binding Site

While the anti-H1 or anti-H2 antibodies discussed above are limited to a single subtype, antibodies C05 and S139/1 remarkably have achieved some level of heterosubtypic reactivity and can bind multiple HA strains from both phylogenetic groups, including the H1, H2, H3, and other divergent subtypes (Ekiert et al. 2012; Lee et al. 2012). Antibody S139/1 was selected from H3N2 immunized mice, and was the first reported heterosubtypic antibody that mapped to the receptor binding site, possessing reactivity against H1, H2, H3, H5, H9, and H13 subtypes (Yoshida et al. 2009). The crystal structure of S139/1 in complex with the HA reveals that the antibody reaches into the receptor binding site using HCDR2 (Lee et al. 2012). Binding and neutralization studies confirmed that S139/1 does indeed have heterosubtypic activity, albeit with narrow specificity within each subtype. Nonetheless, these results suggest that divergent isolates across subtypes and groups can share a similar receptor binding site epitope.

Antibody C05 was isolated from phage libraries constructed from the immune repertoires of individuals who had been infected with seasonal H1N1 influenza viruses (Ekiert et al. 2012). C05 has potent neutralizing activity against H1, H2, H3, and H9 viruses and has a broader breadth of recognition within these subtypes as compared to S139/1. Unlike all other receptor binding site-targeted antibodies described thus far, C05 binds the HA exclusively through the heavy chain. The majority of the interactions are mediated through an exceptionally long HCDR3, which is inserted into the receptor binding site. Since the antibody essentially uses a single antibody loop, the C05 epitope on HA is very compact. As such, C05 makes minimal contacts with variable residues around the receptor binding site, which affords the antibody its broad reactivity spectrum.

2.2 Enhanced Affinity Through Avidity

Due to the large footprints of antibodies compared with sialosides on the HA, antibodies to the HA head inevitably contact variable residues outside of the receptor binding pocket that limits their overall breadth of recognition. One way that these receptor binding site-targeted antibodies appear to accommodate this limitation is by enhanced affinity through avidity. Although monovalent Fab (fragment antigen binding) bind with reasonable affinity to some strains, the enhanced avidity of bivalent IgG (immunoglobulin G) increases the breadth of recognition to additional strains and subtypes where Fab binding is relatively weak. This feature has been seen for a number of the receptor binding site-targeted antibodies such as S139/1, where the monovalent Fab binds weakly to non-H3 isolates but the bivalent IgG substantially increases its affinity, positively correlating with neutralizing activity (Lee et al. 2012). Therefore, antibodies making relatively low affinity Fab interactions with the receptor binding site can have significant antiviral activity when enhanced by avidity, thereby extending the breadth of neutralization to highly divergent influenza virus strains and subtypes. It appears that avidity is a general feature for other receptor binding site-targeted antibodies as observed for C05, 5J8, and CH65 (Ekiert et al. 2012; Hong et al. 2013). Thus, to gain broad recognition against the receptor binding site, it may be favorable for the Fab portion of the antibody to have intermediate specificity for a number of HA strains to account for the variability of the residues in and around the receptor binding site, which can then be rescued by bivalent binding of the IgG.

2.3 Receptor Mimicry by Antibodies

The HA recognizes the chemical features of the sialic acid receptor (e.g., the acetamide, carboxylate, and glycerol groups) using highly conserved residues in different regions of the binding pocket. In accordance, the receptor binding site-targeted antibodies take advantage of these highly conserved HA residues and have found ways of mimicking portions of the glycan receptor using amino acid residues. Striking trends in recognition of the receptor binding site are now becoming apparent as more structural details of these antibodies are uncovered.

The portion of the pocket that is occupied by the acetamide group of sialic acid is almost absolutely conserved across all HAs and is formed by the hydrophobic residues Trp153 and Leu194 (some strains use a similarly placed hydrophobic Ile194). As such, nearly all receptor binding site-targeted antibodies commonly insert a hydrophobic amino acid in this acetamide-binding pocket. There appears to be some freedom in the nature of the hydrophobic amino acid that can be placed here, as some antibodies use large aromatic side chains such as a phenylalanine (the anti-H2 antibodies 2G1 and 8M2), tyrosine (anti-H2 antibody 8F8 and anti-H3 antibody HC19), or tryptophan (heterosubtypic antibody C05) (Fig. 3a) whereas other antibodies insert smaller hydrophobic side chains such as valine or proline (anti-H1 antibodies CH65 and CH67 or 5J8, respectively). These structures reveal a compelling conserved strategy used by these antibodies to insert amino acids with similar properties into a hydrophobic pocket in the HA receptor binding site.

In another region of the receptor binding site, sialic acid inserts its carboxylate into a polar pocket that is adjacent to the pocket for the acetamide moiety. The carboxylate forms specific hydrogen bonds with the main-chain backbone of the 130 loop as well as the side chain of a highly conserved Ser136 or Thr136. Antibodies HC19, HC63, CH65, CH67, and 5J8 mimic this interaction by insertion of an aspartic acid carboxylate into the pocket, which closely overlaps with and utilizes the same hydrogen bonding interactions as the sialic acid receptor (Fig. 3b) (Barbey-Martin et al. 2002; Fleury et al. 1998; Hong et al. 2013; Schmidt et al. 2013; Whittle et al. 2011). However, only a few antibodies insert an aspartic acid into this pocket; other antibodies use an isoleucine, such as S139/1 (Lee et al. 2012), or even the HCDR3 backbone, such as C05 (Ekiert et al. 2012), instead.

Although these receptor binding site-targeted antibodies mimic the acetamide and carboxylate moieties of the receptor, they do not directly contact the region of the binding pocket occupied by the glycerol moiety of sialic acid. As there is only room typically for a single antibody loop to enter into the binding groove, the extent of receptor mimicry therefore may have some spatial limitations. Only antibodies 1F1, 8M2, and C05 approach the pocket for the glycerol moiety of sialic acid (Ekiert et al. 2012; Tsibane et al. 2012; Xu et al. 2013), but do not have the same binding mode and hydrogen bonding interactions to the conserved HA residues as the glycerol moiety.

In summary, the recent identification and structural characterization of a variety of neutralizing antibodies to influenza virus have surprisingly revealed that the

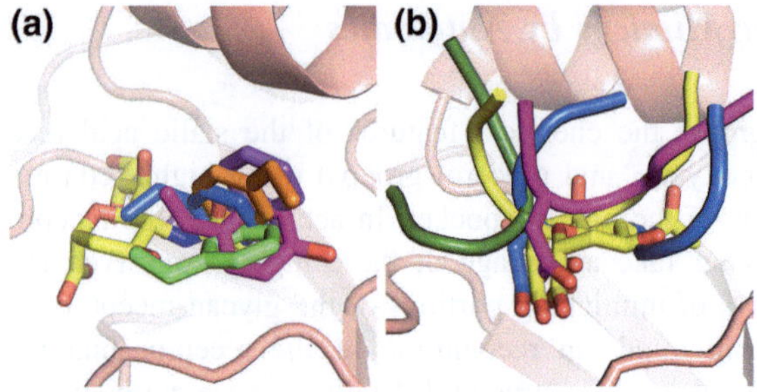

Fig. 3 Common trends in HA receptor binding site-targeted antibodies. **a** Antibodies HC19 (*magenta* PDB 2VIR), C05 (*purple* PDB 4FP8), 8F8 (*blue* PDB 4HF5), 8M2 (*orange* PDB 4HFU), and 2G1 (*green* PDB 4HG4) use hydrophobic residues to target the receptor binding site that would be occupied by the acetamide moiety of sialic acid. **b** Antibodies HC19 (*magenta* PDB 2VIR), HC63 (*dark green* PDB 1KEN), CH65 (*blue* PDB 3SM5), and 5J8 (*yellow* PDB 4M5Z) use an Asp residue to insert a carboxylate in the receptor binding site that would be occupied by the carboxylate of sialic acid

receptor binding site can indeed be considered a viable target on the HA head for bnAbs. The small footprint of the receptor binding site for a glycan makes it much more difficult to target considering the larger footprint of an antibody. Notwithstanding, it is remarkable that these antibodies have now been found to share similar motifs for recognition of the receptor binding site despite deriving from different mouse or human germline genes as well as possessing differing specificities for influenza strains and subtypes. The combination of the recurrent binding motifs of these receptor binding site bnAbs is likely of value for design of small molecule drugs and therapeutics.

3 HA Stem-Reactive Antibodies

Traditional antigenic sites were only mapped to the head and, therefore, it was a popular belief that the membrane-proximal HA stem was not targeted by the humoral immune response. Antibody C179, which was isolated from mice immunized with an H2N2 virus, was the first reported discovery of a putative stem-targeted in 1993 that had heterosubtypic neutralizing activity against group 1 H1, H2, H5, and H6 HAs (Okuno et al. 1993; Smirnov et al. 1999). Escape mutants were isolated along the HA stem and away from the HA head and, unlike the HA head-targeted antibodies, C179 did not block receptor binding but rather inhibited the HA fusion activity (Okuno et al. 1993). However, the influenza field largely overlooked this discovery and a structure of this antibody in complex with HA remained elusive for two decades (Fig. 4a) (Dreyfus et al. 2013). It was also unknown whether stem-targeted antibodies similar to C179 circulated in the human immune repertoire and, thus, whether it had any relevance to eliciting human antibodies with similar activity. Thus, while antibody discovery and

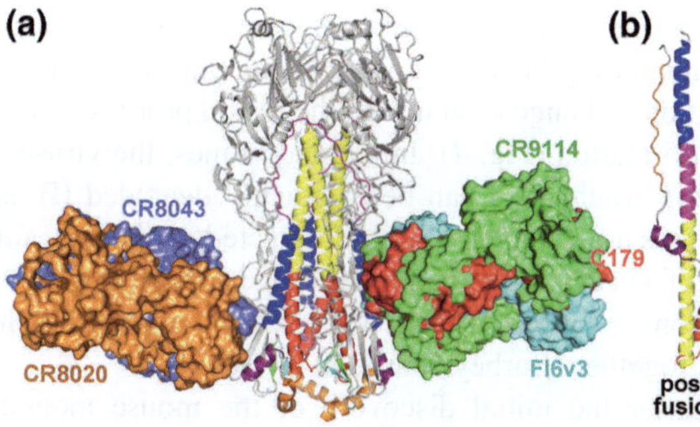

Fig. 4 Recognition of the HA stem. **a** Antibodies CR9114 (*green* PDB 4FQI), C179 (*red* PDB 4HLZ), and FI6v3 (*cyan* PDB 3ZTJ) bind distinct but slightly overlapping epitopes in the HA stem compared with CR8020 (*orange* PDB 3SDY) and CR8043 (*blue* PDB 4NM8). These stem-targeted antibodies inhibit the postfusion conformation (PDB 1QU1) that is triggered at low pH, shown in (**b**). [Partially adapted from (Julien et al. 2012)]

characterization against the HA head was ongoing, the importance of broadly neutralizing or any neutralizing antibodies to the HA stem would be underappreciated and would not be investigated further for many years.

3.1 Group 1 HA Recognition

Nearly 15 years after the initial discovery of C179, several stem-targeted antibodies were identified from human combinatorial antibody libraries (Ekiert et al. 2009; Kashyap et al. 2008; Sui et al. 2009; Throsby et al. 2008). Like C179, these antibodies bind antigenically diverse group 1 HAs. Interestingly, the heavy chains of this large panel of antibodies had very high sequence similarity with one another and are encoded by the V_H1-69 germline gene. Furthermore, as they undergo very limited somatic hypermutation, such an antibody response could potentially be more readily elicited by vaccination. The structures of two of these antibodies, CR6261 and F10, in complex with HA revealed that these human antibodies bound a highly conserved epitope in the membrane-proximal stem that is shared among group 1 HAs (10 of the 16 known HA subtypes at the time) (Ekiert et al. 2009; Sui et al. 2009). Both antibodies approach at a similar, but not identical, angle to bind the shared HA epitope and the interactions are mediated solely through the antibody heavy chains. In particular, both antibodies insert the hydrophobic tip of their HCDR2 loops, a hallmark of the V_H1-69 germline sequence, into a hydrophobic pocket in the HA stem. The epitope consists of a helical region of the stem composed of HA2 and some HA1 residues and has exceptional sequence conservation as it is comprised of key elements of the fusion machinery. However, the viruses can still bind to host cells, since the HA receptor binding sites are not blocked, and subsequently enter the cell via endosomal compartments. In particular, residues in this stem epitope are involved in the rearrangements from the pre-fusion to post-fusion conformation during the fusion process and, thus, these antibodies block the low pH conformational changes and inhibit the fusion process by locking the HA in its pre-fusion conformation (Fig. 4). In the endosomes, the viruses are effectively trapped by CR6261 where they can be eventually degraded (Brandenburg et al. 2013). These features are unique to the stem-targeted antibodies, although HC63 is the only example of a head-targeted antibody that can prevent both receptor binding and the low pH conformational change by cross-linking the HA heads of neighboring protomers together (Barbey-Martin et al. 2002).

Two decades after the initial discovery of the mouse monoclonal antibody C179, its crystal structure confirmed that it indeed is a stem-targeted antibody (Dreyfus et al. 2013). C179 binds a similar epitope as CR6261 and F10, but uses a completely different approach angle. Both heavy and light chains mediate interactions with the HA. Similarities can be drawn between C179 and the V_H1-69 antibodies, as they both use hydrophobic residues (HCDR3 for C179, HCDR2 for CR6261 and F10) to complement the hydrophobic groove of the HA and block the low pH conformational changes. As such, these structures reveal recurring modes of recognition against a broadly neutralizing and highly conserved epitope at the HA stem.

3.2 Group 2 HA Recognition

The identification of the V_H1-69 antibodies that target the HA stem of nearly all group 1 viruses raised hope for the possibility of antibody-based therapy or broader-spectrum influenza vaccine. Yet, these V_H1-69 antibodies do not have activity against group 2 HAs, including H3 viruses that currently circulate in humans. In a major advance, two group 2 targeted bnAbs, called CR8020 and CR8043, were isolated by Crucell from memory B cells of healthy donors and have heterosubtypic neutralizing activity in vitro and protect mice from lethal challenge from H3 and H7 viruses (Ekiert et al. 2011; Friesen et al. 2014). The two antibodies were isolated from a single donor and both target a common epitope lower down on the HA stem distinct from the group 1 antibodies (Fig. 4a). Interestingly, CR8020 and CR8043 derive from different germline genes (V_H1-18 and V_H1-3, respectively) and use different sets of heavy and light chain interactions and alternative angles of approach to target the HA. Moreover, the antibodies have distinct escape mutation sensitivities indicating that there may be versatility in targeting the CR8020 and CR8043 epitopes. Similar to the group 1 targeted antibodies, CR8020 and CR8043 bind key elements of the HA fusion machinery and prevent the conformational changes of the HA that occur low pH. The antibodies also inhibit the maturation process of the HA by blocking the proteolytic cleavage of the HA0 precursor to the mature HA1/HA2 (Ekiert et al. 2011; Friesen et al. 2014). Thus, the identification and structural characterization of these bnAbs have determined a second site of vulnerability on the HA stem.

3.3 Pan-Influenza A and Type B Recognition

Structural characterization of the group 1 and the group 2 heterosubtypic stem-targeted antibodies have defined neutralizing epitopes that can be exploited for therapeutics as well as vaccine design. In a further remarkable breakthrough, bnAb FI6v3 was identified and found to cross the group 1 and group 2 barrier (Corti et al. 2011). FI6v3 was isolated from single plasma cells of human donors with activity against nearly all subtypes of influenza type A. It is encoded by the V_H3-30 germline gene but surprisingly recognizes a similar epitope as the V_H1-69 group 1 specific bnAbs but approaches at a completely different angle to the HA. The FI6v3 binding mode more closely resembles C179 as it uses both heavy and light chains mediate the interactions with the HA and inserts its HCDR3 loop into the hydrophobic groove of the HA stem. The longer HCDR3 has a number of aromatic residues that emulate the binding of the aromatic and nonpolar residues of the hydrophobic HCDR2 of the V_H1-69 antibodies. A unique feature of FI6v3 is that it can contact the uncleaved fusion peptide in the neighboring HA protomer using its light chain, suggesting that it may also prevent HA maturation (Corti et al. 2011).

However, to have the ultimate universal flu vaccine, an antibody response must be elicited across flu type A as well as both lineages of type B. In another unprecedented discovery, bnAb CR9114 was isolated by Crucell using combinatorial display libraries from human B cells and was found to have activity against all subtypes of influenza type A as well as both lineages of type B viruses (Dreyfus et al. 2012). CR9114 is a V_H1-69 encoded antibody and its binding mode highly resembles that of CR6261 and F10, in that it targets a nearly identical epitope in the HA stem solely through its heavy chains and approaches the HA using a similar angle of approach as CR6261. Yet, CR9114 can also recognize group 2 HAs, whereas the CR6261 and F10 V_H1-69 antibodies cannot cross the HA group barrier despite the high sequence conservation of this epitope across all HA subtypes. It has been suggested that a glycan at Asn38 conserved among group 2 HAs sterically interferes with binding by these antibodies (Ekiert et al. 2009; Sui et al. 2009). CR9114 as well as FI6v3 appear to be able to push the glycan away to enable access to the HA protein surface. It is extraordinary that these pan-influenza antibodies recognize a similar epitope as the group 1 stem-targeted antibodies, yet acquire even greater reactivity, coping with both glycan and some amino acid diversity in and around the epitope. Further investigation of this epitope by other bnAbs may provide additional insight into molecular details of weak spots on the HA.

4 Conclusions and Future Directions

Remarkably, the rapid discovery of bnAbs against the influenza virus did not truly take off until 2008. Since then, an explosion in the discovery and characterization of such bnAbs has advanced the field tremendously and given hope that a “universal” flu vaccine may indeed be possible. Structural characterization of antibody-HA complexes by x-ray crystallography and EM has now defined supersites of vulnerability in the HA stem and in the HA head, particularly in and around the receptor binding site.

The recent identification and elucidation of receptor binding site-targeted antibodies have now proven that the HA head can indeed elicit an antibody response with a broader level of cross-reactivity than previously believed. Although these antibodies can have varying levels of activity, the combination of some of these antibodies can provide nearly complete coverage against particular subtypes. For instance, CH65 and CH67 have activity against many seasonal H1 isolates whereas 5J8 can also bind pandemic H1 strains. By combining these three antibodies, perhaps by linking two Fab arms together to create a bispecific antibody with one Fab arm as CH65 or CH67 and the other arm as 5J8 (Ridgway et al. 1996), it may be possible to generate an IgG with near pan-H1 reactivity.

Other putative receptor binding site-targeted antibodies have broad-spectrum activity. For instance, F045-092 reportedly has pan-H3 reactivity (Ohshima et al. 2011) and structural characterization of the F045-092-HA complex reveals that the antibody utilizes receptor mimicry and avidity to achieve its broad breadth of recognition (PMID 24717798). CR8033 neutralizes both flu B lineages (Dreyfus et al. 2012) and currently only. EM reconstructions of the CR8033-HA complex are available. Higher resolution studies of CR8033 in complex with the HA, in conjunction with the pan-H1 and pan-H3 receptor binding site-targeted antibodies, will provide the structural framework for recognition of all subtypes and types of influenza viruses that currently circulate in humans.

The discovery of stem-targeted antibodies with broadly neutralizing activity against group 1 and/or 2 influenza A viruses (Corti et al. 2011; Dreyfus et al. 2013; Ekiert et al. 2009, 2011; Friesen et al. 2014; Kashyap et al. 2008, 2010; Sui et al. 2009; Throsby et al. 2008; Wyrzucki et al. 2014) as well as B viruses (Dreyfus et al. 2012) has truly reinvigorated the influenza research community and raised hopes for the development of antibody-based immunotherapy and long-lasting, universal vaccines for influenza. Structures of these antibody-HA complexes have defined two principal, highly conserved epitopes on the HA stem. Rather than blocking receptor binding, these antibodies can prevent HA maturation as well as the low pH conformational change necessary for fusion of viral and host cell membranes. Some of these antibodies also prevent the release of nascent virions and thus prevent spread of the virus (Brandenburg et al. 2013; Dreyfus et al. 2012). However, despite the detailed efficacy of these bnAbs to neutralize viruses in vitro and in vivo, some concerns have been raised on the accessibility of the membrane-proximal stem epitopes of the densely clustered HA on the surface of viruses. Cryoelectron tomography of viruses with bnAb C179 has now visually confirmed that the HA stem epitope can indeed be accessed by stem-targeted bnAbs (Harris et al. 2013).

The structural characterization of antibody-HA complexes has provided exclusive insight into strategies to harness and employ potent bnAb responses. For instance, vaccination with synthetic peptides that mimic the long α-helix of the HA stem has been reported to provide protection in mice from challenges with H3N2,

H1N1, and H5N1 viruses (Wang et al. 2010). An alternative vaccine strategy through the use of chimeric HAs, where different HA heads are linked to the same HA stem, can bias the immune response towards the conserved stem after consecutive immunization with different chimeric HAs (Hai et al. 2012; Krammer et al. 2013). Perhaps this method can also be applied to generate broader-spectrum antibodies that are more selective to the conserved residues in the receptor binding site, while avoiding the variable loops outside of the pocket. Self-assembling nanoparticles have been engineered to display multiple HA spikes and have been shown to elicit bnAb response against the receptor binding site as well as the stem of the HA (Kanekiyo et al. 2013). To focus elicitation against the stem, headless HA constructs have also been engineered that can bind stem-targeted antibodies (Lu et al. 2014; Mallajosyula et al. 2014). By coupling these headless HAs or similar rational immunogen designs onto self-assembling particles, it may be possible to focus a V_H1-69 germline encoded bnAb response solely against the stem, as was similarly performed against the CD4 binding site of the HIV-1 envelope glycoprotein (Jardine et al. 2013).

The structural details of the bnAbs in complex with the HA have also served as a foundation for the computational design of de novo proteins against the stem (Fleishman et al. 2011; Whitehead et al. 2012). Individual residues of the stem-targeted bnAb CR6261 that form favorable interactions along the hydrophobic groove of the HA were grafted onto protein scaffolds. Crystal structures show that the designs do indeed match the computational model even down to the level of side chain rotamer conformations. Moreover, these designs have antiviral activity and similarly block the low pH conformational change of the HA. In theory, this design method can also extend to design small proteins that target the receptor binding site by combining the recurring themes of recognition, such as receptor mimicry as well as avidity.

In summary, the discovery and structural characterization of receptor binding site and stem-targeted antibodies has shifted the paradigm and outlook for vaccine design against influenza virus. These structures provide a wealth of information that furthers our understanding of how the HA can be targeted and has defined two main supersites of vulnerability and one of two other possible sites (Fig. 1). Recurrent motifs of recognition have been observed both in the receptor binding site and stem epitopes that have directed innovative design of immunogens capable of eliciting broad spectrum antibodies. The road ahead is certainly bright for a new frontier in the structured-based discovery of broad-spectrum vaccines, immunogens, and therapeutics against influenza viruses.

References

Barbey-Martin C, Gigant B, Bizebard T, Calder LJ, Wharton SA, Skehel JJ, Knossow M (2002) An antibody that prevents the hemagglutinin low pH fusogenic transition. Virology 294:70–74

Brandenburg B, Koudstaal W, Goudsmit J, Klaren V, Tang C, Bujny MV, Korse HJ, Kwaks T, Otterstrom JJ, Juraszek J, van Oijen AM, Vogels R, Friesen RH (2013) Mechanisms of hemagglutinin targeted influenza virus neutralization. PLoS One 8:e80034

Bright RA, Shay DK, Shu B, Cox NJ, Klimov AI (2006) Adamantane resistance among influenza A viruses isolated early during the 2005–2006 influenza season in the United States. JAMA 295:891–894

Bullough PA, Hughson FM, Skehel JJ, Wiley DC (1994) Structure of influenza haemagglutinin at the pH of membrane fusion. Nature 371:37–43

Caton AJ, Brownlee GG, Yewdell JW, Gerhard W (1982) The antigenic structure of the influenza virus A/PR/8/34 hemagglutinin (H1 subtype). Cell 31:417–427

CDC (2010) Centers for Disease Control and Prevention (CDC). Estimates of deaths associated with seasonal influenza—United States, 1976–2007. Morb Mortal Wkly Rep 59:1057–1062

Chen H, Yuan H, Gao R, Zhang J, Wang D, Xiong Y, Fan G, Yang F, Li X, Zhou J, Zou S, Yang L, Chen T, Dong L, Bo H, Zhao X, Zhang Y, Lan Y, Bai T, Dong J, Li Q, Wang S, Zhang Y, Li H, Gong T, Shi Y, Ni X, Li J, Zhou J, Fan J, Wu J, Zhou X, Hu M, Wan J, Yang W, Li D, Wu G, Feng Z, Gao GF, Wang Y, Jin Q, Liu M, Shu Y (2014) Clinical and epidemiological characteristics of a fatal case of avian influenza A H10N8 virus infection: a descriptive study. Lancet 383(9918):714–721

Chen J, Lee KH, Steinhauer DA, Stevens DJ, Skehel JJ, Wiley DC (1998) Structure of the hemagglutinin precursor cleavage site, a determinant of influenza pathogenicity and the origin of the labile conformation. Cell 95:409–417

Cho KJ, Hong KW, Kim SH, Seok JH, Kim S, Lee JH, Saelens X, Kim KH (2014) Insight into highly conserved H1 subtype-specific epitopes in influenza virus hemagglutinin. PLoS One 9:e89803

Corti D, Lanzavecchia A (2013) Broadly neutralizing antiviral antibodies. Annu Rev Immunol 31:705–742

Corti D, Voss J, Gamblin SJ, Codoni G, Macagno A, Jarrossay D, Vachieri SG, Pinna D, Minola A, Vanzetta F, Silacci C, Fernandez-Rodriguez BM, Agatic G, Bianchi S, Giacchetto-Sasselli I, Calder L, Sallusto F, Collins P, Haire LF, Temperton N, Langedijk JP, Skehel JJ, Lanzavecchia A (2011) A neutralizing antibody selected from plasma cells that binds to group 1 and group 2 influenza A hemagglutinins. Science 333:850–856

de Jong MD, Tran TT, Truong HK, Vo MH, Smith GJ, Nguyen VC, Bach VC, Phan TQ, Do QH, Guan Y, Peiris JS, Tran TH, Farrar J (2005) Oseltamivir resistance during treatment of influenza A (H5N1) infection. N Engl J Med 353:2667–2672

Dreyfus C, Ekiert DC, Wilson IA (2013) Structure of a classical broadly neutralizing stem antibody in complex with a pandemic H2 influenza virus hemagglutinin. J Virol 87:7149–7154

Dreyfus C, Laursen NS, Kwaks T, Zuijdgeest D, Khayat R, Ekiert DC, Lee JH, Metlagel Z, Bujny MV, Jongeneelen M, van der Vlugt R, Lamrani M, Korse HJ, Geelen E, Sahin O, Sieuwerts M, Brakenhoff JP, Vogels R, Li OT, Poon LL, Peiris M, Koudstaal W, Ward AB, Wilson IA, Goudsmit J, Friesen RH (2012) Highly conserved protective epitopes on influenza B viruses. Science 337:1343–1348

Ekiert DC, Bhabha G, Elsliger MA, Friesen RH, Jongeneelen M, Throsby M, Goudsmit J, Wilson IA (2009) Antibody recognition of a highly conserved influenza virus epitope. Science 324:246–251

Ekiert DC, Friesen RH, Bhabha G, Kwaks T, Jongeneelen M, Yu W, Ophorst C, Cox F, Korse HJ, Brandenburg B, Vogels R, Brakenhoff JP, Kompier R, Koldijk MH, Cornelissen LA, Poon LL, Peiris M, Koudstaal W, Wilson IA, Goudsmit J (2011) A highly conserved neutralizing epitope on group 2 influenza A viruses. Science 333:843–850

Ekiert DC, Kashyap AK, Steel J, Rubrum A, Bhabha G, Khayat R, Lee JH, Dillon MA, O'Neil RE, Faynboym AM, Horowitz M, Horowitz L, Ward AB, Palese P, Webby R, Lerner RA, Bhatt RR, Wilson IA (2012) Cross-neutralization of influenza A viruses mediated by a single antibody loop. Nature 489:526–532

Ekiert DC, Wilson IA (2012) Broadly neutralizing antibodies against influenza virus and prospects for universal therapies. Curr Opin Virol 2:134–141

Fleishman SJ, Whitehead TA, Ekiert DC, Dreyfus C, Corn JE, Strauch EM, Wilson IA, Baker D (2011) Computational design of proteins targeting the conserved stem region of influenza hemagglutinin. Science 332:816–821

Fleury D, Barrere B, Bizebard T, Daniels RS, Skehel JJ, Knossow M (1999) A complex of influenza hemagglutinin with a neutralizing antibody that binds outside the virus receptor binding site. Nat Struct Biol 6:530–534

Fleury D, Daniels RS, Skehel JJ, Knossow M, Bizebard T (2000) Structural evidence for recognition of a single epitope by two distinct antibodies. Proteins 40:572–578

Fleury D, Wharton SA, Skehel JJ, Knossow M, Bizebard T (1998) Antigen distortion allows influenza virus to escape neutralization. Nat Struct Biol 5:119–123

Friesen RH, Lee PS, Stoop EJ, Hoffman RM, Ekiert DC, Bhabha G, Yu W, Juraszek J, Koudstaal W, Jongeneelen M, Korse HJ, Ophorst C, Brinkman-van der Linden EC, Throsby M, Kwakkenbos MJ, Bakker AQ, Beaumont T, Spits H, Kwaks T, Vogels R, Ward AB, Goudsmit J, Wilson IA (2014) A common solution to group 2 influenza virus neutralization. Proc Natl Acad Sci U S A 111:445–450

Gao R, Cao B, Hu Y, Feng Z, Wang D, Hu W, Chen J, Jie Z, Qiu H, Xu K, Xu X, Lu H, Zhu W, Gao Z, Xiang N, Shen Y, He Z, Gu Y, Zhang Z, Yang Y, Zhao X, Zhou L, Li X, Zou S, Zhang Y, Li X, Yang L, Guo J, Dong J, Li Q, Dong L, Zhu Y, Bai T, Wang S, Hao P, Yang W, Zhang Y, Han J, Yu H, Li D, Gao GF, Wu G, Wang Y, Yuan Z, Shu Y (2013) Human infection with a novel avian-origin influenza A (H7N9) virus. N Engl J Med 368:1888–1897

Hai R, Krammer F, Tan GS, Pica N, Eggink D, Maamary J, Margine I, Albrecht RA, Palese P (2012) Influenza viruses expressing chimeric hemagglutinins: globular head and stalk domains derived from different subtypes. J Virol 86:5774–5781

Harris AK, Meyerson JR, Matsuoka Y, Kuybeda O, Moran A, Bliss D, Das SR, Yewdell JW, Sapiro G, Subbarao K, Subramaniam S (2013) Structure and accessibility of HA trimers on intact 2009 H1N1 pandemic influenza virus to stem region-specific neutralizing antibodies. Proc Natl Acad Sci U S A 110:4592–4597

Hong M, Lee PS, Hoffman RM, Zhu X, Krause JC, Laursen NS, Yoon SI, Song L, Tussey L, Crowe JE Jr, Ward AB, Wilson IA (2013) Antibody recognition of the pandemic H1N1 Influenza virus hemagglutinin receptor binding site. J Virol 87:12471–12480

Iba Y, Fujii Y, Ohshima N, Sumida T, Kubota-Koketsu R, Ikeda M, Wakiyama M, Shirouzu M, Okada J, Okuno Y, Kurosawa Y, Yokoyama S (2014) Conserved neutralizing epitope at globular head of hemagglutinin in H3N2 influenza viruses. J Virol 88(13):7130–7144

Jardine J, Julien JP, Menis S, Ota T, Kalyuzhniy O, McGuire A, Sok D, Huang PS, MacPherson S, Jones M, Nieusma T, Mathison J, Baker D, Ward AB, Burton DR, Stamatatos L, Nemazee D, Wilson IA, Schief WR (2013) Rational HIV immunogen design to target specific germline B cell receptors. Science 340:711–716

Julien JP, Lee PS, Wilson IA (2012) Structural insights into key sites of vulnerability on HIV-1 Env and influenza HA. Immunol Rev 250:180–198

Kanekiyo M, Wei CJ, Yassine HM, McTamney PM, Boyington JC, Whittle JR, Rao SS, Kong WP, Wang L, Nabel GJ (2013) Self-assembling influenza nanoparticle vaccines elicit broadly neutralizing H1N1 antibodies. Nature 499:102–106

Kashyap AK, Steel J, Oner AF, Dillon MA, Swale RE, Wall KM, Perry KJ, Faynboym A, Ilhan M, Horowitz M, Horowitz L, Palese P, Bhatt RR, Lerner RA (2008) Combinatorial antibody libraries from survivors of the Turkish H5N1 avian influenza outbreak reveal virus neutralization strategies. Proc Natl Acad Sci U S A 105:5986–5991

Kashyap AK, Steel J, Rubrum A, Estelles A, Briante R, Ilyushina NA, Xu L, Swale RE, Faynboym AM, Foreman PK, Horowitz M, Horowitz L, Webby R, Palese P, Lerner RA, Bhatt RR (2010) Protection from the 2009 H1N1 pandemic influenza by an antibody from combinatorial survivor-based libraries. PLoS Pathog 6:e1000990

Kiso M, Mitamura K, Sakai-Tagawa Y, Shiraishi K, Kawakami C, Kimura K, Hayden FG, Sugaya N, Kawaoka Y (2004) Resistant influenza A viruses in children treated with oseltamivir: descriptive study. Lancet 364:759–765

Kong L, Lee JH, Doores KJ, Murin CD, Julien JP, McBride R, Liu Y, Marozsan A, Cupo A, Klasse PJ, Hoffenberg S, Caulfield M, King CR, Hua Y, Le KM, Khayat R, Deller MC, Clayton T, Tien H, Feizi T, Sanders RW, Paulson JC, Moore JP, Stanfield RL, Burton DR,

Ward AB, Wilson IA (2013) Supersite of immune vulnerability on the glycosylated face of HIV-1 envelope glycoprotein gp120. Nat Struct Mol Biol 20:796–803
Krammer F, Pica N, Hai R, Margine I, Palese P (2013) Chimeric hemagglutinin influenza virus vaccine constructs elicit broadly protective stalk-specific antibodies. J Virol 87:6542–6550
Krause JC, Tsibane T, Tumpey TM, Huffman CJ, Albrecht R, Blum DL, Ramos I, Fernandez-Sesma A, Edwards KM, Garcia-Sastre A, Basler CF, Crowe JE Jr (2012) Human monoclonal antibodies to pandemic 1957 H2N2 and pandemic 1968 H3N2 influenza viruses. J Virol 86:6334–6340
Krause JC, Tsibane T, Tumpey TM, Huffman CJ, Basler CF, Crowe JE Jr (2011) A broadly neutralizing human monoclonal antibody that recognizes a conserved, novel epitope on the globular head of the influenza H1N1 virus hemagglutinin. J Virol 85:10905–10908
Lee PS, Yoshida R, Ekiert DC, Sakai N, Suzuki Y, Takada A, Wilson IA (2012) Heterosubtypic antibody recognition of the influenza virus hemagglutinin receptor binding site enhanced by avidity. Proc Natl Acad Sci U S A 109:17040–17045
Lu Y, Welsh JP, Swartz JR (2014) Production and stabilization of the trimeric influenza hemagglutinin stem domain for potentially broadly protective influenza vaccines. Proc Natl Acad Sci U S A 111:125–130
Martin J, Wharton SA, Lin YP, Takemoto DK, Skehel JJ, Wiley DC, Steinhauer DA (1998) Studies of the binding properties of influenza hemagglutinin receptor-site mutants. Virology 241:101–111
Molinari NA, Ortega-Sanchez IR, Messonnier ML, Thompson WW, Wortley PM, Weintraub E, Bridges CB (2007) The annual impact of seasonal influenza in the US: measuring disease burden and costs. Vaccine 25:5086–5096
Mallajosyula VV, Citron M, Ferrara F, Lu X, Callahan C, Heidecker GJ, Sarma SP, Flynn JA, Temperton NJ, Liang X, Varadarajan R (2014) Influenza hemagglutinin stem-fragment immunogen elicits broadly neutralizing antibodies and confers heterologous protection. Proc Natl Acad Sci U S A 111(25):E2514–E2523. doi:10.1073/pnas.1402766111.
Nabel GJ, Wei CJ, Ledgerwood JE (2011) Vaccinate for the next H2N2 pandemic now. Nature 471:157–158
Ohshima N, Iba Y, Kubota-Koketsu R, Asano Y, Okuno Y, Kurosawa Y (2011) Naturally occurring antibodies in humans can neutralize a variety of influenza virus strains, including H3, H1, H2, and H5. J Virol 85:11048–11057
Okuno Y, Isegawa Y, Sasao F, Ueda S (1993) A common neutralizing epitope conserved between the hemagglutinins of influenza A virus H1 and H2 strains. J Virol 67:2552–2558
Ridgway JB, Presta LG, Carter P (1996) 'Knobs-into-holes' engineering of antibody CH3 domains for heavy chain heterodimerization. Protein Eng 9:617–621
Salzberg S (2008) The contents of the syringe. Nature 454:160–161
Schmidt AG, Xu H, Khan AR, O'Donnell T, Khurana S, King LR, Manischewitz J, Golding H, Suphaphiphat P, Carfi A, Settembre EC, Dormitzer PR, Kepler TB, Zhang R, Moody MA, Haynes BF, Liao HX, Shaw DE, Harrison SC (2013) Preconfiguration of the antigen-binding site during affinity maturation of a broadly neutralizing influenza virus antibody. Proc Natl Acad Sci U S A 110:264–269
Skehel JJ, Bayley PM, Brown EB, Martin SR, Waterfield MD, White JM, Wilson IA, Wiley DC (1982) Changes in the conformation of influenza virus hemagglutinin at the pH optimum of virus-mediated membrane fusion. Proc Natl Acad Sci U S A 79:968–972
Smirnov YA, Lipatov AS, Gitelman AK, Okuno Y, Van Beek R, Osterhaus AD, Claas EC (1999) An epitope shared by the hemagglutinins of H1, H2, H5, and H6 subtypes of influenza A virus. Acta Virol 43:237–244
Stevens J, Corper AL, Basler CF, Taubenberger JK, Palese P, Wilson IA (2004) Structure of the uncleaved human H1 hemagglutinin from the extinct 1918 influenza virus. Science 303:1866–1870
Sui J, Hwang WC, Perez S, Wei G, Aird D, Chen LM, Santelli E, Stec B, Cadwell G, Ali M, Wan H, Murakami A, Yammanuru A, Han T, Cox NJ, Bankston LA, Donis RO, Liddington RC,

Marasco WA (2009) Structural and functional bases for broad-spectrum neutralization of avian and human influenza A viruses. Nat Struct Mol Biol 16:265–273

Sun X, Shi Y, Lu X, He J, Gao F, Yan J, Qi J, Gao GF (2013) Bat-derived influenza hemagglutinin H17 does not bind canonical avian or human receptors and most likely uses a unique entry mechanism. Cell Rep 3:769–778

Throsby M, van den Brink E, Jongeneelen M, Poon LL, Alard P, Cornelissen L, Bakker A, Cox F, van Deventer E, Guan Y, Cinatl J, ter Meulen J, Lasters I, Carsetti R, Peiris M, de Kruif J, Goudsmit J (2008) Heterosubtypic neutralizing monoclonal antibodies cross-protective against H5N1 and H1N1 recovered from human IgM+ memory B cells. PLoS One 3:e3942

Tong S, Zhu X, Li Y, Shi M, Zhang J, Bourgeois M, Yang H, Chen X, Recuenco S, Gomez J, Chen LM, Johnson A, Tao Y, Dreyfus C, Yu W, McBride R, Carney PJ, Gilbert AT, Chang J, Guo Z, Davis CT, Paulson JC, Stevens J, Rupprecht CE, Holmes EC, Wilson IA, Donis RO (2013) New world bats harbor diverse influenza A viruses. PLoS Pathog 9:e1003657

Tsibane T, Ekiert DC, Krause JC, Martinez O, Crowe JE Jr, Wilson IA, Basler CF (2012) Influenza human monoclonal antibody 1F1 interacts with three major antigenic sites and residues mediating human receptor specificity in H1N1 viruses. PLoS Pathog 8:e1003067

Wang TT, Tan GS, Hai R, Pica N, Ngai L, Ekiert DC, Wilson IA, Garcia-Sastre A, Moran TM, Palese P (2010) Vaccination with a synthetic peptide from the influenza virus hemagglutinin provides protection against distinct viral subtypes. Proc Natl Acad Sci U S A 107:18979–18984

Weis W, Brown JH, Cusack S, Paulson JC, Skehel JJ, Wiley DC (1988) Structure of the influenza virus haemagglutinin complexed with its receptor, sialic acid. Nature 333:426–431

Whitehead TA, Chevalier A, Song Y, Dreyfus C, Fleishman SJ, De Mattos C, Myers CA, Kamisetty H, Blair P, Wilson IA, Baker D (2012) Optimization of affinity, specificity and function of designed influenza inhibitors using deep sequencing. Nat Biotechnol 30:543–548

Whittle JR, Zhang R, Khurana S, King LR, Manischewitz J, Golding H, Dormitzer PR, Haynes BF, Walter EB, Moody MA, Kepler TB, Liao HX, Harrison SC (2011) Broadly neutralizing human antibody that recognizes the receptor-binding pocket of influenza virus hemagglutinin. Proc Natl Acad Sci U S A 108:14216–14221

Wiley DC, Wilson IA, Skehel JJ (1981) Structural identification of the antibody-binding sites of Hong Kong influenza haemagglutinin and their involvement in antigenic variation. Nature 289:373–378

Wilson IA, Skehel JJ, Wiley DC (1981) Structure of the haemagglutinin membrane glycoprotein of influenza virus at 3 Å resolution. Nature 289:366–373

Wyrzucki A, Dreyfus C, Kohler I, Steck M, Wilson IA, Hangartner L (2014) Alternative recognition of the conserved stem epitope in influenza a virus hemagglutinin by a VH3-30-encoded heterosubtypic antibody. J Virol 88(12):7083–7092

Xu R, Ekiert DC, Krause JC, Hai R, Crowe JE Jr, Wilson IA (2010) Structural basis of preexisting immunity to the 2009 H1N1 pandemic influenza virus. Science 328:357–360

Xu R, Krause JC, McBride R, Paulson JC, Crowe JE Jr, Wilson IA (2013) A recurring motif for antibody recognition of the receptor-binding site of influenza hemagglutinin. Nat Struct Mol Biol 20:363–370

Yoshida R, Igarashi M, Ozaki H, Kishida N, Tomabechi D, Kida H, Ito K, Takada A (2009) Cross-protective potential of a novel monoclonal antibody directed against antigenic site B of the hemagglutinin of influenza A viruses. PLoS Pathog 5:e1000350

Zhu X, Guo YH, Jiang T, Wang YD, Chan KH, Li XF, Yu W, McBride R, Paulson JC, Yuen KY, Qin CF, Che XY, Wilson IA (2013a) A unique and conserved neutralization epitope in H5N1 influenza viruses identified by an antibody against the A/Goose/Guangdong/1/96 hemagglutinin. J Virol 87:12619–12635

Zhu X, Yu W, McBride R, Li Y, Chen LM, Donis RO, Tong S, Paulson JC, Wilson IA (2013b) Hemagglutinin homologue from H17N10 bat influenza virus exhibits divergent receptor-binding and pH-dependent fusion activities. Proc Natl Acad Sci U S A 110:1458–1463

Skin Immunization with Influenza Vaccines

Ioanna Skountzou and Richard W. Compans

Abstract Problems with existing influenza vaccines include the strain specificity of the immune response, resulting in the need for frequent reformulation in response to viral antigenic drift. Even in years when the same influenza strains are prevalent, the duration of immunity is limited, and results in the need for annual revaccination. The immunogenicity of the present split or subunit vaccines is also lower than that observed with whole inactivated virus, and the vaccines are not very effective in high risk groups such as the young or the elderly. Vaccine coverage is incomplete, due in part to concerns about the use of hypodermic needles for delivery. Alternative approaches for vaccination are being developed which address many of these concerns. Here we review new approaches which focus on skin immunization, including the development of needle-free delivery systems which use stable dry formulations and induce stronger and longer-lasting immune responses.

Contents

I. Skountzou (✉) · R.W. Compans
Department of Microbiology and Immunology and Emory Vaccine Center, Emory University School of Medicine, CNR Building, 1518 Clifton Road, Atlanta, GA 30322, USA
e-mail: iskount@emory.edu

R.W. Compans
e-mail: rcompan@emory.edu

Current Topics in Microbiology and Immunology (2015) 386: 343–369
DOI: 10.1007/82_2014_407

Published Online: 20 July 2014

1 Introduction

Over 200 years ago, Edward Jenner demonstrated that delivery of live cowpox virus to human skin resulted in transient skin lesions, and gave rise to protective immunity against subsequent exposure to smallpox virus (Riedel 2005). This procedure was further developed over the subsequent centuries, and the term **vaccination** was adapted, reflecting the use of the cowpox-related virus **vaccinia** for smallpox immunization. A global vaccination campaign against smallpox resulted in its eradication, which was declared by the WHO in 1980, and is recognized as one of the greatest achievements in medicine (Riedel 2005). During the course of this project, a variety of devices was developed and used for delivery of the smallpox vaccine to the skin, and they have been described in detail in other recent reviews (Weniger and Glenn 2013). In addition to smallpox vaccination, skin immunization has been widely used for delivery of the Bacille Calmette-Guerin (BCG) vaccine for tuberculosis (Hoft et al. 2008). Experimental studies of intradermal vaccine delivery have also been carried out with a number of other vaccines for infectious disease prevention, including clinical trials as well as studies in experimental animals, and have been recently reviewed (Kim et al. 2011). The high current interest in this approach for vaccination reflects its potential immunological as well as logistical advantages, as discussed in this review for influenza immunization. In addition to improving immune responses, acceptability of vaccination by the public is likely to be enhanced by avoiding the use of hypodermic needles. A more complete overview of research on intradermal immunization has been recently published as Volume 351 of this series (Teunissen et al. 2012).

A number of early studies were carried out with inactivated influenza vaccines using intradermal delivery with the goal of using reduced doses of vaccine (Bruyn et al. 1949b; Glazier et al. 1956; Hilleman et al. 1958; Tauraso et al. 1969; Weller et al. 1948) and in several studies it was observed that lower doses were sufficient to elicit the same immune response when compared with subcutaneous injection. The approach for intradermal delivery used in these studies was developed by Mantoux (Mantoux 1909), who used a hypodermic needle inserted at an angle to deliver antigen just beneath the dermis. However this approach is technically difficult and requires trained personnel, and it has not been widely employed in many recent vaccination programs.

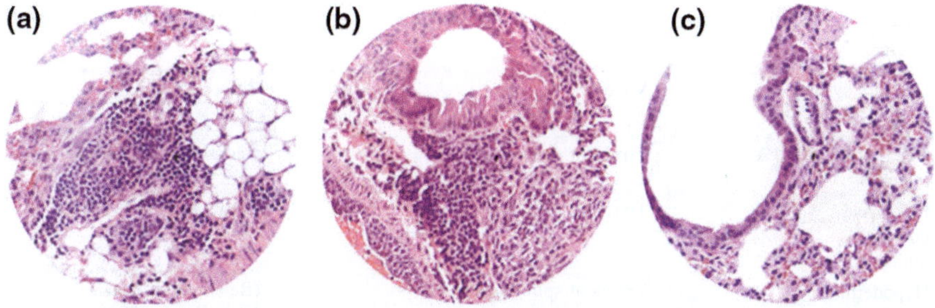

Fig. 1 Lung histopathological examination after lethal infection. Lung tissue sections from naïve, subcutaneously immunized and microneedle immunized mice challenged with$10xLD_{50}$ of live virus six months after immunization were stained with hematoxylin and eosin stain. The histopathology of the lung tissues collected upon challenge of immunized or unimmunized mice 6 months post immunization showed clear signs of profound pulmonary inflammation in the unimmunized infected (**a**) or subcutaneously immunized animals (**b**). Peribronchial and intra-alveolar inflammation was accompanied by significant pulmonary edema and cellular infiltration mainly consisting of neutrophils. The group of microneedle immunized mice did not show any signs of inflammation (**c**)

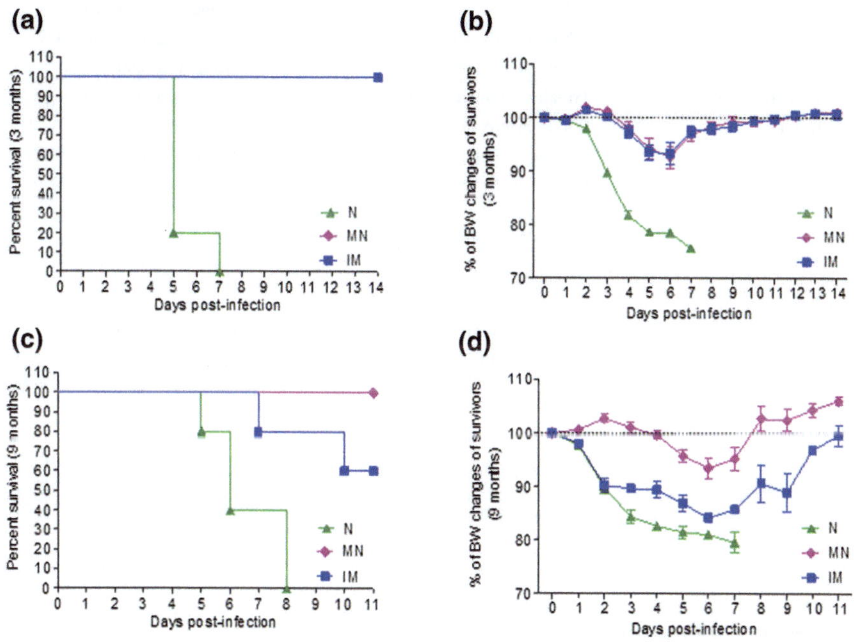

Fig. 2 Protective efficacy against H1N1 A/Brisbane/59/2007 lethal infection. Body weight changes and survival rates were recorded after lethal challenge with $5xLD_{50}$ of live A/Brisbane/59/2007 virus in microneedle (MN) and intramuscularly (IM) immunized and naïve mice at 3 months (**a**, **b**) and nine months (**c**, **d**) post-vaccination. *N* naïve mice. Data represent the mean ± SEM

Table 1 Examples of delivery systems for skin immunization with influenza vaccines in various species

Delivery system	Vaccine	Reference
Human		
Needle-free jet injector	Trivalent split vaccine	(Jackson et al. 2001)
Epidermal powder injection	Trivalent split vaccine	(Dean and Chen 2004)
Hypodermic needle (Mantoux method)	Trivalent split vaccine	(Belshe et al. 2007; Kunzi et al. 2009)
Hollow microneedle (30 gauge) (BD Soluvia)	Trivalent split vaccine	(Laurent et al. 2007), (Icardi et al. 2012)
Epidermal (topical) application	Tetragrip (Tetanus-influenza)	(Combadiere et al. 2010)
Mouse		
Coated metal microneedles	Monovalent subunit vaccine	(Koutsonanos et al. 2012)
	H_1N_1 VLPs	(Quan et al. 2010a)
	H_5N_1 VLPs	(Song et al. 2010a)
	Whole inactivated H_3N_2	(Koutsonanos et al. 2009)
	Whole inactivated H_1N_1	(Zhu et al. 2009)
Nanopatch™	Trivalent subunit vaccine	(Fernando et al. 2010)
Dissolving microneedles	Whole inactivated H_1N_1	(Sullivan et al. 2010)
	Trivalent subunit vaccine	(Kommareddy et al. 2012)
Permeability enhancers	Whole inactivated H_1N_1	(Skountzou et al. 2006)
Blank microneedles and topical application	Influenza subunit vaccine	(Ding et al. 2009)
Electroporation	Recombinant H_5 HA	(Garg et al. 2007)
Epidermal powder injection	Trivalent split vaccine	(Chen et al. 2003)
Guinea Pig		
Coated microneedles	Trivalent subunit vaccine	(Kommareddy et al. 2013)
Dry skin patch	Trivalent split vaccine	(Frolov et al. 2008)
Rat		
Microneedles	Trivalent split vaccine	(Alarcon et al. 2007)
Chicken		
Jet injector H5 DNA vaccine Inactivated recombinant vaccine		
Non-Human Primate		
Epidermal powder injection	Trivalent vaccine	(Chen et al. 2003)

In this review, we have focused on recent studies using alternative approaches for skin delivery of influenza vaccines. These studies have employed a number of different methods for vaccine delivery, examples of which are listed in Table 1. We have included studies using whole inactivated virus, which was widely used until the 1970s, as well as split or subunit vaccines which were subsequently developed using detergent-disrupted virus. Influenza vaccine has been an antigen of choice for many studies of intradermal vaccination, in part because the vaccine is well characterized and widely used, and because animal models are available to evaluate the resulting immune responses as well as the protective efficacy. The results have revealed significant immunological advantages for this route of vaccine delivery. In addition, skin immunization could provide an approach to overcome some of the limitations and problems with current influenza vaccines, including the limited duration of immunity and the problems in conferring effective protection to high risk groups, such as young children and adults over 65 years old (Osterholm et al. 2012).

2 Human Studies

The first studies that explored alternative vaccination routes with inactivated influenza vaccine were carried out in human volunteers by Francis and Magill in 1937, in a series of experiments designed to induce neutralizing antibody production against type A influenza virus grown in tissue culture. The authors showed a significant rise in circulating strain-specific antibody, a booster effect in case of pre-existing immunity and persistence of immune responses up to 5 months (Francis and Magill 1937). Van Gelder et al. reported that intracutaneous delivery of 1/10 of the normal dose of concentrated inactivated influenza type A and B viruses resulted in a rapid and considerable rise in the serum anti-hemagglutinin titers, which was greater than that observed with a subcutaneous dose, and proposed that this vaccine delivery approach should be further studied to determine its protective effect against influenza (Van Gelder et al. 1947). Importantly the authors also observed lower incidence of generalized reactions to the vaccine in the group which received intradermal inoculations. In the spring of the same year an influenza epidemic occurred in Boston, which led Weller et al. to carry out intradermal vaccination in a group of adult hospital personnel. The investigators could not reproduce the dose-sparing effect of intradermal inoculation or the increasing titers reported by Van Gelder, suggesting that these results may be due to differences in vaccine concentration. They confirmed that the local reactions to intradermal vaccination were mild and that systemic reactions were rare (Weller et al. 1948). The need for a single vaccine dose, important for mass vaccinations, was emphasized by Bruyn et al who did not find significant differences between one or two doses of influenza A and B vaccines delivered intradermally in adults or children. Their data did not show differences between responses to intradermal vs. subcutaneous immunization (Bruyn et al. 1949a). Subsequent studies by

Glazier et al on intradermal vaccination of children with inactivated influenza A and B viruses demonstrated effectiveness and dose sparing compared to subcutaneous immunization. The authors also observed rises in titers with booster doses either one week or 5–7 months after primary immunization (Glazier et al. 1956).

The emergence of the Asian flu pandemic (1957–1958) and the urgent need for mass vaccination provided a reason for re-visiting the issue of dose sparing. Boger and Liu reported that intradermal vaccination did not offer any advantages in terms of dose sparing and suggested that subcutaneous immunization in humans should be the recommended vaccination route (Boger and Liu 1957). In contrast Hilleman et al demonstrated that intradermal delivery of 1/10 dose of egg grown A/Japan/305/57 vaccine induced similar antibody responses in human volunteers as the full dose given subcutaneously. The seasonal polyvalent vaccine did not induce cross-reactive responses to A/Japan/305/57 virus, but cross-reactive antibody could be observed with high vaccine doses against A/Swine/30 and A/Hawaii/305/56 suggesting sharing of common antigens. Based on the seroconversion rates elicited after intradermal vaccination, the authors suggested that this route offers considerable advantage in conserving vaccine during periods of shortages as well as reducing the cost for vaccination (Hilleman et al. 1958). The difference between the 1957 and 1958 studies may be related to age differences of vaccinees. Boger and Liu recruited volunteers aged over 70 in order to determine effects of pre-existing immunity that could offer cross-protection against the novel H3N2 influenza subtype, whereas Hilleman et al carried out their studies in healthy adults.

Ten years later the appearance of the Hong Kong pandemic (1968–1969) resulted in a subsequent vaccine shortage, and caused re-evaluation of humoral immune responses following subcutaneous and intradermal inoculation vaccination. Tauraso et al. used vaccine purified by zonal centrifugation for the first time, and tested vaccine efficacy in healthy adult volunteers. Based on their findings of a significant dose sparing (1/5 dose when compared to the subcutaneous dose) the authors suggested that intradermal inoculation would be a reasonable alternative for mass vaccinations. Additional interesting results from this study were the finding of a 4-fold seroconversion after 2 vaccine doses, and an inverse relationship between antibody response and pre-immunization titers; also, individuals 65 years or older developed antibody responses more rapidly than younger age-groups based on a 4-fold or greater rise in antibody and the geometric mean ratio in sera at intervals after vaccination (Tauraso et al. 1969).

With the emergence of a swine flu variant infecting humans in 1976, a national vaccination campaign was initiated in the U.S. Brown et al. reported that among the 18–24 year-old age group, persons who did not have pre-existing immunity against the A/New Jersey/31/76 (HswINI), when vaccinated intradermally with whole-virus vaccine at 1/5 dose than those immunized intramuscularly (40 HA units/0.1-ml dose vs. 200 HA units/0.5-ml dose) exhibited lower HAI titers, and repeated vaccinations did not offer an immunological advantage. In contrast, vaccinees over the age of 24 without detectable homologous immunity had comparable serologic responses to intradermal or intramuscular vaccination. Persons infected with influenza virus prior to vaccination exhibited an immediate antibody response indicative of a secondary type of response. The antibody responses after intradermal vaccination were lower for those vaccinees with pre-existing immunity, and in a younger age group. In older age groups who were vaccinated either intradermally or intramuscularly, only the ID group needed a booster dose (Brown et al. 1977). As a result of mild side effects of intradermal influenza vaccine delivery and the lack of systematic advantages of this route compared to conventional intramuscular inoculation, such as dose sparing, the intradermal route lost its appeal. In addition, other factors such as the inadequate purification of whole inactivated influenza virus, uncertainties about the inactivation process and the termination of the vaccination program due to a media frenzy related to Guillain-Barré syndrome (GBS) among persons receiving swine flu immunizations, attention shifted to newer and safer vaccine formulations such as subunit and split inactivated influenza vaccines (Sencer and Millar 2006). Currently, inactivated trivalent influenza vaccines (TIVs) include the unadjuvanted whole virion, split virus, subunit, virosomes containing subunit antigens, or adjuvanted subunit vaccines.

In 1960 Aaron Ismach designed jet injectors for mass vaccinations aiming to controlled vaccine or drug delivery in the skin (Ismach 1960). Jet injectors are a type of syringe using a high-pressure narrow jet of liquid instead of a hypodermic needle to penetrate the epidermis. Studies in healthy young adults showed that the device caused higher levels of pain and local reactions following vaccination, while there was no dose sparing or improvement of humoral responses (Jackson et al. 2001). A similar approach was attempted by Chen using the PowderJect ND5.2 delivery system for powdered trivalent influenza vaccine delivery in the epidermis, targeting Langerhans cells (Chen et al. 2004). A phase I clinical trial comparing intramuscular and epidermal (EPI) immunization reported no differences in systemic reactogenicity or any severe site reactions, and equivalent or superior immune responses were elicited in EPI-immunized groups as compared to groups immunized intramuscularly (Dean and Chen 2004). Due to potential risks of pathogen transmission during applications, the World Health Organization no longer recommends jet injectors for vaccination (WHO 2005). As of today no influenza vaccines are licensed in the United States for administration via jet-injector (FDA 2011).

Several studies have been carried out using intradermal injection of trivalent subunit vaccines with hypodermic needles (Belshe et al. 2004; Beran et al. 2009; Auewarakul et al. 2007), and a stronger immune response or dose-sparing effect was observed in some of the studies. Subsequently, a device was developed by Becton Dickinson (Soluvia™) for intradermal immunization using a prefilled syringe and a 30 gauge, 1.5mm-long needle, which limits the depth of penetration of the needle (Laurent et al. 2007). A number of clinical trials have been carried out using this device to deliver trivalent detergent-split vaccine, and have been recently reviewed (Icardi et al. 2012; Ansaldi et al. 2012). The device offers improved reproducibility and ease of delivery compared with the Mantoux technique. BD Soluvia™ has been licensed for use in Europe and the U.S for Sanofi Pasteur's Fluzone® for active immunization of adults aged between 18 and 64 years. The reduced-antigen-content ID vaccine (9 μg hemagglutinin per strain) is as immunogenic as standard-dose IM influenza vaccine; it is safe and well tolerated by patients, which could result in an improvement in vaccine coverage by including individuals who fear injection with standard hypodermic needles (Icardi et al. 2012).

NanoPass Technologies LTD developed a single-use device for painless intradermal delivery (MicronJet) to deliver drugs and vaccines. Microneedles are manufactured by using MEMS (Micro Electro Mechanical Systems) technology and were made of pure silicon crystals in the shape of micro-pyramidal needles. Prospective randomized trials in healthy adults who received a 6 μg or a 3 μg dose of hemagglutinin per strain by intradermal injection of seasonal influenza vaccine with the MicronJet device demonstrated humoral immune responses similar to those elicited by the full-dose 15 μg intramuscular vaccination. The microneedle injection device used in this study was found to be effective, safe, and reliable (Van Damme et al. 2009). A follow up prospective randomized trial on elderly and chronically ill adults delivering reduced dose ID TIV (3 or 9 μg of hemagglutinin (HA) per strain) by MicronJet600^{TM} demonstrated dose sparing and improved seroconversion and seroprotection when compared to the full vaccine dose (15 μg) delivered intramuscularly as measured by hemagglutination inhibition (HAI) and neutralizing antibody titers (Hung et al. 2012). The data support further investigation of this approach for intradermal immunization with vaccines of low immunogenicity.

Most of the above studies in humans have been focused on the issue of dose sparing, which has become relatively less important because of the availability of a more reliable vaccine supply. Relatively little information has been obtained on other potential advantages such as quality and duration of the immune response, breadth of immunity, or induction of mucosal or cellular responses. Recently, Combadiere et al. demonstrated the superiority of transcutaneous immunization (TC) with inactivated influenza vaccine in the induction of CD8+ T cell responses in randomized Phase I Clinical Trials (Combadiere et al. 2010).

All human vaccine studies described above have employed intradermal delivery of influenza vaccines with needle-based devices but it is generally accepted that there are many concerns related to unsafe practices and pathogen transmission involving needles. In addition there is a large percentage of children and adults who suffer from distress or fear of injections (Giudice and Campbell 2006), resulting in reluctance to receive immunizations. Another major hurdle in expanding vaccination coverage is the need to maintain vaccines at low temperatures. The need for *cold chain* to preserve vaccine potency mandates a 2–8 °C temperature range for vaccine storage from the time that they are manufactured until they are given to patients (Atkinson et al. 2002; Weir and Hatch 2004) . Needle-phobia, discomfort and reactogenicity of particular vaccines (Moylett and Hanson 2004) directed research to discovery of novel immunization approaches such as lyophilized vaccines delivered in the form of patches (Glenn et al. 2003). An alternative vaccine formulation independent of the *cold chain* is a promising approach for rapid distribution to remote areas of the world without the appropriate infrastructure to establish effective mass vaccination strategies and lead to a reduction in the costs of vaccine distribution.

3 Animal Studies

3.1 Mice

3.1.1 Potency of Immune Responses and Dose Sparing

Inactivated, Subunit and VLP Vaccines

Delivery of inactivated whole influenza virus with topical application on the skin was demonstrated in the mouse model (Skountzou et al. 2006). Despite its large size the virus could transverse the skin after mild pre-treatment and induce influenza-specific hemagglutination inhibition and neutralizing antibody titers in serum as well as salivary and fecal IgA. Lung viral titers were assessed as an indicator of protection after intranasal challenge with mouse adapted homologous virus. Effective clearance of virus in vaccinated animals as compared to unvaccinated infected controls within 8 days was attributed to robust humoral and cellular immune responses. Despite the encouraging data it was evident that this approach for transcutaneous immunization required higher vaccine doses and multiple immunizations, suggesting the need for improved delivery of antigen for dose sparing.

To overcome the limitations of non-invasive skin vaccination methods, while avoiding the concerns about hypodermic needles, minimally invasive methods to administer vaccine to the skin have been developed, primarily using very small hollow or solid needles. Most research on minimally invasive skin vaccination has involved the use of microneedles, which are long enough to cross the stratum corneum barrier and to reliably remain within the skin for targeted delivery, but short enough to avoid pain (Gill et al. 2008). There are four different types of microneedles that have been studied for vaccine delivery: hollow, solid, coated, and dissolving microneedles. Because this approach directly and actively deposits vaccine in the skin, it can deliver vaccine doses faster and more reliably than non-invasive vaccinations (Kim et al. 2012).

Metal microneedle arrays coated with low (3 μg) or higher (10 μg) doses of inactivated A/Aichi/2/68 (H3N2) influenza virus elicited substantial influenza-specific neutralizing antibodies in BALB/c mouse sera after a single immunization (Koutsonanos et al. 2009). Interestingly, mice vaccinated cutaneously or intramuscularly with the low vaccine dose showed similar titers whereas humoral responses to cutaneous immunization were significantly higher with increased vaccine doses. All vaccinated groups were fully protected upon challenge with

$5xLD_{50}$ of mouse adapted Aichi virus. Virus clearance from the lungs was complete by day 4 in mice that received the high vaccine dose. Microneedle vaccination induced a broad spectrum of immune responses including CD4+ and CD8+ responses in the spleen and draining lymph nodes, a high frequency of antibody-secreting cells in the lung and induction of virus-specific memory B-cells. The similarity in results observed after IM and MN immunization demonstrated that microneedle immunization was as effective as intramuscular vaccination (Koutsonanos et al. 2009). Similarly, Zhu et al observed that mice immunized by a single dose of H1N1 inactivated influenza virus (A/PR/8/34) coated on MNs were effectively protected against lethal challenge by a very high dose ($100xLD_{50}$) of mouse-adapted influenza virus A/PR/8/34 (Zhu et al. 2009).

Skin immunization with microneedles fabricated using a biocompatible polymer (PVP, polyvinylpyrollidone) encapsulating 6μg of inactivated whole influenza virus vaccine (A/PR/8/34) with trehalose were inserted and dissolved in the skin within minutes with at least 80 % antigen delivery. Challenge of mice with $5xLD_{50}$ of homologous virus showed a showed a 10^3-fold-decrease in lung viral titers in intramuscularly immunized mice compared to unimmunized infected mice, whereas microneedle-immunized mice showed a dramatic 10^6 -fold decrease in lung viral titers. Levels of IFN-γ, IL-12p70 and IL-21 in the lung induced after polyclonal re-stimulation were higher in the intramuscular compared to the microneedle group, suggesting stronger local Th1 response upon challenge. In contrast, influenza virus MHC Class I and II restricted T cell responses were increased in spleen of microneedle-immunized groups, indicative of increased recall CD4+ and CD8+ T cell responses (Sullivan et al. 2010).

Even without causing cell death in the epidermis, skin immunization is superior to intramuscular delivery in dose sparing. A very low dose of (A/PR/8/34 H1N1) VLPs (0.3μg) delivered with metal microneedles induced significantly superior protective immunity, which included binding and functional antibodies as well as complete protection against a high dose lethal infection with the homologous virus, whereas IM immunization provided only partial (40%) protection (Quan et al. 2010a). Furthermore a single immunization with metal microneedles coated with a very low dose (0.2 μg) of A/Vietnam/1203/04 H5N1 virus (H5 VLPs) induced high levels of antibodies and provided complete protection against $20xLD_{50}$ lethal challenge without apparent disease symptoms. In contrast, intramuscular injection with the same vaccine dose showed low levels of antibodies and provided only 60 % protection accompanied by severe body weight loss (Song et al. 2010a).

Influenza vaccines have a limited shelf-life even when stored at 4 °C. Quan et al found that the integrity of A/PR/8/34 influenza virus, as measured by hemagglutination activity, was significantly damaged during metal microneedle coating at room temperature. The addition of trehalose to the vaccine formulation resulted in retention of functional integrity and vaccine potency as shown in mouse studies. Both intramuscular and microneedle skin immunization with un-stabilized vaccine yielded weaker protective immune responses including viral antibodies, protective efficacies, and recall immune responses to influenza virus, whereas a single microneedle-based vaccination using stabilized influenza vaccine was superior to intramuscular immunization in controlling virus replication as well as in inducing rapid recall immune responses post-challenge (Quan et al. 2009). Addition of trehalose to the coating formulation was found to protect the antigen and retention of 48–82 % antigen activity for all three major subtypes of seasonal influenza: H1N1, H3N2 and B. Influenza vaccine coated in the presence of trehalose also exhibited thermal stability, such that activity loss was independent of temperature over the range of 4–37 °C for 24 h (Kim et al. 2010a). In the absence of trehalose hemagglutinin activity decreased below 10 % after 1 h and was not detected after 1 month of drying, respectively. Addition of trehalose maintained HA activity above 60 % after drying and above 20 % after 1 month storage at 25 °C. Loss of HA activity generally correlated with increased virus particle aggregation. Administration of microneedles coated with trehalose-stabilized influenza vaccine yielded high serum IgG antibody titers even after 1 month storage, and all animals survived lethal challenge infection with minimal weight loss (Kim et al. 2011). Choi et al. reported that crystallization and phase separation of the dried coating matrix are important factors affecting long-term stability of influenza vaccine-coated microneedles (Choi et al. 2012). The partial viral activity loss observed in the trehalose-containing formulation was hypothesized to result from osmotic pressure-induced vaccine destabilization. Inclusion of a viscosity enhancer, carboxymethyl cellulose, overcame this effect and full vaccine activity was retaned on washed or plasma-cleaned titanium surfaces (Choi et al. 2013).

Similarly, addition of trehalose in vaccine coating formulations stabilized influenza VLPs containing HA and M1 proteins from A/PR/8/34 virus, demonstrating preservation of hemagglutinin antigen. A single dose of stabilized influenza VLPs induced 100 % protection against challenge infection with a high lethal dose (20xLD_{50}) of homologous virus. In contrast, unstabilized influenza VLPs, as well as intramuscularly injected vaccines, provided inferior immunity and only partial protection ($\leq$40%). These results correlated with influenza specific neutralizing antibody titers and antibody secreting cells detected in spleen and bone marrow (Quan et al. 2010b). Optimizing the coating formulation required balancing the factors affecting the coating dose and vaccine antigen stability. Vaccine stability, as measured by an in vitro hemagglutination assay, was increased by formulation with higher concentration of trehalose or other stabilizing carbohydrate compounds and lower concentration of carboxymethylcellulose (CMC) or other viscosity-enhancing compounds (Kim et al. 2010b).

Matsuo et al. developed dissolving microneedle arrays, called MicroHyala (MH), as a transcutaneous immunization device, that co-polymerized sodium hyaluronate with influenza antigens dissolved in aqueous solution. The length of microneedles was either 300 μm (MH300) or 800 μm (MH800), and the arrays contained over 200 microneedles/cm^2. TCI vaccination efficacy was compared to that of conventional immunization systems, such as subcutaneous immunization (SC), intradermal immunization (ID), intramuscular immunization (IM), and intranasal immunization (IN). Influenza-specific IgG or HAI titers elicited by TCI delivery of unadjuvanted vaccine were similar to intramuscular or intradermal immunization in the presence or absence of Alum as an adjuvant. These data were correlated with survival studies where all ID, IM and TCI groups survived lethal challenge with homologous virus and showed no lung pathology (Matsuo et al. 2012).

The skin epidermis consists mainly of keratinocytes, melanocytes, and Langerhans cells (LCs) (Skountzou and Kang 2009). Langerhans cells are present in all layers of the epidermis and are in close proximity to the *stratum corneum* (Banchereau and Steinman 1998). These are immature APCs produced from bone marrow precursors that reach and populate the skin through the peripheral circulation (Romani et al. 1985). Fernando et al took advantage of the densely packed cell layer and designed a Nanopatch, which contains an array of densely packed projections (21025/cm^2) (110 micron in length), that were dry-coated with vaccine. They observed that the Nanopatches could deliver a seasonal influenza vaccine (Fluvax® 2008) in 2 min and that by physically targeting vaccine directly to these antigen presenting cells they induced protective levels of functional antibody responses in mice, comparable to the vaccine delivered intramuscularly with a needle and syringe, but with less than 1/100th of the delivered antigen (Fernando et al. 2010; Raphael et al. 2010). The impressive dose sparing effect observed with the Nanopatch suggested that it resulted from cell death in proximity to sites of antigen deposition in the skin, resulting in enhancement of immunogenicity (Depelsenaire et al. 2014).

Vectored Vaccines

Few studies have been done using skin immunization with recombinant vectored vaccines for influenza virus. However, a replication-defective adenovirus recombinant encoding the influenza A/PR/8/34 HA has been evaluated in human volunteers (Van Kampen et al. 2005). The recombinant vaccine was administered intranasally or applied to the abdominal skin after shaving, followed by gentle brushing with a soft-bristle toothbrush for 30 strokes. After the topical application of vaccine, the administration site was covered with a Tegaderm™ patch. The adenovirus-vectored nasal and epicutaneous influenza vaccines were both well tolerated by human volunteers. However the intranasally administered vaccine induced stronger immune responses than those observed in the cohort which received the epicutaneous vaccination.

Universal Influenza Vaccines

Current influenza vaccines induce immune responses which are highly strain-specific, resulting in the need to change the composition in order to protect against variant strains which emerge to escape from preexisting immunity. In addition, current vaccines would provide little or no protection against emergence of a new antigenic subtype, which could result in a global pandemic. It is therefore of high interest to identify conserved antigens and use them to develop vaccines which are broadly cross-reactive with multiple subtypes of influenza A viruses. It is known that the viral internal proteins, such as NP and M1, are more highly conserved. They do not elicit neutralizing antibodies, but can contribute to protective immunity by eliciting cross-reactive T-cell responses (Yewdell et al. 1985). However, most efforts to develop universal vaccines have focused on conserved epitopes on the external surface of the virion. The membrane-proximal HA stalk domain is highly conserved, and is a promising target for universal vaccine design. A growing body of evidence has emerged to support the idea that a stalk-based vaccine is capable of eliciting neutralizing antibodies with broad-cross protective efficacy (Wrammert et al. 2011). However it is not normally exposed to the immune system because it is covered by the globular HA head domain.

A second conserved antigen on the viral surface is the short external domain of the M2 protein, a trans-membrane protein which serves as an ion channel and also functions in viral assembly. This protein is present at low levels in the virion, and does not usually elicit an immune response by vaccination or infection. However it has been possible to design modified forms of the M2 external domain (M2e), some of which elicit protective immune responses when used as vaccines. A fusion protein of the TLR5-agonist domains of the flagellin protein from *Salmonella typhimurium* and multiple repeats of influenza M2e has been constructed, and evaluated as a vaccine in a mouse model using alternative immunization routes (Wang et al. 2014). It was found that skin immunization using metal microneedles coated with the fusion protein elicited strong systemic as well as mucosal immunity, and the protective efficacy induced by microneedle immunization was found to be much better than that observed with IM immunization.

Recombinant Protein Vaccines

Since most currently available influenza vaccines consist of solubilized viral protein antigens, recombinant subunit influenza vaccine was also tested for its immunogenic properties when delivered to the skin by coated microneedles. BALB/c vaccinated via metal microneedle delivery with a stabilized recombinant trimeric soluble hemagglutinin (sHA) derived from A/Aichi/2/68 (H3) virus had significantly higher immune responses than did mice vaccinated with unmodified sHA and they were fully protected against a lethal challenge with influenza virus. Analysis of post-challenge lung titers showed that MN-immunized mice had completely cleared the virus from their lungs, in contrast to mice given the same vaccine by a standard subcutaneous route (Weldon et al. 2011).

DNA Vaccines

Early studies of immunization using DNA plasmids to elicit immune responses to the encoded proteins employed coating the plasmids onto gold particles, which were administered by various routed including the delivery into skin by electroporation

(Wolff et al. 1990) or by high velocity gene gun injection (Jackson et al. 2001). In studies comparing different immunization routes using a DNA plasmid encoding the influenza HA protein (Fynan et al. 1993a, b), it was observed that using a gene gun to deliver DNA-coated gold beads to the epidermis of mice was a more effective route than intramuscular injection. Gene gun delivery of DNA vaccines encoding proteins of H1N1 or H3N2 influenza viruses induced protective immune responses in ferrets against challenge infection with heterologous influenza drift strains (Bragstad et al. 2011). Influenza DNA vaccines have also been shown to induce protective immunity in a phase 1 clinical trial (Jones et al. 2009).

Because of the high molecular weight and viscosity of seasonal or avian influenza DNA vaccines, they can also be used for coating of microneedles in the absence of other excipients such as carboxymethylcellulose or detergents (Kim et al. 2013; Song et al. 2012). It was found that delivery of microneedle-coated seasonal influenza HA-encoding DNA vaccines to the skin conferred dose sparing effects and induced improved protection in mice against subsequent virus challenge, when compared to IM immunization with the same DNA plasmids (Song et al. 2012).

3.1.2 Duration of Immunity

A concern about the present seasonal influenza vaccines is that they elicit a relatively short duration of immunity, which wanes 6–8 months after immunization (Albrecht et al. 2014). Therefore, it is of interest to determine whether an alternative vaccination route could confer improved duration of immunity.

Prime-boost skin vaccination with metal microneedles coated with H5 VLPs containing the hemagglutinin (HA) of A/Vietnam/1203/04 demonstrated higher levels of virus specific neutralizing antibodies as well as B and T cell responses up to 8 months after vaccination compared to the same antigen delivered intramuscularly and conferred 100 % protection against lethal challenge with the wild-type A/Vietnam/1203/04 virus 16 weeks after vaccination (Song et al. 2010b). In the case of seasonal influenza (H1N1 A/PR/8/34) VLPs a single dose was sufficient to confer long-term protective efficacy of influenza after skin vaccination using microneedle patches coated with the vaccine. Microneedle vaccination of mice in the skin induced 100 % protection against lethal challenge infection with influenza A/PR/8/34 virus for at least 14 months, that correlated with humoral systemic and mucosal influenza virus-specific immune responses that were maintained for over a year (Quan et al. 2013).

In another study 5 μg of pandemic swine origin inactivated A/California/04/2009 influenza virus delivered once to BALB/c mice either with metal microneedles or subcutaneously elicited similar serum IgG and hemagglutination inhibition titers and 100% protection against lethal viral challenge 6 weeks after vaccination. However, six months after vaccination, the subcutaneous group exhibited a 60 % decrease in functional antibody titers and extensive lung inflammation after challenge with $10\times LD_{50}$ of homologous virus, whereas the microneedle group maintained high functional antibody titers and IFN-γ levels, inhibition of viral replication, and no signs of lung inflammation after challenge. Microneedle vaccination conferred complete protection against lethal challenge as well as high numbers of bone marrow plasma cells and spleen antibody-secreting cells (Koutsonanos et al. 2011).

A single 3 μg dose of the subunit A/Brisbane/59/2007 vaccine with metal microneedles conferred complete protection against 5xLD_{50} of mouse-adapted virus at 4, 12 and 36 weeks post-vaccination whereas intramuscular immunization conferred completed protection only at 4 and 12 weeks post vaccination (Koutsonanos et al. 2012). The decreased protection at the later time correlated with lower IgG2a titers and a 38 % drop of HAI titers below to levels 40 in the intramuscularly vaccinated group after 9 months, whereas all mice in the microneedle vaccinated group retained HAI titers above protective levels (HAI>40). The maintenance of these high levels of functional antibody titers throughout a period of nine months can be attributed to the higher number of influenza-specific antibody secreting cells (long-lived bone marrow plasma cells) detected in the microneedle immunized group.

3.1.3 Breadth of Immunity

The continuous antigenic drift of influenza viruses mandates frequent changes of the vaccine composition. The need for annual revaccination against influenza is a burden on the healthcare system, leads to low vaccination coverage rates, and makes timely vaccination difficult against pandemic strains such as during the 2009 H1N1 influenza pandemic. Using a DNA vaccine encoding A/PR/8/34 influenza hemagglutinin that increases the viscosity of a coating formulation together with inactivated virus vaccine of the same strain, Kim et al succeeded in generation of robust immune responses and cross-protective immunity in mice (Kim et al. 2013).

Microneedles coated with a recombinant fusion protein comprised of *S. typhimurium* Phase I flagellin (FliC) and the conserved extracellular domain of the membrane-bound matrix protein 2 (M2e) from human influenza A viruses elicited strong humoral as well as mucosal antibody responses, and conferred complete protection against homo- and heterosubtypic lethal virus challenges (A/PR8, H1N1 and A/Philippines, H3N2) three months after vaccination (Wang et al. 2014). These results provide encouraging evidence that skin immunization can be effective in enhancing the breadth of immunity to influenza viruses.

3.1.4 Target Cells for Skin Immunization

As discussed above, the skin epidermis contains densely packed LCs and keratinocytes, whereas dermis which lies beneath the epidermis is largely populated by dermal dendritic cells (DDCs) that are distinct from the epidermal Langerhans cells populations based on their surface markers. LCs express differential levels of

CD11b, CD205 int/high and more specifically CD207 (Langerin) while DCs express CD11b high, and CD205 low/int and are CD207 negative (Itano et al. 2003; Valladeau et al. 2000). Additionally, these two populations are characterized by differences in chemokine receptor expression, especially during the maturation and migration of LCs from tissues to draining lymph nodes (Locati et al. 2000; Sozzani et al. 2000). The presence of two types of antigen presenting cells, LCs and DDCs, classify the skin as an immunological organ (Romani et al. 2012). Additionally, the expression of Toll-like receptors (TLRs) on LCs, DDCs, and keratinocytes make it an ideal target for vaccine delivery (Abdelsadik and Trad 2011). These two types of APCs, in combination with other immunologically active cells residing in the skin including LC-like DCs, monocytes, and macrophages (Dupasquier et al. 2004), recognize and take up the antigen upon delivery in the skin, and migrate while undergoing maturation to the proximal lymph nodes where they prime naïve T and B cells thus initiating and shaping the adaptive immune responses. Both LCs and DDCs are involved in the process of T cell activation. Studies have demonstrated that in the absence of a stimulus, epidermal LCs and dermal DCs express low levels of major histocompatibility antigens (Banchereau and Steinman 1998).

Epidermal powder immunization (EPI) of mice with an influenza vaccine elicited consistently a higher hemagglutination inhibition (HAI) antibody titers than intramuscular (IM) injection using the same dose of vaccine. Controlled vaccine delivery to skin antigen-presenting cells increases the local innate immune responses and facilitates antigen presentation to naïve T and B lymphocytes which reside in the draining lymph nodes adjacent to site of delivery. The epidermal Langerhans cells (LCs) at the site of EPI were found to play an important role in the immune responses because depletion of LCs from the immunization site prior to EPI caused a significant reduction in the antibody response. Transfer of LCs isolated from the EPI sites to naive mice induced a robust antigen-specific antibody response (Chen et al. 2004). In ex vivo experiments using freshly excised human skin, Pearton et al delivered H1 (A/PR/8/34) and H5 (A/VietNam/1203/04) VLPs with solid metal microneedles to the skin epidermis and they demonstrated 80 % deposition of the coating within 60s of insertion. They further showed a dramatic reduction of CD207$^+$ (Langerin$^+$) cells in the epidermal sheaths within 48h of vaccine delivery, which simulated activation and migration of Langerhans cells (LCs) in the human skin environment (Pearton et al. 2010a, b). Gene expression mapping, ontological analysis, and qPCR revealed up-regulation of genes responsible for key immunomodulatory processes and host responses, including cell recruitment, activation, migration, and T cell interaction following either ID or microneedle injection of VLPs; the response from the microneedles being more subtle (Pearton et al. 2013).

Detailed in vivo studies in the mouse model showed that metal microneedle delivery of inactivated influenza virus (A/PR/8/34) significantly increased interleukin 1β (IL-1β), macrophage inflammatory protein 1 alpha (MIP-1α), macrophage inflammatory protein 2 (MIP-2), tumor necrosis factor alpha (TNF-α), and monocyte chemoattractant protein 1 (MCP-1) (del Pilar Martin et al. 2012).

Although these cytokines were also induced upon insertion of blank microneedles, their levels were further increased by immunization using microneedles coated with influenza vaccine. Dendritic ($CD11c^+$) cells that emigrated from the vaccinated skin showed high expression levels of the cell surface markers MHC II and CD205 and, more than 50 % had increased expression of the co-stimulatory markers CD40 and CD86 suggesting activation and maturation of skin-derived dendritic cells (Sparber et al. 2010). This phenotype is required for T cell priming, and such cells are likely to contribute to the strong immune response observed with microneedle vaccination.

3.2 *Guinea Pigs*

Guinea pigs are an attractive model for skin immunization studies due to the similar thickness of guinea pig and human skin. Transcutaneous immunization of guinea pigs on the abdomen after skin pre-treatment with an abrasion device to disrupt the stratum corneum with a patch containing a trivalent inactivated influenza vaccine in a wet fresh formulation or a dried, stabilized formulation showed that the dry patch was as effective as a wet patch in inducing serum anti-influenza IgG and HAI antibodies. The immunological potency of the vaccine product was not affected by one-year storage at 4 or 25 °C (Frolov et al. 2008). Moreover the dry patch could tolerate unexpected environmental stresses such as those that may be encountered during shipping and distribution (low-to-high temperatures of −20/25 and −20/40 °C). Because of its effectiveness in vaccine delivery and its superior thermostability characteristics, the dry TIV patch represented a major advance for needle-free influenza vaccination.

Using 3M's solid Microstructured Transdermal System (sMTS), Kommareddy et al vaccinated guinea pigs with the 2008/2009 seasonal vaccine. The antibody titers to influenza virus were comparable to those observed with trivalent vaccine administered intramuscularly. The coated antigens were stable for at least 8 weeks upon storage at 4 °C and room temperature, and also when subjected to freeze-thaw conditions (Kommareddy et al. 2013).

3.3 *Rats*

Influenza vaccine dose sparing was demonstrated with a delivery system from BD Technologies using hollow microneedles 1 mm long, affixed to a conventional syringe (Alarcon et al. 2007). Rats were selected for the study because of their thicker skin, which ensured reliable deposit of vaccine intradermally. Delivery of the whole inactivated virus provided up to 100-fold dose sparing compared to intramuscular injection. Intradermal delivery of the trivalent human vaccine also enabled at least 10-fold dose sparing for the H1N1 strain, and elicited levels of response across a dose range similar to those of intramuscular injection for the H3N2 and B strains. Furthermore, at least fivefold dose sparing from intradermal delivery was shown in animals immunized with multiple doses of DNA plasmid vaccine.

3.4 Chickens

The continuing outbreaks of highly pathogenic avian influenza (HPAI) H5N1 in avian species increase the risk of reassortment and adaptation of the virus to humans, limit the capacity of egg-based vaccine production, and have severe economic repercussions. In chickens, protection was observed against heterologous strains of HPAI H5N1 after vaccination with a trivalent H5 serotype DNA vaccine with doses as low as 5 μg DNA given twice or 3 times by a needle-free (Agro-Jet®) device. The vaccination elicited comparable responses to intramuscular immunization with hypodermic needles (Rao et al. 2008). Comparable immune responses were also observed between subcutaneous and Agro-Jet injector delivery of a water-in-oil emulsion of inactivated, recombinant H5N3 virus suspended in a proprietary adjuvant mixture (Poulvac Flufend I AI H5N3 RG) (Ogunremi et al. 2013).

3.5 Non-human Primates

Rhesus macaques, which have an immune system and skin structure similar to humans, were used to further evaluate the immunogenicity of the influenza vaccine following epidermal powder immunization (EPI) with an influenza vaccine. Administration of unadjuvanted vaccine by EPI elicited HAI titers in the monkeys which were comparable to intramuscular injection. EPI with an influenza vaccine and QS-21 adjuvant significantly improved serum hemagglutination inhibition (HAI) titers when compared with antigen alone administered by EPI or by intramuscular (IM) injection using a needle and syringe (Chen et al. 2003).

4 Skin Immunization with Adjuvanted Vaccines

Both circulating and mucosal antibodies are considered important for protection against infection by influenza virus in humans and animals. However, current inactivated vaccines administered by intramuscular injection using a syringe and needle elicit primarily circulating antibodies. As discussed above, a number of recent studies have demonstrated that skin immunization with influenza vaccines, using a variety of devices, results in immune responses which are superior to those observed using unadjuvanted vaccines administered by other immunization routes. However there has been limited information on the effects of adjuvants using this route of immunization.

Serum antibody responses to influenza vaccine following epidermal powder immunization (EPI) of mice were enhanced by co-delivery of cholera toxin (CT), a synthetic oligodeoxynucleotide containing immunostimulatory CpG motifs (CpG DNA), or the combination of these two adjuvants. A single dose of influenza vaccine containing CT or CT and CpG DNA conferred complete protection against lethal challenges with A/PR/8/34, whereas a prime and boost immunizations were required for protection in the absence of an adjuvant (Chen et al. 2001b). Co-delivery of influenza vaccine with CpG-DNA as adjuvant elicited Th1 type response whereas EPI with alum adsorbed DT promoted a predominantly IgG1 subclass antibody response, indicating that the use of appropriate adjuvants can produce an augmented antibody response and desirable cellular immune responses (Chen et al. 2001a). Depletion of LCs from the immunization site prior to EPI caused a significant reduction in the antibody response. Chen et al reported that skin immunization with EPI induced cytokine production by the target site cells important for the augmented immune responses and that LTR72, a genetically detoxified heat-labile toxin from Escherichia coli with a strong adjuvant effect in EPI, was found to bind to the keratinocytes of the epidermis, but not the LCs, and caused the production of elevated TNF-alpha and IL-12 cytokines in emigrating epidermal cells (Chen et al. 2004).

EPI of rhesus macaques with the 2000–2001 seasonal influenza vaccine and QS-21 adjuvant elicited significantly higher serum hemagglutination inhibition (HI) titers than antigen alone administered by EPI or by intramuscular (IM) injection using a needle and syringe (Chen et al. 2003).

Application of an adjuvant to the skin has also been used to enhance the response to an injected influenza vaccine in young and aged mice (Guebre-Xabier et al. 2004) as well as in elderly human vaccinees (Frech et al. 2005). A trivalent liposomal vaccine was administered to patients by IM injection, and a skin patch containing the heat labile enterotoxin from E. coli was applied to stratum corneum-disrupted skin near the site of immunization in a subgroup of the patients. The adjuvant patch enhanced the seroconversion rate in the elderly patients to a level similar to that observed in healthy adult vaccinees.

Transcutaneous immunization of mice with whole inactivated influenza virus in the presence of cholera toxin (CT), a potent adjuvant for TCI, significantly enhanced immune responses against influenza virus antigen. Pretreatment of mouse skin with permeability enhancers/immunomodulators oleic acid (OA) and retinoic acid (RA) elicited increased levels of influenza virus-specific binding and neutralizing antibodies to levels equivalent to those induced by intranasal immunization with inactivated influenza virus. Oleic acid and particularly retinoic acid treatments differentially affected the pattern of cytokine production upon stimulation with influenza viral antigen and provided enhanced long-lasting protection (Martin Mdel et al. 2010; Skountzou et al. 2006).

Transdermal immunization by use of the PassPort system that creates 80 micropores within a 1-cm^2 area with a disposable filament attached to an applicator containing 3 μg of baculovirus-expressed H5 rHA protein from the A/Hong Kong/156/97 (H5N1; HK/156) virus either alone or with 25 μg of CpG oligodeoxynucleotide (TLR9 ligand) demonstrated complete protection following challenge with 10xLD_{50} or 50xLD_{50} H5N1 virus. In contrast 30 μg of R-848 (resiquimod hydrochloride, a TLR7 ligand) did not enhance the protective immune responses (Garg et al. 2007).

Some currently used adjuvants are lipid-based, and would be expected to interfere with formulations used to produce coated or dissolving microneedles. The use of toll-like receptor (TLR) ligands as adjuvants was investigated using microneedle delivery of an influenza subunit vaccine in mice (Weldon et al. 2012). The subunit vaccine alone was compared with vaccine coadministered with the TLR ligands, imiquimod or poly(I:C), individually or in combination. The inclusion of poly(I:C) did not enhance immune responses when compared to the non-adjuvanted vaccine. However the imiquimod-adjuvanted vaccine elicited higher levels of virus-specific antibodies and increased hemagglutination inhibition titers, as well as inducing a robust IFN-g cellular response. These responses correlated with improved protection to challenge infection when compared to microneedle immunization with influenza subunit vaccine alone, as well as reduced viral replication levels in the lungs.

In another study, the plant-derived saponin Quil-A was used as an adjuvant with influenza vaccine in mice. The anti-influenza IgG and HAI responses induced by very low antigen doses, 6.5 ng of vaccine, were similar to responses induced by IM injection using 900-fold higher doses of vaccine, demonstrating a potent dose-sparing effect by delivery of the antigen and adjuvant to skin (Fernando et al. 2012).

5 Conclusions and Future Directions

Skin immunization has generated a high level of interest because of its immunological advantages, including the induction of stronger and longer-lasting immunity when compared with conventional intramuscular immunization. A number of delivery systems are at various stages of development, and studies are in progress in various animal models and to a lesser extent, in clinical trials. In addition to its immunological advantages, skin vaccination also offers potential logistical advantages. Dried vaccine formulations are used in many approaches, and provide enhanced vaccine stability which can enable global vaccine distribution without the need for maintaining a cold chain, with a resulting decrease in cost. A particularly noteworthy feature is the avoidance of hypodermic needles, thus enhancing the acceptability of vaccination by subjects who presently remain unvaccinated because of fear of the pain associated with needle sticks. Devices are also being developed which would be suitable for self-administration of vaccines, and a recent study (Norman et al. 2014) has provided evidence that this approach could significantly enhance influenza vaccination coverage by improving patient acceptability.

Whereas there have been many studies of new approaches in animal models, only a limited number have been advanced to clinical studies. More rapid progress in such studies is anticipated in future. Other aspects which remain largely undeveloped include the use of adjuvants and identification of novel adjuvants which are specifically designed to enhance responses to skin immunization. There is also very limited information on the ability of skin immunization to elicit mucosal immune responses, which are known to provide the most effective means of preventing infection by influenza viruses.

Acknowledgements We thank Ms. Erin-Joi Collins for her valuable assistance in the preparation and submission of this manuscript. Research by the authors was supported in part by the U.S. Department of Health and Human Services contract HHSN272201400006C (NIAID Centers of Excellence for Influenza Research and Surveillance) and the National Institutes of Health grant U01EB012495 (M. Prausnitz, PI).

References

Abdelsadik A, Trad A (2011) Toll-like receptors on the fork roads between innate and adaptive immunity. Hum Immunol 72:1188–1193. doi:10.1016/j.humimm.2011.08.015

Alarcon JB, Hartley AW, Harvey NG, Mikszta JA (2007) Preclinical evaluation of microneedle technology for intradermal delivery of influenza vaccines. Clin Vaccine Immunol 14:375–381. doi:10.1128/CVI.00387-06

Albrecht CM, Sweitzer NK, Johnson MR, Vardeny O (2014) Lack of persistence of influenza vaccine antibody titers in patients with heart failure. J Card Fail 20:105–109. doi:10.1016/j.cardfail.2013.12.008

Ansaldi F, Valle L, de Florentiis D, Parodi V, Murdaca G, Bruzzone B, Durando P, Setti M, Icardi G (2012) Phase 4 randomized trial of intradermal low-antigen-content inactivated influenza vaccine versus standard-dose intramuscular vaccine in HIV-1-infected adults. Hum Vaccin Immunother 8:1048–1052. doi:10.4161/hv.20347

Atkinson WL, Pickering LK, Schwartz B, Weniger BG, Iskander JK, Watson JC (2002) General recommendations on immunization. Recommendations of the Advisory Committee on Immunization Practices (ACIP) and the American Academy of Family Physicians (AAFP). MMWR Recomm Rep 51:1–35

Auewarakul P, Kositanont U, Sornsathapornkul P, Tothong P, Kanyok R, Thongcharoen P (2007) Antibody responses after dose-sparing intradermal influenza vaccination. Vaccine 25:659–63. doi:10.1016/j.vaccine.2006.08.026

Banchereau J, Steinman RM (1998) Dendritic cells and the control of immunity. Nature 392:245–252

Belshe RB, Newman FK, Cannon J, Duane C, Treanor J, Van Hoecke C, Howe BJ, Dubin G (2004) Serum antibody responses after intradermal vaccination against influenza. N Engl J Med 351:2286–94. doi:10.1056/NEJMoa043555

Belshe RB, Newman FK, Wilkins K, Graham IL, Babusis E, Ewell M, Frey SE (2007) Comparative immunogenicity of trivalent influenza vaccine administered by intradermal or intramuscular route in healthy adults. Vaccine 25:6755–6763. doi:10.1016/j.vaccine.2007.06.066

Beran J, Ambrozaitis A, Laiskonis A, Mickuviene N, Bacart P, Calozet Y, Demanet E, Heijmans S, Van Belle P, Weber F, Salamand C (2009) Intradermal influenza vaccination of healthy adults using a new microinjection system: a 3-year randomised controlled safety and immunogenicity trial. BMC Med 7:13. doi:10.1186/1741-7015-7-13

Boger WP, Liu OC (1957) Subcutaneous and intradermal vaccination with Asian influenza vaccine. J Am Med Assoc 165:1687–1689

Bragstad K, Martel CJ, Thomsen JS, Jensen KL, Nielsen LP, Aasted B, Fomsgaard A (2011) Pandemic influenza 1918 H1N1 and 1968 H3N2 DNA vaccines induce cross-reactive immunity in ferrets against infection with viruses drifted for decades. Influenza Other Respir Viruses 5:13–23. doi:10.1111/j.1750-2659.2010.00177.x

Brown H, Kasel JA, Freeman DM, Moise LD, Grose NP, Couch RB (1977) The immunizing effect of influenza A/New Jersey/76 (Hsw1N1) virus vaccine administered intradermally and intramuscularly to adults. J Infect Dis 136(Suppl):S466–471

Bruyn HB, Meiklejohn G, Brainerd H (1949a) Influenza vaccine; a study of serologic responses and incidence of reactions following subcutaneous and intradermal inoculation. Am J Dis Child 77:149–163

Bruyn HB, Meiklejohn G, Brainerd HD (1949b) Influenza vaccination; a comparison of antibody response obtained by various methods of administration. J Immunol 62:1–11

Chen D, Erickson CA, Endres RL, Periwal SB, Chu Q, Shu C, Maa YF, Payne LG (2001a) Adjuvantation of epidermal powder immunization. Vaccine 19:2908–2917

Chen D, Weis KF, Chu Q, Erickson C, Endres R, Lively CR, Osorio J, Payne LG (2001b) Epidermal powder immunization induces both cytotoxic T-lymphocyte and antibody responses to protein antigens of influenza and hepatitis B viruses. J Virol 75:11630–11640

Chen D, Endres R, Maa YF, Kensil CR, Whitaker-Dowling P, Trichel A, Youngner JS, Payne LG (2003) Epidermal powder immunization of mice and monkeys with an influenza vaccine. Vaccine 21:2830–2836

Chen D, Burger M, Chu Q, Endres R, Zuleger C, Dean H, Payne LG (2004) Epidermal powder immunization: cellular and molecular mechanisms for enhancing vaccine immunogenicity. Virus Res 103:147–153. doi:10.1016/j.virusres.2004.02.027

Choi HJ, Yoo DG, Bondy BJ, Quan FS, Compans RW, Kang SM, Prausnitz MR (2012) Stability of influenza vaccine coated onto microneedles. Biomaterials 33:3756–3769. doi:10.1016/j.biomaterials.2012.01.054

Choi HJ, Bondy BJ, Yoo DG, Compans RW, Kang SM, Prausnitz MR (2013) Stability of whole inactivated influenza virus vaccine during coating onto metal microneedles. J Control Release 166:159–171. doi:10.1016/j.jconrel.2012.12.002

Combadiere B, Vogt A, Mahe B, Costagliola D, Hadam S, Bonduelle O, Sterry W, Staszewski S, Schaefer H, van der Werf S, Katlama C, Autran B, Blume-Peytavi U (2010) Preferential amplification of CD8 effector-T cells after transcutaneous application of an inactivated influenza vaccine: a randomized phase I trial. PLoS One 5:e10818. doi:10.1371/journal.pone.0010818

Dean HJ, Chen D (2004) Epidermal powder immunization against influenza. Vaccine 23:681–686. doi:10.1016/j.vaccine.2004.06.041

del Pilar Martin M, Seth S, Koutsonanos DG, Jacob J, Compans RW, Skountzou I (2010) Adjuvanted influenza vaccine administered intradermally elicits robust long-term immune responses that confer protection from lethal challenge. PLoS One 5:e10897. doi:10.1371/journal.pone.0010897

del Pilar Martin M, Weldon WC, Zarnitsyn VG, Koutsonanos DG, Akbari H, Skountzou I, Jacob J, Prausnitz MR, Compans RW (2012) Local response to microneedle-based influenza immunization in the skin. MBio 3:e00012–12. doi:10.1128/mBio.00012-12

Depelsenaire AC, Meliga SC, McNeilly CL, Pearson FE, Coffey JW, Haigh OL, Flaim CJ, Frazer IH, Kendall MA (2014) Colocalization of cell death with antigen deposition in skin enhances vaccine immunogenicity. J Invest Dermatol. doi:10.1038/jid.2014.174

Ding Z, Verbaan FJ, Bivas-Benita M, Bungener L, Huckriede A, van den Berg DJ, Kersten G, Bouwstra JA (2009) Microneedle arrays for the transcutaneous immunization of diphtheria and influenza in BALB/c mice. J Control Release 136:71–78. doi:10.1016/j.jconrel.2009.01.025

Dupasquier M, Stoitzner P, van Oudenaren A, Romani N, Leenen PJ (2004) Macrophages and dendritic cells constitute a major subpopulation of cells in the mouse dermis. J Invest Dermatol 123:876–879. doi:10.1111/j.0022-202X.2004.23427.x

FaDA (FDA) (2011) FDA updated communication on use of jet injectors with inactivated influenza vaccines. Food and Drug Administration, Washington, DC

Fernando GJ, Chen X, Prow TW, Crichton ML, Fairmaid EJ, Roberts MS, Frazer IH, Brown LE, Kendall MA (2010) Potent immunity to low doses of influenza vaccine by probabilistic guided micro-targeted skin delivery in a mouse model. PLoS One 5:e10266. doi:10.1371/journal.pone.0010266

Fernando GJ, Chen X, Primiero CA, Yukiko SR, Fairmaid EJ, Corbett HJ, Frazer IH, Brown LE, Kendall MA (2012) Nanopatch targeted delivery of both antigen and adjuvant to skin synergistically drives enhanced antibody responses. J Control Release 159:215–221. doi:10.1016/j.jconrel.2012.01.030

Francis T, Magill TP (1937) The antibody response of human subjects vaccinated with the virus of human influenza. J Exp Med 65:251–259

Frech SA, Kenney RT, Spyr CA, Lazar H, Viret JF, Herzog C, Gluck R, Glenn GM (2005) Improved immune responses to influenza vaccination in the elderly using an immunostimulant patch. Vaccine 23:946–950. doi:10.1016/j.vaccine.2004.06.036

Frolov VG, Seid RC Jr, Odutayo O, Al-Khalili M, Yu J, Frolova OY, Vu H, Butler BA, Look JL, Ellingsworth LR, Glenn GM (2008) Transcutaneous delivery and thermostability of a dry trivalent inactivated influenza vaccine patch. Influenza Other Respir Viruses 2:53–60. doi:10.1111/j.1750-2659.2008.00040.x

Fynan EF, Robinson HL, Webster RG (1993a) Use of DNA encoding influenza hemagglutinin as an avian influenza vaccine. DNA Cell Biol 12:785–789

Fynan EF, Webster RG, Fuller DH, Haynes JR, Santoro JC, Robinson HL (1993b) DNA vaccines: protective immunizations by parenteral, mucosal, and gene-gun inoculations. Proc Natl Acad Sci USA 90:11478–11482

Garg S, Hoelscher M, Belser JA, Wang C, Jayashankar L, Guo Z, Durland RH, Katz JM, Sambhara S (2007) Needle-free skin patch delivery of a vaccine for a potentially pandemic influenza virus provides protection against lethal challenge in mice. Clin Vaccine Immunol 14:926–928. doi:10.1128/CVI.00450-06

Gill HS, Denson DD, Burris BA, Prausnitz MR (2008) Effect of microneedle design on pain in human volunteers. Clin J Pain 24:585–594. doi:10.1097/AJP.0b013e31816778f9, 00002508-200809000-00005

Giudice EL, Campbell JD (2006) Needle-free vaccine delivery. Adv Drug Deliv Rev 58:68–89

Glazier MM, Benenson AS, Wheeler RE (1956) Active immunization with influenza virus A and B in infants and children. Pediatrics 17:482–488

Glenn GM, Kenney RT, Ellingsworth LR, Frech SA, Hammond SA, Zoeteweij JP (2003) Transcutaneous immunization and immunostimulant strategies: capitalizing on the immunocompetence of the skin. Expert Rev Vaccines 2:253–267

Guebre-Xabier M, Hammond SA, Ellingsworth LR, Glenn GM (2004) Immunostimulant patch enhances immune responses to influenza virus vaccine in aged mice. J Virol 78:7610–7618. doi:10.1128/JVI.78.14.7610-7618.2004

Hilleman MR, Flatley FJ, Anderson SA, Luecking ML, Levinson DJ (1958) Antibody response in volunteers to Asian influenza vaccine. J Am Med Assoc 166:1134–1140

Hoft DF, Blazevic A, Abate G, Hanekom WA, Kaplan G, Soler JH, Weichold F, Geiter L, Sadoff JC, Horwitz MA (2008) A new recombinant bacille Calmette-Guerin vaccine safely induces significantly enhanced tuberculosis-specific immunity in human volunteers. J Infect Dis 198:1491–1501. doi:10.1086/592450

Hung IF, Levin Y, To KK, Chan KH, Zhang AJ, Li P, Li C, Xu T, Wong TY, Yuen KY (2012) Dose sparing intradermal trivalent influenza (2010/2011) vaccination overcomes reduced immunogenicity of the 2009 H1N1 strain. Vaccine 30:6427–6435. doi:10.1016/j.vaccine.2012.08.014

Icardi G, Orsi A, Ceravolo A, Ansaldi F (2012) Current evidence on intradermal influenza vaccines administered by Soluvia licensed micro injection system. Hum Vaccin Immunother 8:67–75. doi:10.4161/hv.8.1.18419

Ismach A (1960) Jet injector. http://www.scienceheroes.com/index.php?option=com_content&view=article&id=166&Itemid=165

Itano AA, McSorley SJ, Reinhardt RL, Ehst BD, Ingulli E, Rudensky AY, Jenkins MK (2003) Distinct dendritic cell populations sequentially present antigen to CD4 T cells and stimulate different aspects of cell-mediated immunity. Immunity 19:47–57

Jackson LA, Austin G, Chen RT, Stout R, DeStefano F, Gorse GJ, Newman FK, Yu O, Weniger BG, Vaccine Safety Datalink Study G (2001) Safety and immunogenicity of varying dosages of trivalent inactivated influenza vaccine administered by needle-free jet injectors. Vaccine 19:4703–4709

Jones S, Evans K, McElwaine-Johnn H, Sharpe M, Oxford J, Lambkin-Williams R, Mant T, Nolan A, Zambon M, Ellis J, Beadle J, Loudon PT (2009) DNA vaccination protects against an influenza challenge in a double-blind randomised placebo-controlled phase 1b clinical trial. Vaccine 27:2506–2512. doi:10.1016/j.vaccine.2009.02.061

Kim YC, Quan FS, Compans RW, Kang SM, Prausnitz MR (2010a) Formulation and coating of microneedles with inactivated influenza virus to improve vaccine stability and immunogenicity. J Control Release 142:187–95. doi: 10.1016/j.jconrel.2009.10.013, S0168-3659(09)00708-1

Kim YC, Quan FS, Compans RW, Kang SM, Prausnitz MR (2010b) Formulation of microneedles coated with influenza virus-like particle vaccine. AAPS PharmSciTech 11:1193–1201. doi:10.1208/s12249-010-9471-3

Kim YC, Quan FS, Compans RW, Kang SM, Prausnitz MR (2011) Stability kinetics of influenza vaccine coated onto microneedles during drying and storage. Pharm Res 28:135–144. doi:10.1007/s11095-010-0134-6

Kim YC, Jarrahian C, Zehrung D, Mitragotri S, Prausnitz MR (2012) Delivery systems for intradermal vaccination. Curr Top Microbiol Immunol 351:77–112. doi:10.1007/82_2011_123

Kim YK, Eun BW, Kim NH, Kang EK, Lee BS, Kim DH, Lim JS (2013) Comparison of immunogenicity and reactogenicity of split versus subunit influenza vaccine in Korean children aged 6-35 months. Scand J Infect Dis 45:460–468. doi:10.3109/00365548.2012.755267

Kommareddy S, Baudner BC, Oh S, Kwon SY, Singh M, O'Hagan DT (2012) Dissolvable microneedle patches for the delivery of cell-culture-derived influenza vaccine antigens. J Pharm Sci 101:1021–1027. doi:10.1002/jps.23019

Kommareddy S, Baudner BC, Bonificio A, Gallorini S, Palladino G, Determan AS, Dohmeier DM, Kroells KD, Sternjohn JR, Singh M, Dormitzer PR, Hansen KJ, O'Hagan DT (2013) Influenza subunit vaccine coated microneedle patches elicit comparable immune responses to intramuscular injection in guinea pigs. Vaccine 31:3435–3441. doi:10.1016/j.vaccine.2013.01.050

Koutsonanos DG, del Pilar Martin M, Zarnitsyn VG, Sullivan SP, Compans RW, Prausnitz MR, Skountzou I (2009) Transdermal influenza immunization with vaccine-coated microneedle arrays. PLoS One 4:e4773. doi:10.1371/journal.pone.0004773

Koutsonanos DG, del Pilar Martin M, Zarnitsyn VG, Jacob J, Prausnitz MR, Compans RW, Skountzou I (2011) Serological memory and long-term protection to novel H1N1 influenza virus after skin vaccination. J Infect Dis 204:582–591. doi:10.1093/infdis/jir094

Koutsonanos DG, Vassilieva EV, Stavropoulou A, Zarnitsyn VG, Esser ES, Taherbhai MT, Prausnitz MR, Compans RW, Skountzou I (2012) Delivery of subunit influenza vaccine to skin with microneedles improves immunogenicity and long-lived protection. Sci Rep 2:357. doi:10.1038/srep00357

Kunzi V, Klap JM, Seiberling MK, Herzog C, Hartmann K, Kursteiner O, Kompier R, Grimaldi R, Goudsmit J (2009) Immunogenicity and safety of low dose virosomal adjuvanted influenza vaccine administered intradermally compared to intramuscular full dose administration. Vaccine 27:3561–3567. doi:10.1016/j.vaccine.2009.03.062

Laurent PE, Bonnet S, Alchas P, Regolini P, Mikszta JA, Pettis R, Harvey NG (2007) Evaluation of the clinical performance of a new intradermal vaccine administration technique and associated delivery system. Vaccine 25:8833–8842. doi:10.1016/j.vaccine.2007.10.020, S0264-410X(07)01156-5

Locati M, Allavena P, Sozzani S, Mantovanii A (2000) Shaping and tuning of the chemokine system by regulation of receptor expression and signaling: dendritic cells as a paradigm. J Neuroimmunol 107:174–177

Mantoux C (1909) Tuberculin intradermo reactions in the treatment of tuberculosis: Intradermi-tuberculisation. Comptes Rendus Hebdomadaires Des Seances De L Academie Des Sci 148:996–998

Matsuo K, Hirobe S, Yokota Y, Ayabe Y, Seto M, Quan YS, Kamiyama F, Tougan T, Horii T, Mukai Y, Okada N, Nakagawa S (2012) Transcutaneous immunization using a dissolving microneedle array protects against tetanus, diphtheria, malaria, and influenza. J Control Release 160:495–501. doi:10.1016/j.jconrel.2012.04.001

Moylett EH, Hanson IC (2004) Mechanistic actions of the risks and adverse events associated with vaccine administration. J Allergy Clin Immunol 114:1010–20; quiz 1021

Norman JJ, Arya JM, McClain MA, Frew PM, Meltzer MI, Prausnitz MR (2014) Microneedle patches: usability and acceptability for self-vaccination againt influenza. Vaccine. 32(16):1856–62. doi: 10.1016/j.vaccine.2014.01.076. Epub 2014 Feb 11. PMID: 24530146 [PubMed - in process]

Ogunremi O, Pasick J, Berhane Y (2013) Needle-free delivery of an inactivated avian influenza H5N3 virus vaccine elicits potent antibody responses in chickens. Can J Vet Res 77:309–313

Osterholm MT, Kelley NS, Sommer A, Belongia EA (2012) Efficacy and effectiveness of influenza vaccines: a systematic review and meta-analysis. Lancet Infect Dis 12:36–44. doi:10.1016/S1473-3099(11)70295-X

Pearton M, Kang SM, Song JM, Anstey AV, Ivory M, Compans RW, Birchall JC (2010a) Changes in human Langerhans cells following intradermal injection of influenza virus-like particle vaccines. PLoS One 5:e12410. doi:10.1371/journal.pone.0012410

Pearton M, Kang SM, Song JM, Kim YC, Quan FS, Anstey A, Ivory M, Prausnitz MR, Compans RW, Birchall JC (2010b) Influenza virus-like particles coated onto microneedles can elicit stimulatory effects on Langerhans cells in human skin. Vaccine 28:6104-13. doi: 10.1016/j.vaccine.2010.05.055, S0264-410X(10)00764-4

Pearton M, Pirri D, Kang SM, Compans RW, Birchall JC (2013) Host responses in human skin after conventional intradermal injection or microneedle administration of virus-like-particle influenza vaccine. Adv Healthc Mater 2:1401–1410. doi:10.1002/adhm.201300006

Quan FS, Kim YC, Yoo DG, Compans RW, Prausnitz MR, Kang SM (2009) Stabilization of influenza vaccine enhances protection by microneedle delivery in the mouse skin. PLoS One 4:e7152. doi:10.1371/journal.pone.0007152

Quan FS, Kim YC, Compans RW, Prausnitz MR, Kang SM (2010a) Dose sparing enabled by skin immunization with influenza virus-like particle vaccine using microneedles. J Control Release 147:326–332. doi:10.1016/j.jconrel.2010.07.125

Quan FS, Kim YC, Vunnava A, Yoo DG, Song JM, Prausnitz MR, Compans RW, Kang SM (2010b) Intradermal vaccination with influenza virus-like particles by using microneedles induces protection superior to that with intramuscular immunization. J Virol 84:7760-9. doi:10.1128/JVI.01849-09JVI.01849-09

Quan FS, Kim YC, Song JM, Hwang HS, Compans RW, Prausnitz MR, Kang SM (2013) Long-term protective immunity from an influenza virus-like particle vaccine administered with a microneedle patch. Clin Vaccine Immunol. doi:10.1128/CVI.00251-13

Rao S, Kong WP, Wei CJ, Yang ZY, Nason M, Styles D, DeTolla LJ, Panda A, Sorrell EM, Song H, Wan H, Ramirez-Nieto GC, Perez D, Nabel GJ (2008) Multivalent HA DNA vaccination protects against highly pathogenic H5N1 avian influenza infection in chickens and mice. PLoS One 3:e2432. doi:10.1371/journal.pone.0002432

Raphael AP, Prow TW, Crichton ML, Chen X, Fernando GJ, Kendall MA (2010) Targeted, needle-free vaccinations in skin using multilayered, densely-packed dissolving microprojection arrays. Small 6:1785–1793. doi:10.1002/smll.201000326

Riedel S (2005) Edward Jenner and the history of smallpox and vaccination. Proc (Bayl Univ Med Cent) 18:21–25

Romani N, Tschachler E, Schuler G, Aberer W, Ceredig R, Elbe A, Wolff K, Fritsch PO, Stingl G (1985) Morphological and phenotypical characterization of bone marrow-derived dendritic Thy-1-positive epidermal cells of the mouse. J Invest Dermatol 85:91s–95s

Romani N, Flacher V, Tripp CH, Sparber F, Ebner S, Stoitzner P (2012) Targeting skin dendritic cells to improve intradermal vaccination. Curr Top Microbiol Immunol 351:113–138. doi:10.1007/82_2010_118

Sencer DJ, Millar JD (2006) Reflections on the 1976 swine flu vaccination program. Emerg Infect Dis 12:29–33. doi:10.3201/eid1201.051007

Skountzou I, Kang SM (2009) Transcutaneous immunization with influenza vaccines. Curr Top Microbiol Immunol 333:347–368. doi:10.1007/978-3-540-92165-3_17

Skountzou I, Quan FS, Jacob J, Compans RW, Kang SM (2006) Transcutaneous immunization with inactivated influenza virus induces protective immune responses. Vaccine 24:6110–6119. doi:10.1016/j.vaccine.2006.05.014

Song JM, Kim YC, Barlow PG, Hossain MJ, Park KM, Donis RO, Prausnitz MR, Compans RW, Kang SM (2010a) Improved protection against avian influenza H5N1 virus by a single vaccination with virus-like particles in skin using microneedles. Antiviral Res 88:244–247. doi:10.1016/j.antiviral.2010.09.001

Song JM, Kim YC, Lipatov AS, Pearton M, Davis CT, Yoo DG, Park KM, Chen LM, Quan FS, Birchall JC, Donis RO, Prausnitz MR, Compans RW, Kang SM (2010b) Microneedle delivery of H5N1 influenza virus-like particles to the skin induces long-lasting B- and T-cell responses in mice. Clin Vaccine Immunol 17:1381–1389. doi:10.1128/CVI.00100-10

Song JM, Kim YC, O E Compans RW, Prausnitz RW, Kang (2012) DNA vaccination in the skin using microneedles improves protection against influenza. Mol Ther 20:1472–1480. doi:10.1038/mt.2012.69

Sozzani S, Allavena P, Vecchi A, Mantovani A (2000) Chemokines and dendritic cell traffic. J Clin Immunol 20:151–260

Sparber F, Tripp CH, Hermann M, Romani N, Stoitzner P (2010) Langerhans cells and dermal dendritic cells capture protein antigens in the skin: possible targets for vaccination through the skin. Immunobiology 215:770–779. doi:10.1016/j.imbio.2010.05.014

Sullivan SP, Koutsonanos DG, del Pilar Martin M, Lee JW, Zarnitsyn V, Choi SO, Murthy N, Compans RW, Skountzou I, Prausnitz MR (2010) Dissolving polymer microneedle patches for influenza vaccination. Nat Med 16:915–920. doi:10.1038/nm.2182

Tauraso NM, Gleckman R, Pedreira FA, Sabbaj J, Yahwak R, Madoff MA (1969) Effect of dosage and route of inoculation upon antigenicity of inactivated influenza virus vaccine (Hong Kong strain) in man. Bull World Health Organ 41:507–516

Teunissen MBM (2012) Intradermal Immunization. Current topics in microbiology and immunology, vol 351

Valladeau J, Ravel O, Dezutter-Dambuyant C, Moore K, Kleijmeer M, Liu Y, Duvert-Frances V, Vincent C, Schmitt D, Davoust J, Caux C, Lebecque S, Saeland S (2000) Langerin, a novel C-type lectin specific to Langerhans cells, is an endocytic receptor that induces the formation of Birbeck granules. Immunity 12:71–81

Van Damme P, Oosterhuis-Kafeja F, Van der Wielen M, Almagor Y, Sharon O, Levin Y (2009) Safety and efficacy of a novel microneedle device for dose sparing intradermal influenza vaccination in healthy adults. Vaccine 27:454–459. doi:10.1016/j.vaccine.2008.10.077

Van Gelder DW, Greenspan FS, Dufresne NE (1947) Influenza vaccination; comparison of intracutaneous and subcutaneous methods. U S Nav Med Bull 47:197–206

Van Kampen KR, Shi Z, Gao P, Zhang J, Foster KW, Chen DT, Marks D, Elmets CA, Tang DC (2005) Safety and immunogenicity of adenovirus-vectored nasal and epicutaneous influenza vaccines in humans. Vaccine 23:1029–1036. doi:10.1016/j.vaccine.2004.07.043

Wang BZ, Gill HS, He C, Ou C, Wang L, Wang YC, Feng H, Zhang H, Prausnitz MR, Compans RW (2014) Microneedle delivery of an M2e-TLR5 ligand fusion protein to skin confers broadly cross-protective influenza immunity. J Control Release 178:1–7. doi:10.1016/j.jconrel.2014.01.002

Weir E, Hatch K (2004) Preventing cold chain failure: vaccine storage and handling. Cmaj 171:1050

Weldon WC, del Pilar Martin MP, Zarnitsyn V, Wang B, Koutsonanos D, Skountzou I, Prausnitz MR, Compans RW (2011) Microneedle vaccination with stabilized recombinant influenza virus hemagglutinin induces improved protective immunity. Clin Vaccine Immunol 18:647–654. doi:10.1128/CVI.00435-10

Weldon WC, Zarnitsyn VG, Esser ES, Taherbhai MT, Koutsonanos DG, Vassilieva EV, Skountzou I, Prausnitz MR, Compans RW (2012) Effect of adjuvants on responses to skin immunization by microneedles coated with influenza subunit vaccine. PLoS One 7:e41501. doi:10.1371/journal.pone.0041501

Weller TH, Cheever FS, Enders JF (1948) Immunologic reactions following the intradermal inoculation of influenza A and B vaccine. Proc Soc Exp Biol Med 67:96–101

Weniger BG, Glenn GM (2013) Cutaneous vaccination: antigen delivery into or onto the skin. Vaccine 31:3389–3391. doi:10.1016/j.vaccine.2013.05.048

WHO (WHO) (2005) Solutions: Choosing Technologies for Safe Injections. Accessed 2011-05-06 2011

Wolff JA, Malone RW, Williams P, Chong W, Acsadi G, Jani A, Felgner PL (1990) Direct gene transfer into mouse muscle in vivo. Science 247:1465–1468

Wrammert J, Koutsonanos D, Li GM, Edupuganti S, Sui J, Morrissey M, McCausland M, Skountzou I, Hornig M, Lipkin WI, Mehta A, Razavi B, Del Rio C, Zheng NY, Lee JH, Huang M, Ali Z, Kaur K, Andrews S, Amara RR, Wang Y, Das SR, O'Donnell CD, Yewdell JW, Subbarao K, Marasco WA, Mulligan MJ, Compans R, Ahmed R, Wilson PC (2011) Broadly cross-reactive antibodies dominate the human B cell response against 2009 pandemic H1N1 influenza virus infection. J Exp Med 208:181–93. doi: 10.1084/jem.20101352, S0166-3542(10)00705-9

Yewdell JW, Bennink JR, Smith GL, Moss B (1985) Influenza A virus nucleoprotein is a major target antigen for cross-reactive anti-influenza A virus cytotoxic T lymphocytes. Proc Natl Acad Sci USA 82:1785–1789

Zhu Q, Zarnitsyn VG, Ye L, Wen Z, Gao Y, Pan L, Skountzou I, Gill HS, Prausnitz MR, Yang C, Compans RW (2009) Immunization by vaccine-coated microneedle arrays protects against lethal influenza virus challenge. Proc Natl Acad Sci USA 106:7968–7973. doi:10.1073/pnas.0812652106

Mucosal Immunization and Adjuvants

Hideki Hasegawa, Elly van Reit and Hiroshi Kida

Abstract The goal of the influenza vaccine is to prevent influenza virus infection and control the yearly seasonal epidemic and pandemic. However, the presently available parenteral influenza vaccine induces only systemic humoral immunity, which does not prevent influenza virus infection on the mucosal surface. Secretary IgA antibodies play an important role in preventing natural infection. Moreover, the IgA antibody response mediates cross-protection against variant viruses in animal models. Thus, a mucosal influenza vaccine that induces mucosal immunity would be a powerful tool to protect individuals from the influenza virus. Although the function of the mucosal immune system, especially in the respiratory tract, is not completely understood, there are several studies underway to develop mucosal influenza vaccines. Here, we will review current knowledge concerning the induction of IgA, the role of B-cell production of influenza virus specific IgA antibodies in anti-influenza immunity, and the role of humoral memory responses induced upon vaccination.

Contents

H. Hasegawa (✉) · E.van Reit
Department of Pathology, National Institute of Infectious Diseases, Toyama 1-23-1, Shinjuku, Tokyo 162-8640, Japan
e-mail: hasegawa@nih.go.jp

H. Kida
Research Center for Zoonosis Control, Hokkaido University, Sapporo, Japan

Current Topics in Microbiology and Immunology (2015) 386: 371–380
DOI: 10.1007/82_2014_402

Published Online: 12 July 2014

1 Introduction

Influenza viruses belong to the *Orthomyxoviridae* family, which is categorized into three genera, namely *influenzavirus A*, *B*, and *C*. *Influenzavirus A* comprise several subtypes based on the unique combination of two surface proteins, hemagglutinin (HA) and neuraminidase (NA). The seasonal influenza A virus infects millions of individuals each year, with the highest risk of complications occurring in young, elderly, and immunocompromised patients. For example, influenzavirus A can lead to fatal encephalopathy in infants and pneumonia in the elderly.

In addition, the avian and/or swine influenzavirus A has caused a pandemic every few decades by emerging each time as a genetically novel virus. The most recent pandemic in 2009 was caused by the influenzavirus A (H1N1) pdm09 of swine origin. Cases of highly pathogenic avian influenzavirus A H5N1 and H7N9 infection and fatal pneumonia have been also reported, with many individuals developing acute respiratory distress syndrome (ARDS) (La Gruta et al. 2007).

Vaccination is the most effective method to control both seasonal and newly evolved pandemic strains of the influenza virus. However, currently used parenteral influenza vaccines are only effective against strains that are closely antigenic to the vaccine strains. Thus, the yearly seasonal vaccine contains multiple influenza virus strains, including influenza virus A strains H1N1 and H3N2, and influenza virus B strain. However, there is an urgent need for improved cross-protection because antigenic mismatches between seasonal vaccines and circulating virus strains. It is also difficult to predict the newly evolved strains such as A/H5N1 and A/H7N9. Ideally, a universal influenza vaccine that induces a strong and long-lasting memory response and cross-protects against drifted variants, as well as against several subtypes of the influenza virus, which induce hetero-subtypic immunity, should be developed. While mucosal secretary IgA (S-IgA) antibodies show cross-protection against variant influenza viruses in mouse models, rational design of IgA antibody-inducing vaccines has so far been hampered by a lack of knowledge about local and tissue-specific immune responses and IgA antibody function (Matzinger and Kamala 2011). Consequently, the importance of IgA antibodies in immunity and the mechanisms by which IgA antibody responses are induced and maintained are just beginning to be established (Brandtzaeg 2007). In this review, we discuss the different mechanisms involved in the induction of S-IgA antibodies during influenza virus infection and vaccination and provide insight into how this information could be used to improve vaccine design.

2 The Use of Secretary IgA Antibodies for the Prevention of Influenza Virus Infection

The respiratory mucosal surface is the first line of defense against influenza virus infection. For example, pre-existing S-IgA antibodies on the surface of mucosal epithelial cells can eliminate a pathogen before it infects respiratory epithelial cells, thereby providing immediate immunity (Renegar et al. 2004) in a process defined as immune exclusion (Stokes et al. 1975). S-IgA antibodies can also disarm viruses within infected secretory epithelial cells and redirect antigens to the lumen after they have entered the lamina propria (Brandtzaeg 2007). All of these responses are non-inflammatory in nature because, unlike IgG antibodies, IgA antibodies do not fix complement and do not activate the inflammatory complement pathway (Yel 2010). Therefore, a strong S-IgA response is critical for prevention of influenza virus infection especially in case of pathogenic strains for their severe clinical outcomes. Although it is difficult to study the functions of S-IgA and serum antibodies independently, mucosal vaccination and influenza virus infection in knockout mice, which lack poly Ig receptor expression and fail to secrete IgA antibodies from the mucosal surface, show that S-IgA antibodies protect against both homologous and heterologous influenza virus strains (Asahi et al. 2002, 2004). Moreover, transfer of S-IgA antibodies from respiratory tract washings from immunized to naïve mice has been shown to protect against challenge with a homologous or drifted strain (Tamura et al. 1991). Several studies in mice also have shown induction of strong homosubtypic, as well as modest heterosubtypic, cross-protective IgA antibodies.

Since the influenza vaccine is generally administered intramuscularly or subcutaneously, S-IgA antibodies are generally not produced in large quantities; however, intranasal and intradermal influenza vaccinations can produce an effective IgA antibody response (Amorij et al. 2010). The most common route for the influenza virus to enter the host is via the respiratory tract. Therefore, intranasal immunization is the most widely explored route of mucosal vaccination against influenza. FluMist® (MedImmune, LLC), a live attenuated influenza virus vaccine, is the only nasal vaccine on the market. However, the rational design of S-IgA vaccines has been hampered by a lack of knowledge on the mechanisms by which IgA antibodies are induced (Brandtzaeg 2007).

3 The Characteristics of IgA Antibodies

After IgG, IgA is the second most abundant isotype in the serum; however, approximately 70 % of all antibodies in mucosae are IgA (Macpherson et al. 2008). In the human serum, IgA antibodies are present mostly as monomeric IgA_1 (Yel 2010), while S-IgA antibodies are found as dimeric IgA_2, although tri- and tetrameric molecules also exist. These polymeric IgA antibodies consist of monomeric IgA molecules connected by one or more J (Joining) chains. After binding to the secretory component (SC), the ectodomain of the polymeric Ig receptor (pIgR), the polymeric IgA is secreted as S-IgA antibodies. Since the cross-protective characteristics of nasal IgA antibodies depend on the polymeric nature of IgA, understanding the molecular structure, development, and function of these higher order polymeric IgA antibodies may be important for the rational design of cross-protective vaccines (Taylor and Dimmock 1985; Song et al. 1995; Renegar et al. 1998).

IgA_2 antibodies develop mostly at sites colonized by a wide range of microbiota, including urogenital and distal intestinal tracts. For example, intestinal bacteria instruct dendritic cells (DC) to produce IgA antibodies (Massacand et al. 2008). IgA antibodies are also present in the respiratory tract, which is not populated with many commensals; however, the predominant isotype is IgA_1.

And IgA_1- specific proteases can cleave bonds within human IgA1 molecules, but these specific bonds are only present in IgA molecules in higher primates and not in the mouse (Weiser et al. 2003).

4 IgA Antibody Production in Mucosal Tissues

The inductive site of the mucosal immune system can be divided in two different sites, namely inductive and effector sites. The inductive site includes mucosa-associated lymphatic tissue (MALT), and local and regional draining lymph nodes. Antigens are directly taken from the mucosal surface with an important role of microfold (M) cells and antigen-presenting cells (APC). Antigen-specific antibody producing B-cells can be developed at two different inductive sites, namely extrafollicular and germinal centres (GC), and their induction involves T-cell-dependent or -independent mechanisms (Cerutti 2008). The GC is a specialized environment that supports affinity maturation, which is mediated by activation-induced deaminase (AID) induced somatic hypermutation (Honjo et al. 2004). In addition, AID participates in the production of the preferred antibody class by influencing class switch recombination (CSR) of the heavy chain (Honjo et al. 2004; Zaheen and Martin 2010). Most IgA memory B-cells (BMem) and long-lived IgA plasma cells develop in the GC of peripheral lymphoid organs and that step requires T-cell help via CD40L (CD154) and TGFβ1. T-cell-independent B-cell class switching in the GC might be mediated by interactions with (DC) and stromal cells, including follicular DC (Puga et al. 2010).

At extrafollicular mucosal sites, antibodies can develop both with and without the help of T-cells, with the latter process involving B-cell activating factor (BAFF) and a proliferation-inducing ligand (APRIL) (Chen and Cerutti 2010; Rothaeusler and Baumgarth 2010). Although hypermutation, which is necessary for affinity maturation, is minimal at these sites (MacLennan et al. 2003), antigen-specific antibody producing B-cells at this site can prevent reinfection (Lee et al. 2005) generate an IgG- and IgA-producing BMem subset (Berkowska et al. 2011).

IgA CSR mechanisms have been studied mostly in the gut where they are influenced by specific environmental factors that are mainly created by commensal bacteria and their products (Massacand et al. 2008). While the respiratory tract is not populated with as many commensals as the intestinal tract, it would appear to be protected from the influenza virus by commensals in the gut because CD4 and CD8 T-cell number and the IgA antibody response were reduced in mice treated with an antibiotic. Immunity against the influenza virus was restored by nasal administration of lipopolysaccharides (LPS) but also by rectal administration of

Toll-like receptor (TLR) agonists (e.g., LPS, CpG, polyI:C) (Ichinohe et al. 2011). These findings indicate that signals from distal mucosal regions can support immune priming in the mucosal effector in the respiratory tract. Additional studies are needed to determine whether distal regions contribute to immunity in the respiratory tract.

5 Innate Sensing and Mucosal Adjuvants

Influenza viruses activate pattern recognition receptors belonging to several different families, namely the TLR family, the RIG-I like receptor (RLR) family, the Nod-like receptor (NLR) family (Pang and Iwasaki 2011), and the C-type lectin family (Londrigan et al. 2011). To improve vaccine efficacy, members of the pattern recognition receptor family, which are not activated by influenza virus infection, can be employed. For example, flagellin, which activates TLR5, promotes IgA production and heterosubtypic protection when incorporated into the membrane of influenza virus-like particles (Wang et al. 2010). Similarly, PolyI:PolyC$_{12}$U, activating TLR3, has been shown to induce heterosubtypic protection through IgA antibodies after administration of an intranasal vaccine (Ichinohe et al. 2007). Moreover, the TLR3 ligand acts synergistically with the TLR-2 ligand zymosan (Ainai et al. 2010).

Recently, several models have demonstrated the importance of TLR signaling in CSR. Early studies have shown only two signals to induce CSR in naïve B-cells, namely, the presentation of antigenic peptides on MHC class II molecules after antigen binding to the B-cell receptor, and the activation of these B-cells via cytokines and the interaction of CD40-CD40L with antigen-specific T-cells. Presently, TLR signaling is thought to involve an important third signal (Bekeredjian-Ding and Jego 2009). A recent study has shown that MyD88 can induce a protective immune response during primary, but not secondary, influenza virus infection. The IgA level in MyD88-/-TRIF-/- mice is reduced in the saliva during secondary infection; however, in serum and nasal wash, the level, which was induced in a TLR-independent manner, is similar to those in wild type mice (Seo et al. 2010). Furthermore, TLRs play a role in both T-cell-dependent and -independent IgA responses in mucosal and systemic antibody levels (Bessa et al. 2009).

Some APCs such as plasmacytoid DCs (pDC), Tip-DCs (TNF and Inducible nitric oxygen species (iNOS) Producing DC) and LAPCs have been reported to with the IgA response. In addition, pDCs trigger the anti-influenza response by inducing type 1 interferon, Th1, and cytotoxic responses and enhancing B-cell expansion and differentiation into CD27 high plasmablasts upon TLR7 stimulation (Douagi et al. 2009). pDCs are also necessary for optimal mucosal IgA and serum IgG production after primary, but not secondary, booster influenza vaccination, live attenuated virus vaccination, and inactivated whole virus or split virus vaccination. By contrast, pDCs are not needed to induce an immune response to a live virus (Koyama et al. 2010).

Upon infection of highly pathogenic influenza virus strains, Tip-DCs produce large concentrations of both tumor necrosis factor (TNF) and nitric oxide (NO), which results in tissue damage (Aldridge et al. 2009). However, controlled concentrations of NO induce TGF-βRII expression by B-cells, thereby enabling T-cell dependent IgA class switching. MyD88 signaling downstream of TLR2, 4, and/or 9, which is critical for the induction of iNOS, facilitates T-cell-independent IgA secretion in BAFF- and APRIL-dependent manners (Tezuka et al. 2007).

Late-activator APC (LAPC), a newly identified APC, may play an important role in the immune response several days after influenza virus infection. While the influenza virus activates DCs at approximately 3 days after infection and induces Th1-type responses, the LAPC is activated at approximately 8 days after infection. This results in the induction of a Th2-type response, production of IgA, IgG_1 and IgG_2 antibodies, and downregulation of the anti-viral Th1-type response (Yoo et al. 2010).

6 Mucosal Vaccine Design

Currently used seasonal influenza vaccines are produced based on the prediction of strains that might cause an epidemic in the following season. These vaccines are generally injected intramuscularly or subcutaneously, and are expected to reduce the severity of the disease caused by specific strains that are homologous to the vaccine strain. These vaccines neither induce cross-protection against the heterologous strain nor prevent infection because they largely induce neutralizing IgG antibodies in the serum. On the other hand, influenza vaccines currently under design aim to induce broader cross-protection and are referred to as ‘universal influenza vaccines’. The more diverse and broader cross-protective immune response induced by natural infection than by current parenteral vaccinations suggests the induction of several possible immunological effectors that add to cross-protection. Furthermore, individuals of different genders, ages, and genetic backgrounds respond differently to vaccines; thus, they may rely on different immune mediators for their protection (Nayak et al. 2010; McKinstry et al. 2011).

While infection with the natural influenza virus is superior to vaccination in inducing cross-protection against infection by mutated viruses within a particular subtype of the A-type virus in humans (Hoskins et al. 1976, 1979; Couch and Kasel 1983), an inactivated whole virus particle vaccine has been shown to be more immunogenic than split vaccines. This is in agreement with the general view that the effectiveness and safety of vaccines are usually inversely correlated.

Both inactivated whole virion vaccines and split seasonal vaccines can induce protective immune responses against the homologous virus (Greenbaum et al. 2004). While heterosubtypic immunity is not observed after administration of an ether-split vaccine, an inactivated whole virion vaccine can induce broad heterosubtypic immunity (Takada et al. 2003). The stronger immunogenicity of the inactivated whole virion vaccine in mice is likely due to the stimulation of innate immunity by genomic single-stranded RNA via TLR7 (Diebold et al. 2004; Lund et al. 2004). Since most viruses produce dsRNA during replication (Jacobs and Langland 1996), synthetic dsRNA can likely act as a partial molecular mimic of viral infection.

This has been confirmed in a previous study where intranasal administration of an ether-split vaccine from PR8 (a H1N1 influenza virus strain) and poly(I:C), a TLR3 agonist adjuvant, induced a strong anti-HA IgA and IgG response in nasal washes and serum, respectively, while vaccination without poly(I:C) induced a weak response. In addition, administration of either an A/Beijing (H1N1) or A/Yamagata (H1N1) vaccine, which are antigenically different from A/PR8, in the presence of poly(I:C) confered complete protection against A/PR8 virus challenge in a mouse model of nasal infection, indicating that intranasal vaccination with poly(I:C) adjuvant confers cross-protection against variant viruses (Ichinohe et al. 2005). Safety issue of the adjuvant is very important. One of dsRNA poly(I:C_{12}U)(Ampligen) which are clinically safe were recently shown to be a potent inducer of innate immune responses (Caskey et al. 2011). This dsRNA, poly(I:C12U)(Ampligen), was investigated as a dsRNA adjuvant for intranasal avian influenza vaccines (Ichinohe et al. 2009).

The stronger immunogenicity produced by the live virus than by the whole inactivated virus may be caused by a mechanism that does not involve stimulation of TLR7 or 3. For example, other receptors, or a different biodistribution or kinetic profile may be involved. For inactivated vaccine the former might be mimicked by using a ligand for TLRs as an adjuvant, the latter two might possibly be mimicked by the use of different carriers for the antigens that will influence kinetics as well as biodistribution (Bachmann and Jennings 2010).

While investigators continue to understand infections caused by the influenza virus, the ultimate goal is to produce a vaccine that can overcome natural infections. This might be achieved by carefully selecting highly conservative domains within influenza membrane proteins and using them as vaccines in combination with several adjuvants which could activate a broad spectrum of tissues and cells.

A recent clinical study reported that intranasal administration of a whole inactivated influenza virus without adjuvant but with a prime-booster induced high levels of nasal neutralizing antibodies that consisted primarily of polymeric IgA (Ainai et al. 2013). It is not clear whether the absence of adjuvant was not important for eliciting the antibody response in these subjects who would have had a cross-protective memory resulting from a history of infections and/or vaccinations.

In conclusion, the induction of IgA antibodies after vaccination can enhance the immune response by introducing a local immune response, which adds to cross-protection, balances pro-inflammatory responses, and increases the diversity of immunological memory. The fact that IgA antibodies alone cannot induce complete protection after heterosubtypic infection may be an advantage because partial protection by IgA antibodies can reduce the viral load and provide time for immune system priming. In this way, innate, humoral, and cellular responses are activated, resulting in the strongest renewal of immunological memory. This ensures the best possible preparedness for the next influenza virus encountered.

Acknowledgments E. van Riet is a recipient of a Postdoctoral Fellowship for Foreign Researchers from the Japan Society for the Promotion of Science. Our research is supported by grants from the Ministry of Health, Labour and Welfare, "H23-Shinkou-Ippan-015". We also would like to acknowledge all the scientists whose work we could not cite due to restrictions on the number of references.

References

Ainai A, Ichinohe T et al (2010) Zymosan enhances the mucosal adjuvant activity of poly(I:C) in a nasal influenza vaccine. J Med Virol 82(3):476–484

Ainai A, Tamura S et al (2013) Intranasal vaccination with an inactivated whole influenza virus vaccine induces strong antibody responses in serum and nasal mucus of healthy adults. Hum Vaccin Immunother 9(9):1962–1970

Aldridge JR Jr, Moseley CE et al (2009) TNF/iNOS-producing dendritic cells are the necessary evil of lethal influenza virus infection. Proc Natl Acad Sci U S A 106(13):5306–5311

Amorij JP, Hinrichs W et al (2010) Needle-free influenza vaccination. Lancet Infect Dis 10(10):699–711

Asahi-Ozaki Y, Yoshikawa T et al (2004) Secretory IgA antibodies provide cross-protection against infection with different strains of influenza B virus. J Med Virol 74(2):328–335

Asahi Y, Yoshikawa T et al (2002) Protection against influenza virus infection in polymeric Ig receptor knockout mice immunized intranasally with adjuvant-combined vaccines. J Immunol 168(6):2930–2938

Bachmann MF, Jennings GT (2010) Vaccine delivery: a matter of size, geometry, kinetics and molecular patterns. Nat Rev Immunol 10(11):787–796

Bekeredjian-Ding I, Jego G (2009) Toll-like receptors–sentries in the B-cell response. Immunology 128(3):311–323

Berkowska MA, Driessen GJ et al (2011) Human memory B cells originate from three distinct germinal center-dependent and -independent maturation pathways. Blood 118(8):2150–2158

Bessa J, Jegerlehner A et al (2009) Alveolar macrophages and lung dendritic cells sense RNA and drive mucosal IgA responses. J Immunol 183(6):3788–3799

Brandtzaeg P (2007) Induction of secretory immunity and memory at mucosal surfaces. Vaccine 25(30):5467–5484

Caskey M, Lefebvre F et al (2011) Synthetic double-stranded RNA induces innate immune responses similar to a live viral vaccine in humans. J Exp Med 208(12):2357–2366

Cerutti A (2008) The regulation of IgA class switching. Nat Rev Immunol 8(6):421–434

Chen K, Cerutti A (2010) Vaccination strategies to promote mucosal antibody responses. Immunity 33(4):479–491

Couch RB, Kasel JA (1983) Immunity to influenza in man. Annu Rev Microbiol 37:529–549

Diebold SS, Kaisho T et al (2004) Innate antiviral responses by means of TLR7-mediated recognition of single-stranded RNA. Science 303(5663):1529–1531

Douagi I, Gujer C et al (2009) Human B cell responses to TLR ligands are differentially modulated by myeloid and plasmacytoid dendritic cells. J Immunol 182(4):1991–2001

Greenbaum E, Engelhard D et al (2004) Mucosal (SIgA) and serum (IgG) immunologic responses in young adults following intranasal administration of one or two doses of inactivated, trivalent anti-influenza vaccine. Vaccine 22(20):2566–2577

Honjo T, Muramatsu M et al (2004) AID: how does it aid antibody diversity? Immunity 20(6):659–668

Hoskins TW, Davies JR et al (1976) Influenza at Christ's Hospital: March, 1974. Lancet 1(7951):105–108

Hoskins TW, Davies JR et al (1979) Assessment of inactivated influenza-A vaccine after three outbreaks of influenza A at Christ's Hospital. Lancet 1(8106):33–35

Ichinohe T, Ainai A et al (2009) PolyI:polyC12U adjuvant-combined intranasal vaccine protects mice against highly pathogenic H5N1 influenza virus variants. Vaccine 27(45):6276–6279

Ichinohe T, Pang IK et al (2011) Microbiota regulates immune defense against respiratory tract influenza A virus infection. Proc Natl Acad Sci U S A 108(13):5354–5359

Ichinohe T, Tamura S et al (2007) Cross-protection against H5N1 influenza virus infection is afforded by intranasal inoculation with seasonal trivalent inactivated influenza vaccine. J Infect Dis 196(9):1313–1320

Ichinohe T, Watanabe I et al (2005) Synthetic double-stranded RNA poly(I:C) combined with mucosal vaccine protects against influenza virus infection. J Virol 79(5):2910–2919

Jacobs BL, Langland JO (1996) When two strands are better than one: the mediators and modulators of the cellular responses to double-stranded RNA. Virology 219(2):339–349

Koyama S, Aoshi T et al (2010) Plasmacytoid dendritic cells delineate immunogenicity of influenza vaccine subtypes. Sci Transl Med 2(25):25ra24

La Gruta NL, Kedzierska K et al (2007) A question of self-preservation: immunopathology in influenza virus infection. Immunol Cell Biol 85(2):85–92

Lee BO, Rangel-Moreno J et al (2005) CD4 T cell-independent antibody response promotes resolution of primary influenza infection and helps to prevent reinfection. J Immunol 175(9):5827–5838

Londrigan SL, Turville SG et al (2011) N-linked glycosylation facilitates sialic acid-independent attachment and entry of influenza A viruses into cells expressing DC-SIGN or L-SIGN. J Virol 85(6):2990–3000

Lund JM, Alexopoulou L et al (2004) Recognition of single-stranded RNA viruses by Toll-like receptor 7. Proc Natl Acad Sci U S A 101(15):5598–5603

MacLennan IC, Toellner KM et al (2003) Extrafollicular antibody responses. Immunol Rev 194:8–18

Macpherson AJ, McCoy KD et al (2008) The immune geography of IgA induction and function. Mucosal Immunol 1(1):11–22

Massacand JC, Kaiser P et al (2008) Intestinal bacteria condition dendritic cells to promote IgA production. PLoS ONE 3(7):e2588

Matzinger P, Kamala T (2011) Tissue-based class control: the other side of tolerance. Nat Rev Immunol 11(3):221–230

McKinstry KK, Strutt TM et al (2011) Hallmarks of CD4 T cell immunity against influenza. J Intern Med 269(5):507–518

Nayak JL, Richards KA et al (2010) Analyses of the specificity of CD4 T cells during the primary immune response to influenza virus reveals dramatic MHC-linked asymmetries in reactivity to individual viral proteins. Viral Immunol 23(2):169–180

Pang IK, Iwasaki A (2011) Inflammasomes as mediators of immunity against influenza virus. Trends Immunol 32(1):34–41

Puga I, Cols M et al (2010) Innate signals in mucosal immunoglobulin class switching. J Allergy Clin Immunol 126(5): 889–895, quiz 896–887

Renegar KB, Jackson GD et al (1998) In vitro comparison of the biologic activities of monoclonal monomeric IgA, polymeric IgA, and secretory IgA. J Immunol 160(3):1219–1223

Renegar KB, Small PA Jr et al (2004) Role of IgA versus IgG in the control of influenza viral infection in the murine respiratory tract. J Immunol 173(3):1978–1986

Rothaeusler K, Baumgarth N (2010) B-cell fate decisions following influenza virus infection. Eur J Immunol 40(2):366–377

Seo SU, Kwon HJ et al (2010) MyD88 signaling is indispensable for primary influenza A virus infection but dispensable for secondary infection. J Virol 84(24):12713–12722

Song W, Vaerman JP et al (1995) Dimeric and tetrameric IgA are transcytosed equally by the polymeric Ig receptor. J Immunol 155(2):715–721

Stokes CR, Soothill JF et al (1975) Immune exclusion is a function of IgA. Nature 255(5511):745–746

Takada A, Matsushita S et al (2003) Intranasal immunization with formalin-inactivated virus vaccine induces a broad spectrum of heterosubtypic immunity against influenza A virus infection in mice. Vaccine 21(23):3212–3218

Tamura S, Funato H et al (1991) Cross-protection against influenza A virus infection by passively transferred respiratory tract IgA antibodies to different hemagglutinin molecules. Eur J Immunol 21(6):1337–1344

Taylor HP, Dimmock NJ (1985) Mechanism of neutralization of influenza virus by secretory IgA is different from that of monomeric IgA or IgG. J Exp Med 161(1):198–209

Tezuka H, Abe Y et al (2007) Regulation of IgA production by naturally occurring TNF/iNOS-producing dendritic cells. Nature 448(7156):929–933

Wang BZ, Xu R et al (2010) Intranasal immunization with influenza VLPs incorporating membrane-anchored flagellin induces strong heterosubtypic protection. PLoS ONE 5(11):e13972

Weiser JN, Bae D et al (2003) Antibody-enhanced pneumococcal adherence requires IgA1 protease. Proc Natl Acad Sci U S A 100(7):4215–4220

Yel L (2010) Selective IgA deficiency. J Clin Immunol 30(1):10–16

Yoo JK, Galligan CL et al (2010) Identification of a novel antigen-presenting cell population modulating antiinfluenza type 2 immunity. J Exp Med 207(7):1435–1451

Zaheen A, Martin A (2010) Induction and assessment of class switch recombination in purified murine B cells. J Vis Exp (42), pii: 2130. doi:10.3791/2130

B Cell Responses to Influenza Infection and Vaccination

Christopher Chiu, Ali H. Ellebedy, Jens Wrammert and Rafi Ahmed

Abstract Although vaccines against influenza are widely available, control of the disease remains elusive. In part, this is due to the inability of current vaccines to induce durable, broadly protective immune responses. Prevention of influenza depends primarily on effective antibody responses that block virus entry. Following infection, high-affinity IgA antibodies are generated in the respiratory tract that lead to immune exclusion, while IgG prevents systemic spread. These are effective and long-lasting but also exert immune pressure. Mutation of the antigenic determinants of influenza therefore rapidly leads to emergence of novel variants that evade previously generated protective responses. Not only do vaccines suffer from this strain-specific limitation, but also they are suboptimal in their ability to induce durable immunity. However, recent evidence has demonstrated the possibility of inducing broadly cross-reactive antibody responses. Further understanding of the ways in which high-titer, long-lived antibody responses directed against such cross-reactive epitopes can be induced would lead to the development of novel vaccines that may remove the requirement for recurrent vaccination.

C. Chiu
Centre for Respiratory Infection, National Heart and Lung Institute, Imperial College London, London W2 1PG, UK

A.H. Ellebedy · R. Ahmed
Emory Vaccine Center, Emory University School of Medicine, Atlanta, GA 30322, USA

A.H. Ellebedy · R. Ahmed (✉)
Department of Microbiology and Immunology, Emory University School of Medicine, G211, 1510 Clifton Road, Atlanta, GA 30322, USA
e-mail: rahmed@emory.edu

J. Wrammert
Department of Pediatric Infectious Disease, Department of Hematology and Oncology, Emory University School of Medicine, Atlanta, GA 30322, USA

Current Topics in Microbiology and Immunology (2015) 386: 381–398
DOI: 10.1007/82_2014_425

Published Online: 6 September 2014

Contents

1 Introduction

Despite the widespread availability of influenza vaccines and their place in the vaccination programs of most high-income nations, control of influenza infection remains a major unresolved health issue. As well as the logistic difficulties associated with vaccine delivery and uptake, the fundamental biology of influenza virus raises hurdles that current vaccination strategies are unable to overcome. Furthermore, our understanding of the mechanisms underlying the generation of durable immunity is still incomplete. Until it becomes possible to manufacture vaccines that induce immune responses that match or even improve upon those following natural infection, it is likely that influenza will continue as one of the foremost causes of morbidity and mortality worldwide.

Protection from infection depends on the induction of effective immunological memory. While cellular immunity may have the capacity to clear influenza virus and reduce disease severity, B cells and antibodies are the major mechanism by which prevention of re-infection occurs. However, the propensity for influenza to escape via mutation under immune pressure means that this protection is short-lived and strain-specific. Current vaccines not only suffer from this limitation but also exhibit limited durability of protection even in the absence of strain variation. Annual re-vaccination is therefore required. However, recent evidence suggests that antibodies can be generated that have the capacity to recognize multiple influenza strains. More detailed understanding of how high-affinity long-lasting antibodies against influenza can be generated in the appropriate compartments and the ways in which broadly cross-reactive antibodies can be encouraged may assist in the development of the so-called universal influenza vaccine.

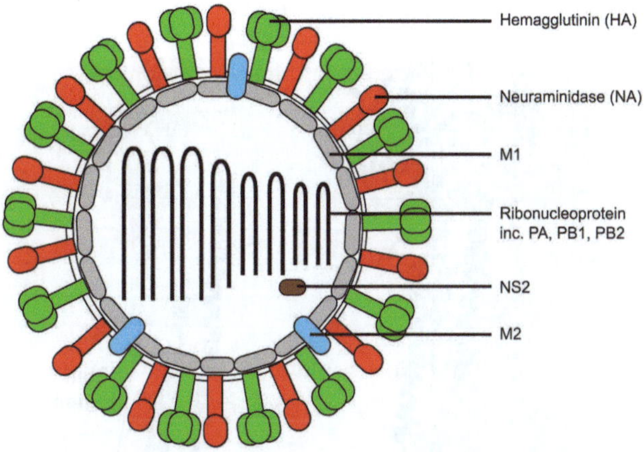

Fig. 1 Schematic of the influenza virion. Influenza is an enveloped RNA virus. Its major surface proteins are hemagglutinin (shown in *red*) and neuraminidase (*green*) with the M2 protein (*blue*) forming a transmembrane ion channel. The capsid is composed of the M1 protein (*gray*) and contains a few copies of NS2 (*brown*) and the eight segments of negative-sense RNA complexed as ribonucleoprotein with NP, PB1, PB2, and PA

2 Targets of Humoral Immunity in Influenza

Influenza belongs to the family *Orthomyxoviridae* and consists of an enveloped capsid containing an eight-segment RNA genome (Fig. 1) (Fields et al. 2007). Two major glycoproteins are expressed on the surface of influenza, hemagglutinin (HA), and neuraminidase (NA). Both are targets of humoral immunity. HA binds to sialic acid, facilitating viral attachment and entry following membrane fusion in the late endosome (Skehel and Wiley 2000). NA cleaves sialic acid and allows virus particles to escape the host cell in which they have been generated (Mitnaul et al. 2000). HA-specific antibodies are therefore capable of preventing infection of cells and are believed to be the primary method by which prevention of infection occurs.

The HA polypeptide, which complexes as a homotrimer, is composed of a globular head (HA1 domain) and a stalk (largely comprised of the HA2 domain) linked to the transmembrane region (Fig. 2). Most anti-HA antibodies are directed against the head and exert immune pressure so that viruses with mutations in this area capable of evading antibody recognition are selected. Over time, at least 18 influenza A HA subtypes have arisen, which are classified into two phylogenetic groups: group 1 includes subtypes expressing H1, H2, and H5, while group 2 contains H3 and H7. Similarly, there are 9 NA subtypes in influenza A, again falling in two groups. The NA head forms a homotetramer, and the stalk is joined to a short cytoplasmic tail via the hydrophobic transmembrane region.

Since RNA polymerase causes rapid mutation within both HA and NA, antigenic drift can quickly give rise to new strains, thus causing epidemics (Yewdell et al. 1979). In addition, the shuffling of the influenza genome allows wholesale re-assortment of its segments so that antigenic shift may occur. New strains may

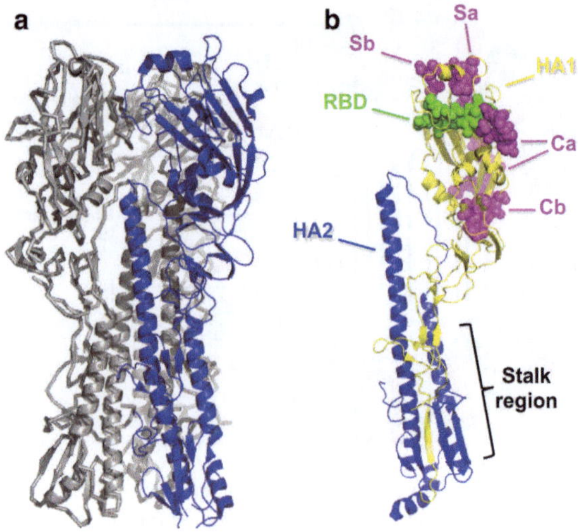

Fig. 2 A structural view of the H1 hemagglutinin from A/PR8/34 (H1N1). **a** Depiction of hemagglutinin as a trimer (with one monomer colored *blue*) and **b** the monomer. Each monomer is composed of two subunits: HA1 (*yellow*) and HA2 (*blue*). Within the HA1 subunit, well-defined neutralizing epitopes within the globular head region (Sa, Sb, Ca, and Cb) are shown in magenta (Caton et al. 1982). The receptor-binding domain (*RBD*) is shown in *green*. The HA stalk domain is formed by the N- and C-terminal domains of HA1 plus the ectodomain part of HA2

therefore arise expressing novel HA and NA variants to which existing antibodies are unable to react on a population level, thus giving rise to influenza pandemics. The humoral response to influenza in most individuals is therefore characterized by a complex mixture of responses originating from encounters with previous as well as contemporary influenza strains.

3 Humoral Correlates of Protection in Influenza

Antibodies alone have long been known to have the capacity to prevent influenza infection. This may be seen after parenteral or intranasal administration of antibodies in animal models (Henle et al. 1941; Gerhard et al. 1997) or in the neonatal period following transfer of maternal IgG (Zinkernagel 2001; Zaman et al. 2008). Recent studies during the influenza A(H1N1)2009 pandemic have also implicated their protective role against fulminant disease (Guihot et al. 2014). They are therefore the most frequently used correlate of protection and are the primary mechanism by which most currently available vaccines aim to mediate protection. Vaccine development has relied largely on antibody-mediated surrogate correlates of protection to assist in the licensing of new products and a number of techniques have been used to define responses of adequate magnitude in this regard.

At the simplest level, enzyme-linked immunosorbent assay (ELISA) may be used to measure antibodies that possess virus-binding capacity (Grund et al. 2011). However, ELISA cannot assess the functional efficacy of antibodies. Historically, the most frequently used measure of serum antibody function has therefore been the hemagglutination inhibition (HAI) assay (Black et al. 2011; Ohmit et al. 2011). This relies on the sialic acid-binding capacity of influenza virions, which causes the agglutination of erythrocytes. Antibodies that interfere with the receptor-binding site of HA can therefore inhibit hemagglutination, and their titers may be used to correlate with likelihood of protection. HAI assays are inexpensive, are easy to carry out, and have been validated extensively in studies of seasonal influenza. Seroconversion is conventionally defined as a >four-fold increase while seroprotection is expressed as an HAI titer >1:40. These definitions are used for influenza vaccine licensing. However, the minimum seroprotection level only equates to around 50 % reduction in infection risk on the basis of experimental challenge and epidemiological studies in adults. Furthermore, prevention of hemagglutination measures only one of a number of mechanisms by which antibody can act and fails to assess Fc-mediated activity among others.

Microneutralization assays can examine neutralization of virus infectivity in cell culture by plaque reduction or other methods and have been found both to be more sensitive and more direct a measure of functional activity (Grund et al. 2011). However, these are less well validated with regard to their use as measures of vaccine efficacy. Standardization of these assay protocols has been problematic and inter-laboratory reproducibility remains an issue (Stephenson et al. 2009).

4 The Generation of Antigen-Specific B Cells and Antibodies in Influenza Infection

Studies in the late 1960s and 1970s defined the durability and subtype specificity of the immunity generated by influenza infection (Couch and Kasel 1983). Classic experiments involving experimental human challenge infections demonstrated homotypic immunity that lasted many years and these were shown to correlate with antibody levels. Studies primarily in mouse models have since sought to elucidate the mechanisms underlying the protective immunity provided by B cells.

Influenza infection occurs principally in the respiratory tract due to tropism conferred by the HA–sialic acid interaction (Thompson et al. 2006). Systemic spread is unusual except in cases of severe infection, highly pathogenic strains, or failure of immune control (Yen et al. 2009; Choi et al. 2012). In the respiratory tract, "natural" IgM antibodies, which are polyspecific and produced by a small subset of B cells, B-1 cells, may play a role in preventing influenza infection independent of B cell receptor ligation (Choi and Baumgarth 2008). However, priming of naïve B cells is believed to occur when they migrate through regional lymphoid tissues where dendritic cells present influenza antigens transported there

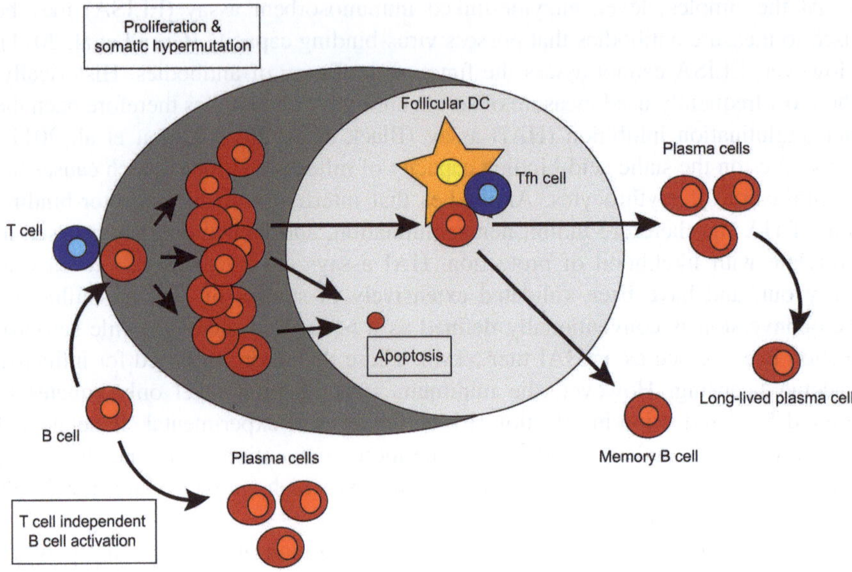

Fig. 3 Generation of antibody-secreting and memory B cells in the germinal center. B cells are activated following encounter with professional antigen-presenting cells displaying viral antigen. Cognate interactions with T follicular helper cells promote the formation of germinal centers in which somatic hypermutation, affinity maturation, and the generation of antigen-secreting cells and memory B cells occur

from the respiratory tract (Pape et al. 2007; Batista and Harwood 2009). This occurs at two main anatomical sites: draining mediastinal lymph nodes or mucosa-associated lymphoid tissue (MALT) (van Riet et al. 2012). Here, recognition of antigen by the B cell receptor induces a program of transcriptional changes that starts the differentiation process and causes the B cell to move to the edge of the lymphoid follicle (Garside et al. 1998).

If the B cell expresses the transcriptional repressor Blimp-1 at this point, it immediately proceeds toward antibody-secreting cell (ASC) differentiation with a short-lived phenotype (Shaffer et al. 2002). This leads to rapid generation of an early local antibody response but does not allow for affinity maturation. Extrafollicular responses such as these can be T cell independent via the involvement of B cell-activating factor (BAFF) and a proliferation-inducing ligand (APRIL) produced by DCs (GeurtsvanKessel et al. 2009).

The classical T cell-dependent differentiation pathway, however, depends on the B cell making contact with specialized CD4+ T follicular helper (Tfh) cells that recognize cognate antigen presented by the B cell via MHC class II (Fig. 3). Tfh cells express CD40L and cytokines including IL-4, IFN-γ, and TGF-β that induce immunoglobulin class switching (McHeyzer-Williams et al. 2012). This irreversible recombination event causes the immunoglobulin isotype to switch from IgM to IgG or IgA. For the production of high-affinity ASCs and effective MBC differentiation,

Bcl-6 is up-regulated, leading to further interaction with Tfh cells in the follicular core and participation in the germinal center (GC) reaction (McHeyzer-Williams et al. 2001). Within the GC, Tfh cells and B cells interact via ICOS/ICOSL, PD-1/PD-L1, CD28/B7, and SLAM/SAP, leading to IL-21 secretion and promotion of B cell survival, somatic hypermutation, and affinity maturation (King et al. 2008). These result in the generation of high-affinity antibody-secreting plasma cells and MBCs, the latter having a long-lived phenotype but no antibody-producing capacity.

Studies in humans have primarily focused on the B cell responses in peripheral blood. Most adults will have been infected or vaccinated with influenza multiple times, and secondary responses are therefore the most commonly examined. During natural infection with influenza A(H1N1)pdm09, virus-specific plasmablasts are readily detected at a frequency of approximately 1,000 IgG-secreting cells per million PBMCs using B cell ELISpot assay at 7–10 days after symptom onset (Wrammert et al. 2011; Lee et al. 2011). The kinetics of these responses have been studied in more detail in the experimental human challenge model, where infection with seasonal influenza H1N1 A/Brisbane/59/07 led to an expansion of ASCs peaking at an average of 166 IgG+ ASCs per million PBMCs around 7 days post-inoculation, correlating with viral shedding and symptoms (Huang et al. 2014). Influenza-specific MBCs were significantly induced by 28 days post-inoculation and were all found in the class-switched IgM-negative population.

Once the infection is cleared, the majority of ASCs undergo apoptosis, while a small proportion go on to further differentiate into long-lived plasma cells (LLPCs) (Chu and Berek 2013). These travel to long-term survival niches such as the bone marrow where they persist and are responsible for ongoing production of antibody. MBCs, which may be found circulating in blood and at peripheral sites, remain poised to respond to re-encounter with antigen in order to rapidly proliferate and differentiate, once again producing ASCs capable of boosting antibody levels.

5 The Generation of Mucosal IgA+ B Cell Responses

Since influenza primarily involves the respiratory mucosa, IgA+ B cells are a major component of the response to infection. Secretory IgA is the principal isotype found at the mucosal surface and is one of the major mechanisms by which immune exclusion (i.e., early immunity capable of preventing infection itself) occurs. This has been demonstrated in IgA knockout mice, which are poorly protected against influenza infection (Asahi et al. 2002). Conversely, transfer of IgA via respiratory secretions can confer protection in naïve mice (Asahi-Ozaki et al. 2004). Furthermore, there is evidence that some cross-protective immunity is provided by antibodies of this isotype as passive intranasal transfer of anti-HA IgA confers some protection against non-homologous strains (Tamura et al. 1991).

At the draining mediastinal lymph nodes, canonical T cell-dependent B cell responses occur and the provision of Tfh signals via CD40L and TGF-β1 leads to class switching to IgA. Here, B cell differentiation and proliferation can also occur in the absence of cognate T cell interactions and IgA+ B cell responses in particular may be less reliant on cognate T cell help. In MHC class II- and CD40-deficient animals, antibody responses to influenza can be generated in the absence of cognate signaling, with IgA+ plasma cells formed even when IgM and IgG responses are abrogated (Sangster et al. 2003). Again, extra-follicular B cell activation can occur in the absence of any T cell help through DC-derived BAFF and APRIL.

These mechanisms can also take place in the respiratory tract itself, where IgA-secreting B cells are preferentially generated in MALT. These secondary lymphoid tissues include lymphoid aggregates in the oronasopharynx (Waldeyer's ring) and bronchus-associated lymphoid tissue (BALT) (Kunisawa et al. 2008). In addition, tertiary lymphoid aggregates may also form during the course of infection. These inducible structures (iBALT) contain follicles and T cell areas, with GC reactions leading to the generation of ASCs and MBCs (Moyron-Quiroz et al. 2004, 2006). These sites may represent preferential compartments in which IgA+ GC B cells are formed, with the frequency of GC B cells peaking later here than in the draining lymph nodes (Boyden et al. 2012). In addition, GCs at mucosal sites may be present for much longer than in secondary lymphoid tissues, with their persistence potentially driven by the presence of antigen beyond the acute period (Baumgarth et al. 2008).

Respiratory mucosa also represents a site for the persistence of LLPCs that function to produce long-term mucosal antibody (Jones and Ada 1986). This may take place at several anatomical locations, with antibody-producing plasma cells found in murine nasal-associated lymphoid tissue for at least 18 months following infection with influenza (Liang et al. 2001). In addition, selective depletion of CD11c+ DCs leads to failure for iBALT to be maintained with an associated reduction of IgA and IgA+ plasma cells, suggesting that prolonged local IgA production may be dependent on iBALT persistence (GeurtsvanKessel et al. 2009).

In the gut, innate signals including TLR ligation have been shown to be important in IgA+ B cell activation and the formation of lymphoid structures, with enhancement and modulation affected by the microbiome (Pabst 2012). Similarly, in the lung, it is increasingly understood that that innate signaling is important in the generation of respiratory B cell responses. Although the respiratory microbiome is more limited than that of the gut, it nevertheless contributes bacterial components that enhance and modulate both innate and adaptive immune responses (Abt et al. 2012). Furthermore, following B cell receptor engagement, pattern recognition receptors including TLR9 and TLR10 are up-regulated on human B cells, providing additional signals that increase immunoglobulin production and are the likely basis for adjuvant effects (Bernasconi et al. 2003).

Thus, the B cell response to influenza infection is generated at several anatomical sites with multiple layers of redundancy, leading to high levels of respiratory IgA that promotes immune exclusion. Furthermore, responses in regional secondary lymphoid tissues generate systemic IgG that may prevent disseminated infection. Durable immunity occurs via T cell-dependent mechanisms and is optimized by the integration of inflammatory signals including those provided by TLRs. This results in the generation of MBCs able to rapidly respond on secondary infection and LLPCs that survive in niches within the respiratory mucosa as well as bone marrow, thus providing long-term protection. Of note, however, these mechanisms have been primarily elucidated in animal models and studies of respiratory mucosal responses in humans remain limited.

6 Replicating the B Cell Response to Natural Infection by Vaccination

Despite this, protective humoral immune responses represent a benchmark for vaccine-induced immunity and vaccinologists have therefore sought to replicate the features of immune protection following natural infection. Two types of influenza vaccine currently exist: inactivated influenza vaccine (IIV) and live attenuated influenza vaccinelive attenuated influenza vaccine (LAIV). IIV relies primarily on the generation of HA-specific neutralizing antibodies while LAIV also induces mucosal immune responses and cellular immunity. Both types of vaccine induce highly strain-specific protection, and seasonal vaccines are therefore formulated as trivalent or quadrivalent, with current vaccines containing HAs from H1N1, H3N2, and one or two influenza B strains. If vaccine strains are well matched with circulating strains that season, vaccine efficacy is estimated to be 65–85 % while mismatch leads to reduced efficacy of as little as 40–50 % (Tricco et al. 2013). Furthermore, the durability of vaccine-induced protection is poor compared to infection with an estimated half-life for HAI titers of less than a year (Wright et al. 2008). Therefore, currently available influenza vaccines are suboptimal, sharing the same limitations with regard to subtype-specific immunity as natural infection with shorter duration of protection. This, coupled with low vaccine uptake, has led to poor coverage in most populations.

The acute response to IIV delivered intramuscularly is characterized by rapid proliferation of ASCs that arise from naïve B cells and/or MBCs with similarities to that seen following infection. Our work in healthy adults showed that this peaks around 7 days post-vaccination and is short-lived, returning to pre-vaccination levels within a week. By B cell ELISpot, the peak frequency of IgG-producing ASCs in response to the monovalent pandemic A(H1N1)2009 influenza vaccine showed substantial variability between individuals but was, on average, 520 per million PBMCs (+/−SEM 253) (Li et al. 2012). These cells exhibit an activated proliferating phenotype, with high expression of HLA-DR and Ki-67, and their frequencies correlate with the increment in serum antibody as measured by HAI, indicating that acutely generated ASCs are responsible for "seroconversion". During infection, IgA-producing ASCs are at least as frequent as IgG due to the mucosal site of infection, but there is evidence that intramuscular vaccination is also able to partially recall these responses (Sasaki et al. 2011; Fink 2012; Li et al. 2012). However, following IIV, most ASCs secrete IgG with as little as 10 times fewer IgA+ ASCs and little or no IgM production, implying that in adults, the response to vaccination is dominated by secondary recall of IgG+ memory responses (Sasaki et al. 2011).

LAIV consists of cold-adapted influenza strains that is unable to replicate at the higher temperatures found in the lower respiratory tract. Immunity is therefore focused on the nasal mucosa, and systemic responses are modest (Cao et al. 2014). However, efficacy in children is better than IIV, suggesting the effective role of local immune responses in protection from infection (Ambrose et al. 2011). In contrast, the effectiveness of LAIV falls with increasing age and is therefore not licensed for older adults, reflecting the effect of pre-existing mucosal immunity that prevents the productive infection required for LAIV efficacy. Following LAIV, the frequency of ASCs induced is significantly smaller than following IIV and this correlates with lower vaccine-specific serum ELISA titers (Sasaki et al. 2014). However, IgA+ ASCs make up a greater proportion of the plasmablast response than IgG+ cells consistent with the route of administration. Differences are also seen in the induction of innate signals that might contribute to the response, with LAIV stimulating a later up-regulation of interferon-signaling genes than IIV (Cao et al. 2014). Interestingly, both IgG- and IgA-producing MBCs are only consistently detected in blood following TIV, suggesting that these cells when locally stimulated might remain associated with the respiratory tract (Sasaki et al. 2007).

7 Unresolved Problems Remaining with Influenza Vaccination

Despite the fact that B cell responses exhibit superficially similar characteristics to those seen following infection, the durability of vaccine-induced responses is comparatively poor. In addition, the protection conferred remains highly strain-specific. Although the more recently developed LAIV has been shown to induce both T cells and IgA-producing B cells with cross-reactive potential, epidemiological evidence has not supported the idea that these vaccines confer clinically significant cross-protection (Belshe et al. 1998; Hoft et al. 2011; Sasaki et al. 2014). Furthermore, vaccine efficacy in frankly or relatively immunosuppressed populations, such as older adults, is especially poor. Since these are high-risk groups in whom the burden of mortality is the greatest, these unresolved issues represent important areas for further study and development.

8 Overcoming Immunosenescence to Improve Protection

Clinically important antigenic drift and shift do not occur at constant rates. For example, since the emergence of the most recent pandemic influenza A strain in 2009, this has remained the predominant circulating strain of H1N1. An influenza vaccine that could confer protection beyond a single influenza season would therefore be valuable in increasing vaccine coverage. This is an even greater issue in elderly adults whose immune responses in general are blunted and in whom the relative reduction in hospitalization conferred by influenza vaccination can be as little as 27 % (Nichol et al. 2007). Improvements in vaccine immunogenicity are therefore urgently required.

The proportion of older adults continues to increase worldwide as life spans extend and birth rates fall. Between 1975 and 2000, there was almost a doubling of individuals aged over 60 years and this increase is accelerating (http://www.un.org/esa/population/publications/worldageing19502050/). With advancing age, the frequency of ASCs decreases, with defects in GC formation, decreased capacity for affinity maturation and decreased survival of long-lived B cell subsets (Haq and McElhaney 2014). B cell responsiveness to vaccination is therefore impaired, with fewer plasmablasts generated following IIV in the elderly leading to significantly reduced increments in HAI titer compared with young adults (Sasaki et al. 2011).

A number of approaches are currently being explored in an attempt to enhance immunogenicity. The simplest strategy has been an increased dose formulation of IIV that has been shown to increase rates of seroconversion/seroprotection (Chen et al. 2011). Also already in use are adjuvanted influenza vaccines, the first of which licensed for use in older adults was the oil-in-water emulsion, MF59 (O'Hagan et al. 2007). Antibody responses to MF59-adjuvanted influenza vaccine are enhanced, allowing antigen dose-sparing and potentially increasing cross-reactive responses. This probably acts through innate myeloid cells, increasing antigen uptake and expression of chemoattractants including CCL2. More recently, alternative delivery methods have been explored including intradermal administration that may enhance vaccine-induced responses (Koutsonanos et al. 2013). Despite these approaches, the induction of long-lasting antibody and B cell responses by influenza vaccination is still suboptimal but may be improved by additional understanding of the biology of antibody generation.

9 Avenues to Overcoming Strain-Specific Immunity to Influenza

In April 2009, a novel strain (influenza A/California/04/2009) emerged with a genome re-assorted from genetic segments originating in swine, avian, and human viruses (Novel Swine-Origin Influenza A (H1N1) Virus Investigation Team 2009). This spread rapidly causing a pandemic and emphasizing that antigen shift is capable of generating strains to which there is no herd immunity in spite of widespread vaccination and experience of serial influenza HA and NA antigens. Current vaccine manufacturing techniques cannot produce vaccines against newly emergent pandemic strains quickly enough. Therefore, an ideal vaccine would be able to induce broadly cross-protective immunity so that even highly divergent viruses with pandemic potential would be recognized by preexisting immunity. However, this remains an elusive goal.

It is commonly understood that cross-protective immune responses occur by recognition of conserved antigenic regions, which are restrained by their structure and/or function from significant divergence. Thus, most or all strains of a pathogen would possess these epitopes and an immune response directed against them would protect broadly. This is widely seen in T cell responses, where antigen processing of non-structural proteins such as nucleoprotein allows T cells to recognize conserved epitopes, although the clinical efficacy of vaccines seeking to induce these has not yet been proven (Powell et al. 2013).

Until recently, it was believed that antibodies capable of preventing influenza infection were universally directed against the globular head regions of HA and NA. These were thought to recognize highly glycosylated regions that had little restriction in terms of mutation and rapidly underwent antigenic drift. These epitopes would be easily accessible on the surface of the virion so these antibodies would be highly effective in neutralizing and opsonizing the virus but would be useless following antigenic change. However, it has become increasingly clear that relatively conserved regions in both the head and the stem of HA can represent targets for the induction of cross-reactive antibodies.

10 Broadly Cross-Reactive Stem-Binding Antibodies

In the early 1990s, Okuno et al. (1993) first described broadly cross-reactive antibodies in mice that recognized the relatively conserved HA stem. These were described as being able to neutralize virus infection but had no HAI activity, blocking virus entry rather than aggregating virus particles. However, their existence in humans remained unproven until the advent of high-throughput technologies. Such methods, including phage display and high-throughput screening of immortalized MBCs, have demonstrated broadly cross-reactive stem-binding antibodies in some individuals (Throsby et al. 2008; Ekiert et al. 2009; Sui et al. 2009; Corti et al. 2010). One monoclonal antibody (mAb) has even been found that can neutralize all known influenza A subtypes from both group 1 and group 2 (Corti et al. 2011). Usage of the heavy chain variable region gene VH1-69 is commonly over-represented and the structural mechanisms underlying this are being elucidated (Avnir et al. 2014) (Fig. 2). However, all found that broadly cross-reactive stem-binding antibodies existed at extremely low frequencies and did not exist in every individual. Their clinical relevance, especially since heterosubtypic immunity is not seen in the population, was therefore unclear.

Following natural infection with the pandemic A(H1N1)2009 virus, we were surprised to see that not only were these antibodies easily detectable but that in some patients they dominated the antibody response, making up over a third of HA-specific mAbs (Wrammert et al. 2011). These appeared to be similar antibodies to those described in other systems and demonstrated no HAI activity despite being able to bind and neutralize virus. All shared the VH1-69 gene usage and were cross-protective. Their preponderance following pandemic A(H1N1)2009 infection was attributed to the presence of the entirely novel HA head to which few memory responses were directed (Fig. 4). Instead, the relatively few MBCs that recognized

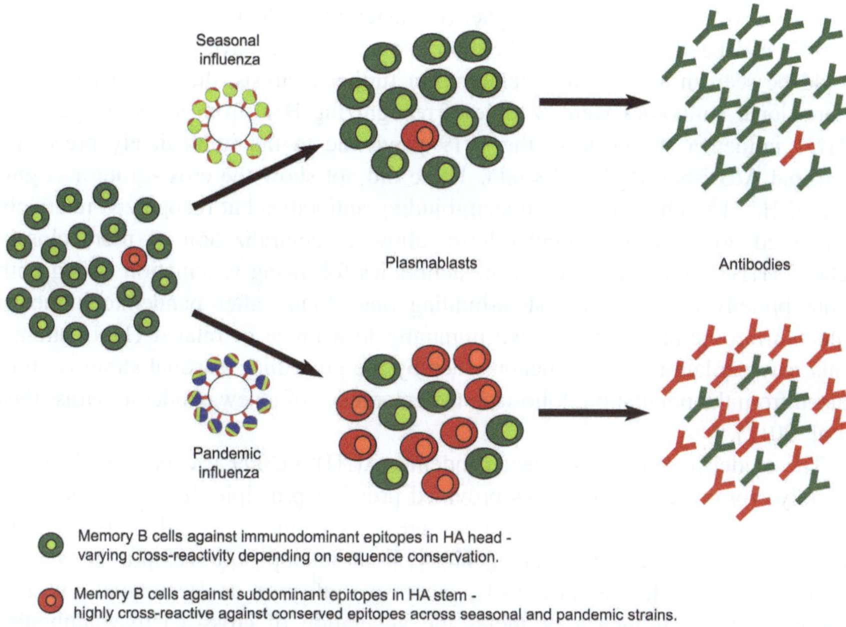

Fig. 4 The antibody response following exposure to seasonal versus pandemic influenza virus strains. All adults have influenza-specific memory B cells primarily recognizing epitopes from the HA head from recent seasonal strains (shown in *green*). Since these change relatively little year to year by antigenic drift, the same anti-head memory B cells are repeatedly boosted by infection or vaccination and come to dominate the repertoire. Memory B cells that recognize highly conserved epitopes in the head and stem (*red*) therefore remain in the minority. However, most of these previously immunodominant epitopes in the HA head are replaced in a pandemic strain (*blue*), leaving only the conserved epitopes in the stem and head. Cross-reactive memory B cells specific for these epitopes are therefore rapidly recruited into the response and come to dominate it. Naïve responses to the novel epitopes in the head are primed more slowly and therefore make a relatively small contribution to the new response. This figure was adapted from Li et al. (2012)

the HA stem (which displayed reactivity against the conserved but subdominant epitope) were preferentially stimulated and outgrew head-specific responses. In the context of seasonal influenza, this minority population would have a low probability of being recruited into the response, thus explaining the rarity of stem-binding antibodies in earlier analyses.

11 Cross-Reactive Antibody Responses to Vaccination and the "Universal" Influenza Vaccine

These antibodies were also seen following pandemic A(H1N1)2009 vaccination, albeit at lower frequencies (Li et al. 2012). Although broadly cross-reactive stem-binding antibodies were only found in a minority of individuals after immunization, they were still found at a much higher frequency than when pre-pandemic memory B cells had been screened. Furthermore, some cross-reactive antibody responses could be seen in almost all vaccinees. On further analysis, the majority of these monoclonal antibodies were capable of recognizing HAs from a diverse panel of H1N1 influenza strains from the 1919 pandemic to the immediately preceding seasonal A/Brisbane/59/2007 strain. These did not show the cross-group recognition of H3 HAs characteristic of stem-binding antibodies but recognized relatively conserved areas of the globular head, allowing neutralization of more closely related H1N1 strains only. Thus, the antibodies following vaccination (along with more broadly cross-reactive stem-binding ones found after pandemic influenza infection) conferred cross-reactive immunity to a range of related H1N1 strains. This may explain the phenomenon whereby the preceding seasonal strain is eliminated from the population, following the emergence of a new pandemic virus (Pica et al. 2012).

The evidence that monovalent pandemic A(H1N1)2009 vaccine could induce broadly cross-reactive antibodies provided proof of principle that these responses could be achieved. Several strategies are now being explored, coupled with improvements in vaccine immunogenicity, in an attempt to develop a "universal" influenza vaccine. In animal models, successive infection or vaccination with differing strains of influenza promotes the generation of cross-reactive antibodies (Wang et al. 2010; Wei et al. 2010). This has been achieved by sequential DNA vaccination of diverse H1 or H3 strains and recapitulates the events that occur when a pandemic strain emerges, with repeated stimulation of MBCs against the HA stem potentially allowing accumulation of these responses to a protective level. Alternatively, stem-specific responses may be encouraged by vaccinating against this region alone using novel stem-only immunogens without the interference that the HA head might cause (Steel et al. 2010).

12 Conclusion

The B cell response to influenza infection represents a complex multi-stage process that requires the coordination of many signals in several anatomical locations. In natural infection, this provides enduring immunity against the infecting strain. However, the antigenic variability of influenza overcomes this and natural immunity cannot confer heterotypic protection. While current vaccines seek to replicate some features of the natural immune response, these remain suboptimal. However, the recent discovery of the nature of broadly cross-reactive antibodies and the ways in which they can be induced offers renewed possibility of a "universal" vaccine that will do away with the need for annual re-vaccination.

References

Abt MC, Osborne LC, Monticelli LA et al (2012) Commensal bacteria calibrate the activation threshold of innate antiviral immunity. Immunity 37:158–170. doi:10.1016/j.immuni.2012.04.011

Ambrose CS, Levin MJ, Belshe RB (2011) The relative efficacy of trivalent live attenuated and inactivated influenza vaccines in children and adults. Influenza Other Respir Viruses 5:67–75. doi:10.1111/j.1750-2659.2010.00183.x

Asahi Y, Yoshikawa T, Watanabe I et al (2002) Protection against influenza virus infection in polymeric Ig receptor knockout mice immunized intranasally with adjuvant-combined vaccines. J Immunol 168:2930–2938. doi:10.4049/jimmunol.168.6.2930

Asahi-Ozaki Y, Yoshikawa T, Iwakura Y et al (2004) Secretory IgA antibodies provide cross-protection against infection with different strains of influenza B virus. J Med Virol 74:328–335. doi:10.1002/jmv.20173

Avnir Y, Tallarico AS, Zhu Q et al (2014) Molecular signatures of hemagglutinin stem-directed heterosubtypic human neutralizing antibodies against influenza A viruses. PLoS Pathog 10: e1004103. doi:10.1371/journal.ppat.1004103

Batista FD, Harwood NE (2009) The who, how and where of antigen presentation to B cells. Nat Rev Immunol 9:15–27. doi:10.1038/nri2454

Baumgarth N, Choi YS, Rothaeusler K et al (2008) B cell lineage contributions to antiviral host responses. Curr Top Microbiol Immunol 319:41–61

Belshe R, Mendelman P, Treanor J et al (1998) The efficacy of live attenuated, cold-adapted, trivalent, intranasal influenzavirus vaccine in children. N Engl J Med 338:1405–1412

Bernasconi NL, Onai N, Lanzavecchia A (2003) A role for Toll-like receptors in acquired immunity: up-regulation of TLR9 by BCR triggering in naive B cells and constitutive expression in memory B cells. Blood 101:4500–4504. doi:10.1182/blood-2002-11-3569

Black S, Nicolay U, Vesikari T et al (2011) Hemagglutination inhibition antibody titers as a correlate of protection for inactivated influenza vaccines in children: Pediatr Infect Dis J 30:1081–1085. doi:10.1097/INF.0b013e3182367662

Boyden AW, Legge KL, Waldschmidt TJ (2012) Pulmonary infection with influenza A virus induces site-specific germinal center and T follicular helper cell responses. PLoS ONE 7: e40733. doi:10.1371/journal.pone.0040733

Cao RG, Suarez NM, Obermoser G et al (2014) Differences in antibody responses between trivalent inactivated influenza vaccine and live attenuated influenza vaccine correlate with the kinetics and magnitude of interferon signaling in children. J Infect Dis jiu079. doi:10.1093/infdis/jiu079

Caton AJ, Brownlee GG, Yewdell JW, Gerhard W (1982) The antigenic structure of the influenza virus A/PR/8/34 hemagglutinin (H1 subtype). Cell 31:417–427. doi:10.1016/0092-8674(82)90135-0

Chen WH, Cross AS, Edelman R et al (2011) Antibody and Th1-type cell-mediated immune responses in elderly and young adults immunized with the standard or a high dose influenza vaccine. Vaccine 29:2865–2873. doi:10.1016/j.vaccine.2011.02.017

Choi S-M, Xie H, Campbell AP et al (2012) Influenza viral RNA detection in blood as a marker to predict disease severity in hematopoietic cell transplant recipients. J Infect Dis 206:1872–1877. doi:10.1093/infdis/jis610

Choi YS, Baumgarth N (2008) Dual role for B-1a cells in immunity to influenza virus infection. J Exp Med 205:3053–3064. doi:10.1084/jem.20080979

Chu VT, Berek C (2013) The establishment of the plasma cell survival niche in the bone marrow. Immunol Rev 251:177–188. doi:10.1111/imr.12011

Corti D, Suguitan AL, Pinna D et al (2010) Heterosubtypic neutralizing antibodies are produced by individuals immunized with a seasonal influenza vaccine. J Clin Invest 120:1663–1673. doi:10.1172/JCI41902 (41902 [pii])

Corti D, Voss J, Gamblin SJ et al (2011) A neutralizing antibody selected from plasma cells that binds to Group 1 and Group 2 influenza A hemagglutinins. Science. doi:10.1126/science.1205669 (science.1205669 [pii])

Couch RB, Kasel JA (1983) Immunity to influenza in man. Annu Rev Microbiol 37:529–549. doi:10.1146/annurev.mi.37.100183.002525

Ekiert DC, Bhabha G, Elsliger MA et al (2009) Antibody recognition of a highly conserved influenza virus epitope. Science 324:246–251. doi:10.1126/science.1171491 (1171491 [pii])

Fields BN, Knipe DM, Howley PM (2007) Fields' virology, 5th edn. Knipe DM, Howley PM (editors-in-chief), Griffin DE (et al) (associate editors). Wolters Kluwer/Lippincott Williams & Wilkins, Philadelphia

Fink K (2012) Origin and function of circulating plasmablasts during acute viral infections. Front Immunol. doi:10.3389/fimmu.2012.00078

Garside P, Ingulli E, Merica R et al (1998) Visualization of specific B and T lymphocyte interactions in the lymph node. Science 281:96–99

Gerhard W, Mozdzanowska K, Furchner M et al (1997) Role of the B-cell response in recovery of mice from primary influenza virus infection. Immunol Rev 159:95–103

GeurtsvanKessel CH, Willart MAM, Bergen IM et al (2009) Dendritic cells are crucial for maintenance of tertiary lymphoid structures in the lung of influenza virus–infected mice. J Exp Med 206:2339–2349. doi:10.1084/jem.20090410

Grund S, Adams O, Wählisch S, Schweiger B (2011) Comparison of hemagglutination inhibition assay, an ELISA-based micro-neutralization assay and colorimetric microneutralization assay to detect antibody responses to vaccination against influenza A H1N1 2009 virus. J Virol Methods 171:369–373. doi:10.1016/j.jviromet.2010.11.024

Guihot A, Luyt C-E, Parrot A et al (2014) Low titers of serum antibodies inhibiting hemagglutination predict fatal fulminant influenza A(H1N1) 2009 infection. Am J Respir Crit Care Med. doi:10.1164/rccm.201311-2071OC

Haq K, McElhaney JE (2014) Immunosenescence: influenza vaccination and the elderly. Curr Opin Immunol 29:38–42. doi:10.1016/j.coi.2014.03.008

Henle W, Stokes Jr J, Shaw DR (1941) Passive immunization of mice against human influenza virus by the intranasal route. J Immunol 40:201–212

Hoft DF, Babusis E, Worku S et al (2011) Live and inactivated influenza vaccines induce similar humoral responses, but only live vaccines induce diverse T-Cell responses in young children. J Infect Dis 204:845–853. doi:10.1093/infdis/jir436

Huang K-YA, Li CK-F, Clutterbuck E et al (2014) Virus-specific antibody secreting cell, memory B-cell, and sero-antibody responses in the human influenza challenge model. J Infect Dis jit650. doi:10.1093/infdis/jit650

Jones PD, Ada GL (1986) Influenza virus-specific antibody-secreting cells in the murine lung during primary influenza virus infection. J Virol 60:614–619

King C, Tangye SG, Mackay CR (2008) T follicular helper (TFH) cells in normal and dysregulated immune responses. Annu Rev Immunol 26:741–766

Koutsonanos DG, Compans RW, Skountzou I (2013) Targeting the Skin for microneedle delivery of influenza vaccine. In: Katsikis PD, Schoenberger SP, Pulendran B (eds) Crossroads between innate and adaptive immunity IV. Springer, New York, pp 121–132

Kunisawa J, Nochi T, Kiyono H (2008) Immunological commonalities and distinctions between airway and digestive immunity. Trends Immunol 29:505–513. doi:10.1016/j.it.2008.07.008

Lee FE-H, Halliley JL, Walsh EE et al (2011) Circulating human antibody-secreting cells during vaccinations and respiratory viral infections are characterized by high specificity and lack of bystander effect. J Immunol 186:5514–5521. doi:10.4049/jimmunol.1002932

Li G-M, Chiu C, Wrammert J et al (2012) Pandemic H1N1 influenza vaccine induces a recall response in humans that favors broadly cross-reactive memory B cells. Proc Natl Acad Sci 109:9047–9052. doi:10.1073/pnas.1118979109

Liang B, Hyland L, Hou S (2001) Nasal-associated lymphoid tissue is a site of long-term virus-specific antibody production following respiratory virus infection of mice. J Virol 75:5416–5420. doi:10.1128/JVI.75.11.5416-5420.2001

McHeyzer-Williams LJ, Driver DJ, McHeyzer-Williams MG (2001) Germinal center reaction. Curr Opin Hematol 8:52–59

McHeyzer-Williams M, Okitsu S, Wang N, McHeyzer-Williams L (2012) Molecular programming of B cell memory. Nat Rev Immunol 12:24–34. doi:10.1038/nri3128

Mitnaul LJ, Matrosovich MN, Castrucci MR et al (2000) Balanced hemagglutinin and neuraminidase activities are critical for efficient replication of influenza A virus. J Virol 74:6015–6020

Moyron-Quiroz JE, Rangel-Moreno J, Hartson L et al (2006) Persistence and responsiveness of immunologic memory in the absence of secondary lymphoid organs. Immunity 25:643–654. doi:10.1016/j.immuni.2006.08.022

Moyron-Quiroz JE, Rangel-Moreno J, Kusser K et al (2004) Role of inducible bronchus associated lymphoid tissue (iBALT) in respiratory immunity. Nat Med 10:927–934. doi:10.1038/nm1091

Nichol KL, Nordin JD, Nelson DB et al (2007) Effectiveness of influenza vaccine in the community-Dwelling Elderly. N Engl J Med 357:1373–1381. doi:10.1056/NEJMoa070844

Novel Swine-Origin Influenza A (H1N1) Virus Investigation Team et al (2009) Emergence of a novel swine-origin influenza A (H1N1) virus in humans. N Engl J Med 360:2605–2615. doi:10.1056/NEJMoa0903810

O'Hagan DT, Wack A, Podda A (2007) MF59 is a safe and potent vaccine adjuvant for flu vaccines in humans: what did we learn during its development? Clin Pharmacol Ther 82:740–744. doi:10.1038/sj.clpt.6100402

Ohmit SE, Petrie JG, Cross RT et al (2011) Influenza hemagglutination-inhibition antibody titer as a correlate of vaccine-induced protection. J Infect Dis 204:1879–1885

Okuno Y, Isegawa Y, Sasao F, Ueda S (1993) A common neutralizing epitope conserved between the hemagglutinins of influenza A virus H1 and H2 strains. J Virol 67:2552–2558

Pabst O (2012) New concepts in the generation and functions of IgA. Nat Rev Immunol 12:821–832. doi:10.1038/nri3322

Pape KA, Catron DM, Itano AA, Jenkins MK (2007) The humoral immune response is initiated in lymph nodes by B cells that acquire soluble antigen directly in the follicles. Immunity 26:491–502. doi:10.1016/j.immuni.2007.02.011

Pica N, Hai R, Krammer F et al (2012) Hemagglutinin stalk antibodies elicited by the 2009 pandemic influenza virus as a mechanism for the extinction of seasonal H1N1 viruses. Proc Natl Acad Sci 109:2573–2578. doi:10.1073/pnas.1200039109

Powell TJ, Peng Y, Berthoud TK et al (2013) Examination of influenza specific T cell responses after influenza virus challenge in individuals vaccinated with MVA-NP+M1 vaccine. PLoS ONE 8:e62778. doi:10.1371/journal.pone.0062778

Sangster MY, Riberdy JM, Gonzalez M et al (2003) An early CD4+ T cell–dependent immunoglobulin a response to influenza infection in the absence of key cognate T–B interactions. J Exp Med 198:1011–1021. doi:10.1084/jem.20021745

Sasaki S, Holmes TH, Albrecht RA et al (2014) Distinct cross-reactive B-cell responses to live attenuated and inactivated influenza vaccines. J Infect Dis jiu190. doi:10.1093/infdis/jiu190

Sasaki S, Jaimes MC, Holmes TH et al (2007) Comparison of the influenza virus-specific effector and memory B-cell responses to immunization of children and adults with live attenuated or inactivated influenza virus vaccines. J Virol 81:215–228. doi:10.1128/JVI.01957-06

Sasaki S, Sullivan M, Narvaez CF et al (2011) Limited efficacy of inactivated influenza vaccine in elderly individuals is associated with decreased production of vaccine-specific antibodies. J Clin Invest 121:3109–3119. doi:10.1172/JCI57834

Shaffer AL, Lin KI, Kuo TC et al (2002) Blimp-1 orchestrates plasma cell differentiation by extinguishing the mature B cell gene expression program. Immunity 17:51–62

Skehel JJ, Wiley DC (2000) Receptor binding and membrane fusion in virus entry: the influenza hemagglutinin. Annu Rev Biochem 69:531–569. doi:10.1146/annurev.biochem.69.1.531

Steel J, Lowen AC, T Wang T et al (2010) Influenza virus vaccine based on the conserved hemagglutinin stalk domain. MBio. doi:10.1128/mBio.00018-10

Stephenson I, Heath A, Major D et al (2009) Reproducibility of serologic assays for influenza virus A (H5N1). Emerg Infect Dis 15:1250–1259. doi:10.3201/eid1508.081754

Sui J, Hwang WC, Perez S et al (2009) Structural and functional bases for broad-spectrum neutralization of avian and human influenza A viruses. Nat Struct Mol Biol 16:265–273

Tamura S-I, Funato H, Hirabayashi Y et al (1991) Cross-protection against influenza A virus infection by passively transferred respiratory tract IgA antibodies to different hemagglutinin molecules. Eur J Immunol 21:1337–1344. doi:10.1002/eji.1830210602

Thompson CI, Barclay WS, Zambon MC, Pickles RJ (2006) Infection of human airway epithelium by human and avian strains of influenza A virus. J Virol 80:8060–8068. doi:10.1128/JVI.00384-06

Throsby M, van den Brink E, Jongeneelen M et al (2008) Heterosubtypic neutralizing monoclonal antibodies cross-protective against H5N1 and H1N1 recovered from human IgM+ memory B cells. PLoS One 3:e3942. doi:10.1371/journal.pone.0003942

Tricco AC, Chit A, Soobiah C et al (2013) Comparing influenza vaccine efficacy against mismatched and matched strains: a systematic review and meta-analysis. BMC Med 11:153. doi:10.1186/1741-7015-11-153

Van Riet E, Ainai A, Suzuki T, Hasegawa H (2012) Mucosal IgA responses in influenza virus infections; thoughts for vaccine design. Vaccine 30:5893–5900. doi:10.1016/j.vaccine.2012.04.109

Wang TT, Tan GS, Hai R et al (2010) Broadly protective monoclonal antibodies against H3 influenza viruses following sequential immunization with different hemagglutinins. PLoS Pathog 6:e1000796. doi:10.1371/journal.ppat.1000796

Wei CJ, Boyington JC, McTamney PM et al (2010) Induction of broadly neutralizing H1N1 influenza antibodies by vaccination. Science 329:1060–1064. doi:10.1126/science.1192517 (science.1192517 [pii])

Wrammert J, Koutsonanos D, Li G-M et al (2011) Broadly cross-reactive antibodies dominate the human B cell response against 2009 pandemic H1N1 influenza virus infection. J Exp Med 208:181–193. doi:10.1084/jem.20101352

Wright PF, Sannella E, Shi JR et al (2008) Antibody responses after inactivated influenza vaccine in young children. Pediatr Infect Dis J 27:1004–1008. doi:10.1097/INF.0b013e31817d53c5

Yen H-L, Aldridge JR, Boon ACM et al (2009) Changes in H5N1 influenza virus hemagglutinin receptor binding domain affect systemic spread. Proc Natl Acad Sci 106:286–291. doi:10.1073/pnas.0811052106

Yewdell JW, Webster RG, Gerhard WU (1979) Antigenic variation in three distinct determinants of an influenza type A haemagglutinin molecule. Nature 279:246–248

Zaman K, Roy E, Arifeen SE et al (2008) Effectiveness of maternal influenza immunization in mothers and infants. N Engl J Med 359:1555–1564. doi:10.1056/NEJMoa0708630

Zinkernagel RM (2001) Maternal antibodies, childhood infections, and autoimmune diseases. N Engl J Med 345:1331–1335. doi:10.1056/NEJMra012493

Memory CD4 T Cells in Influenza

Kyra D. Zens and Donna L. Farber

Abstract Influenza A virus is a significant cause of morbidity and mortality worldwide, particularly among young children and the elderly. Current vaccines induce neutralizing antibody responses directed toward highly variable viral surface proteins, resulting in limited heterosubtypic protection to new viral serotypes. By contrast, memory CD4 T cells recognize conserved viral proteins and are cross-reactive to multiple influenza strains. In humans, virus-specific memory CD4 T cells were found to be the protective correlate in human influenza challenge studies, suggesting their key role in protective immunity. In mouse models, memory CD4 T cells can mediate protective responses to secondary influenza infection independent of B cells or CD8 T cells, and can influence innate immune responses. Importantly, a newly defined, tissue-resident CD4 memory population has been demonstrated to be retained in lung tissue and promote optimal protective responses to an influenza infection. Here, we review the current state of results regarding the generation of memory CD4 T cells following primary influenza infection, mechanisms for their enhanced efficacy in protection from secondary challenge including their phenotype, localization, and function in the context of both mouse models and human infection. We also discuss the generation of memory CD4 T cells in response to influenza vaccines and its future implications for vaccinology.

K.D. Zens · D.L. Farber
Columbia Center for Translational Immunology, Columbia University Medical Center, 650 West 168th Street, BB15, New York, NY 10032, USA

K.D. Zens · D.L. Farber (✉)
Department of Microbiology and Immunology, Columbia University Medical Center, 650 West 168th Street, BB15, New York, NY 10032, USA
e-mail: df2396@cumc.columbia.edu

D.L. Farber
Department of Surgery, Columbia University Medical Center, 650 West 168th Street, BB15, New York, NY 10032, USA

Current Topics in Microbiology and Immunology (2015) 386: 399–421
DOI: 10.1007/82_2014_401

Published Online: 9 July 2014

Contents

1 Introduction

Infection with Influenza A viruses results in moderate to severe acute respiratory illness and is a significant cause of morbidity and mortality worldwide, particularly in children under 5 and adults over 65 (Thompson et al. 2006). In addition, the annual economic burden associated with influenza infection in the United States is more than $85 billion dollars (Molinari et al. 2007). Although vaccines for influenza are available, due to many factors including variations in influenza strains and variable induction of protective immune responses in vaccine recipients, current vaccines are not completely protective against infections with seasonal strains and are ineffective at protecting against emerging new or pandemic strains (Osterholm et al. 2012). Therefore, identifying the immune mechanisms underlying the host response to infection is a priority in the rational design of future vaccines and therapeutics for influenza.

Current influenza vaccines promote protective immunity to infection through the generation of neutralizing antibody responses to hemagglutinin (HA) and neuraminidase (NA) viral surface glycoproteins. Due to a combination of antigenic drift and shift, HA and NA proteins exhibit profound variations in protein sequences and antigenicity in different influenza strains. As a result, antibody responses typically provide limited cross-protection against new viral serotypes, leading to the requirement for new vaccine formulations annually. Immunity that is cross-protective between influenza strains expressing distinct HA and NA serotypes is termed heterosubtypic immunity. Importantly, CD4 and CD8 memory T cells generated following influenza infection have been demonstrated to mediate heterosubtypic immune responses to distinct viral strains via the targeting of conserved viral proteins (Liang et al. 1994; Epstein et al. 1997; Woodland et al. 2001). Thus, the targeted generation of virus-specific memory T cell responses by vaccines could represent a way to achieve durable, cross-protective immunity to influenza.

Both CD4 and CD8 T cells play important roles in the adaptive immune response to influenza infection. However, in contrast to CD8 T cells, which are limited to cytotoxic killing of virally-infected cells, CD4 T cells play much more diverse roles in response to infection. Effector CD4 cells are capable of providing help necessary for both CD8 T cells and B cells to achieve their full functional potential, as well as mediating direct effector functions through cytolysis of influenza-infected cells. Following influenza infection, virus-specific CD4 T cells are maintained as long-lived memory populations with an enhanced capacity to protect against secondary infection, due to their ability to respond more rapidly and robustly upon antigen encounter. In addition, in contrast to naïve cells, which remain in lymphoid tissues, memory cells localize at peripheral sites, poised to respond to secondary challenges at the site of infection. In mouse models of influenza infection, memory CD4 T cells have been shown to mediate protective responses independently of B and CD8 T cells (Teijaro et al. 2010). Additionally, CD4 memory T cell responses are the protective correlate in vivo in human influenza challenge studies (Wilkinson et al. 2012). Furthermore, that memory CD4 T cells can be cross reactive to multiple influenza strains (Lee et al. 2008; Richards et al. 2010) makes them an attractive target for vaccine development strategies. In this review we discuss the general properties of memory CD4 T cells, including their generation, phenotype, localization and function in the context of influenza infection in both mouse models and humans. We will also discuss how tissue distribution influences T cell-mediated protection and how the generation of tissue-targeted memory CD4 T cells is a potentially robust strategy for promoting protection from influenza infections.

2 Primary CD4 T Cell Responses to Influenza Infection

The generation of memory CD4 T cells following exposure to influenza begins with the activation of naïve CD4 T cells. Influenza infection is confined to the lung, and primary replication takes place within the epithelial cells of the respiratory tract expressing α (2,6) sialic acid linked membrane glycoproteins (Couceiro et al. 1993). During primary exposure, respiratory epithelial cells within the lung become infected and release inflammatory cytokines and chemokines including tumor necrosis factor-α (TNF-α), type-I interferons (IFN), interleukin-6 (IL-6), IFN-γ-inducible protein-10 (IP-10), and monocyte chemoattractant protein-1 (MCP-1, also known as CCL2), which in turn recruit innate immune effectors and antigen presenting cells (APCs) to the site of infection (Sanders et al. 2010). Within the infected lung, dendritic cells (DCs) take up viral particles and influenza-derived antigens, which trigger DC activation, maturation, and migration from the lung to the draining mediastinal lymph node (MLN) (Fig. 1a).

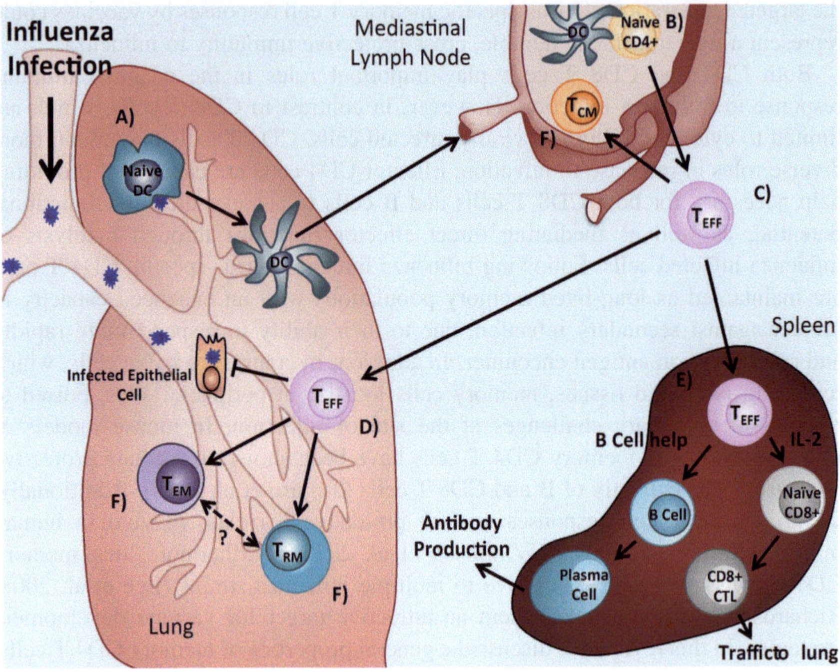

Fig. 1 Overview of the primary CD4 T cell response and memory generation following an influenza infection. **a** Following influenza infection, naïve DCs in the lung take up virus and virally-derived particles, driving their maturation and migration to the lung-draining lymph node. **b** Mature, activated DCs activate influenza-specific naïve CD4 T cells trafficking through the lymph nodes. **c** CD4 effector cells traffic to the lung and can also reach the spleen via the circulation. **d** Effectors in the lung secrete effector cytokines and directly lyse virally-infected epithelial cells. **e** CD4 effectors also activate B cells and CD8 T cells in lymphoid tissues, allowing them to assume effector functions. **f** Responding effectors are retained as long-lived memory populations at diverse sites

Mature naïve T cells express lymphoid homing receptors, including CD62L (also known as L-selectin) and CCR7, which direct their migration and entry into secondary lymphoid tissues. Here, influenza-specific naïve CD4 T cells interact with mature DCs bearing viral antigens and are activated (Fig. 1b). Newly activated T cells proliferate and begin to acquire effector functions, including the ability to produce effector cytokines which direct other immune functions. It is well established that the cytokine environment promotes the differentiation of activated CD4 T cells into different types of effector T helper (Th) cells, with Th1, Th2, Th17, T follicular helper (Tfh) and T regulatory (Treg) subsets being the most well-characterized (O'Shea and Paul 2010). Influenza infection is generally associated with Th1-type responses producing IFN-γ along with TNF-α and IL-2, as well as a robust antibody response (Gerhard et al. 1997), involving Tfh and Th2-type CD4 effector cells.

Concomitant with effector differentiation, activated T cells alter the expression of homing molecules, allowing them to migrate from the lymph nodes to peripheral tissues, such as the lung, during influenza infection (Fig. 1c). These changes include downregulation of CD62L and CCR7 and upregulation of the adhesion molecule CD44 and the integrin lymphocyte function-associated antigen-1 (LFA-1, a dimer of CD11a and CD18). Peak levels of activated CD4 effector T cells in the lung are reached 10–15 days post influenza infection (Fig. 1d). Here, virus-specific CD4 cells secrete effector cytokines and a subset of these cells can also direct cytolysis of virally infected cells. Effector CD4 T cells also play roles in the activation and maturation of virus-specific B and CD8 T cells necessary for clearance of primary influenza infection in the lung-draining lymph nodes and the spleen (Fig. 1e).

3 Generation of Memory CD4 T Cells in Influenza Infection

Following resolution of primary infection, a subset of these responding virus-specific CD4 T cells are retained as long-lived memory T cells which can persist for the life of the animal, conveying protective immunity upon secondary pathogen encounter (Fig. 1f). Mechanisms underlying the transition from primary effectors to memory T cells have been an area of intense study, although this process remains incompletely understood (for reviews, see Kaech et al. 2002; Sallusto et al. 2004; Kaech and Wherry 2007). In the context of influenza infection, roles for antigen persistence and cytokine signaling in memory CD4 T cell generation have been specifically investigated.

During primary influenza infection in mouse models, the virus is cleared between 7 and 10 days post infection (Allan et al. 1990). However, viral antigens have been found to persist up to 28 days post infection (Jelley-Gibbs et al. 2005; Zammit et al. 2006). Importantly, the level of antigenic stimulation during infection has been shown to influence the development of memory CD4 T cells. Transfer of naïve CD4 T cells into hosts infected with influenza during acute infection or weeks following viral clearance resulted in both transferred populations converting to memory CD4 T cells (Jelley-Gibbs et al. 2005). Interestingly, transfer of naive CD4 T cells during early phases of infection resulted in robust expansion and effector generation, with only a small fraction persisting as memory T cells, while transfer of naive CD4 T cells during later phases of infection resulted in modest expansion of intermediately activated effectors, which were more efficiently maintained as memory cells (Jelley-Gibbs et al. 2005). Moreover, the acquisition of effector functions per se, may not be necessary for the generation of memory CD4 T cells, as populations of influenza-specific CD4 T cells primed for short periods of time and lacking effector function were still able to develop into memory cells (Moulton et al. 2006).

Memory CD4 T cells may require cognate TCR signals for their maintenance, as long-term functional maintenance of CD4 memory T cells requires MHC class II expression (Kassiotis et al. 2002; De Riva et al. 2007) and additional TCR stimulation (Seddon et al. 2003; Bushar et al. 2010). Together, these findings provide evidence for a key role of TCR stimulation at different phases of memory CD4 T cell development.

Another key factor required for memory CD4 T cell generation is the presence of homeostatic and survival cytokines such as IL-7 and IL-15. Naïve CD4 and CD8 T cells express IL-7R which is required for their survival and homeostatic proliferation (Rathmell et al. 2001; Tan et al. 2001). After T cell activation, IL-7R is downregulated; however, IL-7R is again expressed at high levels on memory CD4 and CD8 cells (Kaech et al. 2003; Huster et al. 2004). In CD8 T cells, both IL-7 and IL-15 signaling have been shown to contribute to memory formation. Memory CD8 precursor populations can be identified by high expression of IL-7R and low expression of the co-inhibitory receptor killer cell lectin-like receptor G1 (KLRG1) (Kaech et al. 2003; Joshi et al. 2007). As of yet, analogous memory CD4 T cell precursor markers have not yet been identified. However, IL-7 signaling does appear to be necessary for the transition from effector to memory in CD4 cells in an influenza infection model, as memory CD4 cells fail to develop in IL-7-deficient hosts (Li et al. 2003). Roles for IL-15 and continued IL-7 signaling in the long-term survival and homeostatic proliferation CD4 memory T cells have also been described (Kondrack et al. 2003; Li et al. 2003; Lenz et al. 2004; Purton et al. 2007). Together, these findings indicate roles for both TCR and cytokine signals in memory CD4 T cell persistence.

4 Heterogeneity of Memory CD4 T Cells

4.1 Circulating Central and Effector Memory Subsets

Memory CD4 T cells are a heterogeneous population in terms of phenotype, function and localization (Table 1). Like effector T cells, all memory CD4 T cells retain high-level expression of CD44 and human cells generally continue to express the CD45RO isoform. However, memory T cells are heterogeneous in their expression of CD62L and CCR7 which lead to the delineation of two memory subsets: $CD62L^{+}/CCR7^{+}$ lymphoid homing, central memory (Tcm); and $CD62L^{-}/CCR7^{-}$ effector memory (Tem) cells present in peripheral tissues (Sallusto et al. 1999; Masopust et al. 2001). The lymphoid versus peripheral tissue homing properties of these subsets have been confirmed for mouse memory CD4 T cells (Reinhardt et al. 2001) and specifically in the context of influenza infection (Ahmadzadeh and Farber 2002; Bingaman et al. 2005). Following influenza infection, virus-specific CD4 Tem are more predominant in peripheral tissues, including the lungs and CD4 Tcm are more predominant in the lymph nodes. Both populations are present in the spleen (Bingaman et al. 2005). Influenza-specific

Table 1 Phenotype of naïve, effector, and memory CD4 T subsets

Property	Naïve	Effector	Tcm	Tem	Trm
CD44	Low	High	Intermediate	High	High
CD62L	High	Low	High	Low	Low
CCR7	High	Low	High	Low	Low
CD45 Isoform (Humans Only)	CD45RA	CD45RO	CD45RO	CD45RO/ CD45RA (Temra)	CD45RO
CD69	Low	High	Low	Low	High
CD103	–	–	–	–	–[a]
Migratory properties	Lymphoid tissues, circulation	Peripheral tissues	Lymphoid tissues	Peripheral tissues	Resident in peripheral tissue

[a] Present in CD8 Trm

CD4 Tem and Tcm from the spleen are capable of producing IL-2 and effector cytokines after stimulation, while the proliferative capacity of Tcm is slightly greater than the Tem subset (Bingaman et al. 2005).

4.2 Tissue Resident Memory Subsets

In addition to Tem and Tcm subsets, a distinct population of non-circulating CD4 memory T cells has been identified to persist in the lung long-term after infection. These lung-resident memory CD4 T cells are analogous to populations of non-circulating memory CD8 T cells, designated tissue-resident memory T cells (Trm), that have been found to persist long-term in peripheral tissues including the brain, skin, gut and lung (Gebhardt et al. 2009; Liu et al. 2010; Masopust et al. 2010; Wakim et al. 2012; Wu et al. 2013). Phenotypically, CD4 Trm can be distinguished from circulating Tem and Tcm by upregulated CD69 and CD11a expression (Teijaro et al. 2011; Turner et al. 2013). CD8 Trm also express CD69 as well as the integrin CD103, the alpha chain of the $\alpha E\beta 7$ integrin (Mueller et al. 2013), which is not significantly upregulated by CD4 Trm (Sathaliyawala et al. 2013).

In contrast to Tem and Tcm populations, which circulate throughout the peripheral and secondary lymphoid tissues, respectively, recent studies have highlighted the tissue-specific nature of the Trm subset. In mouse models of influenza infection, a population of virus-specific CD4 Trm persists in the lungs for long periods following infection (Teijaro et al. 2011). When lung CD4 Trm are transferred to secondary recipients, they preferentially recirculate back to the lungs, suggesting that this subset has an intrinsic mechanism for specific homing and/or retention in the lung (Teijaro et al. 2011). Influenza-specific CD4 and CD8 Trm populations have also been identified in human lung tissue (Lee et al. 2011; Piet et al. 2011; Sathaliyawala et al. 2013; Turner et al. 2013).

The tissue-specific localization of Trm T cells seems to be dependent on the site of infection. In humans, influenza-specific CD8 T cells were only found within the lung Trm subset while memory CD8 T cells specific for the systemic virus Cytomegalovirus (CMV) were distributed in both lung and spleen (de Bree et al. 2005; Turner et al. 2013). In another study, lung-derived CD4 Trm, but not CD4 cells derived from skin or blood, responded to stimulation with influenza virus, further supporting the site-specific localization of this population (Purwar et al. 2011).

Studies have demonstrated the functional importance of lung-resident CD4 Trm populations in mediating optimal protection from reinfection with respiratory pathogens and, more specifically, from influenza infection (Hogan et al. 2001; Teijaro et al. 2011). Functional studies of lung-derived CD4 Trm have demonstrated that these cells rapidly acquire effector functions and respond vigorously to a secondary stimulation with influenza virus (Purwar et al. 2011; Turner et al. 2013). Importantly, in an influenza infection model, lung-resident HA-specific memory CD4 T cells mediated enhanced viral clearance and survival to lethal influenza infection when transferred to secondary recipients, whereas spleen-derived HA-specific memory CD4 T cells did not confer significant protection (Teijaro et al. 2011).

5 Mechanisms for Tissue Trafficking and Retention

An important question with potential applications in vaccine design is how the homing and retention of activated effector and memory T cell populations occur. Currently, the mechanisms mediating lung trafficking and retention in activated and memory T cells are incompletely understood. However, the process can be delineated into three steps: imprinting, homing, and retention, as schematically outlined in Fig. 2.

Imprinting Imprinting is a process by which DCs in the tissue-draining lymph nodes induce the expression of chemokine receptors and integrins and drive tissue-specific homing of activated T cells (Fig. 2a). Imprinting of skin and gut tissue-homing CD4 T cells has been demonstrated in several studies (Mora et al. 2003, 2005; Dudda et al. 2004). Recently, T cell migration to the lung during influenza infection was shown to be mediated by CCR4 expression, driven by lung DCs (Mikhak et al. 2013). CCR4 binds the chemokine ligands MCP-1 and RANTES (also known as CCL5), which are expressed by infected epithelial cells in the lung during influenza infection (Matsukura et al. 1998; Julkunen et al. 2000), and MIP-1α (also known as CCL3), which is also expressed in influenza infection and is necessary for normal viral clearance (Cook et al. 1995; Sprenger et al. 1996). Importantly, lung DC-imprinted T cells protected against influenza more effectively than gut or skin DC-imprinted T cells. However, another study found that intranasal immunization with *Salmonella typhimurium*-derived antigens resulted in the

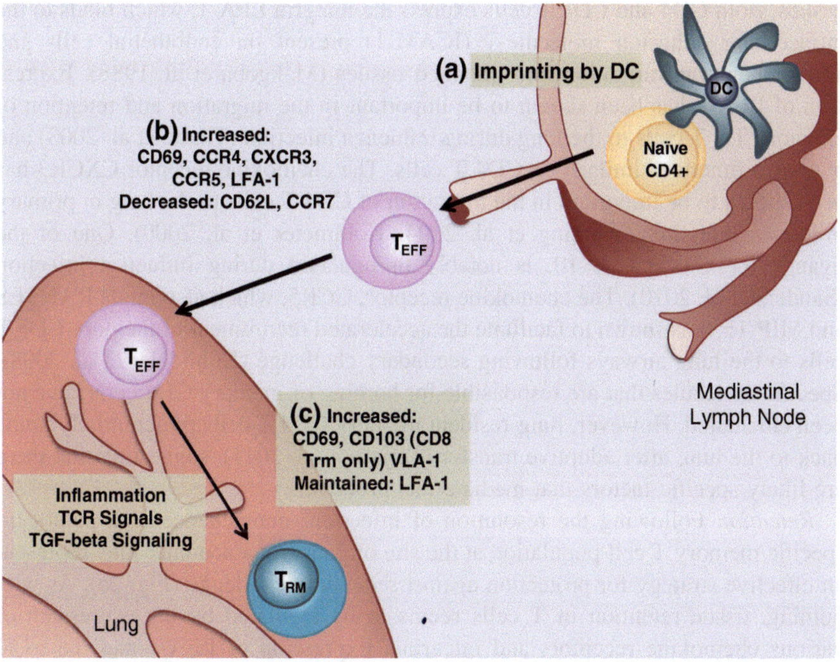

Fig. 2 DC imprinting, tissue homing, and tissue retention in effector and memory CD4 T cells. **a** Following influenza infection, naïve CD4 T cells are activated in the lung-draining lymph node by lung-derived DCs which also imprint homing receptor expression, allowing T cells to traffic to the lung. **b** Newly activated effectors reduce expression of CD62L and CCR7, allowing egress from the lymph node. In addition, lung homing molecules including CCR4, CXCR3, CCR5 and LFA-1 are upregulated, allowing cells to traffic to the lung by following a chemokine gradient. Integrins, such as LFA-1, facilitate tissue entry. **c** Activated effectors remain in the lung via expression of integrins, including LFA-1 and VLA-1. Factors such as inflammation and TCR signaling may trigger an increased expression of CD69, though it is not clear. Expression of CD103 by CD8 Trm is triggered by TGF-β signaling

generation of gut-homing T cells, suggesting that imprinting in the draining lymph node is not the only factor responsible for T cell tissue homing (Ruane et al. 2013). Other factors, such as inflammation or the presence of various pathogen-associated molecular patterns (PAMPs) during DC activation, may also influence this process.

Homing In the context of infection, tissue homing refers to the trafficking of antigen-specific T cells to inflamed peripheral tissues. This process depends on expression of chemokine receptors and integrins by T cells, which promote their chemokine-directed migration and transmigration into inflamed tissues, respectively. The expression of tissue-homing molecules likely depends on the site and type of infection, and is driven, at least in part, by DC imprinting. During influenza infection, several molecules have been implicated in the trafficking of activated T cells to the lung (Fig. 2b). After initial infection, downregulation of CD62L and CCR7 allows activated T cells to exit the lymph nodes and traffic to the peripherial tissues. Both CD4 and CD8 T cells express the integrin LFA-1, which binds to the intracellular adhesion molecule-1 (ICAM-1) present on endothelial cells and allows their transmigration into inflamed tissues (Makgoba et al. 1988). Expression of LFA-1 has been shown to be important in the migration and retention of effector CD8 T cells to the lung during influenza infection (Thatte et al. 2003) and may also function similarly in CD4 T cells. The chemokine receptor CXCR3 has been shown to be important in the migration of CD4 T cells to the lung in primary influenza infection (Wareing et al. 2004; Kohlmeier et al. 2009). One of the ligands for CXCR3, IP-10, is notably upregulated during influenza infection (Sanders et al. 2010). The chemokine receptor, CCR5, which also binds RANTES and MIP-1α, was shown to facilitate the accelerated recruitment of memory CD8 T cells to the lung airways following secondary challenge (Kohlmeier et al. 2008). Specific molecules that are responsible for homing of memory CD4 cells have not been elucidated. However, lung-resident memory CD4 T cells preferentially home back to the lung after adoptive transfer (Teijaro et al. 2011), suggesting that there are likely specific factors that mediate this process.

Retention Following the resolution of infection, maintenance of a pathogen-specific memory T cell population at the site of pathogen encounter may represent an effective strategy for protection against secondary challenge (Fig. 2c). As with homing, tissue retention of T cells seems to be regulated by the expression of various chemokine receptors and integrins. Expression of LFA-1 and the $\alpha 1\beta 1$ integrin very late antigen-1 (VLA-1, a dimer of CD49a and CD29), which binds collagen, were shown to contribute to retention of memory CD8 T cells in the lung following influenza infection (Thatte et al. 2003; Ray et al. 2004), although their role in memory CD4 T cell retention is unclear. CD4 Trm were recently described to express high levels of the LFA-1 subunit CD11a (Teijaro et al. 2011; Turner et al. 2013), suggesting that integrins may also mediate memory CD4 T cell retention in the lung.

Recently, the Trm-specific markers CD69 and CD103 were shown to contribute to Trm maintenance in tissues. During T cell activation, CD69 suppresses the expression of sphingosine 1-phosphate receptor type 1 (S1PR1), preventing lymph node egress (Shiow et al. 2006). Interestingly, a recent study found that CD8 Trm cells do not express S1PR1 and that forced expression of S1PR1 prevented the establishment of Trm cells (Skon et al. 2013). As CD69 suppresses S1PR1, these results suggest that increased CD69 expression on Trm cells may represent a non-canonical role for this molecule in retention of activated T cells in peripheral tissues. For CD103, a role in tissue homing has been previously demonstrated via its ability to bind to E-cadherin on epithelial cells (Cepek et al. 1994). Expression of CD103 by lung memory CD8 T cells was shown to be induced by TGF-β during influenza infection (Yu et al. 2013). Importantly, CD103-deficient CD8 T cells are inefficiently retained in the lungs following influenza infection, suggesting an important role for CD103 in the establishment of lung-resident CD8 Trm populations (Lee et al. 2011). Although CD4 Trm do not express CD103 at high levels (Sathaliyawala et al. 2013), expression of other integrins, such as LFA-1, may function in the tissue retention of this subset.

Table 2 Mechanisms of protection against influenza infection mediated by primary effector and memory CD4 T cells

Factor	Primary effector	Memory effector
Response to antigen stimulation	Delayed	Immediate
Need for APC costimulation	Required	Not required
Location of activation	Draining lymph nodes (MLN)	Local (Lung)
Effector cytokine secretion (IFN-γ, etc.)	++	+++
Innate immune cell help	–	+++
B cell help[a]	++	+++
CD8 T cell help[a]	+++	Possibly
Cytolytic ability	++	++

[a] Transferred CD4 memory are able to protect from influenza infection independent of these factors, but the presence of B and/or CD8 T cells results in enhanced protection, while protection mediated by naïve CD4 T cells requires either B cells or CD8 T cells

6 Memory CD4 T Cell Function in Influenza

While CD4-mediated B cell and CD8 T cell help has been demonstrated to be important in generating optimal primary responses to influenza infection, in the absence of both B and CD8 T cells, CD4 T cells alone are not sufficient, nor are they required, for viral clearance (Graham and Braciale 1997; Mozdzanowska et al. 2000; Gerhard 2001). In contrast, memory CD4 cells can direct viral clearance in the absence of B cells or CD8 T cells (Teijaro et al. 2010; McKinstry et al. 2012). However, protection was enhanced by the presence of naïve B cells or CD8 T cells and maximized when both were present (McKinstry et al. 2012).

Like primary effector CD4 T cells, memory CD4 T cells have the potential to play diverse roles in coordinating secondary responses including providing CD8 and B cell help as well as exerting independent effector functions. However, two key factors in the superior protective capacity of memory versus naive CD4 T cells are their localization and enhanced function. In contrast to naive cells, memory CD4 T cells are comprised of subsets localized to both the lymphoid (Tcm) and peripheral tissues (Tem and Trm). In the lymphoid tissues, memory CD4 cells are able to enhance B cell responses, and may enhance CD8 T responses. Localization to sites of pathogen encounter, combined with reduced requirements for activation, allow memory CD4 T cells to rapidly respond to secondary infection. In addition, memory cells are able to secrete an expanded array of cytokines, which supports inflammatory responses and innate immune cell recruitment to the lung. Finally, memory CD4 T cells possess cytolytic activity, allowing them to directly kill virally infected cells in the lung. Memory CD4 T cell responses in secondary influenza infection are described in the following sections and are summarized in Table 2.

6.1 Helper Functions in Lymphoid Tissues

The generation of neutralizing antibodies directed toward the viral surface glycoproteins HA and NA during an influenza infection is a major mechanism of protection in both the primary and secondary responses to infection, as well the mechanism by which current influenza vaccines provide protective immunity. It is well established that CD4 T cell help is essential for the production of class-switched antibodies by antigen-specific B cells and the generation of plasma cells (Crotty 2011). The CD4 T cells that provide help to B cells are referred to as T follicular helper (Tfh) cells. Although it has been established that Tfh cells are important in primary antibody responses, it is less clear whether there is a distinct set of memory Tfh cells and whether they play a role in the response to heterosubtypic influenza infection. Memory CD4 T cells can enable B cells to expand and class-switch more rapidly than do naïve CD4 T cells (MacLeod et al. 2011). In addition, a circulating population of memory CD4 T cells expressing CXCR5 in human blood was shown to induce antibody production from naïve B cells (Morita et al. 2011). It has also been demonstrated that the presence of such Tfh-like populations in the blood after influenza vaccination in humans correlates with the generation of virus-specific antibody responses (Bentebibel et al. 2013; Spensieri et al. 2013). To address whether a specific memory Tfh population exists, a recent study demonstrated that the adoptive transfer of CXCR5-positive antigen-specific memory CD4 T cell populations promoted the enhanced formation of germinal center B cells following infection with LCMV, providing evidence for the existence of a distinct Tfh-committed CD4 memory T cell population (Hale et al. 2013). Taken together, these findings suggest that memory CD4 cells play an important role in providing signals for B cell responses, and that this may be mediated by a specific Tfh-committed memory population poised to reacquire their lineage-specific effector functions and promote strain-specific antibody production upon heterosubtypic infection.

A role for CD4 T cell help in the generation of pathogen-specific CD8 memory T cells that can respond upon secondary infection has been well established (Shedlock and Shen 2003; Sun and Bevan 2003). The need for CD4 help in the generation of CD8 memory has also been demonstrated during the primary response to influenza infection (Belz et al. 2002); however, specific roles for memory CD4 T cells in the generation, maintenance or reactivation of CD8 memory have not been established. Memory CD4 T cells are able to mediate protection against lethal influenza infection in the absence of CD8 T cells, and transfer of memory CD4 T cells does not promote recruitment of CD8 T cells into the lung after infection (Teijaro et al. 2010, 2011). However, viral clearance is enhanced in B cell-deficient mice receiving memory CD4 T cells when naïve CD8 T cells are present compared to CD8-depleting conditions (McKinstry et al. 2012). Similarly, reconstitution of severe combined immunodeficiency (SCID) hosts, which lack both B and T cells, with either naïve CD8 T cells, memory CD4 T cells or a combination of both, demonstrated that co-transfer provided greater protection than either population alone (McKinstry et al. 2012), suggesting that memory CD4 T cells may play some role in helping naïve CD8 T cells.

6.2 Independent Effector Mechanisms in the Lung

6.2.1 Cytokine Production

Memory CD4 T cells, in contrast to naïve CD4 T cells, are known to rapidly produce multiple inflammatory cytokines and chemokines in response to TCR stimulation, resulting in the recruitment of macrophages, natural killer (NK) and other innate effector cells. These cells, in turn, produce additional cytokines which further support the inflammatory response. In response to secondary influenza challenge, primed mice or mice receiving memory CD4 cells upregulate factors including IFN-γ, TNF-α, IL-6, IL-12, CXCL9 and CXCL10 compared to naive animals (Strutt et al. 2010). This enhanced production of cytokines and chemokines correlates with early viral control during secondary infection (Strutt et al. 2010).

The most well-characterized memory CD4 response in influenza infection is production of the Th1-type cytokine IFN-γ. In contrast to naïve CD4 T cells, which slowly begin to upregulate IFN-γ production driven by T-bet days after TCR stimulation, the production of IFN-γ by memory CD4 T cells occurs rapidly via an NF-kB-mediated transcriptional program (Lai et al. 2011). In primary influenza infection, IFN-γ is not required for protection from infection and the development of CTL or antibody responses were not reduced in IFN-γ knockout mice compared to wild-type (Graham et al. 1993). However, memory CD4 T cell-mediated protection to influenza challenge is dependent on IFN-γ as neutralization of IFN-γ production abrogates protection (Bot et al. 1998; Teijaro et al. 2010; McKinstry et al. 2012). In addition, in human influenza challenge studies, early responses to virus infection were characterized by CD4-mediated production of IFN-γ (Wilkinson et al. 2012). Taken together, these results demonstrate the importance of memory CD4-mediated production of IFN-γ in secondary responses to influenza.

Mechanisms for IFN-γ-mediated protection during infection are not completely understood. IFN-γ has been shown to be involved in the activation and recruitment of innate immune populations such as macrophages and NK cells. In one study, administration of IFN-γ at early stages of influenza infection stimulated NK cell proliferation, function and number in the lungs and protected infected mice from death in a NK cell-dependent manner (Weiss et al. 2010).

Interleukin-10 (IL-10) is an anti-inflammatory cytokine broadly produced by both innate and adaptive immune cell types (Saraiva and O'Garra 2010). During acute influenza infection, IL-10 is produced in the lungs by virus-specific CD4 and CD8 effector T cells (Sun et al. 2009). Expression of IL-10 in this context seems to be important in limiting inflammation and lung pathology. Interestingly, mice deficient for IL-10 display increased survival after challenge with lethal doses of influenza compared to wild-type mice (McKinstry et al. 2009). Another study has suggested that increased protection to influenza infection in IL-10-deficient mice is the result of enhanced virus-specific antibody production (Sun et al. 2010). Memory CD4 cells, although able to enhance viral clearance, do not protect from lung pathology associated with infection (Teijaro et al. 2010). Interestingly, studies have demonstrated that CD4 memory T cells produce less IL-10 than do primary effectors (Dong et al. 2007; McKinstry et al. 2007). The decreased IL-10 response may contribute to enhanced viral clearance after secondary infection while failing to limit pulmonary pathology.

A role for IL-17 in influenza infection is less clearly defined. It is typically associated with allergic-type responses and the promotion of inflammation (Korn et al. 2009). Overall, most sources agree that IL-17 likely contributes to immune pathology and mice deficient in the IL-17 receptor display delayed weight loss and reduced total protein and lactate dehydrogenase activity in bronchoalveolar lavage (BAL) samples compared to wild-type mice suggesting reduced pathology (Crowe et al. 2009). However, IL-17 has previously been shown to play roles in the immune response to several different lung infections (Ye et al. 2001a; Umemura et al. 2007; Murdock et al. 2013). The transfer of in vitro generated Th17-polarized TCR-transgenic CD4 memory cells protected mice from lethal influenza infection as effectively as Th1-polarized memory cells (McKinstry et al. 2012), suggesting that Th17 responses may contribute to positive outcome in influenza infection. Furthermore, IL-17-secreting, influenza-specific CD4 memory T cells have been described in human lung tissue (Sathaliyawala et al. 2013). Although no mechanism for this protection has been established, IL-17 promotes neutrophil recruitment in the lung (Ye et al. 2001b), which could contribute to protection.

6.2.2 Perforin-Dependent Cytolytic Activity

The cytotoxic role of CD8 T cells in influenza infections is well established (Topham et al. 1997), consistent with its role in many different infection systems. There is increasing evidence that effector and memory CD4 T cells can also mediate cytotoxic responses in influenza infection. A subset of influenza-specific effector CD4 T cells with cytolytic activity was identified some time ago (Graham et al. 1994) and later found to be mediated by a perforin-dependent mechanism (Appay et al. 2002). In vitro primed and in vivo generated CD4 effectors were able to kill influenza-specific peptide-coated targets in cytolytic assays and were capable of protecting against lethal influenza infection (Brown et al. 2006, 2012). Cytolytic memory CD4 T cells may also mediate protective immunity to influenza infection as perforin-deficient memory CD4 T cells exhibited reduced protective capacity during infection (McKinstry et al. 2012). The mechanism by which this protection occurs has not yet been elucidated, however, recent studies have demonstrated that the development of CD4 T cells with cytotoxic potential was dependent on type I interferon signaling and IL-2 mediated induction of the transcription factors T-bet and Blimp-1 (Hua et al. 2013).

7 Implications for Vaccines

As discussed above, influenza-specific memory CD4 T cells are capable of mediating protective immune responses to secondary viral challenge (Teijaro et al. 2010; Wilkinson et al. 2012). Furthermore, it is well established that memory CD4 T cells protective against secondary challenge are generated and retained in the host long-term following primary infection (Teijaro et al. 2011; Turner et al. 2013), and are capable of mediating protective heterosubtypic responses to multiple viral strains (Teijaro et al. 2010). By contrast, current influenza vaccines induce neutralizing antibody responses that are only protective to seasonal strains and, therefore, do not provide lasting protection against subsequent infections. Thus, targeting the generation of memory CD4 T cells, and in particular, influenza-specific CD4 Trm in the lung, has the potential to provide durable, long-lasting cross-strain protection against influenza virus.

There is evidence that vaccine type and route of administration affect memory CD4 T cell generation in response to influenza vaccination. In studies comparing inactivated trivalent influenza vaccine (TIV), given intramuscularly, and live attenuated influenza vaccine (LAIV), administered intranasally, the percentage of virus-specific CD4 and CD8 T cells secreting IFN-γ increased significantly after LAIV, but not TIV, immunization in children 5–9 years of age (He et al. 2006). Protection against subsequent influenza infection was also found to be superior following immunization with LAIV as compared to TIV (Belshe et al. 2007). A later study comparing combinations of TIV and LAIV prime and booster vaccinations demonstrated that only vaccine combinations containing LAIV-induced influenza-specific, IFN-γ-producing CD4 memory (Hoft et al. 2011). Thus, LAIV appears to induce stronger virus-specific CD4 responses and is better able to generate CD4 memory than the current inactivated vaccine formulation. Significantly, these findings suggest that both vaccine localization and the ability of virus to replicate within the host may be important for the design of influenza vaccines able to promote development of memory CD4 T cells.

Though current vaccines do not target the development of tissue-homing T cells, strategies that promote this population are under investigation. In one study, intranasal, but not parenteral, delivery of a cancer vaccine was able to inhibit mucosal tumor growth (Sandoval et al. 2013). Importantly, only the intranasal vaccine was able to elicit a CD8 T cell population expressing both CD49a, and CD103, molecules important in lung homing and retention, respectively. These results demonstrate a link between the route of vaccination, T cell tissue homing and the development of protective immune responses (Sandoval et al. 2013). The ability of a vaccine to establish a protective Trm population has also recently been demonstrated. In a herpes simplex virus type 2 model, parenteral vaccination with viral antigens was coupled with topical chemokine application to recruit virus-specific T cells to the genital mucosa. This 'prime and pull' strategy resulted in the establishment of a virus-specific Trm population capable of providing protective immunity (Shin and Iwasaki 2012). The development of vaccines capable of eliciting a Trm population for influenza will likely be the key to the development of lasting, heterosubtypic protection against infection.

8 Conclusion

In contrast to their naïve counterparts, memory CD4 T cells are capable of mediating protective responses to influenza challenge independent of B cells or CD8 T cells. One factor driving the heightened protective capacity of memory CD4 T cells is their peripheral tissue localization, facilitating their rapid response to reinfection in situ. Importantly, a newly defined, tissue-resident CD4 memory population has been demonstrated to be optimally protective against influenza challenge. Memory CD4 T cells also exhibit enhanced effector functions compared to naïve CD4 T cells including the ability to better promote B cell responses, as well as enhanced cytokine recruitment and activation of innate effector cells. Furthermore, that memory CD4 T cells can mediate heterosubtypic immune responses to multiple influenza strains makes them an attractive target in vaccine development strategies. Recent studies have demonstrated that route of vaccine administration and the use of live-attenuated, rather than inactivated virus significantly impact the generation of memory CD4 T cells and protective capacity of vaccines following administration. Significantly, these findings may be important for the design of influenza vaccines able to elicit protective memory CD4 T cells.

Acknowledgments Donna L. Farber is supported by NIH grants AI106697, AI100119, and AI083022.

References

Ahmadzadeh M, Farber DL (2002) Functional plasticity of an antigen-specific memory CD4 T cell population. Proc Natl Acad Sci U S A 99(18):11802–11807

Allan W, Tabi Z, Cleary A, Doherty PC (1990) Cellular events in the lymph node and lung of mice with influenza. Consequences of depleting CD4+ T cells. J Immunol 144(10):3980–3986

Appay V, Zaunders JJ, Papagno L, Sutton J, Jaramillo A, Waters A, Easterbrook P, Grey P, Smith D, McMichael AJ, Cooper DA, Rowland-Jones SL, Kelleher AD (2002) Characterization of CD4(+) CTLs ex vivo. J Immunol 168(11):5954–5958

Belshe RB, Edwards KM, Vesikari T, Black SV, Walker RE, Hultquist M, Kemble G, Connor EM (2007) Live attenuated versus inactivated influenza vaccine in infants and young children. N Engl J Med 356(7):685–696. doi:10.1056/NEJMoa065368

Belz GT, Wodarz D, Diaz G, Nowak MA, Doherty PC (2002) Compromised influenza virus-specific CD8(+)-T-cell memory in CD4(+)-T-cell-deficient mice. J Virol 76(23):12388–12393

Bentebibel SE, Lopez S, Obermoser G, Schmitt N, Mueller C, Harrod C, Flano E, Mejias A, Albrecht RA, Blankenship D, Xu H, Pascual V, Banchereau J, Garcia-Sastre A, Palucka AK, Ramilo O, Ueno H (2013) Induction of ICOS+CXCR3+CXCR5+TH cells correlates with antibody responses to influenza vaccination. Sci Transl Med 5(176):176ra132. doi:10.1126/scitranslmed.3005191

Bingaman AW, Patke DS, Mane VR, Ahmadzadeh M, Ndejembi M, Bartlett ST, Farber DL (2005) Novel phenotypes and migratory properties distinguish memory CD4 T cell subsets in lymphoid and lung tissue. Eur J Immunol 35:3173–3186

Bot A, Bot S, Bona CA (1998) Protective role of gamma interferon during the recall response to influenza virus. J Virol 72(8):6637–6645

Brown DM, Dilzer AM, Meents DL, Swain SL (2006) CD4 T cell-mediated protection from lethal influenza: perforin and antibody-mediated mechanisms give a one-two punch. J Immunol 177(5):2888–2898

Brown DM, Lee S, Garcia-Hernandez Mde L, Swain SL (2012) Multifunctional CD4 cells expressing gamma interferon and perforin mediate protection against lethal influenza virus infection. J Virol 86(12):6792–6803. doi:10.1128/JVI.07172-11

Bushar ND, Corbo E, Schmidt M, Maltzman JS, Farber DL (2010) Ablation of SLP-76 signaling after T cell priming generates memory CD4 T cells impaired in steady-state and cytokine-driven homeostasis. Proc Natl Acad Sci U S A 107(2):827–831. doi:10.1073/pnas.0908126107 0908126107 [pii]

Cepek KL, Shaw SK, Parker CM, Russell GJ, Morrow JS, Rimm DL, Brenner MB (1994) Adhesion between epithelial cells and T lymphocytes mediated by E- cadherin and the alpha E beta 7 integrin. Nature 372(6502):190–193

Cook DN, Beck MA, Coffman TM, Kirby SL, Sheridan JF, Pragnell IB, Smithies O (1995) Requirement of MIP-1 alpha for an inflammatory response to viral infection. Science 269(5230):1583–1585

Couceiro JN, Paulson JC, Baum LG (1993) Influenza virus strains selectively recognize sialyloligosaccharides on human respiratory epithelium; the role of the host cell in selection of hemagglutinin receptor specificity. Virus Res 29(2):155–165

Crotty S (2011) Follicular helper CD4 T cells (TFH). Annu Rev Immunol 29:621–663. doi:10.1146/annurev-immunol-031210-101400

Crowe CR, Chen K, Pociask DA, Alcorn JF, Krivich C, Enelow RI, Ross TM, Witztum JL, Kolls JK (2009) Critical role of IL-17RA in immunopathology of influenza infection. J Immunol 183(8):5301–5310. doi:10.4049/jimmunol.0900995

de Bree GJ, van Leeuwen EM, Out TA, Jansen HM, Jonkers RE, van Lier RA (2005) Selective accumulation of differentiated CD8+ T cells specific for respiratory viruses in the human lung. J Exp Med 202(10):1433–1442

De Riva A, Bourgeois C, Kassiotis G, Stockinger B (2007) Noncognate interaction with MHC class II molecules is essential for maintenance of T cell metabolism to establish optimal memory CD4 T cell function. J Immunol 178(9):5488–5495

Dong J, Ivascu C, Chang HD, Wu P, Angeli R, Maggi L, Eckhardt F, Tykocinski L, Haefliger C, Mowes B, Sieper J, Radbruch A, Annunziato F, Thiel A (2007) IL-10 is excluded from the functional cytokine memory of human CD4+ memory T lymphocytes. J Immunol 179(4):2389–2396

Dudda JC, Simon JC, Martin S (2004) Dendritic cell immunization route determines CD8+ T cell trafficking to inflamed skin: role for tissue microenvironment and dendritic cells in establishment of T cell-homing subsets. J Immunol 172(2):857–863

Epstein SL, Lo CY, Misplon JA, Lawson CM, Hendrickson BA, Max EE, Subbarao K (1997) Mechanisms of heterosubtypic immunity to lethal influenza A virus infection in fully immunocompetent, T cell-depleted, beta2-microglobulin-deficient, and J chain-deficient mice. J Immunol 158(3):1222–1230

Gebhardt T, Wakim LM, Eidsmo L, Reading PC, Heath WR, Carbone FR (2009) Memory T cells in nonlymphoid tissue that provide enhanced local immunity during infection with herpes simplex virus. Nat Immunol 10(5):524–530. doi:10.1038/ni.1718 ni.1718 [pii]

Gerhard W (2001) The role of the antibody response in influenza virus infection. Curr Top Microbiol Immunol 260:171–190

Gerhard W, Mozdzanowska K, Furchner M, Washko G, Maiese K (1997) Role of the B-cell response in recovery of mice from primary influenza virus infection. Immunol Rev 159:95–103

Graham MB, Braciale TJ (1997) Resistance to and recovery from lethal influenza virus infection in B lymphocyte-deficient mice. J Exp Med 186(12):2063–2068

Graham MB, Braciale VL, Braciale TJ (1994) Influenza virus-specific CD4+ T helper type 2 T lymphocytes do not promote recovery from experimental virus infection. J Exp Med 180(4):1273–1282

Graham MB, Dalton DK, Giltinan D, Braciale VL, Stewart TA, Braciale TJ (1993) Response to influenza infection in mice with a targeted disruption in the interferon gamma gene. J Exp Med 178(5):1725–1732

Hale JS, Youngblood B, Latner DR, Mohammed AU, Ye L, Akondy RS, Wu T, Iyer SS, Ahmed R (2013) Distinct memory CD4+ T cells with commitment to T follicular helper- and T helper 1-cell lineages are generated after acute viral infection. Immunity 38(4):805–817. doi:10.1016/j.immuni.2013.02.020

He XS, Holmes TH, Zhang C, Mahmood K, Kemble GW, Lewis DB, Dekker CL, Greenberg HB, Arvin AM (2006) Cellular immune responses in children and adults receiving inactivated or live attenuated influenza vaccines. J Virol 80(23):11756–11766

Hoft DF, Babusis E, Worku S, Spencer CT, Lottenbach K, Truscott SM, Abate G, Sakala IG, Edwards KM, Creech CB, Gerber MA, Bernstein DI, Newman F, Graham I, Anderson EL, Belshe RB (2011) Live and inactivated influenza vaccines induce similar humoral responses, but only live vaccines induce diverse T-cell responses in young children. J Infect Dis 204(6):845–853. doi:10.1093/infdis/jir436

Hogan RJ, Zhong W, Usherwood EJ, Cookenham T, Roberts AD, Woodland DL (2001) Protection from respiratory virus infections can be mediated by antigen-specific CD4(+) T cells that persist in the lungs. J Exp Med 193(8):981–986

Hua L, Yao S, Pham D, Jiang L, Wright J, Sawant D, Dent AL, Braciale TJ, Kaplan MH, Sun J (2013) Cytokine-dependent induction of CD4+ T cells with cytotoxic potential during influenza virus infection. J Virol 87(21):11884–11893. doi:10.1128/JVI.01461-13

Huster KM, Busch V, Schiemann M, Linkemann K, Kerksiek KM, Wagner H, Busch DH (2004) Selective expression of IL-7 receptor on memory T cells identifies early CD40L-dependent generation of distinct CD8+ memory T cell subsets. Proc Natl Acad Sci U S A 101(15):5610–5615. doi:10.1073/pnas.0308054101

Jelley-Gibbs DM, Brown DM, Dibble JP, Haynes L, Eaton SM, Swain SL (2005) Unexpected prolonged presentation of influenza antigens promotes CD4 T cell memory generation. J Exp Med 202(5):697–706

Joshi NS, Cui W, Chandele A, Lee HK, Urso DR, Hagman J, Gapin L, Kaech SM (2007) Inflammation directs memory precursor and short-lived effector CD8(+) T cell fates via the graded expression of T-bet transcription factor. Immunity 27(2):281–295

Julkunen I, Melen K, Nyqvist M, Pirhonen J, Sareneva T, Matikainen S (2000) Inflammatory responses in influenza A virus infection. Vaccine 19(Suppl 1):S32–S37

Kaech SM, Tan JT, Wherry EJ, Konieczny BT, Surh CD, Ahmed R (2003) Selective expression of the interleukin 7 receptor identifies effector CD8 T cells that give rise to long-lived memory cells. Nat Immunol 4(12):1191–1198

Kaech SM, Wherry EJ (2007) Heterogeneity and cell-fate decisions in effector and memory CD8+ T cell differentiation during viral infection. Immunity 27(3):393–405

Kaech SM, Wherry EJ, Ahmed R (2002) Effector and memory T-cell differentiation: implications for vaccine development. Nat Rev Immunol 2(4):251–262

Kassiotis G, Garcia S, Simpson E, Stockinger B (2002) Impairment of immunological memory in the absence of MHC despite survival of memory T cells. Nat Immunol 3(3):244–250

Kohlmeier JE, Cookenham T, Miller SC, Roberts AD, Christensen JP, Thomsen AR, Woodland DL (2009) CXCR3 directs antigen-specific effector CD4+ T cell migration to the lung during parainfluenza virus infection. J Immunol 183(7):4378–4384. doi:10.4049/jimmunol.0902022 jimmunol.0902022 [pii]

Kohlmeier JE, Miller SC, Smith J, Lu B, Gerard C, Cookenham T, Roberts AD, Woodland DL (2008) The chemokine receptor CCR5 plays a key role in the early memory CD8+ T cell response to respiratory virus infections. Immunity 29(1):101–113

Kondrack RM, Harbertson J, Tan JT, McBreen ME, Surh CD, Bradley LM (2003) Interleukin 7 regulates the survival and generation of memory CD4 cells. J Exp Med 198(12):1797–1806

Korn T, Bettelli E, Oukka M, Kuchroo VK (2009) IL-17 and Th17 cells. Annu Rev Immunol 27: 485–517. doi:10.1146/annurev.immunol.021908.132710 10.1146/annurev.immunol.021908.132710 [pii]

Lai W, Yu M, Huang MN, Okoye F, Keegan AD, Farber DL (2011) Transcriptional control of rapid recall by memory CD4 T cells. J Immunol 187(1):133–140. doi:10.4049/jimmunol.1002742 jimmunol.1002742 [pii]

Lee LY, Ha DL, Simmons C, de Jong MD, Chau NV, Schumacher R, Peng YC, McMichael AJ, Farrar JJ, Smith GL, Townsend AR, Askonas BA, Rowland-Jones S, Dong T (2008) Memory T cells established by seasonal human influenza A infection cross-react with avian influenza A (H5N1) in healthy individuals. J Clin Invest 118(10):3478–3490

Lee YT, Suarez-Ramirez JE, Wu T, Redman JM, Bouchard K, Hadley GA, Cauley LS (2011) Environmental and antigen receptor-derived signals support sustained surveillance of the lungs by pathogen-specific cytotoxic T lymphocytes. J Virol 85(9):4085–4094. doi:10.1128/JVI.02493-10

Lenz DC, Kurz SK, Lemmens E, Schoenberger SP, Sprent J, Oldstone MB, Homann D (2004) IL-7 regulates basal homeostatic proliferation of antiviral CD4+ T cell memory. Proc Natl Acad Sci U S A 101(25):9357–9362

Li J, Huston G, Swain SL (2003) IL-7 promotes the transition of CD4 effectors to persistent memory cells. J Exp Med 198(12):1807–1815

Liang S, Mozdzanowska K, Palladino G, Gerhard W (1994) Heterosubtypic immunity to influenza type A virus in mice. Effector mechanisms and their longevity. J Immunol 152(4):1653–1661

Liu L, Zhong Q, Tian T, Dubin K, Athale SK, Kupper TS (2010) Epidermal injury and infection during poxvirus immunization is crucial for the generation of highly protective T cell-mediated immunity. Nat Med 16(2):224–227. doi:10.1038/nm.2078 nm.2078 [pii]

MacLeod MK, David A, McKee AS, Crawford F, Kappler JW, Marrack P (2011) Memory CD4 T cells that express CXCR5 provide accelerated help to B cells. J Immunol 186(5):2889–2896. doi:10.4049/jimmunol.1002955

Makgoba MW, Sanders ME, Ginther Luce GE, Dustin ML, Springer TA, Clark EA, Mannoni P, Shaw S (1988) ICAM-1 a ligand for LFA-1-dependent adhesion of B, T and myeloid cells. Nature 331(6151):86–88. doi:10.1038/331086a0

Masopust D, Choo D, Vezys V, Wherry EJ, Duraiswamy J, Akondy R, Wang J, Casey KA, Barber DL, Kawamura KS, Fraser KA, Webby RJ, Brinkmann V, Butcher EC, Newell KA, Ahmed R (2010) Dynamic T cell migration program provides resident memory within intestinal epithelium. J Exp Med 207(3):553–564. doi:10.1084/jem.20090858 jem.20090858 [pii]

Masopust D, Vezys V, Marzo AL, Lefrancois L (2001) Preferential localization of effector memory cells in nonlymphoid tissue. Science 291(5512):2413–2417

Matsukura S, Kokubu F, Kubo H, Tomita T, Tokunaga H, Kadokura M, Yamamoto T, Kuroiwa Y, Ohno T, Suzaki H, Adachi M (1998) Expression of RANTES by normal airway epithelial cells after influenza virus A infection. Am J Respir Cell Mol Biol 18(2):255–264. doi:10.1165/ajrcmb.18.2.2822

McKinstry KK, Golech S, Lee WH, Huston G, Weng NP, Swain SL (2007) Rapid default transition of CD4 T cell effectors to functional memory cells. J Exp Med 204(9):2199–2211

McKinstry KK, Strutt TM, Buck A, Curtis JD, Dibble JP, Huston G, Tighe M, Hamada H, Sell S, Dutton RW, Swain SL (2009) IL-10 deficiency unleashes an influenza-specific Th17 response and enhances survival against high-dose challenge. J Immunol 182(12):7353–7363. doi:10.4049/jimmunol.0900657

McKinstry KK, Strutt TM, Kuang Y, Brown DM, Sell S, Dutton RW, Swain SL (2012) Memory CD4+ T cells protect against influenza through multiple synergizing mechanisms. J Clin Invest 122(8):2847–2856. doi:10.1172/JCI63689 63689 [pii]

Mikhak Z, Strassner JP, Luster AD (2013) Lung dendritic cells imprint T cell lung homing and promote lung immunity through the chemokine receptor CCR4. J Exp Med 210(9):1855–1869. doi:10.1084/jem.20130091

Molinari NA, Ortega-Sanchez IR, Messonnier ML, Thompson WW, Wortley PM, Weintraub E, Bridges CB (2007) The annual impact of seasonal influenza in the US: measuring disease burden and costs. Vaccine 25(27):5086–5096. doi:10.1016/j.vaccine.2007.03.046

Mora JR, Bono MR, Manjunath N, Weninger W, Cavanagh LL, Rosemblatt M, Von Andrian UH (2003) Selective imprinting of gut-homing T cells by Peyer's patch dendritic cells. Nature 424(6944):88–93

Mora JR, Cheng G, Picarella D, Briskin M, Buchanan N, von Andrian UH (2005) Reciprocal and dynamic control of CD8 T cell homing by dendritic cells from skin- and gut-associated lymphoid tissues. J Exp Med 201(2):303–316

Morita R, Schmitt N, Bentebibel SE, Ranganathan R, Bourdery L, Zurawski G, Foucat E, Dullaers M, Oh S, Sabzghabaei N, Lavecchio EM, Punaro M, Pascual V, Banchereau J, Ueno H (2011) Human blood CXCR5(+)CD4(+) T cells are counterparts of T follicular cells and contain specific subsets that differentially support antibody secretion. Immunity 34(1):108–121. doi:10.1016/j.immuni.2010.12.012 S1074-S7613(10)00491-7 [pii]

Moulton VR, Bushar ND, Leeser DB, Patke DS, Farber DL (2006) Divergent generation of heterogeneous memory CD4 T cells. J Immunol 177(2):869–876. doi:177/2/869 [pii]

Mozdzanowska K, Maiese K, Gerhard W (2000) Th cell-deficient mice control influenza virus infection more effectively than Th- and B cell-deficient mice: evidence for a Th-independent contribution by B cells to virus clearance. J Immunol 164(5):2635–2643

Mueller SN, Gebhardt T, Carbone FR, Heath WR (2013) Memory T cell subsets, migration patterns, and tissue residence. Annu Rev Immunol 31:137–161. doi:10.1146/annurev-immunol-032712-095954

Murdock BJ, Huffnagle GB, Olszewski MA, Osterholzer JJ (2013) IL-17A enhances host defense against cryptococcal lung infection through effects mediated by leukocyte recruitment, activation, and IFN-gamma production. Infect Immun. doi:10.1128/IAI.01477-13

O'Shea JJ, Paul WE (2010) Mechanisms underlying lineage commitment and plasticity of helper CD4+ T cells. Science 327(5969):1098–1102. doi:10.1126/science.1178334

Osterholm MT, Kelley NS, Sommer A, Belongia EA (2012) Efficacy and effectiveness of influenza vaccines: a systematic review and meta-analysis. Lancet Infect Dis 12(1):36–44. doi:10.1016/S1473-3099(11)70295-X

Piet B, de Bree GJ, Smids-Dierdorp BS, van der Loos CM, Remmerswaal EB, von der Thusen JH, van Haarst JM, Eerenberg JP, Ten Brinke A, van der Bij W, Timens W, van Lier RA, Jonkers RE (2011) CD8+ T cells with an intraepithelial phenotype upregulate cytotoxic function upon influenza infection in human lung. J Clin Invest. doi:10.1172/JCI44675 44675 [pii]

Purton JF, Tan JT, Rubinstein MP, Kim DM, Sprent J, Surh CD (2007) Antiviral CD4+ memory T cells are IL-15 dependent. J Exp Med 204(4):951–961. doi:10.1084/jem.20061805

Purwar R, Campbell J, Murphy G, Richards WG, Clark RA, Kupper TS (2011) Resident memory T cells (T(RM)) are abundant in human lung: diversity, function, and antigen specificity. PLoS One 6(1):e16245. doi:10.1371/journal.pone.0016245

Rathmell JC, Farkash EA, Gao W, Thompson CB (2001) IL-7 enhances the survival and maintains the size of naive T cells. J Immunol 167(12):6869–6876

Ray SJ, Franki SN, Pierce RH, Dimitrova S, Koteliansky V, Sprague AG, Doherty PC, de Fougerolles AR, Topham DJ (2004) The collagen binding alpha1beta1 integrin VLA-1 regulates CD8 T cell-mediated immune protection against heterologous influenza infection. Immunity 20(2):167–179

Reinhardt RL, Khoruts A, Merica R, Zell T, Jenkins MK (2001) Visualizing the generation of memory CD4 T cells in the whole body. Nature 410(6824):101–105

Richards KA, Topham D, Chaves FA, Sant AJ (2010) Cutting edge: CD4 T cells generated from encounter with seasonal influenza viruses and vaccines have broad protein specificity and can directly recognize naturally generated epitopes derived from the live pandemic H1N1 virus. J Immunol 185(9):4998–5002. doi:10.4049/jimmunol.1001395

Ruane D, Brane L, Reis BS, Cheong C, Poles J, Do Y, Zhu H, Velinzon K, Choi JH, Studt N, Mayer L, Lavelle EC, Steinman RM, Mucida D, Mehandru S (2013) Lung dendritic cells induce migration of protective T cells to the gastrointestinal tract. J Exp Med 210 (9):1871–1888. doi:10.1084/jem.2012276210.1084/jem.20122762

Sallusto F, Geginat J, Lanzavecchia A (2004) Central memory and effector memory T cell subsets: function, generation, and maintenance. Annu Rev Immunol 22:745–763

Sallusto F, Lenig D, Forster R, Lipp M, Lanzavecchia A (1999) Two subsets of memory T lymphocytes with distinct homing potentials and effector functions [see comments]. Nature 401(6754):708–712

Sanders CJ, Doherty PC, Thomas PG (2010) Respiratory epithelial cells in innate immunity to influenza virus infection. Cell Tissue Res. doi:10.1007/s00441-010-1043-z

Sandoval F, Terme M, Nizard M, Badoual C, Bureau MF, Freyburger L, Clement O, Marcheteau E, Gey A, Fraisse G, Bouguin C, Merillon N, Dransart E, Tran T, Quintin-Colonna F, Autret G, Thiebaud M, Suleman M, Riffault S, Wu TC, Launay O, Danel C, Taieb J, Richardson J, Zitvogel L, Fridman WH, Johannes L, Tartour E (2013) Mucosal imprinting of vaccine-induced CD8(+) T cells is crucial to inhibit the growth of mucosal tumors. Sci Transl Med 5(172):172ra120. doi:10.1126/scitranslmed.3004888

Saraiva M, O'Garra A (2010) The regulation of IL-10 production by immune cells. Nat Rev Immunol 10(3):170–181. doi:10.1038/nri2711

Sathaliyawala T, Kubota M, Yudanin N, Turner D, Camp P, Thome JJ, Bickham KL, Lerner H, Goldstein M, Sykes M, Kato T, Farber DL (2013) Distribution and compartmentalization of human circulating and tissue resident memory T cell subsets. Immunity 38(1):187 197. doi:10.1016/j.immuni.2012.09.020 S1074-7613(12)00521-3 [pii]

Seddon B, Tomlinson P, Zamoyska R (2003) Interleukin 7 and T cell receptor signals regulate homeostasis of CD4 memory cells. Nat Immunol 4(7):680–686

Shedlock DJ, Shen H (2003) Requirement for CD4 T cell help in generating functional CD8 T cell memory. Science 300(5617):337–339

Shin H, Iwasaki A (2012) A vaccine strategy that protects against genital herpes by establishing local memory T cells. Nature 491(7424):463–467. doi:10.1038/nature11522 nature11522 [pii]

Shiow LR, Rosen DB, Brdickova N, Xu Y, An J, Lanier LL, Cyster JG, Matloubian M (2006) CD69 acts downstream of interferon-alpha/beta to inhibit S1P1 and lymphocyte egress from lymphoid organs. Nature 440(7083):540–544. doi:10.1038/nature04606 nature04606 [pii]

Skon CN, Lee JY, Anderson KG, Masopust D, Hogquist KA, Jameson SC (2013) Transcriptional downregulation of S1pr1 is required for the establishment of resident memory CD8(+) T cells. Nat Immunol 14(12):1285–1293. doi:10.1038/ni.2745

Spensieri F, Borgogni E, Zedda L, Bardelli M, Buricchi F, Volpini G, Fragapane E, Tavarini S, Finco O, Rappuoli R, Del Giudice G, Galli G, Castellino F (2013) Human circulating influenza-CD4+ ICOS1+IL-21+ T cells expand after vaccination, exert helper function, and predict antibody responses. Proc Natl Acad Sci U S A 110(35):14330–14335. doi:10.1073/pnas.1311998110

Sprenger H, Meyer RG, Kaufmann A, Bussfeld D, Rischkowsky E, Gemsa D (1996) Selective induction of monocyte and not neutrophil-attracting chemokines after influenza A virus infection. J Exp Med 184(3):1191–1196

Strutt TM, McKinstry KK, Dibble JP, Winchell C, Kuang Y, Curtis JD, Huston G, Dutton RW, Swain SL (2010) Memory CD4+ T cells induce innate responses independently of pathogen. Nat Med 16(5):558–564 (551 p following 564). doi:10.1038/nm.2142 nm.2142 [pii]

Sun J, Madan R, Karp CL, Braciale TJ (2009) Effector T cells control lung inflammation during acute influenza virus infection by producing IL-10. Nat Med 15(3):277–284

Sun JC, Bevan MJ (2003) Defective CD8 T cell memory following acute infection without CD4 T cell help. Science 300(5617):339–342

Sun K, Torres L, Metzger DW (2010) A detrimental effect of interleukin-10 on protective pulmonary humoral immunity during primary influenza A virus infection. J Virol 84(10):5007–5014. doi:10.1128/JVI.02408-09

Tan JT, Dudl E, LeRoy E, Murray R, Sprent J, Weinberg KI, Surh CD (2001) IL-7 is critical for homeostatic proliferation and survival of naive T cells. Proc Natl Acad Sci U S A 98(15): 8732–8737

Teijaro JR, Turner D, Pham Q, Wherry EJ, Lefrancois L, Farber DL (2011) Cutting edge: tissue-retentive lung memory CD4 T cells mediate optimal protection to respiratory virus infection. J Immunol 187(11):5510–5514. doi:10.4049/jimmunol.1102243 jimmunol.1102243 [pii]

Teijaro JR, Verhoeven D, Page CA, Turner D, Farber DL (2010) Memory CD4 T cells direct protective responses to influenza virus in the lungs through helper-independent mechanisms. J Virol 84(18):9217-9226. doi:10.1128/JVI.01069-10 JVI.01069-10 [pii]

Thatte J, Dabak V, Williams MB, Braciale TJ, Ley K (2003) LFA-1 is required for retention of effector CD8 T cells in mouse lungs. Blood 101(12):4916–4922

Thompson WW, Comanor L, Shay DK (2006) Epidemiology of seasonal influenza: use of surveillance data and statistical models to estimate the burden of disease. J Infect Dis 194(Suppl 2):S82–S91. doi:10.1086/507558

Topham DJ, Tripp RA, Doherty PC (1997) CD8+ T cells clear influenza virus by perforin or Fas-dependent processes. J Immunol 159(11):5197–5200

Turner DL, Bickham KL, Thome JJ, Kim CY, D'Ovidio F, Wherry EJ, Farber DL (2013) Lung niches for the generation and maintenance of tissue-resident memory T cells. Mucosal Immunol. doi:10.1038/mi.2013.67 mi201367 [pii]

Umemura M, Yahagi A, Hamada S, Begum MD, Watanabe H, Kawakami K, Suda T, Sudo K, Nakae S, Iwakura Y, Matsuzaki G (2007) IL-17-mediated regulation of innate and acquired immune response against pulmonary *Mycobacterium bovis* bacille Calmette-Guerin infection. J Immunol 178(6):3786–3796

Wakim LM, Woodward-Davis A, Liu R, Hu Y, Villadangos J, Smyth G, Bevan MJ (2012) The molecular signature of tissue resident memory CD8 T cells isolated from the brain. J Immunol 189(7):3462–3471. doi:10.4049/jimmunol.1201305 jimmunol.1201305 [pii]

Wareing MD, Lyon AB, Lu B, Gerard C, Sarawar SR (2004) Chemokine expression during the development and resolution of a pulmonary leukocyte response to influenza A virus infection in mice. J Leukoc Biol 76(4):886–895. doi:10.1189/jlb.1203644

Weiss ID, Wald O, Wald H, Beider K, Abraham M, Galun E, Nagler A, Peled A (2010) IFN-gamma treatment at early stages of influenza virus infection protects mice from death in a NK cell-dependent manner. J Interferon Cytokine Res 30(6):439–449. doi:10.1089/jir.2009.0084

Wilkinson TM, Li CK, Chui CS, Huang AK, Perkins M, Liebner JC, Lambkin-Williams R, Gilbert A, Oxford J, Nicholas B, Staples KJ, Dong T, Douek DC, McMichael AJ, Xu XN (2012) Preexisting influenza-specific CD4(+) T cells correlate with disease protection against influenza challenge in humans. Nat Med 18(2):274–280. doi:10.1038/nm.2612 nm.2612 [pii]

Woodland DL, Hogan RJ, Zhong W (2001) Cellular immunity and memory to respiratory virus infections. Immunol Res 24(1):53–67

Wu T, Hu Y, Lee YT, Bouchard KR, Benechet A, Khanna K, Cauley LS (2013) Lung-resident memory CD8 T cells (TRM) are indispensable for optimal cross-protection against pulmonary virus infection. J Leukoc Biol. doi:10.1189/jlb.0313180

Ye P, Garvey PB, Zhang P, Nelson S, Bagby G, Summer WR, Schwarzenberger P, Shellito JE, Kolls JK (2001a) Interleukin-17 and lung host defense against *Klebsiella pneumoniae* infection. Am J Respir Cell Mol Biol 25(3):335–340. doi:10.1165/ajrcmb.25.3.4424

Ye P, Rodriguez FH, Kanaly S, Stocking KL, Schurr J, Schwarzenberger P, Oliver P, Huang W, Zhang P, Zhang J, Shellito JE, Bagby GJ, Nelson S, Charrier K, Peschon JJ, Kolls JK (2001b) Requirement of interleukin 17 receptor signaling for lung CXC chemokine and granulocyte colony-stimulating factor expression, neutrophil recruitment, and host defense. J Exp Med 194(4):519–527

Yu CI, Becker C, Wang Y, Marches F, Helft J, Leboeuf M, Anguiano E, Pourpe S, Goller K, Pascual V, Banchereau J, Merad M, Palucka K (2013) Human CD1c+ dendritic cells drive the differentiation of CD103+ CD8+ mucosal effector T cells via the cytokine TGF-beta. Immunity 38(4):818–830. doi:10.1016/j.immuni.2013.03.004

Zammit DJ, Turner DL, Klonowski KD, Lefrancois L, Cauley LS (2006) Residual antigen presentation after influenza virus infection affects CD8 T cell activation and migration. Immunity 24(4):439–449

The Effector T Cell Response to Influenza Infection

Matthew M. Hufford, Taeg S. Kim, Jie Sun and Thomas J. Braciale

Abstract Influenza virus infection induces a potent initial innate immune response, which serves to limit the extent of viral replication and virus spread. However, efficient (and eventual) viral clearance within the respiratory tract requires the subsequent activation, rapid proliferation, recruitment, and expression of effector activities by the adaptive immune system, consisting of antibody producing B cells and influenza-specific T lymphocytes with diverse functions. The ensuing effector activities of these T lymphocytes ultimately determine (along with antibodies) the capacity of the host to eliminate the viruses and the extent of tissue damage. In this review, we describe this effector T cell response to influenza virus infection. Based on information largely obtained in experimental settings (i.e., murine models), we will illustrate the factors regulating the induction of adaptive immune T cell responses to influenza, the effector activities displayed by these activated T cells, the mechanisms underlying the expression of these effector mechanisms, and the control of the activation/differentiation of these T cells, in situ, in the infected lungs.

M. M. Hufford (✉) · J. Sun (✉)
Department of Pediatrics, Indiana University School of Medicine, Indianapolis, USA

M. M. Hufford · J. Sun
Department of Microbiology and Immunology, Indiana University School of Medicine, Indianapolis, USA

T. S. Kim (✉) · T. J. Braciale (✉)
The Beirne B. Carter Center for Immunology Research, University of Virginia, Charlottesville, USA
e-mail: tjb2r@virginia.edu

T. S. Kim · T. J. Braciale
The Department of Pathology and Molecular Medicine, University of Virginia, Charlottesville, USA

T. J. Braciale
The Department of Microbiology, Immunology and Cancer Biology University of Virginia, Charlottesville, USA

Current Topics in Microbiology and Immunology (2015) 386: 423–455
DOI: 10.1007/82_2014_397

Published Online: 18 July 2014

Abbreviations

APC	Antigen presenting cell
Bid	BH3 interacting-domain death agonist
Blimp-1	B lymphocyte–induced maturation protein-1
cRDC	Conventional RDC
CTL	Cytotoxic T lymphocyte
DAMP	Damage-associated molecular pattern
DC	Dendritic cell
DLN	Draining lymph node
FADD	Fas-associated death domain (FADD)
FasL	Fas ligand
IAV	Influenza A virus
IFN	Interferon
IL	Interleukin
IRF	IFN Regulatory factor
MIP-1α	Macrophage inflammatory protein-1α
MARCO	Macrophage receptor with collagenous structure
MAVS	Mitochondrial antiviral signaling
MHC	Major histocompatibility complex
Mo-RDC	Monocyte-like RDC
NLR	NOD-like receptor
PAMP	Pathogen-associated molecular pattern
pDC	Plasmacytoid DC
PRR	Pattern recognition receptor
RDC	Respiratory DC
REC	Respiratory epithelial cell
RIG-I	Retnoic acid-inducible gene 1
RLR	Rig-I-like receptor
TCR	T cell receptor
T_H	T helper
TipDC	TNF^+iNOS^+ DC
TLR	Toll-like receptor
TNF	Tumor necrosis factor
TRAIL	TNF-related apoptosis-inducing ligand
TRAIL-DR	TRAIL-death receptor

Contents

1 Introduction

In this section of the volume of Current Topics in Microbiology and Immunology on Influenza Pathogenesis and Control, we focus on the contribution of a specific subset of adaptive immune cells, that is activated T effector cells, to the control of viral replication in the host response to influenza A virus (IAV) infection. These activated T effector cells are classically categorized as $CD8^+$ cytotoxic T lymphocytes (CTLs) and $CD4^+$ T helper (T_H) cells. However, there is evidence for considerable heterogeneity of function among these T lymphocytes subsets, most notably among the T_H cells.

Both T cell subsets have been reported to have regulatory or suppressive activity against other adaptive or innate immune cell types. The most prominent cell type identified with such regulatory activity is the $CD4^+$ T regulatory cell subset which can be directed to either self-constituents and/or foreign molecules such as the IAV gene products. Another important but only more recently appreciated distinct subset of $CD4^+$ T cells is the subset of T cells which regulate B cell activation and germinal center formation in response to infection, the so-called T follicular helper T cell subset.

In this review, we will exclude the $CD4^+$ (and $CD8^+$) T regulatory cells as well as the T follicular helper T cell subset and restrict our focus to "conventional" CTLs and T_H cells which exhibit the capacity to migrate from draining lymph nodes (DLNs) to the site of IAV infection in the lungs. We will systematically review the factors regulating the induction of the effector cells from naïve precursors (and the role of respiratory dendritic cells in this process), expression of effector activities by these activated T cells, and the regulation of the activation and differentiation state of these T effector cells in the IAV-infected lungs.

2 Initiation of Adaptive Immunity

2.1 *Dendritic Cell Networking in the Steady-State and Inflamed Lung*

Because of its continuous encounter with the environment as it carries out its essential role in gas exchange, the respiratory tract is exposed to airborne foreign particles, such as pollutants, allergens, dusts, and microorganisms. The lungs have therefore evolved a variety of strategies to sense, respond to, and cope with these potential 'dangers,' including the establishment of a well-developed network of dendritic cells (DCs). DCs serve as the sentinels of the immune system at body surfaces (e.g., the lungs, skin, and gut), linking the response of innate immune cells and molecular sensors to the induction of adaptive immunity (Banchereau and Steinman 1998). DCs were once thought to be a homogenous population that was difficult to distinguish phenotypically from lung-resident alveolar macrophages. However, recent advances in the development of genetic tools to provide definitive information on DC biology now make it clear that DCs are a heterogenous cell population consisting of distinct DC subsets with discrete functions and with developmental pathways separate from the macrophage lineages (Helft et al. 2010). In the lung, DCs perform a range of tasks including recognition and acquisition of antigens derived from pathogens and allergens, antigen transportation to the regional lymph nodes, and perhaps most importantly, induction of $CD4^+$ or $CD8^+$ T cell immunity (Braciale et al. 2012; Lambrecht and Hammad 2012).

In the unperturbed lung, the DC network is composed of several distinct respiratory DC (RDC) subsets that differ in phenotype, anatomic localization, and function (Table 1). Of these, $CD103^+$ and $CD11b^{hi}$ RDC subsets exhibit several features characteristics of DC found in extralymphoid mucosal sites and are distributed at distinct anatomical sites: primarily intraepithelial localization for $CD103^+$ RDC and submucosal/interstitial distribution for $CD11b^{hi}$ RDC (Sung et al. 2006; del Rio et al. 2007; Edelson et al. 2010). In addition to these major populations, monocyte-like RDC (Mo-RDC) are also readily detectable in the uninflamed lung (Hao et al. 2008; Kim and Braciale 2009). In certain microenvironments within the lung parenchyma (i.e., alveolar septa), so-called conventional RDC (cRDC) (e.g., $CD103^+$ and $CD11b^{hi}$ RDC) and plasmacytoid DC (pDC) are both detectable. The human counterparts of murine $CD103^+$, $CD11b^{hi}$ RDC and pDC have recently been identified in the human lung (Table 1) (Villadangos and Shortman 2010; Neyt and Lambrecht 2013). Thus, several distinct DC subsets strategically positioned at the interface between the lung and the surroundings sense and sample the respiratory tract.

The aforementioned DC subsets are largely identifiable in inflammatory conditions such as viral infections; however, inflammatory mononuclear cells recruited to and infiltrating the inflamed tissues in response to infection (e.g., monocytes) add to the complexity of DC network in the infected lungs since many of them express/upregulate prototypical DC markers such as CD11c, major

Table 1 Major lung DC subsets in mice

DC subset	Mouse surface markers	Transcription factors	Human equivalent surface markers	Labor division	Anatomical distribution
$CD103^+$ RDC	$CD11c^+$	IRF8	$CD11c^+$	Surveillance of airway luminal surface	Associated with epithelium
–	$CD103^+$	Batf3	$BCDA3^+$ (CD141)	Antigen uptake	Above basement membrane
–	$CD11b^{+/-}$	–	$XCR1^-$	Antigen transport to the lymph node	Alveolar septa
–	$Langerin^+$	–	MHC II^{++}	Activation of $CD8^+$ T cells	–
–	$XCR1^+$	–	–	Cross-presentation	–
–	MHC II^{++}	–	–	–	–
CD11bhi RDC	$CD11c^+$	IRF4	$CD11c^+$	Surveillance of parenchymal tissue	Submucoas airways
–	$CD103^-$	–	$BCDA1^+$ (CD1c)	Antigen uptake	Beneath basement membrane
–	$CD11b^{++}$	–	MHC II^{++}	Antigen transport to the lymph node	Parenchyma
–	MHC II^{++}	–	–	Activation of $CD4^+$ T cells	Alveolar septa
–	$SIRP1\alpha^+$	–	–	Chemokine/cytokine production	–
pDCs	$CD11c^+$	E2-2	$CD123^+$	Type I IFN production	Parenchyma
–	Siglec H^+	–	$CD1c^-$	Regulating effectors in the lung	Alveolar septa
–	$Ly6C^+$	–	$BCDA2^+$	–	–
–	$B220^+$	–	MHC II^{++}	–	–
–	$PDCA\text{-}1^+$	–	$BCDA4^+$	–	–
Monocytic RDC (Mo-RDC)	$CD11c^+$	PU.1	–	Chemokine/cytokine production	–
–	$CD103^-$	–	–	TH1 cell priming	Parenchyma
–	$CD11b^{++}$	–	–	–	'Marginated' vasculature
–	MHC $II^{+/-}$	–	–	–	–
–	$Ly6C^{+/-}$	–	–	–	–

histocompatiblity complex (MHC) II and costimulatory markers at various levels (Lin et al. 2008). The potential precursor-product relationship between CD11b^{hi} DCs and Mo-RDC in steady-state as well as inflamed lung remains at present speculative. A DC subset prominent in IAV-infected lung, but minimal in the normal lung, is TNF^{+}iNOS^{+} DC (TipDC) (Aldridge et al. 2009). These DC are likely derived from the circulating Ly6C^{+}CCR2^{+} monocyte subset that are rapidly mobilized to the infected lung upon viral infection and contribute to both the viral control and immunopathology.

2.2 Activation of DCs and Antiviral Innate Immunity in the Lung

Prompt activation of innate antiviral immunity at the site of virus replication is a crucial step toward ultimate control of pathogen replication and a successful host defense against invading pathogens such as IAV. In particular, DC activation is pivotal to initiate adaptive immunity and to ultimately clear infectious virions from the infected lung (Braciale et al. 2012; Neyt and Lambrecht 2013). The recent discovery of several DC subsets in the lung implies that these distinct RDC subsets likely respond differently (i.e., display distinctive as well as overlapping functions) to a given virus; however, most studies investigating respiratory virus infection have not yet fully assimilated the impact of this DC heterogeneity into the cellular/molecular processes underpinning the induction and expression of the host response: an area meriting further detailed investigation.

Resting DCs in the lung can be stimulated by several mechanisms upon IAV infection. Foremost, DCs are equipped with a various innate immune recognition receptors that recognize conserved pathogen-associated molecular patterns (PAMPs). Specific pattern recognition receptors (PRRs) for these PAMPs include Toll-like receptors (TLRs), retinoic acid-inducible gene-1 (RIG-1)-like receptors (RLRs), and NOD-like receptors (NLRs). Several forms of IAV nucleic acids can be recognized by TLR3 (dsRNA) and TLR7/8 (ssRNA) (Yoo et al. 2013). Within the DC compartments, gene array data compiled in the Immunological Genome Project reveal that CD103^{+} RDCs predominately express TLR3, whereas CD11b^{hi} RDCs express TLR2/7. Although the contribution of PRR recognition of viral PAMPs has been well-established in vitro, the relevance of PAMP/PRR interaction to the development of innate and adaptive immunity in vivo after IAV infection is less clear. Neither the absence of TLR3 (Le Goffic et al. 2006) or the RIG-I signaling adaptor mitochondrial antiviral signaling (MAVS) (Koyama et al. 2007) diminishes virus clearance and the adaptive immunity to IAV infection. Furthermore, *Tlr7*$^{-/-}$ or *Tlr7*$^{-/-}$*Mavs*$^{-/-}$ mice are able to mount an effective CTL response and efficiently clear IAV (Heer et al. 2007; Pang et al. 2013a). Paradoxically, TLR7 and RIG-1 signals are required for efficient IAV replication in vivo (Pang et al. 2013b). These studies suggest a considerable complexity among different

PAMPs/PRRs (and the cell types in the lung expressing these PRRs) in their ability to support the induction of antiviral immunity.

Although direct recognition of viral nucleic acids and proteins by PRRs is the primary stimulatory pathway, DC activation through the recognition of nonmicrobial danger signals associated with cellular stress or damage as a result of infection has also been increasingly recognized. Damage-associated molecular patterns (DAMPs) are the host cell constituents released from damaged/dying cells as well as intact cells located within sites of viral replication. Notable DAMPs include nucleotides, heat shock proteins, nuclear proteins (e.g., HMGB1), mitochondrial DNA, cytokines, and reactive oxygen species (Said-Sadier and Ojcius 2012). Virus propagation within the respiratory tract results in the leak of or stimulates the release of DAMPs from intracellular compartments as well as extracellular sources (e.g., extracellular ATP, extracellular matrix components, and uric acids) (Pang and Iwasaki 2011). These DAMPs (also known as 'alarmins' or 'danger signals') serve to alert the host immune system and along with viral PAMPs, are believed to play a crucial role in activating innate immune sentinels such as DC in the airway mucosa in part via an inflammasome-dependent mechanism.

Inflammasomes are large intracellular multiprotein complexes consisting of NLR family members, such as NLRP3 and IPAF. The DAMP-activated NLR protein complex recruits the inflammasome-adaptor protein ASC, which in turn engages caspase-1 leading to caspase-1 activation. Once activated, caspase-1 promotes the maturation of the pro-inflammatory cytokines interleukin (IL)-1β and IL-18 (Said-Sadier and Ojcius 2012). By virtue of their ability to detect and respond to a large range of PAMPs and DAMPs, inflammasomes are an integral part of the host defense to pathogens like IAV. Indeed, IAV-derived ssRNA can, in an NLPR3-dependent manner, activate the inflammasome complex in a variety of cell types including bone marrow-derived DCs or macrophages (Kanneganti et al. 2006). In addition, the IAV-M2 viral protein, a proton-selective ion channel, can serve as an ionophore to promote nucleotide transport into the cell cytosol and directly trigger caspase-1 activation and secretion of IL-1β (Ichinohe et al. 2009). The importance of inflammasome activation to anti-IAV immunity is evident in mice deficient in inflammasome complex-associated molecules, such as NLPR3, IL-1R, caspase-1, or ASC. These mice exhibit sustained, elevated lung viral titers, reduced infiltration of neutrophils and monocytes into the infected lung, an impaired adaptive immune response, and reduced cytokine/chemokine levels compared to infected inflammasome-sufficient mice (Ichinohe et al. 2009; Thomas et al. 2009; Allen et al. 2011). Although reports differ in the extent to which inflammasome impairment affects the host response to respiratory virus infection, the accumulating data overall strongly suggest that activation of the NLRP3-dependent inflammasome and the ensuing activation of the IL-1/IL-1R-mediated signaling defense are critical for the establishment of antiviral innate and adaptive immunity (Pang et al. 2013a). It is likely that additional DAMPs will be identified which are involved in modulating lung DC activation and antiviral immunity during IAV infection.

2.3 Antigen Acquisition and Migration of Lung DCs

After activation in the lung, RDCs carry out two distinct roles in the host response to IAV infection. On one hand, perhaps the most important and unique function of RDC in the infected lung is the capture of antigen derived from IAV for delivery to the DLN. Upon arrival here, the migrant RDCs present the processed viral peptides to IAV-specific T cells to initiate adaptive immunity. On the other hand, the activated DCs release various pro-inflammatory mediators in the infected lung which serve to limit viral replication and spread but when released in excess, enhance disease severity.

The acquisition of IAV antigen in the lung by cRDC prior to their egress from the inflamed lung is most likely achieved by direct infection of RDC. Different DC subsets in both mice and humans differ in susceptibility to IAV infection. In case of IAV H1N1 PR/8 infection in mice, $CD103^+$ RDCs, unlike $CD11b^{hi}$ RDCs, are highly susceptible to infection with this strain in vivo (Hao et al. 2008; Manicassamy et al. 2010; Hargadon et al. 2011). This differential susceptibility among the RDC subsets to IAV infection is in part dependent on DC-intrinsic sensitivity to type 1 interferons (IFN) (Moltedo et al. 2011). DC infection by human IAV fails to release infectious virions likely due to lack of hemagglutinin cleavage by furan enzymes. Furthermore, phagocytic engulfment of cell-free virions or dying/dead infected cells harboring viral antigen (e.g., respiratory epithelial cells and neutrophils) is another feasible mechanism. In addition, antigen acquisition by a membrane nibbling process, known as 'trogocytosis' (Desch et al. 2011), can be employed by activated DCs, although this latter remains to be formally demonstrated during IAV infection. Viral antigen transfer from migrant antigen-bearing RDC to LN-resident DC (i.e., $CD8\alpha^+$ DC) for presentation to naïve T cells (i.e., cross-presentation) has also been reported (Belz et al. 2004). The relative contribution of these various mechanisms of antigen uptake and their impact on antigen presentation efficiency and the subsequent antiviral immune response is currently ill-defined.

Following an inflammatory stimulus like virus infection (see below), the viral antigen-bearing activated RDC migrate to the DLN along a chemokine gradient dependent on expression of the chemokine receptor CCR7 (Kim and Braciale 2009). Although the detailed molecular mechanisms underlying CCR7 upregulation by RDC after IAV infection remains elusive, stimulation through receptors for PAMPs and DAMPs likely play an integral role in promoting DC migration. Stimulation by DAMPs and inflammasome activation can recruit immature DCs and induce their functional maturation, leading them to take up antigens and home to secondary lymphoid organs. After IAV infection of mice deficient in IL-1R signaling, the migration of $CD103^+$ RDC to the DLN is severely impaired, along with a reduction in the total accumulation of inflammatory/immune cells into the DLN and the subsequent impairment of the antiviral CTL and T_H cell responses in the infected lungs (see below). On the other hand, it is noteworthy that persistent or unchecked release of DAMPs (i.e., S100A9) into the local milieu can lead to excessive stimulation of innate immune cells including DCs (Tsai et al. 2014), which can trigger aberrant uncontrolled T cell proliferation (perhaps even self-reactive T cells). Thus, net effects of DAMPs to host immunity are determined by the microenvironment and DAMP concentration.

The complement system is an essential component of innate immunity and bridges between the innate and adaptive immune systems. Similar to viral PAMPs and cellular DAMPs, components of the complement pathway in the lung provide additional immunological cues to DC activation and antiviral immunity to IAV infection. Complements, however, affect DC migration rather than the DC's T cell stimulatory activity (Kandasamy et al. 2013). Mice deficient in complement following IAV infection resulted in diminished lung DC migration (notable in $CD103^+$ RDC compartment) and accumulation into the DLN, contributing to the subsequent impaired anti-IAV T cell response in the infected lungs. Of interest, $CD103^+$ RDC possesses a unique capacity to both sense and produce complement, thereby controlling both its own migration and the migration of $CD11b^+$ RDCs from the infected lung into the MLN.

2.4 Antigen Presentation and T Cell Activation in the DLNs

Efficient viral clearance from the site of infection and establishment of lifelong protective immunity against intracellular pathogens such as viruses requires the activation of CTLs and T_H cells. Naive T cells undergo several distinct phases of immune responses including clonal expansion, acquisition of effector function, migration to the site of infection, and self-renewal (Williams and Bevan 2007). Initial programming of T lymphocyte responses occurs sequentially in lymphoid tissues draining sites of infection where IAV-specific naïve T cells are selected by professional antigen presenting cells (APCs) to proliferate, yielding functionally distinct activated T cell subsets with different functions and fates (Lawrence and Braciale 2004; Yoon et al. 2010).

Among the DC populations present in the DLN of IAV infected mice (i.e., migrant $CD103^+$, $CD11b^{hi}$ and Mo-DC, pDC, $CD8\alpha^{+/-}$ LNDC), the lung-derived migrant $CD103^+$ and $CD11b^{hi}$ RDCs serve as the primary APCs for naïve IAV-specific T cells albeit with different capacities (Kim and Braciale 2009). $CD103^+$ migrant RDCs are the most potent APC for activating CTLs following IAV infection among the DC subsets in the DLN. $CD103^+$ RDCs (but not $CD11b^{hi}$ RDCs) also have the capacity to capture noninfectious virus preparations delivered into the RT, then process and present IAV antigens CTLs (i.e., cross-presentation) (Kim and Braciale 2009; Helft et al. 2012). In keeping with its prominent role in priming antiviral CTLs, selective depletion of langerin-expressing $CD103^+$ RDCs prior to IAV infection (GeurtsvanKessel et al. 2008) or mice constitutively lacking $CD103^+$ RDCs (Batf3-deficient mice) (Helft et al. 2012) results in a severely diminished CTL response and impaired virus clearance from the lungs with subsequent infection. While the mechanistic basis for the potency displayed by

$CD103^+$ RDC to prime CTL activation are under intense instigation, its superior cross-presenting ability (Kim and Braciale 2009; Moltedo et al. 2011; Helft et al. 2012) along with enhanced loading of processed antigen onto MHC I molecules (Ho et al. 2011) have been described. In support of this view, $CD103^+$ DCs (and $CD8\alpha^+$ DC) preferentially express the DC receptor DNGR-1 (CLEC9A), which is implicated in cross-priming (Schreibelt et al. 2012; Zelenay et al. 2012).

Consistent with its dominant role in CTL priming, $CD103^+$ RDC migration and accumulation in the DLN is rigorous at an earlier phase (i.e., up to day 4 post-infection in mice) (Kim and Braciale 2009). Following this initial wave of migration and antigen presentation to CTLs by $CD103^+$ RDC, IAV antigen is continuously replenished and presented to T cells in the DLN by migrant $CD11b^{hi}$ RDCs. This temporal transition of APC to $CD11b^{hi}$ RDC in a greater quantity at later phases could serve as an amplification loop for generating CTLs until the resolution of the acute infection (Ballesteros-Tato et al. 2012). In contrast to migrant cRDC subsets, pDC has been reported to capture viral antigen in the lung, but antigen positive pDCs in the DLN fail to induce CTL responses during sub-lethal IAV infection (GeurtsvanKessel et al. 2008; Wolf et al. 2009). However, pDCs appear to play a role in eliminating virus-specific CTLs in the infected lung via Fas/Fas ligand (FasL) interaction and enhance mortality during lethal infection (Langlois and Legge 2011). Likewise, antigen-bearing Mo-RDC are detected in the DLN; however, they exhibit a minimal, if any, activity to stimulate CTL proliferation (Kim and Braciale 2009).

In contrast to their differing ability to activate naïve IAV-specific $CD8^+$ T cells, migrant $CD103^+$ and $CD11b^{hi}$ RDC subsets both robustly trigger naive $CD4^+$ T cell activation with an equal efficiency (Nakano et al. 2009). In addition, other DC subsets such as Mo-RDC can drive $CD4^+$ T cell differentiation into T_H1 cells, albeit with lower efficiency (Nakano et al. 2009). Thus, lung DC subsets accumulated in the DLN display a differential hierarchy in APC function for the activation of anti-IAV CTL and T_H cells. The distribution of distinct activities among DC subsets in the regulation of the host immune response and IAV pathogenesis is poorly characterized and is of great interest in discovering novel therapeutics and vaccinations.

3 Lymphocyte Migration into the IAV-Infected Lung

T lymphocyte migration into the lung has relatively defined, albeit overlapping, steps: selectin interactions between lymphocytes and the vascular endothelium mediate rolling and tethering stages; firm lymphocyte adhesion onto the lung vascular network is mediated by integrin interactions; and coordinated migration into the respiratory tract is regulated by integrins and chemokine gradients.

IAV-specific lymphocyte migration into nonlymphoid tissues has both specific and nonspecific components (Masopust and Schenkel 2013). The integrin CD11a, which is only upregulated in activated T cells, is required for optimal lung vascular adhesion and retention within the respiratory tract allowing preferential recruitment over naïve cells (Thatte et al. 2003). In addition, RDCs preferentially upregulate the chemokine receptor CCR4 on effector T cells, allowing selected recruitment to the IAV-infected lung, wherein the corresponding ligands CCL17 and CCL22 are produced (Mikhak et al. 2013). However, ICAM-1, the corresponding ligand for CD11a is constitutively expressed in secondary tissues allowing nonspecific recruitment of effector cells (Thatte et al. 2003), and during influenza infection, a large number of IAV-specific CTLs are detected in noninflamed tissues (Lawrence and Braciale 2004). This dichotomy of nonspecific and specific recruitment of activated lymphocytes may allow heightened systemic immunosurveillance on one hand while allowing preferentially, but not stringent, enrichment at the site of infection on the other.

T cell migration into the airways, the principal site of IAV replication, may occur either through T cells transversing the respiratory epithelium from the lung interstitium or direct entry from the circulation. The ability of T cells to migrate into the airways is selective, with CTL recruitment favored over T_H cells due to an unknown mechanism. CTL entry into the airways from the circulation is dependent on IL-15 (Verbist et al. 2011), which is regulated by type I IFN (Mattei et al. 2001). IL-15 can increase CD11a expression (Allavena et al. 1997), and IL-15 itself is chemotactic (Verbist et al. 2011). It is currently unclear which signals are required to promote migration from the lung interstitium into the airways or whether this is a major avenue of migration into the airspace environment.

It is noteworthy that a significant fraction of T lymphocytes (as well as innate immune cells (e.g., neutrophils, monocytes)) localized to the normal/unperturbed lungs are not located within the pulmonary interstitium but rather remain “marginated” within the circulation of the pulmonary vasculature even following lung profusion (Anderson et al. 2012). Therefore following infection, the frequency of innate immune and antigen-specific adaptive immune cells within the “lungs” will need to take into account cell numbers within the airspaces, interstitium, and pulmonary vasculature.

4 Adaptive Immune-Mediated Antiviral Activity in the Lung

The arrival of IAV-specific T_H cells (more precisely $CD4^+$ effector T cells) and $CD8^+$ CTLs into the respiratory tract coincides with a significant impact on overall virus titer. Adaptive immune cells and their products (e.g., immune-modulating cytokines and chemokines, neutralizing antibodies, etc.) act in concert, and in a partly redundant fashion, in ultimately eliminating infectious virus. In the murine model of IAV infection, efficient viral clearance is not solely dependent on T_H cells or CTLs (Eichelberger et al. 1991; Topham et al. 1996a; Topham and Doherty 1998); however, the removal of both cell types (i.e., via acute depletion or genetic deficiency) renders mice incapable of clearing IAV from the respiratory tract (Wells et al. 1981; Topham et al. 1997). Thus, the adaptive immune response to primary IAV infections implements a multifaceted approach to virus elimination not dependent on any one cell type.

The relative contribution of CTLs to optimal IAV clearance has been highlighted with the use of β_2-M deficient mice (i.e., defective in MHC I display and presentation), which have a severe reduction in the number of CTLs. These mice are able to clear IAV in the absence of CTLs albeit with a delay in viral clearance depending on viral strain (Eichelberger et al. 1991; Bender et al. 1992). More so, infection of β_2-M deficient mice with a highly virulent strain of influenza results in reduced survival (Bender et al. 1992). These data indicate IAV-specific CTL effector activity has a significant impact on viral clearance, with the requirement for this effector cell type in experimental models, dependent on the virulence of the influenza stain. While CTLs produce robust levels of cytokines and chemokines upon antigen encounter, the primary contribution of CTLs to IAV clearance is through the cytotoxic elimination of IAV-infected respiratory epithelial cells (RECs) (Lukacher et al. 1984; Hou and Doherty 1995; Topham et al. 1997; Hufford et al. 2011). Due to unhindered access to the respiratory epithelium and their concentration in the airways, CTLs localized to the airspace are likely the primary mediators of eliminating infected RECs; however, there is evidence MHC I is localized basolateral on the respiratory epithelium (Walters et al. 1999), and it may be that CTLs eliminate IAV-infected RECs as they transverse the basement membrane into the airways.

IAV-specific T_H cells are the dominant adaptive immune cell type localized in the lung during the time of IAV clearance. T_H cells express a wide array of soluble mediators (e.g., IFNγ, IL-2, IL-10) (Sun et al. 2009, 2011) and can be cytotoxic (Graham et al. 1994; Brown et al. 2006; Hua et al. 2013). Although T_H cytotoxic mechanisms may contribute to the control of virus replication and elimination (Brown et al. 2006; Hua et al. 2013), T_H cell anti-IAV roles may be primarily indirect through cytokine production and B cell help (Topham et al. 1996a, b; Topham and Doherty 1998).

4.1 T Lymphocyte Cytotoxic Mechanisms

T lymphocytes employ cytotoxic mechanisms to eliminate cells infected with intracellular pathogens such as IAV. The exquisite specificity of T cell-mediated killing is dependent on the interaction between the T cell receptor (TCR) and requisite antigen complexed with MHC on the infected cell. Unlike cytokine production, TCR signaling strength required to elicit cytolysis is minimal (Valitutti et al. 1996; Faroudi et al. 2003; Purbhoo et al. 2004), and killing is unilateral allowing the T effector cell to survive following target cell engagement (Kupfer et al. 1986). This allows a given T lymphocyte to serially eliminate a number of virally infected cells in a short manner of time. Despite this rapid killing, T cell-mediated

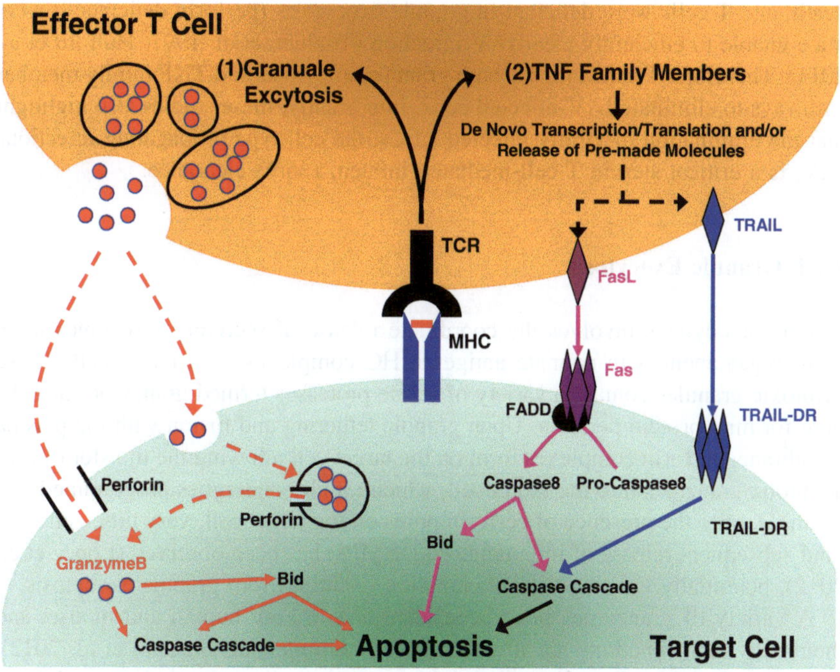

Fig. 1 Effector T cell-mediated cytotoxic pathways during influenza infection: (1) Granuale excytosis is initiated following TCR stimulus resulting in the release of premade cytotoxic granuales onto target cells. The subsequent release of the pore-forming protein perforin and serine proteases (granzymes) activate caspase cascades resulting in target cell apoptosis. (2) TNF-related proteins are upregulated upon TCR stimulus. Binding to their respective ligands on target cells recruits ligand associated death domains which ultimately activate caspase cascades resulting in target cell apoptosis

cytotoxicity exhibits little nonspecific killing. The requirement of specific antigen to elicit cytotoxicity and the polarized release of cytolytic material towards the target cell with the formation of a tight ring of adhesion molecules around the point of release are all thought to limit potential damage in uninfected neighboring cells (Lukacher et al. 1984; Dustin and Long 2010).

T lymphocyte-mediated cytotoxicity is mediated by two distinct mechanisms: (1) granule exocytosis which utilizes the pore-forming protein, perforin, to facilitate the entry of serine proteases and (2) the engagement of tumor necrosis factor (TNF) family members with their respective ligands (Fig. 1). Both pathways initiate apoptotic cascades within the target cell culminating in target cell death (Russell and Ley 2002). In several murine viral infection models, granule exocytosis alone is the principal means of immune-mediated cytotoxic clearance (Kagi et al. 1994; Walsh et al. 1994; Mullbacher et al. 1999); however, perforin-deficient mice have no defect in clearing IAV infection (Topham et al. 1997). Only when RECs lacked the expression of Fas, a TNF family member involved in cell death, and T cells were deficient in granule exocytosis (perforin deficiency) were mice unable to efficiently clear IAV infection (Topham et al. 1997; Hufford et al. 2011). Therefore, T cells employ both granule exocytosis and TNF family member pathways to eliminate IAV-infected cells. Importantly, these studies also highlight that the elimination of virally infected RECs, the cell type propagating infectious IAV, is a critical step in T cell-mediated influenza virus clearance.

4.1.1 Granule Exocytosis

Granule exocytosis involves the coordinate release of secretory lysosomes upon TCR engagement with cognate antigen/MHC complexes on a target cell. These cytotoxic granules contain a variety of serine proteases termed granzymes and the pore-forming protein perforin. Upon granule tethering and fusion with the plasma membrane, perforin complexes form on the target cell allowing the transfer of pro-apoptotic granzmes into the target cell, which rapidly undergoes programmed cell death. Despite the presence of perforin pores on the target cell, very little cell lysis (and subsequent release of inflammatory DAMPs) has been observed (Lopez et al. 2012), potentially limiting the inflammation resulting from granule exocytosis.

A variety of granzymes have been identified in both human and mouse, and their individual functions are ill-defined and controversial (Susanto et al. 2012). Granzyme B, which is well studied, initiates target cell apoptosis by two distinct mechanisms (Waterhouse et al. 2005; Kaiserman et al. 2006; Cullen et al. 2007). In mice, granzyme B preferentially cleaves pro-caspases directly into their pro-apoptotic active form. Human granzyme B mediated apoptosis is largely dependent on cleavage of the BH3 interacting domain death agonist (Bid), thereby initiating the mitochondrial apoptotic pathway and caspase activation. Other granzymes can also initiate cell death but with distinct mechanisms. For example, granzyme K-induced apoptosis is dependent on Bid cleavage but independent of downstream caspase activation (Zhao et al. 2007; Guo et al. 2010).

Granzyme activity is not limited to triggering apoptotic cell death. Granzyme K can disrupt influenza nucleocapsid protein importation into the nucleus thereby inhibiting virus replication in vivo (Zhong et al. 2012). In addition, granzymes have the potential to modify the extracellular matrix (Buzza et al. 2005) and trigger target cell cytokine production (e.g., TNF, IL-1β) (Metkar et al. 2008; Joeckel et al. 2011); however, it is unclear whether these latter functions are pivotal during IAV clearance and subsequent tissue damage.

While individual granzymes have distinct functions, granzyme-mediated cell death is dependent on perforin as evidenced by the inability of perforin-deficient mice to exhibit granule exocytosis (Kagi et al. 1994). Perforin functions by binding to the target cell membrane in a receptor-independent mechanism and forming multimeric complexes (Blumenthal et al. 1984; Voskoboinik et al. 2005). The subsequent pore in the target cell membrane permits the transfer of the constituents of the cytotoxic granules. It is currently unclear whether granzymes passively diffuse through large perforin pores on the target cell membrane surface or through a more active process within endocytic membranes (Lopez et al. 2012; Susanto et al. 2012).Thus, the precise role of perforin in this process remains to be elucidated.

During IAV infection, both T_H cells and CTLs utilize granule excytosis. As mentioned previously, the principal target for CTL-mediated cytolysis is the IAV-infected RECs (Topham et al. 1997; Hufford et al. 2011), whose elimination is essential for successful IAV clearance. The capacity for T_H cells to engage in granule exocytosis has only been recently appreciated. Few RECs express MHC II (Gereke et al. 2009), and MHC II respiratory epithelium deficiency does not influence IAV clearance in murine models (Topham et al. 1996b). However, passive transfer of cytotoxic T_H cells into IAV-infected wild type or B cell-deficient mice can improve host morbidity (Brown et al. 2006; Hua et al. 2013). In addition, the presence of IAV-specific T_H cells correlated with improved disease protection in patients with heterologous influenza infections (Wilkinson et al. 2012), indicating T_H cell-mediated cytolysis may be of significant benefit during subsequent infections.

4.1.2 TNF Family Members

Cytotoxicity can be elicited by a variety of TNF family members, the prototypical example being FasL. Interaction of FasL with its cognate receptor, Fas, is vital in regulating T cell homeostasis, and human deficiencies in Fas signaling result in autoimmune lymphoproliferative syndrome (Roths et al. 1984; Legge and Braciale 2005; Stranges et al. 2007; Imai et al. 2012); however, these interactions can also be critical in eradicating virally infected cells, notably during IAV infections (Topham et al. 1997; Hufford et al. 2011).

TCR engagement with peptide complexed MHC upregulates FasL expression in T lymphocytes. The nature of FasL trafficking to the outer membrane is debatable with evidence indicating FasL deposition is dependent on vesicular traffic of premade FasL molecules onto the outer membrane (Isaaz et al. 1995; Li et al. 1998; Lettau et al. 2006) or de novo transcription/translation following TCR engagement (Lowin et al. 1996). Nonetheless, FasL-mediated cytotoxicity occurs via the oligomerization of the target cell's Fas molecules, which are expressed on the cellular membranes of most cell types, by membrane-bound FasL (Rouvier et al. 1993). FasL is sensitive to metalloproteinase cleavage on the cell surface (Kayagaki et al. 1995), thereby limiting surface exposure and minimizing non-specific cell killing. This soluble form of FasL is a chemoattractant and can induce nonspecific cell death, albeit at much less efficiency as its membrane-bound counterpart (Schneider et al. 1998; Ottonello et al. 1999).

Fas signaling on the target cell's surface requires Fas trimerization, which may or may not precede binding to FasL (Siegel et al. 2000; Dockrell 2003). Upon FasL/Fas engagement, Fas-associated death domain (FADD) binds the death domain of Fas and recruits pro-caspase-8. Caspase 8 proceeds to cleave pro-apoptotic Bid, thereby initiating the mitochondrial apoptotic pathway, and in parallel, converts pro-caspase-3 to caspase 3 leading to a subsequent apoptotic caspase cascade.

Additional TNF family molecules can initiate cytotoxicity, either as soluble factors (i.e., TNF—as discussed later) or membrane-bound ligands (i.e., TNF-related apoptosis-inducing ligand (TRAIL)). TRAIL-induced apoptosis is commonly associated with tumor clearance (Benedict and Ware 2012); however, there is evidence of its importance in viral models (Lum et al. 2001; Kotelkin et al. 2003). TRAIL and its cognate ligand, TRAIL-death receptor (TRAIL-DR), are similar to FasL/Fas in that TRAIL engagement with TRAIL-DR recruits a death complex, thereby initiating an apoptosis cascade (Benedict and Ware 2012). Like FasL, TRAIL also can be present in a soluble form. Nonspecific cell death may be limited because high TRAIL-DR expression is limited to IAV-infected cells compared to noninfected cells (Brincks et al. 2008; Herold et al. 2008), and TRAIL expression in CTLs is partially regulated by TCR stimulus (Ishikawa et al. 2005; Brincks et al. 2008). In murine models, neutralization of TRAIL or the use of TRAIL deficient mice leads to delayed IAV clearance and increased morbidity (Ishikawa et al. 2005; Brincks et al. 2008); however, the significant role for TRAIL in regulating CTL expansion and migration during influenza infection must also be taken into account (Brincks et al. 2011)

4.2 T Cell Soluble Mediators

CTLs and in particular, T_H cells produce a wide array of cytokines and chemokines upon their infiltration into the IAV-infected lung (Fig. 2). The TCR-mediated production of these soluble mediators is important in ultimately orchestrating the elimination of infectious IAV while also minimizing the extant of the resulting inflammation. While impossible to describe all the T cell-derived products, the following subsections highlight pivotal cytokines/chemokines shaping IAV disease.

4.2.1 IFNγ

IFNγ is the most prominent cytokine produced by both IAV-specific T_H cells and CTLs upon entry into the infected lung. While other cell types can produce IFNγ, the peak IFNγ production coincides with the arrival of IAV-specific T_H cells and CTLs into the respiratory tract, and acute removal of both subsets with depleting antibodies effectively eliminates detectable IFNγ (Hufford et al. 2011).

IFNγ can activate immune cells (e.g., macrophages), upregulate immune-modulating molecules (e.g., MHC), and modulate antibody isotype switching. Despite these processes, IFNγ deficiency has no impact on IAV clearance (Graham et al. 1993). It is likely that IFNγ contributes to viral clearance but is not essential due to overlapping antiviral mechanisms. This concept is illustrated in nitric oxide

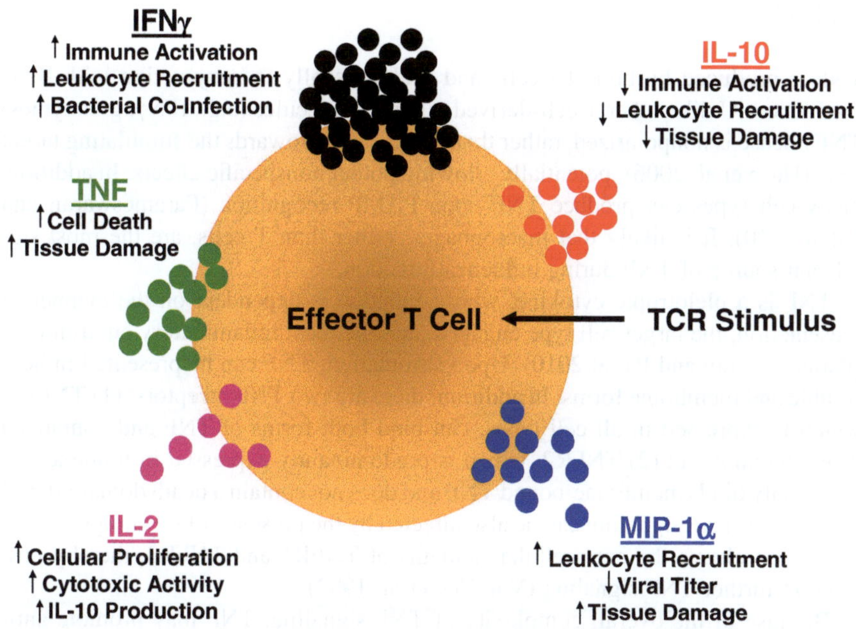

Fig. 2 The major types and functions of soluble mediators produced by effector T cells during IAV infection. Upon entry into the lung and subsequent TCR stimulation, IAV-specific T cells can produce an array of cytokines and chemokines. Major T cell derived soluble factors involved in influenza disease are depicted along with a brief summary of function

synthase knockout mice (unable to synthesize the inflammatory signaling molecule nitric oxide), which require IFNγ for the elimination of IAV (Karupiah et al. 1998). Additionally, absence of IFNγ during murine influenza infections has been demonstrated to affect leukocyte recruitment (Baumgarth and Kelso 1996; Turner et al. 2007), isotype switched antibody levels (Baumgarth and Kelso 1996; Bot et al. 1998), and immunopathology (Wiley et al. 2001).

There is sparse evidence to suggest that IFNγ is a significant contributor to immune-associated tissue damage during IAV infection. Rather, its absence can be linked with reduced tissue damage, likely due to its impact in regulating leukocyte recruitment to the lung (Wiley et al. 2001). However, IFNγ may contribute to the susceptibility to secondary bacterial infections during IAV infection. During IAV infection, alveolar macrophages exhibit decreased expression of the scavenger molecule MARCO (macrophage receptor with collagenous structure) and reduced capacity to phagocytize bacteria (Sun and Metzger 2008). Subsequently, it was demonstrated that acute IFNγ neutralization restores MARCO expression and bacterial ingestion in alveolar macrophages. Furthermore, IAV-infected mice receiving IFNγ neutralizing antibody demonstrated increased resistance to secondary bacterial infection (Sun and Metzger 2008).

4.2.2 TNF

TNF is produced by both T_H cells and CTLs, usually in conjunction with IFNγ production. Unlike other T cell-derived effector molecules (e.g., IFNγ, granzymes) TNF release is nonpolarized, rather than directionally towards the stimulating target cells (Huse et al. 2006), potentially allowing potent nonspecific effects. In addition, many cell types can produce TNF upon PAMP recognition (Parameswaran and Patial 2010). It is likely that macrophages, rather than T cells, are the most significant source of TNF during influenza infection.

TNF is a pleiotropic cytokine, whose function is dependent on the manner of presentation, the target cell type engaged, and the local inflammatory environment (Parameswaran and Patial 2010). Upon stimulation, TNF can be presented in both soluble and membrane forms. In addition, there are two TNF receptors: (1) TNFR1, which is expressed in all cell types, can bind both forms of TNF and contains a death domain; and (2) TNFR2, which is predominantly expressed in immune cell types, only binds membrane-bound TNF and does not contain a death domain (Grell et al. 1995). TNF signaling can be also affected by the presence of metalloproteases, which can cleave the extracellular domains of TNFR1 and TNFR2, thereby prohibiting further TNF signaling (Van Zee et al. 1992).

Because of the overall complexity of TNF signaling, TNF may promote anti-inflammatory (e.g., diminish cytokine production, inhibit phagocytosis, trigger apoptosis) or pro-inflammatory (e.g., stimulate cytokine production, augment cellular proliferation, trigger cellular necrosis) outcomes. A similar dichotomy in function is present during IAV infection. TNF has been demonstrated to reduce CCL2, a chemokine which promotes infiltration of inflammatory monocytes/macrophages into the lung (Damjanovic et al. 2011). In contrast, TNF has been demonstrated to be a significant contributor to immune-mediated tissue damage during IAV infection without any discernable impact on viral clearance (Peper and Van Campen 1995; Hussell et al. 2001; Belisle et al. 2010). It is currently unclear, however, whether the loss of TNF signaling in murine studies, like IFNγ, is compensated by other antiviral mechanisms.

4.2.3 IL-10

Potential sources of IL-10 in the lung during IAV infection are CTLs, T_H cells, and regulatory T cells; however, IL-10 reporter mice (which effectively mark cells undergoing IL-10 gene expression) indicate lung CTLs are the predominant source (Sun et al. 2009). Despite the capacity to make IL-10, these CTLs infiltrating the respiratory tract are not a strict regulatory subset because they readily produce inflammatory cytokines (e.g., IFNγ) and are cytotoxic (Sun et al. 2009). Thus, IL-10 production is concomitant with T cell-mediated antiviral activity, likely to limit rather than effectively prohibit subsequent inflammation.

IL-10 is a potent regulatory cytokine which, upon binding to its receptor, IL-10R, on innate and adaptive immune cells, can downregulate MHC and co-stimulatory molecule expression, modulate inflammatory cytokine expression, and inhibit cellular proliferation (Couper et al. 2008). During IAV infection, acute blockade of IL-10R signaling during T cell-mediated virus clearance results in excessive pulmonary inflammation and injury (Sun et al. 2009). In contract, mice with IL-10 deficiency have reduced viral titers, likely due to enhanced antibody production and T_H cell responses (McKinstry et al. 2009; Sun et al. 2010). Thus, the timing and location of IL-10 production can hamper antiviral immunity (i.e., during adaptive immune activation) or prohibit excessive pulmonary inflammation (i.e., during viral clearance).

4.2.4 MIP-1α

Macrophage inflammatory protein (MIP)-1α (i.e., CCL3) is readily produced by CTLs and T_H cells upon activation (Obaru et al. 1986). Other potential sources include B lymphoctyes, natural killer cells, and myeloid cells (e.g., macrophages, neutrophils, etc.). MIP-1α is a chemokine which, upon binding to its receptors CCR1, CCR3, or CCR5, exerts potent chemotactic and pro-inflammatory effects (Menten et al. 2002). MIP-1α can enhance lymphocyte cytokine production and is a potent recruiter of monocytes, lymphocytes, immature DCs, and activated neutrophils (Karpus et al. 1997; Menten et al. 2002). In IAV-infected MIP-1α deficient mice, viral clearance was delayed, albeit eventually achieved (Cook et al. 1995). Inefficient viral clearance was accompanied with deficient leukocyte recruitment in the lung and reduced tissue damage. Thus, MIP-1α is likely a significant pro-inflammatory soluble mediator necessary for efficient IAV clearance.

5 Regulation of Effector T cell Responses in the Lung

5.1 Local Differentiation of Effector T Cells in the Lung

As discussed previously, IAV-specific CTLs and T_H cells are activated in the DLN. The classical view in immunology is that T cell activation and differentiation into effector T cells are programmed and completed in the DLN; however, recent murine studies have found that upon migration to the IAV-infected lungs, both IAV-specific CTLs and T_H cells undergo extensive phenotypic changes during IAV infection, suggesting that local lung environments can further shape the differentiation of effector T cells (Fig. 3). CTLs activated in the DLN are capable of producing high levels of IFNγ upon antigenic stimulation. Interestingly, compared to CTLs residing in the DLN or spleen, CTLs in the lung downregulate their capacity to produce IFNγ following antigenic stimulation (Fulton et al. 2008), suggesting that lung environment factors restricts the extent of IFNγ production by CTLs to avoid potential collateral damage caused by exuberant IFNγ (Fulton and Varga 2010).

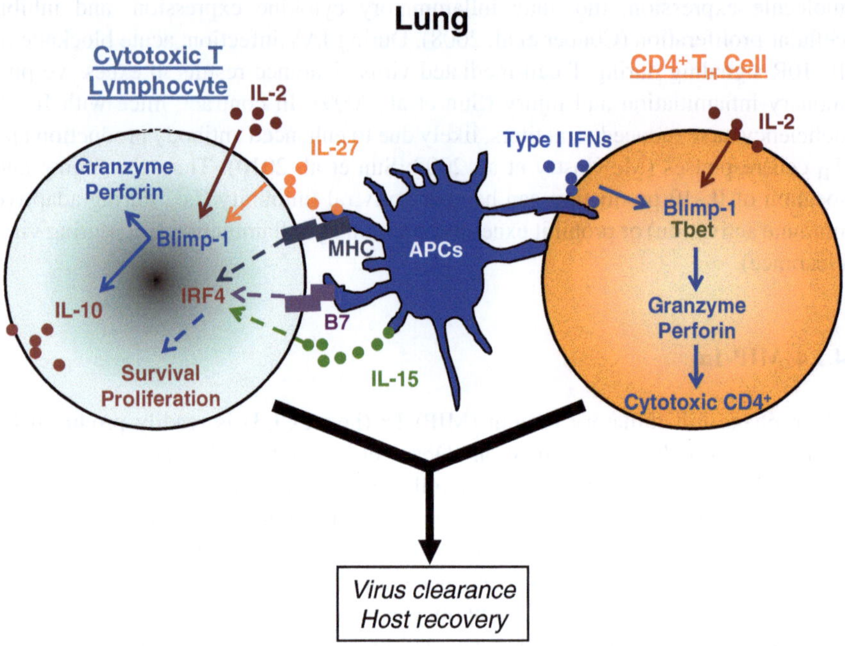

Fig. 3 Lung APCs shape local CTL and CD4$^+$ T$_H$ cell responses by providing essential differentiation, survival, and proliferation signals. Within the DLN, professional APCs and local inflammatory milieu control the early stages of antigen-specific T cell proliferation and differentiation. During influenza infection, there is significant evidence demonstrating that upon arrival into the infected lung after activation in the DLN, effector T cells undergo additional rounds of differentiation and proliferation regulated by APCs present in the respiratory tract and locally produced soluble mediators

Coinciding with their downregulation of effector cytokine IFNγ, CTLs also acquire the ability to produce IL-10 upon migrating into the lung (Sun et al. 2009, 2011). It was demonstrated that lung CTLs, but not LN effector CTLs, produce significant amount of IL-10 following antigenic-stimulation in vitro (Sun et al. 2009, 2011). As discussed previously, IL-10 functions to inhibit exuberant pulmonary inflammation during virus-induced diseases. Thus, these data suggested that CTLs acquire potent regulatory functions (i.e., capacity to produce IL-10) in the lung in response to the IAV-infected environment. The inflammatory cytokine IL-27 plays a critical role in the local instruction of IL-10 production by CTLs (Sun et al. 2011). Compared to DLN, IL-27 message is highly enriched in the infected lungs and the cellular sources of IL-27 appear mainly to be local inflammatory phagocytes including DCs, macrophages, and neutrophils, which are recruited to the lung following IAV infection (Sun et al. 2011). Therefore, lung inflammatory responses caused by virus infection are able to further instruct the continuous differentiation of CTLs for the acquisition of regulatory features.

T_H cells also upregulate IL-10 production upon migration into the lungs, suggesting the same IL-27-dependent mechanisms relates to lung T_H cells as well (Sun et al. 2009). More strikingly, T_H cells in the lungs also acquire the ability to eliminate IAV-infected MHC II^+ cells via granule exocytosis (Brown et al. 2006, 2012; Hua et al. 2013). T_H cells in the DLN, however, express minimum granzyme B and perforin (Brown et al. 2012; Hua et al. 2013), suggesting that the acquisition of cytotoxic molecules in T_H cells requires signals from the local lung environments during IAV infection. Type I IFN (expressed at higher levels in the IAV infected lung compared to the DLN) and IL-2 are required for the expression of cytotoxic molecules in lung T_H cells (Hua et al. 2013). Thus, lung environmental cues modulate the in situ differentiation of T_H cells into cytotoxic T_H cells through type I IFNs.

5.2 *Local Regulation of Proliferation and Survival of Effector T Cells*

Besides shaping the phenotype of T_H cells and CTLs, local APCs and the lung environment also provide essential survival and proliferation signals for lung T_H cells and CTLs. Early studies have identified that CTLs undergo extensive proliferation in the lung following IAV infection (Lawrence and Braciale 2004; McGill and Legge 2009). Interestingly, acute depletion of mononuclear phagocytes (mostly DCs) in the lung following T cell priming abrogated CTL proliferation and impaired antiviral T cell responses (McGill et al. 2008), suggesting that local DC and T cell interaction provides signals for the continuous proliferation of effector T cells in the lung during influenza infection. Interestingly, like the proliferation of T cells during naïve T cell activation, the in situ proliferation of lung CTLs also requires both signal 1 (MHC-peptide stimulation) and signal 2 (B7-CD28 and CD70-CD27 co-stimulation) during IAV infection (Dolfi et al. 2011; van Gisbergen et al. 2011). In addition to providing signals licensing the in situ proliferation of effector T cells, RDCs also provide critical surviving signals for CTLs. Mechanistically, the trans-presentation of IL-15 by RDCs plays a critical role in sustaining the viability of lung antiviral CTLs (McGill et al. 2010). Interestingly, IL-15 trans-presentation to effector T cells is regulated by TSLP signaling in DCs (Yadava et al. 2013). Taken together, these recent data have extended our conventional lymphoid organ-centered view of T cell responses during infection and established that local environmental cues can continuously shape tissue effector T cells phenotype and constantly modulate their function.

5.3 *Molecular Mechanisms Regulating Effector T Cell Responses in the Lung*

5.3.1 Transcriptional Control of Effector T_H Cell Responses in the Lung

T cell activation and effector differentiation are subject to intensive transcriptional control, and various transcription factors have been demonstrated to regulate the transition from naïve T cells to effector T cells (O'Shea and Paul 2010; Zhang and Bevan 2011). Emerging evidence also suggests various transcription factors regulate the extensive phenotypic changes effector T cells exhibit upon their migration into the lung, as well.

B lymphocyte–induced maturation protein-1 (Blimp-1) is a transcription repressor that plays an important role in regulating T and B cell function (Crotty et al. 2010). The expression of Blimp-1 has previously been shown to promote effector T cell migration to the lung and modulate memory T cell generation during IAV infection (Kallies et al. 2009). Interestingly, Blimp-1 is highly expressed in lung T_H cells, compared to their counterparts in the DLN (Hua et al. 2013). Importantly, Blimp-1, whose expression can be orchestrated by IL-2 and type I IFN, is required for the expression of granzyme B and perforin in lung T_H cells as well as their ability to kill target cells (Hua et al. 2013).

Besides Blimp-1, the T-box transcription factor, T-bet, also plays an important role in the development of lung cytotoxic T_H cells during IAV infection (Hua et al. 2013). Like Blimp-1, T-bet expression is upregulated in lung T_H cells by local type I IFN signaling (Hua et al. 2013). Mechanistically, T-bet and Blimp-1 cooperate to regulate the differentiation of cytotoxic T_H cells as T-bet directly binds to cytotoxic molecules and Blimp-1 controls the accessibility of the cytotoxic molecule loci to T-bet (Hua et al. 2013). Thus, local cytokine milieu controls the development of cytotoxic T_H cell development through the upregulation of the transcription factors T-bet and Blimp-1 during IAV infection.

5.3.2 Transcriptional Control of CTL Responses in the Lung

Besides regulating local T_H cell differentiation, Blimp-1 also modulates local CTL responses in the lung during IAV infection. Similar to its function in T_H cells, Blimp-1 promotes cytotoxic molecule expression in lung CTLs (Shin et al. 2009; Sun et al. 2011). Moreover, the production of IL-10 by lung CTLs is critically dependent on Blimp-1 during IAV infection. The ablation of Blimp-1 expression in CTLs specifically abrogate IL-10 but not IFNγ production by CTLs following antigen restimulation (Sun et al. 2011), suggesting that Blimp-1 is uniquely required for the requisition of regulatory function of effector CTLs. Consistent with this result, T cell specific Blimp-1 deficiency is associated with enhanced host inflammation in the airway (Sun et al. 2011). Notably, IL-27, which is highly produced in the lung compared to the DLN, cooperates with IL-2 to induce Blimp-1 expression in CTLs (Sun et al. 2011). Thus, Blimp-1 appears to be a transcription factor that translates local environmental cues into the phenotypic and functional traits of lung effector T_H cell and CTLs during IAV infection. Recently, interferon-regulatory factor (IRF) 4 was shown to play an essential role in regulating both the quality and quantity of CTL responses during IAV infection (Man et al. 2013; Yao et al. 2013). IRF4 acts as a transcriptional activator to promote effector differentiation and as a transcriptional repressor to regulate cell cycle progression and survival, thereby sustaining both the expansion and effector differentiation of CTLs during IAV infection (Yao et al. 2013). Interestingly, the conditional deletion of IRF4 expression in $CD8^+$ T cells specifically impairs the proliferation and survival of lung CTLs (Yao et al. 2013), suggesting that IRF4 is a critical regulator of CTL responses in the lung in vivo. As discussed previously, RDCs can sustain CTL proliferation and survival through the provision of antigen, co-stimulatory molecules, and cytokines. Thus, it is tempting to speculate that local DCs exert their function by promoting IRF4 expression in lung CTLs.

5.4 *In Situ Control of Effector T Cell Activities by Different Types of APCs*

Effector T cells express high levels of mRNAs encoding various effector cytokines and cytotoxic molecules and thus are able to promptly produce these cytokines and cytotoxic molecules following antigenic or mitogenic stimulation. However, it is important to note that effector T cells do not spontaneously secret cytokines or release cytotoxic molecules in vivo without further stimulation due to additional layers of translational control of cytokine expression, possibly to avoid potential self-destruction. Classically, the activities of effector T cells (i.e., production of cytokines and release of cytotoxic molecules) were often monitored through in vitro cytokine staining and degranulation assays following maximally antigenic or mitogenic stimulation. Such methods are efficient to measure the potential of effector T cells to produce cytokines and release cytotoxic molecules but fail to faithfully report the in vivo activities of effector T cells. In an in vivo setting, effector T cells likely interact with multiple target cell types and the strength of antigenic stimulation they receive from these cells could vary drastically. In particular, as noted above, early in vitro analysis demonstrated an expressional hierarchy in the regulation of T cell effector activities in which high-strength antigenic signaling induces the production of cytokine and release of cytotoxic molecules, while weak antigenic stimulation only induces the release of cytotoxic molecules but not the production of cytokines (Valitutti et al. 1996).

During IAV infection, the infected lungs contain many cell types that potentially bear IAV antigen (Kohlmeier and Woodland 2009; Braciale et al. 2012). These cells include both infiltrating lung $CD45^+$ APCs as well as $CD45^-$ RECs.

Interestingly, it was recently demonstrated that the interaction of CTLs with RECs and APCs resulted in differential effector activities by CTLs (Hufford et al. 2011). Using techniques that measure the in vivo release of cytokines through the injection of a reagent inhibiting T cell secretion, Hufford et al found that effector T cells releasing IFNγ primarily reside in the lung interstitium rather than the airways (Hufford et al. 2011). Since the lung interstitium is enriched with APCs, the authors further demonstrated that the interaction of the APCs with effector CTLs triggers the release of both cytokines and cytotoxic molecules, while the interaction of RECs with CTLs primarily induce the release of cytotoxic molecules but not effector cytokines by CTLs (Hufford et al. 2011). One crucial difference between the APC and CD45$^-$ target is the expression of the co-stimulatory ligands, B7-1 and B7-2. Lung APCs express high levels of B7 molecules (which ligate CD28 in the effector CTLs) while RECs express minimal B7 expression (Hufford et al. 2011). Indeed, blockade of the B7-CD28 interaction suppresses IFNγ production by effector CD8 T cells but not their cytotoxic activity or virus clearance in vivo. Thus, the engagement of co-stimulatory receptors on effector CD8$^+$ T cells by APCs provide the additional signal strength necessary for the production of pro-inflammatory cytokines by the T cells (Hufford et al. 2011). In further analysis, the principal population stimulating in vivo release of effector cytokines by CTLs were the lung CD11c$^+$ inflammatory DCs or TipDCs (Aldridge et al. 2009; Neyt and Lambrecht 2013). The acute depletion of CD11c$^+$ cells in the lung drastically abrogate in vivo effector T cell cytokine production (Hufford et al. 2011). Thus, lung DCs controls all the aspects of CTL responses in the lungs including survival, proliferation, differentiation, and effector activities.

Surprisingly, another significant population of lung APCs was neutrophils. Neutrophils were previously demonstrated to be required for the innate defense against IAV infection. Despite their condensed nuclei and low levels of gene transcription, neutrophils can be directly infected with IAV transcribe viral genes, and thus contain significant influenza antigen. In vivo depletion of neutrophils diminished CTL IFNγ production (Hufford et al. 2012). These data demonstrated that neutrophils are required for triggering the maximal effector activities of CTLs in vivo.

The aforementioned results have revealed a potential new layer of effector T cell regulation in vivo: effector T cell activities in the lung are differentially regulated by the strength of interaction with their target cell types. This uncoupling of the release of inflammatory cytokines and the release of cytolytic molecules by effector T cells may be employed in the future to design novel therapeutics for influenza infection (Sun and Braciale 2013). For example, the specific blockade of certain co-stimulatory signals such as B7 may specifically dampen unwanted tissue inflammation by inhibiting the release of pathogenic cytokines from effector T cells but not perturb viral clearance since this blockade regimen specifically retain the ability of effector T cells to clear virus through cytotoxic molecule-dependent mechanisms.

6 Conclusion and Future Avenues of Research

This report has reviewed the current state of knowledge concerning the effector T cell response to IAV infection in the experimental setting. As the findings within demonstrated, our knowledge of the factors regulating the induction of adaptive immune T cell responses to IAV, the effector activities displayed by these activated T cells, the mechanisms underlying the expression of these effector mechanisms, and the control of the activation/differentiation state of these T cells in the infected lungs has progressed dramatically in recent years. While of necessity much of this information has come from studies in experimental nonhuman IAV infections, this work has provided both insight and a focus for current and future research in human IAV infection (Lee et al. 2011).

Although we now understand the broad outline of the events regulating the response of $CD8^{+}$ and $CD4^{+}$ T cells to respiratory virus infections like IAV, there remains both larger fundamental issues concerning the course of the host response during and following virus clearance as well as specific questions related to the role of specific cell types within the uninfected and infected respiratory tract as inducers and regulators of T effector cell activity and as targets for immune recognition. A major gap in our knowledge is the process of restoration of normal pulmonary function following a severe the respiratory tract IAV infection and the contribution (if any) from effector T cells remaining in the lungs following infectious virus clearance. Likewise, the role of specific cell types such as the alveolar macrophages and distinct subsets of RDC both as inducers of effector T cell differentiation and as targets and regulators of T cell effector activity need to be understood. Equally importantly is the need for a deeper understanding, in particular in the human, of the impact of differential susceptibility of various cell types in the respiratory tract to infection by different IAV strains (i.e., both seasonal and pandemic) on disease severity and the outcome of infection. As we look to the prospect of a "universal influenza vaccine," we must also be cognizant of the need to develop novel strategies to control excess inflammation in those individuals unfortunate enough to develop severe life-threatening IAV infection.

References

Aldridge JR Jr, Moseley CE, Boltz DA, Negovetich NJ, Reynolds C, Franks J, Brown SA, Doherty PC, Webster RG, Thomas PG (2009) TNF/iNOS-producing dendritic cells are the necessary evil of lethal influenza virus infection. Proc Natl Acad Sci USA 106:5306–5311

Allavena P, Giardina G, Bianchi G, Mantovani A (1997) IL-15 is chemotactic for natural killer cells and stimulates their adhesion to vascular endothelium. J Leukoc Biol 61:729–735

Allen S, Turner SJ, Bourges D, Gleeson PA, van Driel IR (2011) Shaping the T-cell repertoire in the periphery. Immunol Cell Biol 89:60–69

Anderson KG, Sung H, Skon CN, Lefrancois L, Deisinger A, Vezys V, Masopust D (2012) Cutting edge: intravascular staining redefines lung CD8 T cell responses. J Immunol 189:2702–2706

Ballesteros-Tato A, Leon B, Graf BA, Moquin A, Adams PS, Lund FE, Randall TD (2012) Interleukin-2 inhibits germinal center formation by limiting T follicular helper cell differentiation. Immunity 36:847–856

Banchereau J, Steinman RM (1998) Dendritic cells and the control of immunity. Nature 392:245–252

Baumgarth N, Kelso A (1996) In vivo blockade of gamma interferon affects the influenza virus-induced humoral and the local cellular immune response in lung tissue. J Virol 70:4411–4418

Belisle SE, Tisoncik JR, Korth MJ, Carter VS, Proll SC, Swayne DE, Pantin-Jackwood M, Tumpey TM, Katze MG (2010) Genomic profiling of tumor necrosis factor alpha (TNF-alpha) receptor and interleukin-1 receptor knockout mice reveals a link between TNF-alpha signaling and increased severity of 1918 pandemic influenza virus infection. J Virol 84:12576–12588

Belz GT, Smith CM, Kleinert L, Reading P, Brooks A, Shortman K, Carbone FR, Heath WR (2004) Distinct migrating and nonmigrating dendritic cell populations are involved in MHC class I-restricted antigen presentation after lung infection with virus. Proc Natl Acad Sci USA 101:8670–8675

Bender BS, Croghan T, Zhang L, Small PA Jr (1992) Transgenic mice lacking class I major histocompatibility complex-restricted T cells have delayed viral clearance and increased mortality after influenza virus challenge. J Exp Med 175:1143–1145

Benedict CA, Ware CF (2012) TRAIL: not just for tumors anymore? J Exp Med 209:1903–1906

Blumenthal R, Millard PJ, Henkart MP, Reynolds CW, Henkart PA (1984) Liposomes as targets for granule cytolysin from cytotoxic large granular lymphocyte tumors. Proc Natl Acad Sci USA 81:5551–5555

Bot A, Bot S, Bona CA (1998) Protective role of gamma interferon during the recall response to influenza virus. J Virol 72:6637–6645

Braciale TJ, Sun J, Kim TS (2012) Regulating the adaptive immune response to respiratory virus infection. Nat Rev Immunol 12:295–305

Brincks EL, Katewa A, Kucaba TA, Griffith TS, Legge KL (2008) CD8 T cells utilize TRAIL to control influenza virus infection. J Immunol 181:4918–4925

Brincks EL, Gurung P, Langlois RA, Hemann EA, Legge KL, Griffith TS (2011) The magnitude of the T cell response to a clinically significant dose of influenza virus is regulated by TRAIL. J Immunol 187:4581–4588

Brown DM, Dilzer AM, Meents DL, Swain SL (2006) CD4 T cell-mediated protection from lethal influenza: perforin and antibody-mediated mechanisms give a one-two punch. J Immunol 177:2888–2898

Brown DM, Lee S, Garcia-Hernandez Mde L, Swain SL (2012) Multifunctional CD4 cells expressing gamma interferon and perforin mediate protection against lethal influenza virus infection. J Virol 86:6792–6803

Buzza MS, Zamurs L, Sun J, Bird CH, Smith AI, Trapani JA, Froelich CJ, Nice EC, Bird PI (2005) Extracellular matrix remodeling by human granzyme B via cleavage of vitronectin, fibronectin, and laminin. J Biol Chem 280:23549–23558

Cook DN, Beck MA, Coffman TM, Kirby SL, Sheridan JF, Pragnell IB, Smithies O (1995) Requirement of MIP-1 alpha for an inflammatory response to viral infection. Science 269:1583–1585

Couper KN, Blount DG, Riley EM (2008) IL-10: The master regulator of immunity to infection. J Immunol 180:5771–5777

Crotty S, Johnston RJ, Schoenberger SP (2010) Effectors and memories: Bcl-6 and Blimp-1 in T and B lymphocyte differentiation. Nat Immunol 11:114–120

Cullen SP, Adrain C, Luthi AU, Duriez PJ, Martin SJ (2007) Human and murine granzyme B exhibit divergent substrate preferences. J Cell Biol 176:435–444

Damjanovic D, Divangahi M, Kugathasan K, Small CL, Zganiacz A, Brown EG, Hogaboam CM, Gauldie J, Xing Z (2011) Negative regulation of lung inflammation and immunopathology by TNF-alpha during acute influenza infection. Am J Pathol 179:2963–2976

del Rio ML, Rodriguez-Barbosa JI, Kremmer E, Forster R (2007) CD103- and CD103+ bronchial lymph node dendritic cells are specialized in presenting and cross-presenting innocuous antigen to CD4+ and CD8+ T cells. J Immunol 178:6861–6866
Desch AN, Randolph GJ, Murphy K, Gautier EL, Kedl RM, Lahoud MH, Caminschi I, Shortman K, Henson PM, Jakubzick CV (2011) CD103+ pulmonary dendritic cells preferentially acquire and present apoptotic cell-associated antigen. J Exp Med 208:1789–1797
Dockrell DH (2003) The multiple roles of Fas ligand in the pathogenesis of infectious diseases. Clin Microbiol Infect 9:766–779
Dolfi DV, Duttagupta PA, Boesteanu AC, Mueller YM, Oliai CH, Borowski AB, Katsikis PD (2011) Dendritic cells and CD28 costimulation are required to sustain virus-specific CD8+ T cell responses during the effector phase in vivo. J Immunol 186:4599–4608
Dustin ML, Long EO (2010) Cytotoxic immunological synapses. Immunol Rev 235:24–34
Edelson BT, Kc W, Juang R, Kohyama M, Benoit LA, Klekotka PA, Moon C, Albring JC, Ise W, Michael DG, Bhattacharya D, Stappenbeck TS, Holtzman MJ, Sung SS, Murphy TL, Hildner K, Murphy KM (2010) Peripheral CD103+ dendritic cells form a unified subset developmentally related to CD8alpha+ conventional dendritic cells. J Exp Med 207:823–836
Eichelberger M, Allan W, Zijlstra M, Jaenisch R, Doherty PC (1991) Clearance of influenza virus respiratory infection in mice lacking class I major histocompatibility complex-restricted CD8+ T cells. J Exp Med 174:875–880
Faroudi M, Utzny C, Salio M, Cerundolo V, Guiraud M, Muller S, Valitutti S (2003) Lytic versus stimulatory synapse in cytotoxic T lymphocyte/target cell interaction: manifestation of a dual activation threshold. Proc Natl Acad Sci USA 100:14145–14150
Fulton RB, Varga SM (2010) Editorial: CD8 T cells cut back on calcium intake in the lungs. J Leukoc Biol 87:961–964
Fulton RB, Olson MR, Varga SM (2008) Regulation of cytokine production by virus-specific CD8 T cells in the lungs. J Virol 82:7799–7811
Gereke M, Jung S, Buer J, Bruder D (2009) Alveolar type II epithelial cells present antigen to CD4(+) T cells and induce Foxp3(+) regulatory T cells. Am J Respir Crit Care Med 179:344–355
GeurtsvanKessel CH, Willart MA, van Rijt LS, Muskens F, Kool M, Baas C, Thielemans K, Bennett C, Clausen BE, Hoogsteden HC, Osterhaus AD, Rimmelzwaan GF, Lambrecht BN (2008) Clearance of influenza virus from the lung depends on migratory langerin+CD11b- but not plasmacytoid dendritic cells. J Exp Med 205:1621–1634
Graham MB, Dalton DK, Giltinan D, Braciale VL, Stewart TA, Braciale TJ (1993) Response to influenza infection in mice with a targeted disruption in the interferon gamma gene. J Exp Med 178:1725–1732
Graham MB, Braciale VL, Braciale TJ (1994) Influenza virus-specific CD4+ T helper type 2 T lymphocytes do not promote recovery from experimental virus infection. J Exp Med 180:1273–1282
Grell M, Douni E, Wajant H, Lohden M, Clauss M, Maxeiner B, Georgopoulos S, Lesslauer W, Kollias G, Pfizenmaier K, Scheurich P (1995) The transmembrane form of tumor necrosis factor is the prime activating ligand of the 80 kDa tumor necrosis factor receptor. Cell 83:793–802
Guo Y, Chen J, Shi L, Fan Z (2010) Valosin-containing protein cleavage by granzyme K accelerates an endoplasmic reticulum stress leading to caspase-independent cytotoxicity of target tumor cells. J Immunol 185:5348–5359
Hao X, Kim TS, Braciale TJ (2008) Differential response of respiratory dendritic cell subsets to influenza virus infection. J Virol 82:4908–4919
Hargadon KM, Zhou H, Albrecht RA, Dodd HA, Garcia-Sastre A, Braciale TJ (2011) Major histocompatibility complex class II expression and hemagglutinin subtype influence the infectivity of type A influenza virus for respiratory dendritic cells. J Virol 85:11955–11963
Heer AK, Shamshiev A, Donda A, Uematsu S, Akira S, Kopf M, Marsland BJ (2007) TLR signaling fine-tunes anti-influenza B cell responses without regulating effector T cell responses. J Immunol 178:2182–2191

Helft J, Ginhoux F, Bogunovic M, Merad M (2010) Origin and functional heterogeneity of non-lymphoid tissue dendritic cells in mice. Immunol Rev 234:55–75

Helft J, Manicassamy B, Guermonprez P, Hashimoto D, Silvin A, Agudo J, Brown BD, Schmolke M, Miller JC, Leboeuf M, Murphy KM, Garcia-Sastre A, Merad M (2012) Cross-presenting CD103+ dendritic cells are protected from influenza virus infection. J Clin Invest 122:4037–4047

Herold S, Steinmueller M, von Wulffen W, Cakarova L, Pinto R, Pleschka S, Mack M, Kuziel WA, Corazza N, Brunner T, Seeger W, Lohmeyer J (2008) Lung epithelial apoptosis in influenza virus pneumonia: the role of macrophage-expressed TNF-related apoptosis-inducing ligand. J Exp Med 205:3065–3077

Ho AW, Prabhu N, Betts RJ, Ge MQ, Dai X, Hutchinson PE, Lew FC, Wong KL, Hanson BJ, Macary PA, Kemeny DM (2011) Lung CD103+ dendritic cells efficiently transport influenza virus to the lymph node and load viral antigen onto MHC class I for presentation to CD8 T cells. J Immunol 187:6011–6021

Hou S, Doherty PC (1995) Clearance of Sendai virus by CD8+ T cells requires direct targeting to virus-infected epithelium. Eur J Immunol 25:111–116

Hua L, Yao S, Pham D, Jiang L, Wright J, Sawant D, Dent AL, Braciale TJ, Kaplan MH, Sun J (2013) Cytokine-dependent induction of CD4+ T cells with cytotoxic potential during influenza virus infection. J Virol 87:11884–11893

Hufford MM, Kim TS, Sun J, Braciale TJ (2011) Antiviral CD8+ T cell effector activities in situ are regulated by target cell type. J Exp Med 208:167–180

Hufford MM, Richardson G, Zhou H, Manicassamy B, Garcia-Sastre A, Enelow RI, Braciale TJ (2012) Influenza-infected neutrophils within the infected lungs act as antigen presenting cells for anti-viral CD8(+) T cells. PLoS One 7:e46581

Huse M, Lillemeier BF, Kuhns MS, Chen DS, Davis MM (2006) T cells use two directionally distinct pathways for cytokine secretion. Nat Immunol 7:247–255

Hussell T, Pennycook A, Openshaw PJ (2001) Inhibition of tumor necrosis factor reduces the severity of virus-specific lung immunopathology. Eur J Immunol 31:2566–2573

Ichinohe T, Lee HK, Ogura Y, Flavell R, Iwasaki A (2009) Inflammasome recognition of influenza virus is essential for adaptive immune responses. J Exp Med 206:79–87

Imai M, Watanabe T, Hatta M, Das SC, Ozawa M, Shinya K, Zhong G, Hanson A, Katsura H, Watanabe S, Li C, Kawakami E, Yamada S, Kiso M, Suzuki Y, Maher EA, Neumann G, Kawaoka Y (2012) Experimental adaptation of an influenza H5 HA confers respiratory droplet transmission to a reassortant H5 HA/H1N1 virus in ferrets. Nature 486:420–428

Isaaz S, Baetz K, Olsen K, Podack E, Griffiths GM (1995) Serial killing by cytotoxic T lymphocytes: T cell receptor triggers degranulation, re-filling of the lytic granules and secretion of lytic proteins via a non-granule pathway. Eur J Immunol 25:1071–1079

Ishikawa E, Nakazawa M, Yoshinari M, Minami M (2005) Role of tumor necrosis factor-related apoptosis-inducing ligand in immune response to influenza virus infection in mice. J Virol 79:7658–7663

Joeckel LT, Wallich R, Martin P, Sanchez-Martinez D, Weber FC, Martin SF, Borner C, Pardo J, Froelich C, Simon MM (2011) Mouse granzyme K has pro-inflammatory potential. Cell Death Differ 18:1112–1119

Kagi D, Ledermann B, Burki K, Seiler P, Odermatt B, Olsen KJ, Podack ER, Zinkernagel RM, Hengartner H (1994) Cytotoxicity mediated by T cells and natural killer cells is greatly impaired in perforin-deficient mice. Nature 369:31–37

Kaiserman D, Bird CH, Sun J, Matthews A, Ung K, Whisstock JC, Thompson PE, Trapani JA, Bird PI (2006) The major human and mouse granzymes are structurally and functionally divergent. J Cell Biol 175:619–630

Kallies A, Xin A, Belz GT, Nutt SL (2009) Blimp-1 transcription factor is required for the differentiation of effector CD8(+) T cells and memory responses. Immunity 31:283–295

Kandasamy M, Ying PC, Ho AW, Sumatoh HR, Schlitzer A, Hughes TR, Kemeny DM, Morgan BP, Ginhoux F, Sivasankar B (2013) Complement mediated signaling on pulmonary

CD103(+) dendritic cells is critical for their migratory function in response to influenza infection. PLoS Pathog 9:e1003115

Kanneganti TD, Body-Malapel M, Amer A, Park JH, Whitfield J, Franchi L, Taraporewala ZF, Miller D, Patton JT, Inohara N, Nunez G (2006) Critical role for Cryopyrin/Nalp3 in activation of caspase-1 in response to viral infection and double-stranded RNA. J Biol Chem 281:36560–36568

Karpus WJ, Lukacs NW, Kennedy KJ, Smith WS, Hurst SD, Barrett TA (1997) Differential CC chemokine-induced enhancement of T helper cell cytokine production. J Immunol 158:4129–4136

Karupiah G, Chen JH, Mahalingam S, Nathan CF, MacMicking JD (1998) Rapid interferon gamma-dependent clearance of influenza A virus and protection from consolidating pneumonitis in nitric oxide synthase 2-deficient mice. J Exp Med 188:1541–1546

Kayagaki N, Kawasaki A, Ebata T, Ohmoto H, Ikeda S, Inoue S, Yoshino K, Okumura K, Yagita H (1995) Metalloproteinase-mediated release of human Fas ligand. J Exp Med 182:1777–1783

Kim TS, Braciale TJ (2009) Respiratory dendritic cell subsets differ in their capacity to support the induction of virus-specific cytotoxic CD8+ T cell responses. PLoS One 4:e4204

Kohlmeier JE, Woodland DL (2009) Immunity to respiratory viruses. Annu Rev Immunol 27:61–82

Kotelkin A, Prikhod'ko EA, Cohen JI, Collins PL, Bukreyev A (2003) Respiratory syncytial virus infection sensitizes cells to apoptosis mediated by tumor necrosis factor-related apoptosis-inducing ligand. J Virol 77:9156–9172

Koyama S, Ishii KJ, Kumar H, Tanimoto T, Coban C, Uematsu S, Kawai T, Akira S (2007) Differential role of TLR- and RLR-signaling in the immune responses to influenza A virus infection and vaccination. J Immunol 179:4711–4720

Kupfer A, Singer SJ, Dennert G (1986) On the mechanism of unidirectional killing in mixtures of two cytotoxic T lymphocytes. Unidirectional polarization of cytoplasmic organelles and the membrane-associated cytoskeleton in the effector cell. J Exp Med 163:489–498

Lambrecht BN, Hammad H (2012) Lung dendritic cells in respiratory viral infection and asthma: from protection to immunopathology. Annu Rev Immunol 30:243–270

Langlois RA, Legge KL (2011) Plasmacytoid dendritic cells enhance mortality during lethal influenza infections by eliminating virus-specific CD8 T cells. J Immunol 184:4440–4446

Lawrence CW, Braciale TJ (2004) Activation, differentiation, and migration of naive virus-specific CD8+ T cells during pulmonary influenza virus infection. J Immunol 173:1209–1218

Le Goffic R, Balloy V, Lagranderie M, Alexopoulou L, Escriou N, Flavell R, Chignard M, Si-Tahar M (2006) Detrimental contribution of the Toll-like receptor (TLR)3 to influenza A virus-induced acute pneumonia. PLoS Pathog 2:e53

Lee N, Wong CK, Chan PK, Chan MC, Wong RY, Lun SW, Ngai KL, Lui GC, Wong BC, Lee SK, Choi KW, Hui DS (2011) Cytokine response patterns in severe pandemic 2009 H1N1 and seasonal influenza among hospitalized adults. PLoS One 6:e26050

Legge KL, Braciale TJ (2005) Lymph node dendritic cells control CD8+ T cell responses through regulated FasL expression. Immunity 23:649–659

Lettau M, Qian J, Linkermann A, Latreille M, Larose L, Kabelitz D, Janssen O (2006) The adaptor protein Nck interacts with Fas ligand: Guiding the death factor to the cytotoxic immunological synapse. Proc Natl Acad Sci U S A 103:5911–5916

Li JH, Rosen D, Ronen D, Behrens CK, Krammer PH, Clark WR, Berke G (1998) The regulation of CD95 ligand expression and function in CTL. J Immunol 161:3943–3949

Lin KL, Suzuki Y, Nakano H, Ramsburg E, Gunn MD (2008) CCR2+ monocyte-derived dendritic cells and exudate macrophages produce influenza-induced pulmonary immune pathology and mortality. J Immunol 180:2562–2572

Lopez JA, Brennan AJ, Whisstock JC, Voskoboinik I, Trapani JA (2012) Protecting a serial killer: pathways for perforin trafficking and self-defense ensure sequential target cell death. Trends Immunol 33:406–412

Lowin B, Mattman C, Hahne M, Tschopp J (1996) Comparison of Fas(Apo-1/CD95)- and perforin-mediated cytotoxicity in primary T lymphocytes. Int Immunol 8:57–63

Lukacher AE, Braciale VL, Braciale TJ (1984) In vivo effector function of influenza virus-specific cytotoxic T lymphocyte clones is highly specific. J Exp Med 160:814–826
Lum JJ, Pilon AA, Sanchez-Dardon J, Phenix BN, Kim JE, Mihowich J, Jamison K, Hawley-Foss N, Lynch DH, Badley AD (2001) Induction of cell death in human immunodeficiency virus-infected macrophages and resting memory CD4 T cells by TRAIL/Apo2l. J Virol 75:11128–11136
Man K, Miasari M, Shi W, Xin A, Henstridge DC, Preston S, Pellegrini M, Belz GT, Smyth GK, Febbraio MA, Nutt SL, Kallies A (2013) The transcription factor IRF4 is essential for TCR affinity-mediated metabolic programming and clonal expansion of T cells. Nat Immunol 14:1155–1165
Manicassamy B, Manicassamy S, Belicha-Villanueva A, Pisanelli G, Pulendran B, Garcia-Sastre A (2010) Analysis of in vivo dynamics of influenza virus infection in mice using a GFP reporter virus. Proc Natl Acad Sci USA 107:11531–11536
Masopust D, Schenkel JM (2013) The integration of T cell migration, differentiation and function. Nat Rev Immunol 13:309–320
Mattei F, Schiavoni G, Belardelli F, Tough DF (2001) IL-15 is expressed by dendritic cells in response to type I IFN, double-stranded RNA, or lipopolysaccharide and promotes dendritic cell activation. J Immunol 167:1179–1187
McGill J, Legge KL (2009) Cutting edge: contribution of lung-resident T cell proliferation to the overall magnitude of the antigen-specific CD8 T cell response in the lungs following murine influenza virus infection. J Immunol 183:4177–4181
McGill J, Van Rooijen N, Legge KL (2008) Protective influenza-specific CD8 T cell responses require interactions with dendritic cells in the lungs. J Exp Med 205:1635–1646
McGill J, Van Rooijen N, Legge KL (2010) IL-15 trans-presentation by pulmonary dendritic cells promotes effector CD8 T cell survival during influenza virus infection. J Exp Med 207:521–534
McKinstry KK, Strutt TM, Buck A, Curtis JD, Dibble JP, Huston G, Tighe M, Hamada H, Sell S, Dutton RW, Swain SL (2009) IL-10 deficiency unleashes an influenza-specific Th17 response and enhances survival against high-dose challenge. J Immunol 182:7353–7363
Menten P, Wuyts A, Van Damme J (2002) Macrophage inflammatory protein-1. Cytokine Growth Factor Rev 13:455–481
Metkar SS, Menaa C, Pardo J, Wang B, Wallich R, Freudenberg M, Kim S, Raja SM, Shi L, Simon MM, Froelich CJ (2008) Human and mouse granzyme A induce a proinflammatory cytokine response. Immunity 29:720–733
Mikhak Z, Strassner JP, Luster AD (2013) Lung dendritic cells imprint T cell lung homing and promote lung immunity through the chemokine receptor CCR4. J Exp Med 210:1855–1869
Moltedo B, Li W, Yount JS, Moran TM (2011) Unique type I interferon responses determine the functional fate of migratory lung dendritic cells during influenza virus infection. PLoS Pathog 7:e1002345
Mullbacher A, Hla RT, Museteanu C, Simon MM (1999) Perforin is essential for control of ectromelia virus but not related poxviruses in mice. J Virol 73:1665–1667
Nakano H, Lin KL, Yanagita M, Charbonneau C, Cook DN, Kakiuchi T, Gunn MD (2009) Blood-derived inflammatory dendritic cells in lymph nodes stimulate acute T helper type 1 immune responses. Nat Immunol 10:394–402
Neyt K, Lambrecht BN (2013) The role of lung dendritic cell subsets in immunity to respiratory viruses. Immunol Rev 255:57–67
Obaru K, Fukuda M, Maeda S, Shimada K (1986) A cDNA clone used to study mRNA inducible in human tonsillar lymphocytes by a tumor promoter. J Biochem 99:885–894
O'Shea JJ, Paul WE (2010) Mechanisms underlying lineage commitment and plasticity of helper CD4+ T cells. Science 327:1098–1102
Ottonello L, Tortolina G, Amelotti M, Dallegri F (1999) Soluble Fas ligand is chemotactic for human neutrophilic polymorphonuclear leukocytes. J Immunol 162:3601–3606
Pang IK, Iwasaki A (2011) Inflammasomes as mediators of immunity against influenza virus. Trends Immunol 32:34–41

Pang IK, Ichinohe T, Iwasaki A (2013a) IL-1R signaling in dendritic cells replaces pattern-recognition receptors in promoting CD8(+) T cell responses to influenza A virus. Nat Immunol 14:246–253

Pang IK, Pillai PS, Iwasaki A (2013b) Efficient influenza A virus replication in the respiratory tract requires signals from TLR7 and RIG-I. Proc Natl Acad Sci USA 110:13910–13915

Parameswaran N, Patial S (2010) Tumor necrosis factor-alpha signaling in macrophages. Crit Rev Eukaryot Gene Expr 20:87–103

Peper RL, Van Campen H (1995) Tumor necrosis factor as a mediator of inflammation in influenza A viral pneumonia. Microb Pathog 19:175–183

Purbhoo MA, Irvine DJ, Huppa JB, Davis MM (2004) T cell killing does not require the formation of a stable mature immunological synapse. Nat Immunol 5:524–530

Roths JB, Murphy ED, Eicher EM (1984) A new mutation, gld, that produces lymphoproliferation and autoimmunity in C3H/HeJ mice. J Exp Med 159:1–20

Rouvier E, Luciani MF, Golstein P (1993) Fas involvement in Ca(2+)-independent T cell-mediated cytotoxicity. J Exp Med 177:195–200

Russell JH, Ley TJ (2002) Lymphocyte-mediated cytotoxicity. Annu Rev Immunol 20:323–370

Said-Sadier N, Ojcius DM (2012) Alarmins, inflammasomes and immunity. Biomed J 35:437–449

Schneider P, Holler N, Bodmer JL, Hahne M, Frei K, Fontana A, Tschopp J (1998) Conversion of membrane-bound Fas(CD95) ligand to its soluble form is associated with downregulation of its proapoptotic activity and loss of liver toxicity. J Exp Med 187:1205–1213

Schreibelt G, Klinkenberg LJ, Cruz LJ, Tacken PJ, Tel J, Kreutz M, Adema GJ, Brown GD, Figdor CG, de Vries IJ (2012) The C-type lectin receptor CLEC9A mediates antigen uptake and (cross-)presentation by human blood BDCA3+ myeloid dendritic cells. Blood 119:2284–2292

Shin H, Blackburn SD, Intlekofer AM, Kao C, Angelosanto JM, Reiner SL, Wherry EJ (2009) A role for the transcriptional repressor Blimp-1 in CD8(+) T cell exhaustion during chronic viral infection. Immunity 31:309–320

Siegel RM, Frederiksen JK, Zacharias DA, Chan FK, Johnson M, Lynch D, Tsien RY, Lenardo MJ (2000) Fas preassociation required for apoptosis signaling and dominant inhibition by pathogenic mutations. Science 288:2354–2357

Stranges PB, Watson J, Cooper CJ, Choisy-Rossi CM, Stonebraker AC, Beighton RA, Hartig H, Sundberg JP, Servick S, Kaufmann G, Fink PJ, Chervonsky AV (2007) Elimination of antigen-presenting cells and autoreactive T cells by Fas contributes to prevention of autoimmunity. Immunity 26:629–641

Sun J, Braciale TJ (2013) Role of T cell immunity in recovery from influenza virus infection. Curr Opin Virol 3:425–429

Sun K, Metzger DW (2008) Inhibition of pulmonary antibacterial defense by interferon-gamma during recovery from influenza infection. Nat Med 14:558–564

Sun J, Madan R, Karp CL, Braciale TJ (2009) Effector T cells control lung inflammation during acute influenza virus infection by producing IL-10. Nat Med 15:277–284

Sun K, Torres L, Metzger DW (2010) A detrimental effect of interleukin-10 on protective pulmonary humoral immunity during primary influenza A virus infection. J Virol 84:5007–5014

Sun J, Dodd H, Moser EK, Sharma R, Braciale TJ (2011) CD4+ T cell help and innate-derived IL-27 induce Blimp-1-dependent IL-10 production by antiviral CTLs. Nat Immunol 12:327–334

Sung SS, Fu SM, Rose CE Jr, Gaskin F, Ju ST, Beaty SR (2006) A major lung CD103 (alphaE)-beta7 integrin-positive epithelial dendritic cell population expressing Langerin and tight junction proteins. J Immunol 176:2161–2172

Susanto O, Trapani JA, Brasacchio D (2012) Controversies in granzyme biology. Tissue Antigens 80:477–487

Thatte J, Dabak V, Williams MB, Braciale TJ, Ley K (2003) LFA-1 is required for retention of effector CD8 T cells in mouse lungs. Blood 101:4916–4922

Thomas PG, Dash P, Aldridge JR Jr, Ellebedy AH, Reynolds C, Funk AJ, Martin WJ, Lamkanfi M, Webby RJ, Boyd KL, Doherty PC, Kanneganti TD (2009) The intracellular sensor NLRP3 mediates key innate and healing responses to influenza A virus via the regulation of caspase-1. Immunity 30:566–575

Topham DJ, Doherty PC (1998) Clearance of an influenza A virus by CD4+ T cells is inefficient in the absence of B cells. J Virol 72:882–885

Topham DJ, Tripp RA, Hamilton-Easton AM, Sarawar SR, Doherty PC (1996a) Quantitative analysis of the influenza virus-specific CD4+ T cell memory in the absence of B cells and Ig. J Immunol 157:2947–2952

Topham DJ, Tripp RA, Sarawar SR, Sangster MY, Doherty PC (1996b) Immune CD4+ T cells promote the clearance of influenza virus from major histocompatibility complex class II -/- respiratory epithelium. J Virol 70:1288–1291

Topham DJ, Tripp RA, Doherty PC (1997) CD8+ T cells clear influenza virus by perforin or Fas-dependent processes. J Immunol 159:5197–5200

Tsai SY, Segovia JA, Chang TH, Morris IR, Berton MT, Tessier PA, Tardif MR, Cesaro A, Bose S (2014) DAMP molecule S100A9 acts as a molecular pattern to enhance inflammation during influenza A virus infection: role of DDX21-TRIF-TLR4-MyD88 pathway. PLoS Pathog 10:e1003848

Turner SJ, Olivas E, Gutierrez A, Diaz G, Doherty PC (2007) Disregulated influenza A virus-specific CD8+ T cell homeostasis in the absence of IFN-gamma signaling. J Immunol 178:7616–7622

Valitutti S, Muller S, Dessing M, Lanzavecchia A (1996) Different responses are elicited in cytotoxic T lymphocytes by different levels of T cell receptor occupancy. J Exp Med 183:1917–1921

van Gisbergen KP, Klarenbeek PL, Kragten NA, Unger PP, Nieuwenhuis MB, Wensveen FM, ten Brinke A, Tak PP, Eldering E, Nolte MA, van Lier RA (2011) The costimulatory molecule CD27 maintains clonally diverse CD8(+) T cell responses of low antigen affinity to protect against viral variants. Immunity 35:97–108

Van Zee KJ, Kohno T, Fischer E, Rock CS, Moldawer LL, Lowry SF (1992) Tumor necrosis factor soluble receptors circulate during experimental and clinical inflammation and can protect against excessive tumor necrosis factor alpha in vitro and in vivo. Proc Natl Acad Sci USA 89:4845–4849

Verbist KC, Cole CJ, Field MB, Klonowski KD (2011) A role for IL-15 in the migration of effector CD8 T cells to the lung airways following influenza infection. J Immunol 186:174–182

Villadangos JA, Shortman K (2010) Found in translation: the human equivalent of mouse CD8+ dendritic cells. J Exp Med 207:1131–1134

Voskoboinik I, Thia MC, Fletcher J, Ciccone A, Browne K, Smyth MJ, Trapani JA (2005) Calcium-dependent plasma membrane binding and cell lysis by perforin are mediated through its C2 domain: A critical role for aspartate residues 429, 435, 483, and 485 but not 491. J Biol Chem 280:8426–8434

Walsh CM, Matloubian M, Liu CC, Ueda R, Kurahara CG, Christensen JL, Huang MT, Young JD, Ahmed R, Clark WR (1994) Immune function in mice lacking the perforin gene. Proc Natl Acad Sci U S A 91:10854–10858

Walters RW, Grunst T, Bergelson JM, Finberg RW, Welsh MJ, Zabner J (1999) Basolateral localization of fiber receptors limits adenovirus infection from the apical surface of airway epithelia. J Biol Chem 274:10219–10226

Waterhouse NJ, Sedelies KA, Browne KA, Wowk ME, Newbold A, Sutton VR, Clarke CJ, Oliaro J, Lindemann RK, Bird PI, Johnstone RW, Trapani JA (2005) A central role for Bid in granzyme B-induced apoptosis. J Biol Chem 280:4476–4482

Wells MA, Albrecht P, Ennis FA (1981) Recovery from a viral respiratory infection. I. Influenza pneumonia in normal and T-deficient mice. J Immunol 126:1036–1041

Wiley JA, Cerwenka A, Harkema JR, Dutton RW, Harmsen AG (2001) Production of interferon-gamma by influenza hemagglutinin-specific CD8 effector T cells influences the development of pulmonary immunopathology. Am J Pathol 158:119–130

Wilkinson TM, Li CK, Chui CS, Huang AK, Perkins M, Liebner JC, Lambkin-Williams R, Gilbert A, Oxford J, Nicholas B, Staples KJ, Dong T, Douek DC, McMichael AJ, Xu XN (2012) Preexisting influenza-specific CD4+ T cells correlate with disease protection against influenza challenge in humans. Nat Med 18:274–280

Williams MA, Bevan MJ (2007) Effector and memory CTL differentiation. Annu Rev Immunol 25:171–192

Wolf AI, Buehler D, Hensley SE, Cavanagh LL, Wherry EJ, Kastner P, Chan S, Weninger W (2009) Plasmacytoid dendritic cells are dispensable during primary influenza virus infection. J Immunol 182:871–879

Yadava K, Sichelstiel A, Luescher IF, Nicod LP, Harris NL, Marsland BJ (2013) TSLP promotes influenza-specific CD8+ T-cell responses by augmenting local inflammatory dendritic cell function. Mucosal Immunol 6:83–92

Yao S, Buzo BF, Pham D, Jiang L, Taparowsky EJ, Kaplan MH, Sun J (2013) Interferon regulatory factor 4 sustains CD8(+) T cell expansion and effector differentiation. Immunity 39:833–845

Yoo JK, Kim TS, Hufford MM, Braciale TJ (2013) Viral infection of the lung: Host response and sequelae. J Allergy Clin Immunol 132:1263–1276

Yoon H, Kim TS, Braciale TJ (2010) The cell cycle time of CD8+ T cells responding in vivo is controlled by the type of antigenic stimulus. PLoS One 5:e15423

Zelenay S, Keller AM, Whitney PG, Schraml BU, Deddouche S, Rogers NC, Schulz O, Sancho D, Reis e Sousa C (2012) The dendritic cell receptor DNGR-1 controls endocytic handling of necrotic cell antigens to favor cross-priming of CTLs in virus-infected mice. J Clin Invest 122:1615–1627

Zhang N, Bevan MJ (2011) CD8(+) T cells: foot soldiers of the immune system. Immunity 35:161–168

Zhao T, Zhang H, Guo Y, Fan Z (2007) Granzyme K directly processes bid to release cytochrome c and endonuclease G leading to mitochondria-dependent cell death. J Biol Chem 282:12104–12111

Zhong C, Li C, Wang X, Toyoda T, Gao G, Fan Z (2012) Granzyme K inhibits replication of influenza virus through cleaving the nuclear transport complex importin alpha1/beta dimer of infected host cells. Cell Death Differ 19:882–890

Part III
New Antiviral Discovery

Antiviral Effects of Inhibiting Host Gene Expression

Ralph A. Tripp and S. Mark Tompkins

Abstract RNA interference (RNAi) has been used to probe the virus-host interface to understand the requirements for host-gene expression needed for virus replication. The availability of arrayed siRNA libraries has enabled a genome-scale, high-throughput analysis of gene pathways usurped for virus replication. Results from these and related screens have led to the discovery of new host factors that regulate virus replication. While effective delivery continues to limit development of RNAi-based drugs, RNAi-based genome discovery has led to identification of druggable targets. These validated targets enable rational development of novel antiviral drugs, including the rescue and repurposing of existing, approved drugs. Existing drugs with known cytotoxicity and mechanisms of action can potentially be re-targeted to regulate host genes and gene products needed by influenza to replicate. Drug repositioning is more cost-effective, less time-consuming, and more effective for anti-influenza virus drug discovery than traditional methods. In this chapter, a general overview of RNAi screening methods, host-gene discovery, and drug repurposing is examined with emphasis on utilizing RNAi to identify druggable genes that can be targeted for drug development or repurposing.

Contents

R.A. Tripp (✉) · S. Mark Tompkins
Department of Infectious Disease, University of Georgia, Athens, GA 30602, USA
e-mail: ratripp@uga.edu

S. Mark Tompkins
e-mail: smt@uga.edu

Current Topics in Microbiology and Immunology (2015) 386: 459–477
DOI: 10.1007/82_2014_409

Published Online: 11 July 2014

1 Introduction

The emergence of new strains of avian and swine influenza viruses combined with the emergence of drug-resistant influenza virus strains emphasize the urgent need for developing new antiviral drugs and repurposing or rescuing existing drugs as antiviral agents. Currently, only two classes of antiviral drugs targeting influenza virus are approved for use by the Food and Drug Administration (FDA). The two classes of antiviral drugs are the M2 inhibitors amantadine and rimantadine, and neuraminidase (NA) inhibitors zanamivir and oseltamivir (Fiore et al. 2011; Preziosi 2011). Peramivir, a third NA inhibitor was briefly approved for emergency use as an intravenous antiviral during the 2009 H1N1 pandemic, but that emergency use authorization was terminated in 2010 (http://www.fda.gov). The M2 inhibitors are not recommended for general use due to widespread resistance in circulating H1N1 and H3N2 influenza viruses, and potential resistance to NA inhibitors continues to be a concern (Fiore et al. 2011). A primary strategy for developing influenza virus antivirals has been to screen existing drug libraries of small molecule inhibitors primarily developed as cancer therapeutics, and only recently have rationally-designed drug strategies been employed (Krug and Aramini 2009; Preziosi 2011; Saladino et al. 2010). There are a spectrum of natural compounds being explored as anti-influenza drugs, including NA inhibitors (Grienke et al. 2012) and some of these more promising compounds have been tested in clinical trials (Chen et al. 2007). Today, as the pendulum swings toward rationally designed antivirals, critical to success is a better understanding of the virus-host interface and the exploitation of the knowledge of the role of host genes required for virus replication, computational/in silico approaches in drug design, and the integration of "-omics" in driving anti-influenza drug development.

2 Influenza A Virus and RNAi

2.1 Influenza Virus Lifecycle

Influenza A viruses are segmented, negative-sense RNA viruses that contain 8 gene segments encoding at least 10 proteins. Segments 1–6 encode basic polymerase 2 (PB2), PB1, acidic polymerase (PA), hemagglutinin (HA), nucleoprotein (NP), and neuraminidase (NA), respectively. Segment 7 encodes the matrix capsid protein (M1) and through alternate splicing, the M2 protein. Similarly, segment 8 encodes the non-structural protein (NS1) and nuclear export protein (NEP). Most influenza viruses also encode two additional proteins in alternate open reading frames within the PB1 gene; the PB1-F2 and PB1-N40 proteins (Shaw and Palese 2013). The virion is enveloped with the HA, NA and M2 proteins on the surface of the virion, with the M1 protein providing capsid structure. The segmented genome is encapsidated by NP, with each segment having an associated PA, PB1 and PB2 protein, comprising the ribonucleoprotein (RNP). The 8 RNPs make up the virion core. NEP is found within the virion, however PB1-F2, PB1-N40 and NS1 are non-structural proteins (Shaw and Palese 2013).

As obligate parasites, influenza viruses co-opt and modify cellular processes to produce progeny and alter the host response to infection. Influenza viruses bind to sialic acids on the surface of cellular glycoproteins via the hemagglutinin (HA) protein (Fig. 1). The virion is internalized through several mechanisms, including clatherin-dependent endocytosis and macropinocytosis (Shaw and Palese 2013). As the endosome acidifies, the HA protein undergoes structural changes resulting in fusion of the virion membrane with the endosomal membrane. Concurrently, the M2 protein allows the influx of H+ protons from the endosome into the virus particle dissociating the RNPs from the M1 protein, and allowing release of RNPs into the cell cytoplasm. The viral RNPs are actively transported into the nucleus via a nuclear localization sequence (NLS) on the NP interacting with cellular importin-α. Once in the nucleus, viral mRNA synthesis is initiated by the polymerase complex (PA, PB1, and PB2), utilizing host 5′-capped primers. Virus mRNAs are translocated to the cytoplasm for translation. NP and NS1 proteins are preferentially expressed early during infection reflecting the need for NP to encapsidate newly synthesized genomic and complementary RNAs, (vRNA and cRNA, respectively), and for NS1 to regulate several cellular processes, particularly interferon antiviral responses. The membrane-associated proteins, HA, NA, and M2 are translated, folded, and glycosylated in the ER and Golgi apparatus before transport to the cell surface. The polymerase, NEP and M1 proteins localize in the nucleus, potentially all directing the shift from mRNA expression to the accumulation of vRNAs, i.e., RNPs. M1 and NEP proteins also accumulate in the nucleus, with M1 associating with the vRNA and NP protein of the RNPs and associating with NEP. The NEP interacts with Crm1, enabling export of the RNP-M1 complex from the nucleus (Shaw and Palese 2013). While the maturation and transport of the transmembrane proteins is fairly well-described, the movement of

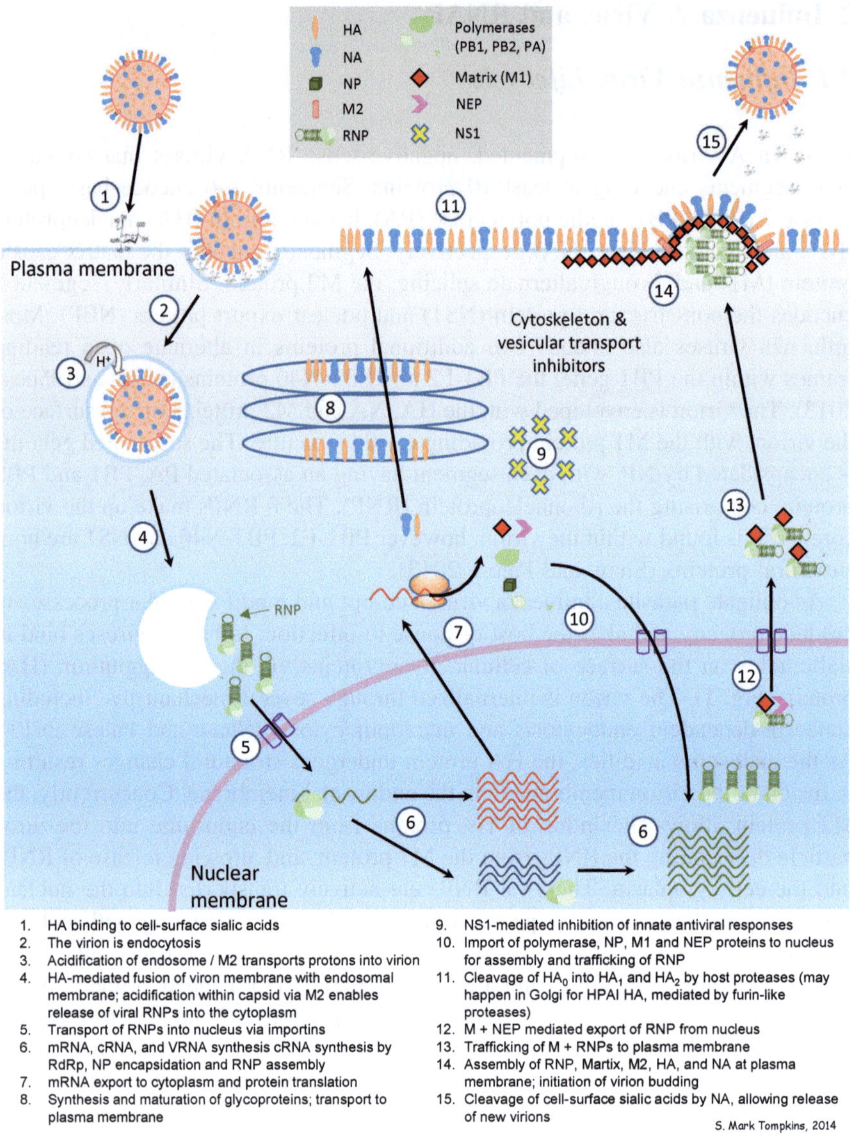

Fig. 1 Influenza virus lifecycle

the M1 and RNP complexes is poorly understood. Both NP and M1 can interact with cytoskeletal proteins, and Rab proteins have been shown to be required for productive infection, but precise mechanisms are not known. Similarly, the mechanism of RNP packaging into budding virions is unclear. While data support a selection process to specifically package one of each segment (PB2, PB1, PA, HA, NP, NA, M, and NS), the precise signals and interactions are not yet known

(Shaw and Palese 2013). Virus budding is cooperatively mediated by the M1, M2, HA and NA proteins, with the M2 protein having a specific role in membrane scission. Finally, the NA protein, which has neuraminidase activity, cleaves the sialic acids from the cell surface and virus glycoproteins, preventing HA binding and aggregation of newly formed virus particles (Shaw and Palese 2013).

2.2 RNAi to Interrogate Gene Function

RNAi is a post-transcriptional gene-silencing mechanism conserved from plants to humans that uses double-stranded RNA (dsRNA) to direct homology-dependent suppression of gene activity. RNAi has been increasingly used to determine host-gene requirements for influenza virus replication and to discover novel therapeutic approaches to control influenza virus (Bakre et al. 2013; Meliopoulos et al. 2012a; Perwitasari et al. 2013a; Watanabe et al. 2010). The pairing of RNAi with genomic sequencing has allowed for the construction of genome-scale RNAi libraries to silence all genes in the host genome, allowing for reduction-of-function studies (Brass et al. 2009; Campeau and Gobeil 2011; Clark and Ding 2006; Hao et al. 2008; Karlas et al. 2010; Konig et al. 2010; Mohr et al. 2010; Perrimon and Mathey-Prevot 2007; Perwitasari et al. 2013a; Shapira et al. 2009; Ward et al. 2012). These types of RNAi platforms allow for systematic functional analyses that was previously impractical, and genome-wide cell-based RNAi high-throughput sequencing (HTS) in mammalian cells has led to novel host-pathway discoveries and the identification of novel and potential targets for the development of prophylactic and therapeutic treatments for virus infection (Mohr et al. 2010; Perrimon and Mathey-Prevot 2007; Perwitasari et al. 2013a).

RNAi silencing of a host gene does not need to be complete as partial gene silencing usually leads to a reduction-of-function in gene pathway that can be assessed using biological endpoint assays that may include an mRNA and/or protein levels, and/or virus titers. Although genome-wide RNAi screens have been successfully used to identify and interrogate critical host genes, these screens have also missed identifying genetic elements having more subtle roles in host pathways. This has occurred primarily because of artificial thresholds set by the investigator to clarify positive hits from false-positives during the RNAi screen, and because certain components of these pathways are expressed at all phases of the host cell being interrogated, and because some genes are not be sufficiently silenced. However, with proper endpoint assay optimization, and the proper controls, these variations are less typically encountered in the RNAi screen.

RNAi screening is also being used to better understand the systems biology surrounding the host cell responses to danger signals and those as they relate to influenza virus infection (Betakova and Svancarova 2013; Haasnoot et al. 2003; Hong-Geller and Micheva-Viteva 2010; Korth et al. 2013; Meliopoulos et al. 2012a; Prussia et al. 2011; Stertz and Shaw 2011; Watanabe et al. 2010). This information is being translated in vivo where applicable, and for influenza virus, has provided a rapid pathway for rescuing and repurposing antiviral drugs (Martinez-Gil et al. 2013; Meliopoulos et al. 2012a; Perwitasari et al. 2013b; Prussia et al. 2011; Prusty et al. 2011; Su et al. 2013).

2.3 Genome-Wide Mammalian Cell-Based RNAi Screening

A genome-wide RNAi HTS assay is typically performed using small-interfering RNAs (siRNAs) transfected into mammalian cells as an arrayed format based on sub-libraries where individual siRNA pools target host gene families such as kinases, proteases, phosphatases, etc; or where single genes are targeted by siRNAs. Three different RNAi mediators have been used to mediate a reduction-of-function in mammalian cell lines, (1) chemically synthesized siRNAs which are $\sim$21 nucleotide (nt) duplexes, (2) vector-expressed short hairpin RNAs (shRNAs), or (3) diverse pools of short dsRNAs prepared by enzymatic digestion of a transcribed long dsRNA by RNaseIII in vitro (Aigner 2006; Clark and Ding 2006; Mohr et al. 2010; Perwitasari et al. 2013a). The most common siRNA delivery system is lipid-mediated transfection although electroporation is becoming common for shRNAs and some dsRNAs (Foged 2012; Jeong et al. 2009; Lares et al. 2010; Shim and Kwon 2010). Pooling of multiple siRNAs targeted against the same gene but at different 'seed sites' in the screening approach has the advantage to lower off-target effects and decrease the number of wells assayed during primary screening compared to multiple individual siRNAs (Chen and Zhang 2012). Given that siRNA or other RNAi mediators can be delivered at a reasonable transfection efficiency to many different cells line of interest, an array of cell-based assays can be used to evaluate endpoints of RNAi efficacy including cell viability, apoptosis, protein expression, transcriptional reporter assays, cell motility, quantitative PCR, virus replication, etc. (Kittler et al. 2007; Kobos et al. 2013; Matsumoto et al. 2007; Theis and Buchholz 2011). In this regard, high content screening (HCS) and image analysis is popular in RNAi screening as it allows a multiparameter approach to visualize and quantitate or monitor multiple parameters in a single screen, a feature that expands the power of RNAi to interrogate gene function (Antczak et al. 2009, 2014; Freeley et al. 2010; Galea and Simpson 2013; Haney 2007; Sundaramurthy et al. 2014).

2.4 The Appropriate Cell Line for HTS

The choice of an appropriate mammalian cell line for viral RNAi screening depends on the biological process being studied, the ability of the virus to infect and replicate in the cell line, the endpoint assays to be used, and HTS requirements such as robustness of signal readout(s). For influenza virus, using adherent, primary, fully differentiated normal human bronchoepithelial cells would be preferential

(Ilyushina et al. 2008; Oshansky et al. 2009, 2011), however, these cell lines are difficult to maintain, grow at the air-liquid interface, are costly, exhibit substantial biological variation, and it remains challenging to efficiently transfect them with siRNA. For these reasons, adherent, immortalized cell lines can provide an advantage providing a homogeneous unlimited resource of cells for screening, and if derived from the human respiratory epithelia, the added benefit of being closer to physiological relevance. Thus, the adherent human type II respiratory epithelial cell line, A549, and related cell line like HEp-2 have proven valuable for RNAi influenza screening (Bakre et al. 2013; Karlas et al. 2010; Konig et al. 2010; Matskevich et al. 2009; Matskevich and Moelling 2007; Meliopoulos et al. 2012a, b; Perwitasari et al. 2013a; Tripp et al. 2013; Tripp and Tompkins 2009).

2.5 Choosing Appropriate Endpoint Assays for HTS

Numerous plate formats, i.e., 96-well or 384-well and related read-out systems are compatible with HTS. The 96-well format allows for medium-to-large-scale HTS while also providing a larger well format for examining biological process and products, as well as a larger sample for analysis of multiple endpoints. In this example, the endpoint assays are specific to identifying host genes critical for influenza virus replication. Typically, the level of virus replication is assessed by qPCR, measuring virus genome or mRNA; hemagglutinin assay (HA), measuring virion release into the supernatant; infectivity assay, measuring infectious particles released into the supernatant (e.g., 50 % tissue culture infectious dose ($TCID_{50}$); cell viability, measuring virus-induce cytopathic effects; or immune staining, for virus protein-antigen (e.g., nucleoprotein (NP) staining) (Bakre et al. 2013; Meliopoulos et al. 2012a; Prussia et al. 2011; Ward et al. 2012). NP staining is often quantified by ELISA or images acquired with high-content microscopy platforms that provide spatial and temporal information about the levels of NP-staining as well as changes in cell morphology, and changes in the localization of proteins (Emery et al. 2011; Mastyugin et al. 2005; Wang and Xie 2007). The major caveat of this high-content analysis (HCA) is the large quantity of data that accumulates that must be stored to be analyzed. A 384-well plate format for HTS screening has the advantage of reducing costs associated with reagents and media, and reducing time associated with plate manipulation, but increases the requirement for automation, as well as limiting potential endpoints in the screen. Genome-wide screens for influenza virus using the 384-well format and NP immune staining have been effectively used (Brass et al. 2009; Karlas et al. 2010), as well as others measuring luciferase activity using a recombinant influenza virus (Hao et al. 2008; Konig et al. 2010). Of note, the two screens utilizing imaging for screening did not utilize high-content analysis—they assessed infected versus uninfected cells. Only one 384-well format genome-wide screen assessed more than one endpoint, and in this regard, evaluated virus infection in A549 cells with NP immune staining and quantifying virus released into supernatants on a separate luciferase reporter cell line (Karlas et al. 2010). Importantly, when designing endpoint assays, the assays employed should be optimized to reduce or eliminate the signal-to-noise ratio and enhance assay reproducibility. The more robust the HTS assay performs, the better the statistical significance when assessing the assay, particularly by the Z-factor method (Haney 2005; Mazur and Kozak 2012; Zhang 2007). The Z-factor is used to measure the statistical separation of the positive from the negative controls and thereby allow for adjusting the HTS parameters used to detect positive hits from the background noise to achieve the maximum sensitivity of the assay.

2.6 Validation of HTS Findings

Following an RNAi screen, the data must be analyzed to identify positive from false-positive hits based on the several features that include deconvoluting pooled siRNA if used in the screen, normalizing data, establishing appropriate thresholds for cutoffs, replicating tests, and validating with new siRNAs targeting a different 'seed site' on the target gene transcript (Meliopoulos et al. 2012a; Parker et al. 2006). Important factors to consider in RNAi screens are (1) perform at least one replicate assay for each sub-library from the primary screen, (2) normalize data to validated positive and negative controls present on every plate in the screen, and (3) set cut-off values for achieving real and significant results. Perhaps validating HTS screening could be improved by incorporating recent innovative '-omics' approaches that can be integrative and multiplex a variety of approaches linked to systems biology, e.g., microarray findings, protein-protein interactions, genomic analyses, transcriptomic analyses, and deep-sequencing. Importantly, the validation should reconcile that the findings are applicable beyond the HTS analysis, i.e., repeat in different cell lines, for different virus strains, and in other assay formats and endpoints. This helps to gain a system-wide understanding of gene networks involved in various replication processes, such as those associated with influenza virus replication, protein processing, and budding.

3 Optimizing RNAi Genome-Wide Screens to Facilitate Drug Rescue and Repurposing

To optimize translational approaches when performing RNAi HTS, it is important to use a cell line that best emulates the natural tropism of the virus being screened, and, ideally for influenza virus, a human type II respiratory epithelial cell line like A549 cells. With regard to conditions, the host cell line is typically transfected with individual siRNA pools per target gene and the cells incubated for 48 h to allow for optimal gene silencing. The silencing of genes is generally confirmed by qPCR. Pending gene silencing, the cells are infected and at appropriate times, i.e.,

24–48 hpi, the gene hits from the screen are determined. The gene hits are validated, as previously noted, by deconvoluting the siRNA pool to individual siRNAs, and/or by using different siRNAs targeting a different 'seed site' on the same gene (Meliopoulos et al. 2012a). Once gene hits are validated, various bioinformatics tools can be employed to determine where the druggable targets, i.e., the genes validated to be required for influenza virus replication, are. Doing this funnels the range of host genes to therapeutic targets and often identifies an upstream key regulator in the host gene pathway co-opted by influenza viruses.

False-positives occur in RNAi screens. This is may be due to off-target effects, the limitations of the efficiency of the screening endpoint assays, and/or the thresholds set by the investigator identifying a positive hit from a negative hit or a null result. False negatives may arise from partial gene knockdown, and/or gene ploidy typically associated with transformed cell lines, e.g., 3N or 4N chromosomes. This caveat can affect HTS screens interpretation, particularly for drug discovery and repurposing, where the dosage of drug produces an unintended or insufficient phenotype. The endpoint assay may also miss potential gene targets by design. For example, one genome-wide HTS screen for influenza gene targets utilized a recombinant influenza virus encoding a luciferase gene in place of the hemagglutinin gene. This enabled easy assay for early events in the virus infection process, but excluded analysis of genes involved in the late stages of the virus lifecycle (Konig et al. 2010; Stertz and Shaw 2011). Despite these caveats, RNAi can be an effective drug target discovery tool, which combines the power of gene silencing with the scale of HTS.

3.1 *Identifying Antiviral Drugs Affecting Influenza Virus Replication*

There are several approaches for rescuing or repurposing available drugs (Law et al. 2013), some that include prediction methods, to others involving RNAi screening for identification of druggable targets (Perwitasari et al. 2013a). Although initial RNAi screening for critical host genes can be cumbersome, it provides a wealth of information regarding host genes and pathways that promote or resist virus replication. Thus, RNAi screening is a desirable first step due to its targeted approach and because it identifies and validates drug targets in a single process, thereby improving confidence in proposed targets for drug discovery or drug repurposing. Typically, database mining is used to find available small molecules or drugs once potential host gene targets have been identified. This approach can be coupled with an initiative launched by NIH/NCATS called "Discovering New Therapeutic Uses for Existing Molecules" which is aimed to facilitate drug repurposing by providing research funds and limited access to pharmaceutical companies' drug compound libraries. There are several databases containing available drugs and their gene targets that are available such as the PROMISCUOUS database which contains >25,000 annotated, withdrawn, or experimental drugs, searchable by name, target, or pathway (Shin et al. 2013), and related drug databases, including ChemSpider, having >28 million searchable structures (Southan 2013), and DrugBank, containing >4,800 drugs, including FDA-approved small molecule inhibitors (Perwitasari et al. 2013a; Rask-Andersen et al. 2011; Shin et al. 2013; Southan 2013). Many of these databases provide systematic collections of compounds, including drug-protein interactions and the associations of proteins with genetic information, such as Swissprot. This allows one to couple this information to pathway analysis databases, such as Ingenuity Pathway Analysis (Thomas and Bonchev 2010), allowing for integrated genome-wide drug assessment and identification strategies.

The question arises as to why legitimate drug targets known to be involved in a particular phenotype might not be identified in an RNAi screen. In addition to the previously described caveats of screen or endpoint design, there are potential genomic explanations, as well. There is host gene redundancy within the genome where RNAi may target only one gene, and copy-number variation and genomic rearrangements in the human genome may also contribute to phenotypic variation (Spielmann and Klopocki 2013). Gene duplication appears to be a common event during evolution (Haraksingh and Snyder 2013), and duplicated genes can gradually change in both sequence and sub-function where one paralog may remain able to perform an activity in the absence of the other (Cooper et al. 2013). RNAi gene-targeting has shown us that functional redundancy is common in many multi-gene families of proteins (Fievet et al. 2013). Similarly, genetic redundancy may explain false-negative results in genome-wide RNAi screens.

4 Host Factors and Drug Targets for Influenza Virus

Identifying druggable genes in the human genome is essential for the identification of novel drug targets and for the rescue or repurposing of existing pharmaceutical products. G protein-coupled receptors (GPCRs) are the most common gene products targeted by the drug industry, (Heng et al. 2013; Rask-Andersen et al. 2011). GPCRs have key roles in cell physiology and homeostasis, in signaling pathways, and many viruses co-opt these pathways for their replication, packaging, and transport to the host cell surface (Cannon 2007; Katano and Sata 2000; Nicholas 2005; Unutmaz et al. 1998). Ligand-gated ion channels, the second largest receptor drug target class, are appealing gene targets (Akk and Steinbach 2011), given the role of the matrix protein-2 (M2) of influenza virus which forms a proton channel in the viral envelope necessary for the release of the viral genome into the host cell cytoplasm (Wang and Chou 2012). The other large classes of drug targets are kinases, phosphatases, and ubiquitinases, which have been predominantly targeted by anticancer drugs (Britten 2013; Micel et al. 2013; Perrotti and Neviani 2013). Several recent studies have shown that identifying critical genes in these host pathways can provide a rapid and safe pathway for rescuing, repurposing and retargeting FDA-approved drugs that are efficacious for influenza

A viruses (Banerjee et al. 2013; Hong-Geller and Micheva-Viteva 2010; Karlas et al. 2010; Konig et al. 2010; Martinez-Gil et al. 2013; Perwitasari et al. 2013a; Ward et al. 2012). Specifically, our recent studies using RNAi screens to identify influenza druggable targets (Table 1) have shown that genes validated as critical for A/WSN/33 (H1N1) influenza virus replication in human A549 cells are ADAMTS7, CPE, DPP3, MST1, and PRSS12, and pathway analysis showed these genes were in global host cell pathways governing inflammation (NF–kB), calcium signaling, and apoptosis (Meliopoulos et al. 2012b). Additionally, 17 human protein kinase genes (NPR2, MAP3K1, DYRK3, EPHA6, TPK1, PDK2, EXOSC10, NEK8, PLK4, SGK3, NEK3, PANK4, ITPKB, CDC2L5 (CDK13), CALM2, PKN3, and HK2) were validated as essential for A/WSN/33 influenza virus replication, and 6 protein kinase genes (CDK13, HK2, NEK8, PANK4, PLK4 and SGK3) were identified as vital for both A/WSN/33 and A/New Caledonia/20/99 influenza virus replication (Bakre et al. 2013). These protein kinase genes were found to affect multiple host pathways and regulated by miRNAs induced during infection. Other studies using different approaches, viruses, and endpoints have identified other host genes important for influenza virus replication (Table 1) (Hao et al. 2008; Karlas et al. 2010; Konig et al. 2010; Martinez-Gil et al. 2013; Perwitasari et al. 2013a; Southan 2013; Su et al. 2013; Ward et al. 2012). Previous analysis of four early genome-wide screens using human cells or Drosophila cells for the screen identified only three genes in common: ARCN1, ATP6AP1 and COPG (Stertz and Shaw 2011). However, if one relaxes the threshold used to screen for hits based on statistical differences, this low number of overlapping genes is increased substantially to >20 genes in common. While the low frequency of overlap across screens has raised questions regarding the validity of genome-wide RNAi screens, there are a variety of potential explanations for the differences in results. For example, differences in cell lines, siRNA libraries, transfection reagents, and timing of the transfection, infection and assay endpoints will affect gene knockdown, the effect of gene knockdown, or possible non-specific effects. Similarly, the use of different viruses (even different strains of a virus) could change results and differences in endpoint assays will clearly limit or allow for identification of different cellular gene targets (Stertz and Shaw 2011). Despite the variances across screens, many screens have successfully identified druggable gene targets (Karlas et al. 2010; Konig et al. 2010; Perwitasari et al. 2013a, b; Ward et al. 2012).

4.1 Host Genes Critical for Influenza Replication Are Not Universal for All Strains

Notably, many host genes determined as critical for one strain or subtype of influenza virus are not found to be critical for replication of related strains or subtypes (Bakre et al. 2013; Karlas et al. 2010; Meliopoulos et al. 2012a). For example, in one RNAi genome-wide HTS study, 287 human host cell genes

Table 1 Arrayed RNAi screens for genes affecting influenza A virus infection

Reference	Primary screening virus	Cells used for primary screen	Genes identified/ Genes screened	Endpoints	Steps in lifecycle[a]
(Hao et al. 2008)	Recombinant A/WSN/33 (H1N1) w/VSV-G pseudotype and NA-Luc)	Drosophila cells	~100/13,071	Luciferase activity in primary culture	3, 5, 6, 7
(Brass et al. 2009)	A/PR/8/34 (H1N1)	Osteosarcoma cells, U2OS	120/17,877	Virus antigen (HA) by immune staining in primary culture	1–8, 11
(Shapira et al. 2009)	A/PR/8/34, A/Udorn/307/72 (H3N2)	HBEC	616/1,745[b]	luciferase activity in secondary culture (infectious virus titer)	1–15
(Karlas et al. 2010)	A/WSN/33	human lung carcinoma, A549	287/22,843	Virus antigen (NP) by immune staining in primary culture; luciferase activity in secondary culture (infectious virus titer)	1–15
(Konig et al. 2010)	Recombinant A/WSN/33 with HA-Luc reporter	human lung carcinoma, A549	295/19,628	Luciferase activity in primary culture	1–7
(Ward et al. 2012)	A/WSN/33	HBEC30-KT cells	235/21,125	Cell viability in primary culture	1–7
(Meliopoulos et al. 2012b)	A/WSN/33	human lung carcinoma, A549	5/481	Secondary culture endpoint dilution (infectious virus titer)	1–15
(Bakre et al. 2013)	A/WSN/33	human lung carcinoma, A549	18/720	Secondary culture endpoint dilution (infectious virus titer)	1–15

[a] See Fig. 1 for steps in virus lifecycle

[b] Targeted screen based on protein–protein interactions

influencing influenza A virus replication were identified, and by using an independent assay it was confirmed that 119 hits inhibited A/WSN/33 (H1N1) and 121 hits inhibited pandemic H1N1 (A/Hamburg/04/2009), with 72 of those genes overlapping for the two viruses. Remarkably, a subset of these common hits was also determined to be essential for the H5N1 highly pathogenic avian influenza virus replication (Karlas et al. 2010). Analysis of these validated host genes showed that most genes were linked to host pathways that affected trafficking of influenza virions to late endosomes early in infection. By knowing which host genes were critical for influenza virus replication, small molecule inhibitors were identified to target these host genes. For example, it was shown that a small molecule inhibitor of CDC-like kinase 1 (CLK1) was able to reduce influenza virus replication by greater than two orders of magnitude, an effect attributed to impaired splicing of the viral M2 messenger RNA (Karlas et al. 2010). These findings, confirmed in primary normal human bronchial epithelial cells (NHBE), highlight the potential of genome-wide RNAi HTS as a method for rapid and accurate dissection of virus–host interactions, allowing for the identification of druggable host gene targets and rescue or repurposing of a broad range of potential anti-influenza virus drugs. It is of interest to note that for almost all RNI genome-wide screens performed to date, most gene hits determined as critical for influenza virus replication appear to function very early after infection; thus, it appears that targeting the early infection processes linked to viral synthesis and nuclear export of viral RNA is perhaps the best approach when looking toward antiviral drugs.

4.2 IFN Antiviral Host Pathways Responding to Influenza Virus Infection

Interferon (IFN) expression is used by infected cells to control virus replication, as well as alert innate and adaptive immune responses to viral infection by features linked to IFN-stimulated genes (ISGs) (Ahmed et al. 2010; Antonelli and Turriziani 2012; Krug and Aramini 2009; Luo 2012; Pazienza et al. 2010). Accordingly, many viruses encode non-structural and other viral proteins that antagonize the effects of IFNs, as well as inhibit transcription and cellular gene expression, translation, and preventing synthesis of antiviral genes. Viral IFN antagonists generally inhibit at least one of three key host pathways, i.e., IRF3, JAK-STAT, and/or the PKR pathways (Audsley and Moseley 2013; Laurent-Rolle et al. 2010; Munoz-Jordan et al. 2005; Varga et al. 2011). The host genes in these pathways include ISGs whose functions are inhibited or sequestered, as well as a range of other host proteins whose function is to regulate IFN and ISG expression, e.g., suppressor of cytokine signaling (SOCS) proteins (Bonjardim et al. 2009; Dalpke et al. 2008; Krebs and Hilton 2000). Drugs that relieve the suppression of the antiviral cytokine pathway are expected to promote antiviral responses to influenza virus infection (Flowers et al. 2004; Pauli et al. 2008; Song and Shuai 1998; Wei et al. 2014).

Table 2 Experimental anti-influenza drugs targeting host proteins/pathways

Target/ inhibitor class	Identified by RNAi?	Inhibitors/agonists	Mechanism of action	References
CAMK2B	Yes	KN-93	Regulate viral RNA transcription	(Konig et al. 2010; Perwitasari et al. 2013b)
CDC25B	Yes	NSC95397	Inhibits CDK1 activity → NS1 function	(Perwitasari et al. 2013b)
CHEK1	Yes	SB218078	Regulation of cell cycle or innate responses (?)	(Ward et al. 2012)
CLK1	Yes	TG003	↓ splicing of viral mRNA	(Karlas et al. 2010)
COX-2	No	Celecoxib	Reduction of inflammation	(Carey et al. 2010)
IKK/NFkB signaling	No	Bay 11-7082	Inhibition of NFkB signaling. ↓ proinflammatory cytokines	(Pinto et al. 2011)
MEK1/2	No	U0126	Block MEK/ERK signaling, ↓ virus replication.	(Pinto et al. 2011; Pleschka et al. 2001)
OAT3	Yes	Probenecid	Block transport of cellular or viral protein	(Perwitasari et al. 2013c)
Proteases	Yes	7-amino-4-methylcoumarin	Block HA cleavage	(Baron et al. 2012; Meliopoulos et al. 2012b; Meyer et al. 2013)
PPAR agonists	No	Gemfibrozil, pioglitazone	↓ inflammation	(Aldridge et al. 2009; Budd et al. 2007)
Rab-family GTPases	Yes	3-IPEHPC	Type II Geranylgeranyl-transferases inhibitor blocks Rab protein modification	(Ward et al. 2012)
Sialic acid	No	Sialidase (DAS181), Fludase	Cleave surface sialic acids	(Malakhov et al. 2006)
V-ATPase	Yes	Diphyllin	Inhibits pH-dependent fusion	(Konig et al. 2010)
XPO1 (CRM1)	No	Leptomycin B, KPT335	Blocks export of RNP from nucleus	(Watanabe et al. 2001), unpublished

4.3 microRNA Screens

Classes of small non-coding RNA molecules which function in the transcriptional and post-transcriptional regulation of gene expression, i.e., microRNAs (miRNAs), are known to comprise more than 2,000 species in the human genome. They are transcribed in the nucleus, forming primary miRNAs, ~2 kb in length. The primary miRNAs are processed by Drosha and Pasha into 70–100 nt stem-loop structures called pre-miRNAs. The pre-miRNAs are exported to the cytoplasm where they are further processed by Dicer into mature double-stranded miRNAs (Dong et al. 2013). miRNAs function similarly to siRNAs where one of the miRNA strands associates with the RNA-induced silencing complex (RISC), and provides specificity for RISC to bind to complimentary mRNA and mediate its degradation. Importantly, the specificity of miRNAs is dictated primarily through a 6-8 nt region of the miRNA called the "seed site." This small region of complementarity enables the miRNA to potentially target numerous mRNAs (Dong et al. 2013; Perwitasari et al. 2013a). With this ability to broadly regulate gene function, miRNAs are likely regulating almost all cellular processes including disease.

miRNA screening tools are commercially available, and similar to genome-wide siRNA libraries, arrays of plates targeting all known miRNAs are available. These miRNA libraries can be made to contain both miRNA mimics and/or miRNA inhibitors allowing for one to probe the loss or gain of function by a given miRNA. miRNA screening is an appealing approach to genome-wide gene screening. However, because of the broad activity of miRNAs, identification of a given phenotype requires perhaps a more robust validation process of the host gene targets. Moreover, the phenotype may not be the result of regulation of translation of a single gene product, but rather an effect linked to partial inhibition of multiple genes (Dong et al. 2013; Perwitasari et al. 2013a).

miRNA screens have been concluded for influenza virus, both as full screens and as focused screens, to better understand miRNA regulation of host genes identified and validated in siRNA screens (Bakre et al. 2013; Meliopoulos et al. 2012b; Ward et al. 2012). miRNA mimics or inhibitors were shown to increase or decrease influenza virus replication, however, the effect was not as profound as what was seen by gene-silencing with an siRNA, a finding consistent with their role in governing gene expression (Bakre et al. 2013; Meliopoulos et al. 2012b; Ward et al. 2012).

While miRNA screening is not as advanced as siRNA screening in practice or interpretation, it is gaining interest not only as a means for initial target identification, but also as a validation tool to correlate with siRNA screen data to help identify high-confidence hits (Perwitasari et al. 2013a). Moreover, miRNAs also represent potential drug targets. For example, miRNA-122 (miR-122) has been shown to be critical for hepatitis C infection. A modified oligonucleotide inhibitor of miR-122 is now in clinical trials and shows efficacy in reducing HCV RNA levels (Gupta et al. 2014; Janssen et al. 2013).

5 Conclusions and Looking Forward

Genome-wide screening for host genes important in influenza virus replication has dramatically changed the landscape of drug development and disease intervention. Recent improvements in RNAi technologies have allowed for better targeting of siRNAs, and in the development of miRNA mimics and inhibitors. Moreover, the successes of targeted and sub-library screening (e.g., kinases, GPCRs, or the druggable genome) support partial screening projects as opposed to full-genome screens. In the case of infectious diseases, and viruses in particular, RNAi screening to identify host genes, that when silenced reduces virus replication, has initiated a renaissance in drug discovery. Precise identification of specific gene targets has enabled the identification of high-quality targets and has provided a better understanding of the virus-host interface, where researchers are considering novel targets previously not associated with the viral replication process.

The large-scale discovery of novel drug targets has also breathed new life into existing FDA-approved and late clinical-stage drugs. The drug development industry has many examples of highly successful drugs licensed for indications other than their original purpose. Azidothymidine (AZT), originally developed as a cancer therapeutic, was approved as the first anti-retroviral drug only 2 years after the first demonstration of its activity against HIV (Perwitasari et al. 2013a).

RNAi screening and the interaction networks generated from these large datasets have also opened up new opportunities for combination drugs. Targeting host processes raises the risk for toxic side effects associated with a given drug. In some cases, a reduction in gene expression or gene product function will have still affect virus replication, albeit incompletely. RNAi screens enable identification of multiple host pathways involved in the virus lifecycle. Partial inhibition of multiple host cell targets can result in additive or potentially synergistic inhibition of virus replication with reduced toxicity. This may be accomplished through use of drug combinations or therapeutic miRNAs. Moreover, host-targeting drugs can also be used in combination with virus-specific antivirals (e.g., NA inhibitors) (Perwitasari et al. 2013c). New programs such as the NIH's NCATS "Discovering New Therapeutic Uses for Existing Molecules" initiative will enable drug repurposing based upon target discovery and validation through RNAi.

References

Ahmed CM, Dabelic R, Martin JP, Jager LD, Haider SM, Johnson HM (2010) J Immunol 185:1103–1113

Aigner A (2006) J Biotechnol 124:12–25

Akk G, Steinbach JH (2011) Anesthesiology 115:1338–1348

Aldridge JR, Moseley CE, Boltz DA, Negovetich NJ, Reynolds C, Franks J, Brown SA, Doherty PC, Webster RG, Thomas PG (2009) Proceedings of the National Academy of Sciences 106:5306–5311

Antczak C, Mahida JP, Singh C, Calder PA, Djaballah H (2014) Comb Chem High Throughput Screen 17:12–24
Antczak C, Takagi T, Ramirez CN, Radu C, Djaballah H (2009) J Biomol Screen 14:956–969
Antonelli G, Turriziani O (2012) Int J Antimicrob Agents 40:95–102
Audsley MD, Moseley GW (2013) World J Virol 2:57–70
Bakre A, Andersen LE, Meliopoulos V, Coleman K, Yan X, Brooks P, Crabtree J, Tompkins SM, Tripp RA (2013) PLoS One 8:e66796
Banerjee I, Yamauchi Y, Helenius A, Horvath P (2013) PLoS One 8:e68450
Baron J, Tarnow C, Mayoli-Nüssle D, Schilling E, Meyer D, Hammami M, Schwalm F, Steinmetzer T, Guan Y, Garten W, Klenk H-D, Böttcher-Friebertshäuser E (2012) J Virol 87(3):1811–1820
Betakova T, Svancarova P (2013) Acta Virol 57:97–104
Bonjardim CA, Ferreira PC, Kroon EG (2009) Immunol Lett 122:1–11
Brass AL, Huang IC, Benita Y, John SP, Krishnan MN, Feeley EM, Ryan BJ, Weyer JL, van der Weyden L, Fikrig E, Adams DJ, Xavier RJ, Farzan M, Elledge SJ (2009) Cell 139:1243–1254
Britten CD (2013) Cancer Chemother Pharmacol 71:1395–1409
Budd A, Alleva L, Alsharifi M, Koskinen A, Smythe V, Mullbacher A, Wood J, Clark I (2007) Antimicrob Agents Chemother 51:2965–2968
Campeau E, Gobeil S (2011) Brief Funct Genomics 10:215–226
Cannon M (2007) Curr Top Microbiol Immunol 312:137–156
Carey MA, Bradbury JA, Rebolloso YD, Graves JP, Zeldin DC, Germolec DR (2010) PLoS One 5:e11610
Chen J, Zhang W (2012) J Chem Phys 137:225102
Chen XY, Wu TX, Liu GJ, Wang Q, Zheng J, Wei J, Ni J, Zhou LK, Duan X, Qiao JQ (2007) Cochrane Database Syst Rev CD004559
Clark J, Ding S (2006) J Biomed Biotechnol 2006:45716
Cooper DN, Krawczak M, Polychronakos C, Tyler-Smith C, Kehrer-Sawatzki H (2013) Hum Genet 132:1077–1130
Dalpke A, Heeg K, Bartz H, Baetz A (2008) Immunobiology 213:225–235
Dong H, Lei J, Ding L, Wen Y, Ju H, Zhang X (2013) Chemical Reviews 113:6207–6233
Emery A, Sorrell DA, Lawrence S, Easthope E, Stockdale M, Jones DO, Zheleva D, Scaerou F, Glover DM (2011) J Biomol Screen 16:925–931
Fievet BT, Rodriguez J, Naganathan S, Lee C, Zeiser E, Ishidate T, Shirayama M, Grill S, Ahringer J (2013) Nat Cell Biol 15:103–112
Fiore AE, Fry A, Shay D, Gubareva L, Bresee JS, Uyeki TM (2011) MMWR Recomm Rep 60:1–24
Flowers LO, Johnson HM, Mujtaba MG, Ellis MR, Haider SM, Subramaniam PS (2004) J Immunol 172:7510–7518
Foged C (2012) Curr Top Med Chem 12:97–107
Freeley M, Bakos G, Davies A, Kelleher D, Long A, Dunican DJ (2010) J Biomol Screen 15:541–555
Galea G, Simpson JC (2013) Methods Cell Biol 118:281–295
Grienke U, Schmidtke M, von Grafenstein S, Kirchmair J, Liedl KR, Rollinger JM (2012) Nat Prod Rep 29:11–36
Gupta P, Cairns MJ, Saksena NK (2014) Virol J 11:64
Haasnoot PC, Cupac D, Berkhout B (2003) J Biomed Sci 10:607–616
Haney SA (2005) IDrugs 8:997–1001
Haney SA (2007) Pharmacogenomics 8:1037–1049
Hao L, Sakurai A, Watanabe T, Sorensen E, Nidom CA, Newton MA, Ahlquist P, Kawaoka Y (2008) Nature 454:890–893
Haraksingh RR, Snyder MP (2013) J Mol Biol 425:3970–3977
Heng BC, Aubel D, Fussenegger M (2013) Biotechnol Adv 31:1676–1694
Hong-Geller E, Micheva-Viteva SN (2010) Curr Drug Discov Technol 7:86–94

Ilyushina NA, Govorkova EA, Gray TE, Bovin NV, Webster RG (2008) PLoS Pathog 4:e1000043
Janssen HL, Reesink HW, Lawitz EJ, Zeuzem S, Rodriguez-Torres M, Patel K, van der Meer AJ, Patick AK, Chen A, Zhou Y, Persson R, King BD, Kauppinen S, Levin AA, Hodges MR (2013) N Engl J Med 368:1685–1694
Jeong JH, Mok H, Oh YK, Park TG (2009) Bioconjug Chem 20:5–14
Karlas A, Machuy N, Shin Y, Pleissner KP, Artarini A, Heuer D, Becker D, Khalil H, Ogilvie LA, Hess S, Maurer AP, Muller E, Wolff T, Rudel T, Meyer TF (2010) Nature 463:818–822
Katano H, Sata T (2000) Jpn J Infect Dis 53:137–155
Kittler R, Pelletier L, Heninger AK, Slabicki M, Theis M, Miroslaw L, Poser I, Lawo S, Grabner H, Kozak K, Wagner J, Surendranath V, Richter C, Bowen W, Jackson AL, Habermann B, Hyman AA, Buchholz F (2007) Nat Cell Biol 9:1401–1412
Kobos R, Nagai M, Tsuda M, Merl MY, Saito T, Lae M, Mo Q, Olshen A, Lianoglou S, Leslie C, Ostrovnaya I, Antczak C, Djaballah H, Ladanyi M (2013) J Pathol 229:743–754
Konig R, Stertz S, Zhou Y, Inoue A, Hoffmann HH, Bhattacharyya S, Alamares JG, Tscherne DM, Ortigoza MB, Liang Y, Gao Q, Andrews SE, Bandyopadhyay S, De Jesus P, Tu BP, Pache L, Shih C, Orth A, Bonamy G, Miraglia L, Ideker T, Garcia-Sastre A, Young JA, Palese P, Shaw ML, Chanda SK (2010) Nature 463:813–817
Korth MJ, Tchitchek N, Benecke AG, Katze MG (2013) Semin Immunol 25:228–239
Krebs DL, Hilton DJ (2000) J Cell Sci 113(Pt 16):2813–2819
Krug RM, Aramini JM (2009) Trends Pharmacol Sci 30:269–277
Lares MR, Rossi JJ, Ouellet DL (2010) Trends Biotechnol 28:570–579
Laurent-Rolle M, Boer EF, Lubick KJ, Wolfinbarger JB, Carmody AB, Rockx B, Liu W, Ashour J, Shupert WL, Holbrook MR, Barrett AD, Mason PW, Bloom ME, Garcia-Sastre A, Khromykh AA, Best SM (2010) J Virol 84:3503–3515
Law GL, Tisoncik-Go J, Korth MJ, Katze MG (2013) Curr Opin Immunol 25:588–592
Luo M (2012) Adv Exp Med Biol 726:201–221
Malakhov MP, Aschenbrenner LM, Smee DF, Wandersee MK, Sidwell RW, Gubareva LV, Mishin VP, Hayden FG, Kim DH, Ing A, Campbell ER, Yu M, Fang F (2006) Antimicrob Agents Chemother 50:1470–1479
Martinez-Gil L, Alamares-Sapuay JG, Ramana Reddy MV, Goff PH, Premkumar Reddy E, Palese P (2013) Antiviral Res 100:29–37
Mastyugin V, McWhinnie E, Labow M, Buxton F (2005) Drug Discov Today Suppl:43–49
Matskevich AA, Jung JS, Schumann M, Cascallo M, Moelling K (2009) J Innate Immun 1:389–394
Matskevich AA, Moelling K (2007) J Gen Virol 88:2627–2635
Matsumoto S, Miyagishi M, Taira K (2007) Methods Mol Biol 360:131–142
Mazur S, Kozak K (2012) RNA Biol 9:624–632
Meliopoulos VA, Andersen LE, Birrer KF, Simpson KJ, Lowenthal JW, Bean AG, Stambas J, Stewart CR, Tompkins SM, van Beusechem VW, Fraser I, Mhlanga M, Barichievy S, Smith Q, Leake D, Karpilow J, Buck A, Jona G, Tripp RA (2012a) FASEB J 26:1372–1386
Meliopoulos VA, Andersen LE, Brooks P, Yan X, Bakre A, Coleman JK, Tompkins SM, Tripp RA (2012b) PLoS One 7:e37169
Meyer D, Sielaff F, Hammami M, Bottcher-Friebertshauser E, Garten W, Steinmetzer T (2013) Biochem J 452:331–343
Micel LN, Tentler JJ, Smith PG, Eckhardt GS (2013) J Clin Oncol 31:1231–1238
Mohr S, Bakal C, Perrimon N (2010) Annu Rev Biochem 79:37–64
Munoz-Jordan JL, Laurent-Rolle M, Ashour J, Martinez-Sobrido L, Ashok M, Lipkin WI, Garcia-Sastre A (2005) J Virol 79:8004–8013
Nicholas J (2005) J Interferon Cytokine Res 25:373–383
Oshansky CM, Krunkosky TM, Barber J, Jones LP, Tripp RA (2009) Viral Immunol 22:147–161
Oshansky CM, Pickens JA, Bradley KC, Jones LP, Saavedra-Ebner GM, Barber JP, Crabtree JM, Steinhauer DA, Tompkins SM, Tripp RA (2011) PLoS One 6:e21183
Parker JS, Roe SM, Barford D (2006) Cold Spring Harb Symp Quant Biol 71:45–50

Pauli EK, Schmolke M, Wolff T, Viemann D, Roth J, Bode JG, Ludwig S (2008) PLoS Pathog 4:e1000196
Pazienza V, Vinciguerra M, Andriulli A, Mangia A (2010) J Gen Virol 91:1678–1686
Perrimon N, Mathey-Prevot B (2007) Genetics 175:7–16
Perrotti D, Neviani P (2013) Lancet Oncol 14:e229–e238
Perwitasari O, Bakre A, Tompkins SM, Tripp RA (2013a) Pharmaceuticals (Basel) 6:124–160
Perwitasari O, Torrecilhas AC, Yan X, Johnson S, White C, Tompkins SM, Tripp RA (2013b) J Virol 87:13775–13784
Perwitasari O, Yan X, Johnson S, White C, Brooks P, Tompkins SM, Tripp RA (2013c) Antimicrob Agents Chemother 57:475–483
Pinto R, Herold S, Cakarova L, Hoegner K, Lohmeyer J, Planz O, Pleschka S (2011) Antiviral Res 92:45–56
Pleschka S, Wolff T, Ehrhardt C, Hobom G, Planz O, Rapp UR, Ludwig S (2001) Nat Cell Biol 3:301–305
Preziosi P (2011) Expert Opin Pharmacother 12:1523–1549
Prussia A, Thepchatri P, Snyder JP, Plemper RK (2011) Int J Mol Sci 12:4027–4052
Prusty BK, Karlas A, Meyer TF, Rudel T (2011) Methods Mol Biol 721:383–395
Rask-Andersen M, Almen MS, Schioth HB (2011) Nat Rev Drug Discov 10:579–590
Saladino R, Barontini M, Crucianelli M, Nencioni L, Sgarbanti R, Palamara AT (2010) Curr Med Chem 17:2101–2140
Shapira SD, Gat-Viks I, Shum BO, Dricot A, de Grace MM, Wu L, Gupta PB, Hao T, Silver SJ, Root DE, Hill DE, Regev A, Hacohen N (2009) Cell 139:1255–1267
Shaw ML, Palese P (2013) Orthomyxoviridae. In: Knipe DM, Howley PM (eds) Fields Virology. Lippincott Williams & Wilkins, Philadelphia, pp 1151–1185
Shim MS, Kwon YJ (2010) FEBS J 277:4814–4827
Shin JH, Kim HU, Kim DI, Lee SY (2013) Biotechnol Adv 31:925–935
Song MM, Shuai K (1998) J Biol Chem 273:35056–35062
Southan C (2013) J Cheminform 5:10
Spielmann M, Klopocki E (2013) Curr Opin Genet Dev 23:249–256
Stertz S, Shaw ML (2011) Microbes Infect 13:516–525
Su WC, Chen YC, Tseng CH, Hsu PW, Tung KF, Jeng KS, Lai MM (2013) Proc Natl Acad Sci U S A 110:17516–17521
Sundaramurthy V, Barsacchi R, Chernykh M, Stoter M, Tomschke N, Bickle M, Kalaidzidis Y, Zerial M (2014) Nat Protoc 9:474–490
Theis M, Buchholz F (2011) Methods 53:424–429
Thomas S, Bonchev D (2010) Hum Genomics 4:353–360
Tripp RA, Mejias A, Ramilo O (2013) Curr Top Microbiol Immunol 372:193–209
Tripp RA, Tompkins SM (2009) Methods Mol Biol 555:43–61
Unutmaz D, KewalRamani VN, Littman DR (1998) Semin Immunol 10:225–236
Varga ZT, Ramos I, Hai R, Schmolke M, Garcia-Sastre A, Fernandez-Sesma A, Palese P (2011) PLoS Pathog 7:e1002067
Wang J, Xie X (2007) Acta Pharmacol Sin 28:1698–1704
Wang JF, Chou KC (2012) Mini Rev Med Chem 12:971–978
Ward SE, Kim HS, Komurov K, Mendiratta S, Tsai PL, Schmolke M, Satterly N, Manicassamy B, Forst CV, Roth MG, Garcia-Sastre A, Blazewska KM, McKenna CE, Fontoura BM, White MA (2012) PLoS One 7:e39284
Watanabe K, Takizawa N, Katoh M, Hoshida K, Kobayashi N, Nagata K (2001) Virus Res 77:31–42
Watanabe T, Watanabe S, Kawaoka Y (2010) Cell Host Microbe 7:427–439
Wei H, Wang S, Chen Q, Chen Y, Chi X, Zhang L, Huang S, Gao GF, Chen JL (2014) PLoS Pathog 10:e1003845
Zhang XD (2007) Genomics 89:552–561

Index

Current Topics in Microbiology and Immunology (2015) 386: 479–404
DOI: 10.1007/978-3-319-11158-2

MIX
Papier aus verantwortungsvollen Quellen
Paper from responsible sources
FSC® C105338

If you have any concerns about our products,
you can contact us on
ProductSafety@springernature.com

In case Publisher is established outside the EU,
the EU authorized representative is:
Springer Nature Customer Service Center GmbH
Europaplatz 3, 69115 Heidelberg, Germany

Printed by Libri Plureos GmbH
in Hamburg, Germany